The Social Determinants of Health Illustrated:

a primer for

Advocates ♦ Healthcare Professionals ♦ Lawmakers

AUTHORS: Eloy Alibin, DO; Kathryn Annand, MD; Sonja Chen, MD; Ariahnna Croskey, DO; Nicole Delos Santos, MD; Naomi Epstein, MD; David Estroff, MD; Joe Eubanks, MA; David Greco, MD; James Lenhart, MD, MPH; Andrea Lynde, DO; Joshua Monson, MD; Sylvia Otto, DO; James Pecsok, MD; Karl Riecken, DO; Andrea Saunders, JD; Jessica Skelton, DO; Laura Whitehill, MD

EDITORS: Stacie Beck, MD; Stephen Cook, MD; Janell Harro, MD; James Lenhart, MD, MPH; Cliff Moeckelmann, MD; Dylan Peterson, MD; Gary Reichard, MD; Eddie Seto, MD; Laila Siddiqui, MD; Carri Jo Timmer, DO; Amanda Wolf, MD

SENIOR EDITOR: James Lenhart, MD, FAAFP, MPH

COMMUNITY HEALTH CARE FEDERALLY QUALIFIED TEACHING HEALTH CENTER

TACOMA, WASHINGTON

In Affiliation with the University of Washington School of Medicine

and the

WWAMI Family Medicine Education Network

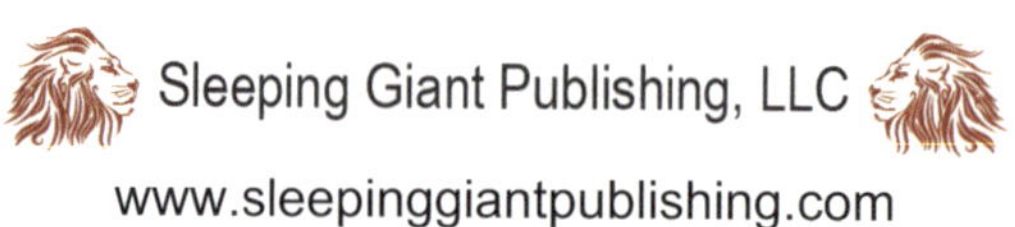

www.sleepinggiantpublishing.com

The Social Determinants of Health Illustrated:

a primer for

Advocates ⬥ Healthcare Professionals ⬥ Lawmakers

Technical Director: Jonathan Sturak

Cover design: Melissa Reed
Designed & printed in the United States of America

ISBN: 978-0-9835277-5-6
Library of Congress Cataloging-in-Publication Data

Be Healthy! Be Happy!™
www.sleepinggiantpublishing.com

Dedication

The Family Physicians and Colleagues for Health Justice dedicate this work to Earl Warren Chief Justice of the U.S. Supreme Court (1953 – 1969) whose judicial opinions gave civil rights leaders legal ground to advance human rights, and marginalized people opportunity for a better life.

Acknowledgements

Gratitude and immeasurable thanks to the following:

Dr. Carri Jo Timmer whose vision provided the authors and editors the protected time as well as organizational resources to bring this work to completion.

The resolute leaders of Community Health Care of Tacoma a Federally Qualified Teaching Health Center for providing the substance to educate the next generation of family physicians in best practices patient care and the importance of health justice.

The authors and editors of this manuscript that embraced the project, rolled up their sleeves and got the work done.

The significant others of the authors and editors who sacrificed personal and family time for execution of this endeavor.

Drs. Marmot, Wilkinson, Dahlgren, Whitehead, and H. Jack Geiger who rightfully lay claim as the fathers of the social medicine.

The past and present U.S. Presidents, Supreme Court Justices, and Congressional leaders that transformed human rights ideologies into substantive legal action.

The Reverand Martin Luthor King, Jr. who gave his life for the cause of civil rights, human rights, and health justice.

Earl Warren Chief Justice of the U.S. Supreme Court (1953 – 1969) whose judicial opinions *(Brown v. Board of Education, Gideon v. Wainwright, Mapp v. Ohio, Miranda v. Arizona, Loving v. Virginia)* gave civil rights leaders legal ground to advance human rights, and marginalized people opportunity for a better life.

To all those who give and have given their blood, sweat, and tears – and sometimes their lives – to ensure that all men *and* women – regardless of race, religion, color, or creed – are created equal.

Contributors

University of Washington Faculty

Stacie Beck, MD University of Washington School of Medicine

Stephen Cook, MD University of California at San Francisco

Janell Harro, MD Michigan State College of Human Medicine

David Estroff, MD Hahnemann Medical College

James Lenhart, MD, MPH University of New Mexico SOM, University of Liverpool MPH

Cliff Moeckelmann, MD Oregon Health Sciences Center

Dylan Peterson, MD University of Maryland School of Medicine

Gary Reichard, MD Loma Linda University School of Medicine

Eddie Seto, MD Texas A & M University Health Science Center

Laila Siddiqui, MD University College Dublin School of Medicine and Medical Science

Carri Jo Timmer, DO Western University of Health Sciences College of Osteopathic Medicine

Amanda Wolf, MD Xavier University School of Medicine

Colleagues for Health Justice

Joe Eubanks, Master of Arts in Leadership, Diversity and Inclusion University of Kansas

Andrea Saunders, JD University of San Francisco School of Law

Resident Authors

Eloy Alibin, DO American University of the Caribbean School of Medicine

Kathryn Annand, MD New York Medical College

Sonja Chen, MD University of Washington School of Medicine

Ariahnna Croskey, DO Michigan State University College of Osteopathic Medicine

Nicole Delos Santos, MD University of Nevada School of Medicine

Naomi Epstein, MD University of South Florida School of Medicine

David Greco, MD University of Michigan School of Medicine

Andrea Lynde, DO Pacific Northwest School of Medicine

Joshua Monson, MD University of Washington School of Medicine

Sylvia Otto, DO Campbell University School of Osteopathic Medicine

James Pecsok, MD Virginia Common Wealth University School of Medicine

Karl Riecken, DO Rocky Vista University College of Osteopathic Medicine

Jessica Skelton, DO A.T. Still University of Health Sciences

Laura Whitehill, MD University College Dublin School of Medicine and Medical Science

Permissions

This work borrows significantly from the publications of many credible organizations like the Centers for Disease Control and Prevention, the Organization for Economic Co-operation and Development, The Commonwealth Fund, The Kaiser Family Foundation, and the Environmental Protection Agency. As well, it leverages the publication of the many scholars producing reliable works published in peer reviewed journals.

In the writing and publication of this manuscript every effort was made to avoid plagiarism and to ensure attribution of intellectual property to respective authors. Indeed, our inclusion of these works honors those responsible for the significant body of reputable published material in the arena of the social determinants of health (SDH).

The collaborating authors in *The Social Determinants of Health Illustrated: a primer for Advocates • Health Professionals • Lawmakers* took care throughout their work to appropriately attribute the intellectual property utilized including graphs, charts, illustrations, photographs, and diagrams. Each manuscript underwent plagiarism scrubbing and correction utilizing Scribbbr https://www.scribbr.com/plagiarism-checker/.

Furthermore, where substantial portions of a publication were utilized, permission was appropriately solicited.

Community Health Care is a not-for-profit 501c2 Federally Qualified Health Center (FQHC) and an ACA Teaching Health Center located in Tacoma, Washington. Our missions include serving the underserved in need of health care and preparing medical school graduates for Board Certification in Family Medicine.

Consistent with that obligation, we profess a responsibility to teach health professionals, social activists, health advocates and law makers the critical importance of understanding, embracing, and advocating for the social determinants of health and health justice.

Claiming some understanding of Fair Use, we submit the following:

1. *The Social Determinants of Health Illustrated: a primer for Advocates • Health Professionals • Lawmakers* is educational.
2. It is not for profit (net revenue from sales funds directly to resident educational expenses).
3. The content is transformational in so much as it *illustrates* the impact of the SDH relying on recent and remote events to give demonstrative life to the non-medical conditions that affect health outcomes.
4. The contents are factual and technical.
5. The authors and editors respect limited use of copyrighted materials.
6. Cited intellectual property promotes and honors original author’s concepts.

Preface

Bitter wind and rain pelted the Pacific Northwest in the early morning of 20 November 2021. Arriving at my destination, I parked in the doctor's lot, donned my white coat, grabbed my stethoscope, and made the way to the hospital entrance – my turn to attend our hospital service and oversee resident patient care.

Having said good morning to the group of sleepy-eyed residents working with me, I went to the doctor's lounge, took my first cup of Starbucks, and sat down at the computer. The census looked typical. On adult medicine 11 patients – 7 acutely ill diagnosed with an array of problems – congestive heart failure, diabetic ketoacidosis, sepsis, gastrointestinal bleeding, exacerbation of chronic obstructive pulmonary disease and the like.

The 4 others presented discharge planning challenges. An otherwise healthy appearing young adult male on day 31 of admission to treat lumbar spine osteomyelitis due to intravenous opioid injections unable to be transferred to a skilled nursing facility (SNF) to complete 42 days of IV antibiotics. SNFs in our region refuse to admit and care for IV drug users. A 67-year-old homeless woman with end stage kidney disease experiencing recurrent admissions for dialysis due to missed appointments for three times weekly therapy owing to lack of reliable transportation. Another elderly female on day 61 of admission with osteoporosis and a fractured humerus prompted by a fall in unsafe living conditions awaiting discharge to an adult family home. And a cantankerous, if not mildly demented 74-year-old male with stable chronic bronchitis unsafe for discharge to his usual residence, at risk for readmission and adamant refusal for placement to a skilled nursing facility or an adult family home.

I took a deep breath and turned my attention to the OB/Newborn service. Three moms and newborns awaited our rounds and preparation for discharge, yet another on the labor deck whose last cervical check showed 7cm centimeters dilatation, zero station, and progressing expectantly through labor with a category I tracing.

The residents and I met up on the post-partum floor and methodically made our way through rounds. Before attending on the third mom and newborn, the social worker buttonholed us at the nursing station to report Child Protective Services was in the room investigating concerns for a domestic violence "situation" – dad toward mom with concern for child abuse in a sibling. To complicate matters, mother's car was "in the shop," she did not have an infant car seat for the newborn and her landlord was threatening eviction for unpaid rent.

Postpartum rounds complete, we headed up to the OB floor for an update on the laboring mom just in time to learn her drug screen came back positive for opioids and meth. Between contractions, mom offered little denial, "I'm a single mom, life's been 'shit' – pardon the expression and I treat my depression with street drugs, it's as simple as that."

Her defenseless and unapologetic explanation helped us understand why she rarely presented for care during pregnancy but didn't mitigate the risks she gambled for her and her unborn child due to sporadic prenatal care. I fought off and avoided any judgmental dialogue knowing that I had no idea what it's like to walk in her shoes and, at the same time, suspicious she's doing the best that she can.

On exam, she'd progressed to 9cm, still at zero station and a category I strip. An effective epidural blocked her pain.

We asked the nurse to alert the newborn ICU for neonatal abstinence syndrome and I headed back to the residents on adult medicine, leaving the labor deck residents to manage the mother.

At the conclusion of refreshingly efficient medicine rounds, Dr. Gabrielson, the senior on OB, texted me that the laboring mom was complete and ready to push. I reminded the medicine residents to communicate our care management strategies for the four stubborn discharges to the case management workers and headed back to L&D.

Mom pushed like a trooper with every contraction and within an hour the head delivered. A potential shoulder dystocia easily reduced and Dr. Gabrielson delivered a beautiful baby boy up on mom's chest and abdomen, skin to skin. APGARs 8/9.

I don't remember who cried longer and louder – mother or baby – but I am pretty certain it was mom.

We gave the couplet some time to bond and breast feed, then returned to check on her and perform the newborn exam. Mom looked comfortable and at peace although on continuous verge of tears. Baby boy was perfect in every respect, and I told her so.

She called him Jamison.

As we swaddled and handed him back to mom, Jamison looked up at me with big wide eyes. I stared back, wondering as I often do, "Jamison what will it be for you? Will you be surrounded by a loving mother and father that care about and protect you? Will there be food on your plate and at every meal? What about a roof over your head and a warm bed in a safe place you call home? How about school? Will you be given the opportunity to attend a good school and beyond that college or a vocational school leading to a decent job and a living wage? I wonder these things, Jamison because I know what we all want in the beginning (and over which you have no control) is the fair chance for a good life. So, I wonder. Will circumstances give you that chance?"

Driving home that evening, I reminisced on the day and under my breath said, "We talk the social determinants of health talk, but it's plain and simple. We don't walk the walk. Maybe it's time to settle in and write the social determinants of health 'call to action' I envisioned more than 10 years ago."

In 2010, I completed a Master of Public Health degree at the University of Liverpool, England, selected based on its reputation for strong academics in social medicine. It turned out to be an excellent choice. I authored my dissertation comparing the health outcomes of the U.S. states of

Mississippi (50th) and Hawaii (1st) which fueled my growing enthusiasm for the social determinants of health.

During the course of study, I adopted the conclusion that an introductory textbook that illustrated the profound effect social determinants have on health outcomes needed to see the light of day. Although we owe deep gratitude to the fathers of social medicine like Dahlgren, Whitehead, Marmot, and Wilkinson, their depositions and treatises elaborate a deep epidemiological dive into the science, creating scholarly arguments difficult for novice learners less equipped to fully comprehend and, most importantly, less likely to provoke urgent need for full throttle advocacy.

My array of experiences over the past 44 years firmly embed the indisputable facts that best practices health outcomes are rooted *not* in the clinician's exam room but rather socially progressive policies that deliver equitable opportunities rooted in health justice for all.

It was not always that way.

My medical education at the University of New Mexico in Albuquerque and residency in Family Medicine at Brown University affiliated hospitals, honed my skills early on and cemented my understanding of what it took to be a caring, responsible family physician in the best interest of the patients I cared for – a dedicated one on one, face to face experience in the exam room. I had little regard for, nor had I ever been exposed to, the dynamics of population health. When evidence-based medicine gripped our vocabulary in the mid-nineties, a new responsibility confronted me – scrutinizing the medical literature for evidence that the prescriptions I wrote and the therapies I recommended were based on patient-oriented, versus disease-oriented medicine. Double blinded, placebo controlled randomized clinical trials and metanalyses of homogeneous investigations – the sine qua non of evidence-based medicine – became my mantra.

The University of North Carolina-Chapel Hill recruited me to Wilmington, North Carolina in 1995 as founding Program Director for an upstart University affiliated residency in Family Medicine. Among the faculty I recruited was Paul Aitken, a family doc bred at NYU-Buffalo and Duke Universities. His pedigree also included a Master of Public Health from Columbia. Now separated by 3000 miles (Dr. Aitken is Chief of Population Health & Associate Dean for Clinical Integration at Stony Brook Medicine, NY), Paul and I are distant colleagues, but it is to Paul I tip my hat for introduction to population health (and led to my enrollment in the MPH program at the University of Liverpool).

In 2014, I joined Community Health Care (CHC) a Federally Qualified Health Center (FQHC) serving the South Puget Sound region's unserved and underserved. The patient population is no stranger to poverty, food insecurity, homelessness, limited access to health care, social injustice, and racism. As family physicians committed to full spectrum care, we treat children and adults throughout the life cycle including pregnancy, labor, and delivery.

In 2020, we confronted a significant challenge. The Board-Certified Rheumatologist that generously volunteered his expertise for treatment of patients with inflammatory joint disease announced his retirement leaving the population we serve without access to care for these crippling disorders. Rheumatologists are in short supply in our region, and most do not accept patients without health insurance. Due to my lifetime interest in musculoskeletal medicine, I offered to train with our volunteer rheumatologist during the last 6 months of his tenure and assumed the care of these patients after his retirement.

This experience has further shaped my population health perspectives. Untreated, rheumatoid arthritis cripples. Damage done is damage done. Hands become useless. Victims are unable to manage their hygiene, dress or lift a cup of coffee to their lips let alone enjoy the fruits of employment. The medications used to treat it most effectively cost $6000 and more monthly. Patients with insurance must arm wrestle (with my assistance) the insurance companies and pharmaceutical giants to get "prior authorization," delaying appropriate care if ever, it is approved.

In addition to patient care, CHC enjoys designation as a Federally Qualified Teaching Health Center. Affiliated with the University of Washington and the nation's premier Family Medicine education network WWAMI (a consortium of 31 Family Medicine residencies spread throughout Washington, Wyoming, Alaska, Montana, and Idaho), CHC is charged with educating the nation's next generation of family physicians. As Associate Program Director, my responsibilities comprise curriculum administration including education in scholarship and research.

The Accreditation Council for Graduate Medical Education (ACGME) makes scholarship a requirement for all residency education programs. Fulfilling my responsibilities and reflecting on my interest in writing a SDH textbook, I had an ah-ha moment and presented it to my boss, Dr. Carri Jo Timmer. "How about a resident rotation that requires each upper-level resident physician to write an essay on a social determinant of health, edited by their faculty advisors, polished to perfection and presented for publication." She embraced the idea. Thus, the creation I envisioned over 10 years before was launched in the spring of 2023.

As my dream straddles the final days leading to its publication, this segment of my professional journey buttresses my knowledge that the abysmal health outcomes in the United States are the result of executive, legislative and judicial neglect, disregard and ignorance for the devastation wrought by poverty, limited education, food insecurity, minimum wage employment, healthcare injustice, racism, and gender inequities.

Coupled with my leadership, the unwavering support of our faculty and the dedicated work of our residents and colleagues enmeshed in this project, here is our call to action.

It is time to walk the walk!

We are the Family Physicians and Colleagues for Health Justice.

James Lenhart, MD, FAAFP, MPH
Senior Editor and Author

The Social Determinants of Health Illustrated: a primer for Advocates • Healthcare Professionals • Lawmakers

Foreword

My career changing exposure to the social determinants of health occurred when I led a medical team in a village in Sierra Leone, West Africa. The village had no running water, no sanitation system, no immunizations, and no access to healthcare. We documented a 50% childhood mortality rate due to deaths from neonatal tetanus, meningitis, malaria, malnutrition, diarrheal illness, whooping cough, and other preventable diseases. The obvious realization was that building a hospital with an intensive care unit would be far less valuable than clean water, sanitary systems, good nutrition, immunizations, access to healthcare and other social resources that are the primary determinants of health. What is not so obvious to many Americans that this book by James Lenhart, M.D. and his colleagues so powerfully illustrates is that health outcomes for U.S. citizens are worse than most other industrialized countries due to a lack of social resources for large portions of our population.

This African village experience spurred me to devote much of my career to care for the underserved with a focus on social as well as medical needs. I practiced and served as the medical director of a County Health Department, a Federally Qualified Health Center and led a highly successful county wide community social and health improvement initiative. As a lead investigator in the Institute for Translational Medicine at the University of Chicago, I launched the Urban Health Initiative to serve the South Side of Chicago, among the poorest of communities in the U.S.

I am therefore honored to write this forward on behalf of the Family Physicians and Colleagues for Health Justice. They have created a distinctive work of scholarship devoted to a cause that is near and dear to my heart. Dr. Lenhart and his colleagues serve on the frontline of medical care for patients who experience the very social disparities they write about. They not only know these patients and their lives, but they have also compiled a thorough, fascinating and at a times heartbreaking body of research, description of political events, and graphic representations that collectively tell a compelling story.

This book serves as an excellent introduction as well as a resource for advocates, health professionals, policymakers and community leaders. Simply skimming the chapters will lead you to surprising facts such as the United States, compared to other high-income countries in the Organization of Economic Co-operation and Development has the highest infant mortality rate, the highest maternal mortality rate, the lowest life expectancy, the highest rates of COVID deaths, and the fewest physicians per capita. For those who wish to take a deeper dive each chapter has an extensive set of references plus recommendations for sentinel readings.

I hope you will choose this valuable resource to raise awareness, to take action, and recognize that a career focused on improving health and health care, as these authors model through this book, serves as a life well lived.

Bernard Ewigman, MD, MSPH
Founding Chair, Department of Family Medicine University of Chicago

Contents

Chapter 1

Introduction

James Lenhart. MD, FAAFP, MPH

"Injustice anywhere is a threat to justice everywhere. We are caught in an inescapable network of mutuality, tied in a single garment of destiny. Whatever affects one directly, affects all indirectly."
- Martin Luther King Jr.

This work aims to light the flame for health justice in the minds, hearts, and souls of all people everywhere, *for without health justice illness persists universally.*

It strives to teach budding health professionals the critical importance of the social determinates of health, *for ignorance of their importance leaves life's calling undone.*

It means to illustrate how, during the past 400 years and continuing to this day, the alleged halls of justice in the United States have trampled people seen as less worthy subjugating them to a life of marginal means, with less educational opportunity, low paying, backbreaking jobs, harsh environmental exposures, food insecurity, water unfit to drink, lack of access to health care and absence of legal resource to right the wrong, *for disregard of inequities perpetuates a system deleterious to national health too long ignored.*

It serves to educate activists, advocates, and lawmakers that the health of our nation is dependent *not* on National Institutes of Health funding for the next state of the art monoclonal antibody, but finding the will and determination to legislate and enact social programs that defy systemic racism, poverty, food insecurity, homelessness, unconscionable minimum wages, toxic environments, contaminated water supplies, unemployment, and suppression of legal options, *for the wealth of our nation thrives under the umbrella of population well-being.*

It leverages recent and remote events to illustrate that what we do and how do it make fundamental and lasting differences, *for if we listen, if we are curious, history always makes the best teacher.*

And it screams from the rooftops that all men *and* women are created equal regardless of race, religion, color, or creed, *for we are endowed by our Creator with certain unalienable rights, that among these are life, liberty, and the pursuit of happiness.*

The Family Physicians and Colleagues For Health Justice comprise a collective of individuals dedicated to the health and well-being of people directly served, the community in which we live and individuals around the globe. Our band is small – 26 family physician faculty and resident physicians caring for underserved patients at Community Health Care, a Federally Qualified Health Center in the barrio of Tacoma, Washington. We count among our peers the expertise of a graduate of the University of San Francisco School of Law impassioned to a career in public service and legal aid, and a Master of Leadership, Diversity, and Inclusion from the University of Kansas with an appetite for public policy demonstrated by his drive to organize against Confederate flag displays at the University of Mississippi.

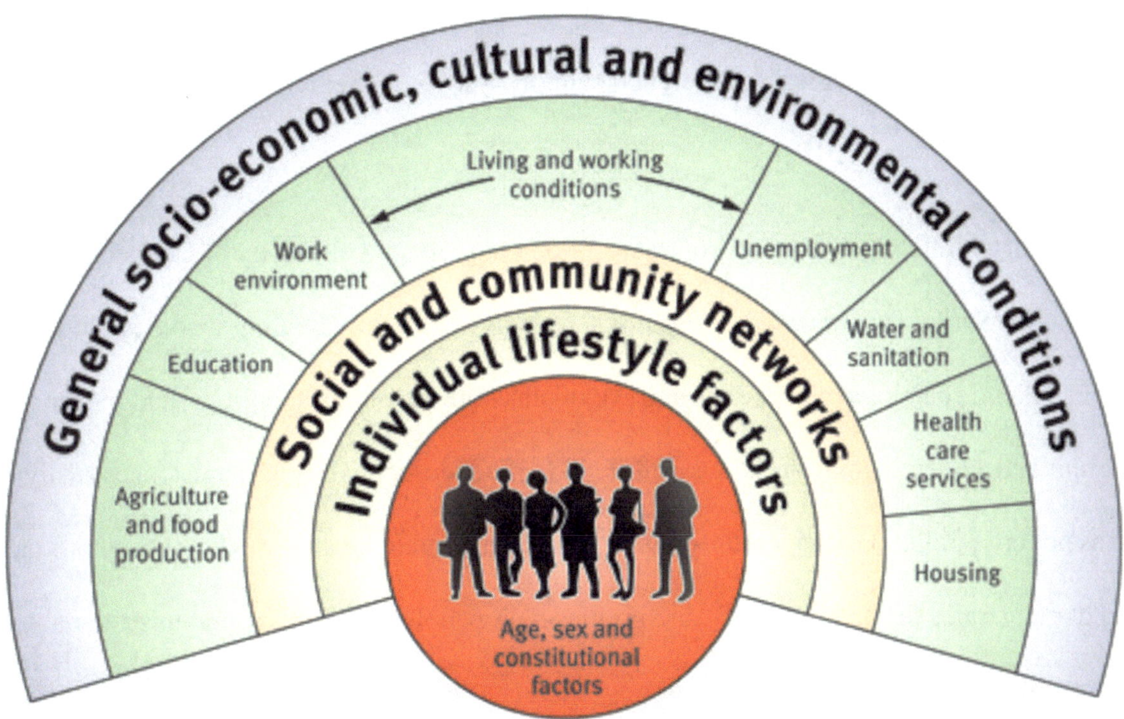

The Social Determinants of Health, Dahlgren and Whitehead 1991.

We stand on the solid shoulders of Drs. Marmot, Wilkinson, Dahlgren, Whitehead, and H. Jack Geiger who rightfully lay claim as the fathers of the social medicine. Indeed, we now celebrate for over thirty years Dahlgren and Whitehead's classic rainbow model illustrated above.

The arc of time marches forward – research, technology, innovation, science, experience, political discourse, and activism act to continuously refine, expand, contract, and redefine our knowledge, and the struggle of implementing change. Marmot and Wilkinson's treatise *Social Determinants of Health* (2006) followed their tidy expose *The Social Determinants of Health: The Solid Facts* (1998) and produced an epidemiological deep dive into the dialogue. Helliwell and Putnam (2004) *The social context of well-being*, Bradshaw (2008) *Determinants of Health and Their Trends*, and Bambra, et al., (2009) *Tackling the wider social determinants of health and health inequalities: evidence from systematic reviews* have made important contributions to social medicine as well. More recently, Davidson's *Social Determinants of Health: A Comparative Approach* 2nd ed. "takes a macro-level look at the many ways in which social factors - such as income, education, employment, gender, and support systems - interact to determine health across the lifespan" (Davidson, 2019).

Kathryn Ratcliff, Assistant Professor of Sociology at the University of Connecticut (2017) authored *The Social Determinants of Health: Looking Upstream.* Creating a somewhat different spin, she takes a sociologic perspective and "explains how the policies, politics, and power behind corporate and governmental decisions and actions produce unhealthy circumstances of living – such as poverty, pollution, dangerous working conditions, and unhealthy modes of food production – and demonstrates that putting profit and politics over people is unhealthy and unsustainable." In so doing, Ratcliff makes a clear case urging activists, policymakers, health professionals, and students in sociology and public health to advocate for healthy public policy.

Parallel with the emerging interest in social medicine, the human genome project launched in 1990, which resulted in the sequencing of the human genome and the birth of exposomics and microbiomics capable of precisely analyzing social determinants of health at the micro level.

Overlay the havoc and divisive nature of political rancor world-wide on the three decades of landmark SDH accomplishments described, the Family Physicians and Colleagues for Health Justice offer this pictograph to illustrate a 21st century dynamic of the social determinants of health.

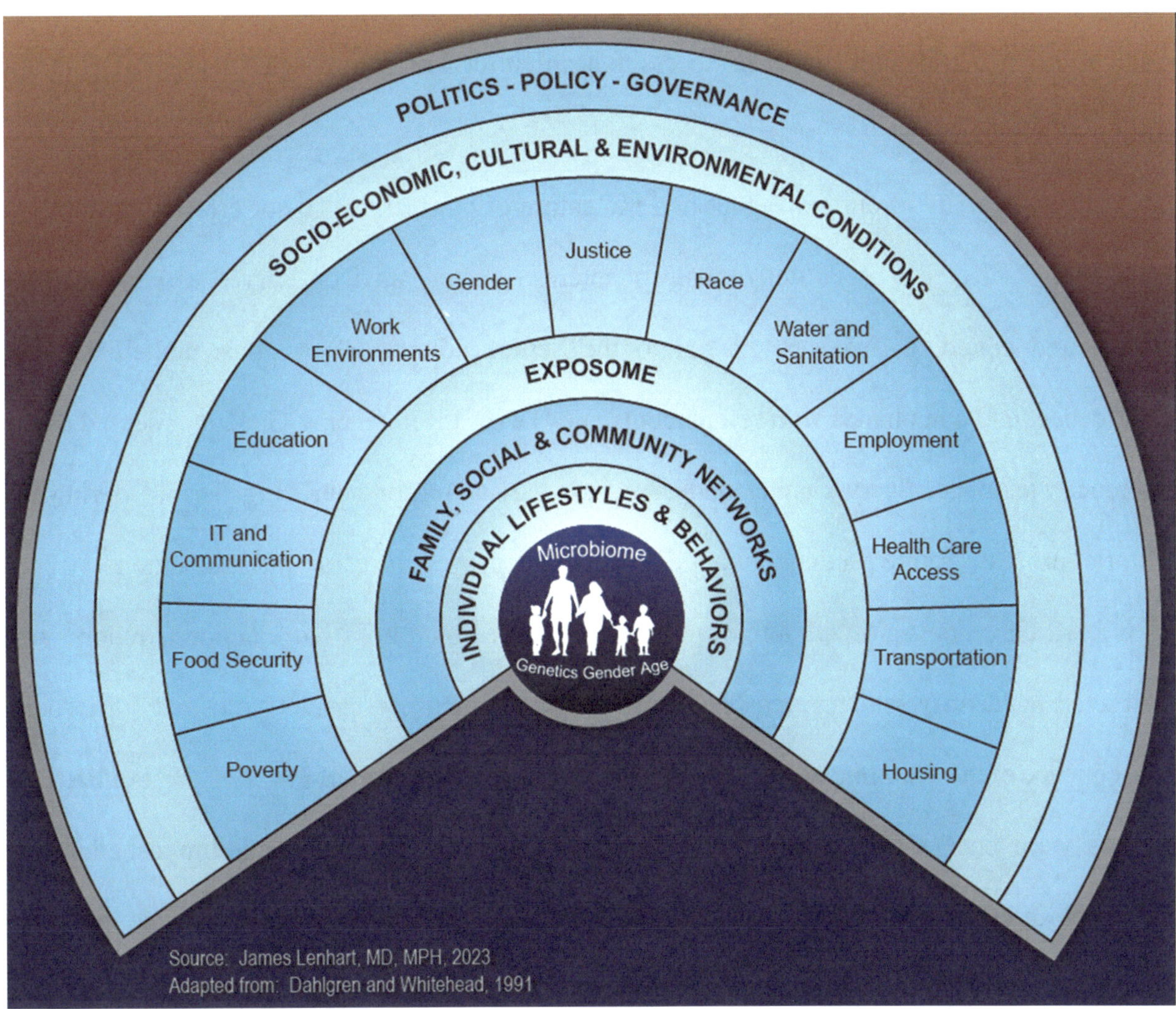

Our modifications to the Dahlgren/Whitehead rainbow include: 1) *politics, policy and governance* pulling up or pressing down on socioeconomic, cultural, and environmental conditions; 2) *justice, race, and gender* with acknowledgement of, and respect for the implications of centuries long discrimination against women, people of color, national origin, and religion; 3) *exposome and microbiome* – as elaborated in Chapter 16, the exposome is "the measure of all of the exposures an individual has in a lifetime and how those exposures relate to health. The exposome represents the totality of exogenous (external) and endogenous (internal) exposures from conception onwards" (Juárez, 2018); and 4) *IT/Communication* – in family physician parlance, "90% of the diagnosis is in history." So, communication coupled with the extraordinary reach of internet communications and access to health information comes to life as an SDH in this edition of the diagram.

The diversity of our colleagues and the nature of our task called for creative uniformity. Each author selected a social determinant of interest. Faculty advisors served as editors. Once drafted and edited, essays were passed to the Senior Editor for revisions, embellishments, congruence, and compliance with referencing. The Harvard Referencing Generator served as the reference template. Every chapter underwent plagiarism scrutiny utilizing Scribbr during the editorial process. Before sending on to press, authors approved the essay for publication.

All chapters begin with a relevant quote, followed by a brief introduction. Authors were instructed to identify salient recent and remote events which persuasively illustrated the social consequence of the determinant, e.g., the U.S. Supreme Court reversal of *Roe v. Wade.* For balance, authors were encouraged to identify experiences that both improved and diminished health outcomes and to expand the consequences in the context of a collateral SDH, e.g., the impact of poverty on food security. The essays conclude with relevant examples of the ways politics, policies and governance affect the determinant.

For those using this treatise as a textbook Questions for Further Consideration follow the body of text, after which those curiously intrigued can take a journey through recommended Sentinel Readings for a Deeper Dive. References, a Lexicon for Listed Terms and Agencies and the Author's Bio Sketch round out each chapters.

Authors relied on published works emanating from the Centers for Disease Control and Prevention (CDC), the Environmental Protection Agency (EPA), Organization for Economic Co-Operation and Development (OECD), the Supreme Court of the United States (SCOTUS), the World Health Organization (WHO), the United States Constitution, the Commonwealth Fund, the Kaiser Family Foundation (KFF), the Library of Congress, the United Nations, and the Gallup Poll. Published peer reviewed scholarship in healthcare, policy, science, and economics discovered through literature search provided important sources of relevant information for authors as well. Authors were instructed to present information free of bias, especially political. While global and international circumstances and comparisons provide important relevant information throughout the text, the focus in each chapter explores and points directly at the support, promotion, abandonment, opposition, and/or neglect for the subject social determinant.

Chapter Summaries

Chapter 2 Justice

Andrea Saunders, J.D. tackled this important essay articulating the juxtaposition of justice versus injustice through the lens of medical ethics, Congressional Acts, and landmark U.S. Supreme Court decisions. For example, the SDH impact of *Plessy v. Ferguson (1896),* which legalized segregation in the United States and *Dandridge v. Williams (1970)* that capped Aid to Families with Dependent Children irrespective of size and need. Pertaining to medical ethics, Saunders explores the various concepts of distributive justice – the tension of distribution according *to each person an equal share* vs. *distribution according to need, effort, contribution, or merit ... I am eligible because I am.* She wraps into the conversation the reality that justice dealt by the highest court in the United States (SCOTUS) is fragile, if not fickle, leveraging obscure case precedents to justify the overturn of previous opinions.

Finally, "Just as medical ethics champion distributive justice in healthcare, social determinants of health must be promulgated with distributive justice in law, policy, and governance. Studies have identified the positive effect of access to legal professionals as a critical facet of community response to intimate partner violence. Communities need access to legal professionals to secure just outcomes, like they need access to medical professionals for clinical care. Access to a fair system of justice is a critical social determinant of health."

Chapter 3 Race

Eubanks paints important historical context pertaining to race as an SDH at the beginning of Chapter 3. Starting with colonial slave owners like Thomas Jefferson and cascading through other influencers like Dr. Samuel Cartwright, Benjamin Gould and Frederick Hoffman, readers begin to understand the ways in which white supremacist ideology took grip in the nation. Concepts of racism in the U.S. are not confined to Black people. The author describes the treatment of persons of Hispanic origin throughout this chapter. He graphically depicts the "management" of Indigenous people, e.g., the Indian Removal Act of 1830 and other actions spawned by the Doctrines of Manifest Destiny and Eminent Domain to shine historical light on nearly two centuries of malignant treatment of Native Americans. The impact of systematic oppression, white supremacy and bias are thoughtfully illustrated showing their detriment well-being, housing, educational attainment, poverty, employment, wages, violence, and personal safety.

This essay concludes with examples of Supreme Court, Congressional and Presidential actions that have and continue to support white supremacy in the United States.

Chapter 4 Gender

When we initiated this project, Dr. Monson made the case for gender as a social determinant of health. His rationale spills out in Chapter 4 providing readers a clear understanding of discrimination wrought by others against women, the LGBTQ+ community and those with gender dysphoria. The plight of women worldwide, the history of Pride, wage and professional discrimination unfolds across the pages. Included in Dr. Monson's dissertation is a discussion of the historic importance of the SCOTUS ruling in *Lawrence v. Texas,* which protects the right of gay people to form intimate relationships and "retain their dignity as persons" (ACLU, 2023).

Chapter 5 Poverty

Who better to author an essay on poverty as a social determinant of health than a woman who personally faced it as a single parent to as disabled child? Dr. Skelton graphically shows the effect of poverty on life expectancy and mortality rates nationally and internationally and explains how poverty impacts quality of life. She reveals that children of poverty are victims of alterations in physical, cognitive, emotional, and social development. Further, she discusses the bearing of poverty on prevalence of obesity, infectious diseases, food insecurity, and domestic violence. In the final segment of the essay, she compares international policies to address poverty using the Organization of Economic Co-operation and Development (OECD) data.

Chapter 6 Food Security

This essay begins by clarifying the concepts of food insecurity, then evolves to a discussion on food insecurity worldwide. Dr. Annand considers the nutritional value of foods and the harms of energy dense, nutrient poor leading to the epidemic of obesity throughout the world, especially in the U.S.

Important to the essay is her dialogue pertaining international food inequality and the direct impact of global conflict on the quantity and quality food available to populations in war torn countries like the Ukraine and African nations as well as the effect of conflict on the worldwide food supply chain using the example of Ukraine given its global prominence in grain exports. Food inequality in the U.S. becomes known showing how poverty, single parent households, food deserts, transportation and minority populations are disproportionately affected.

The essay concludes examining U.S. government programs that mitigate food insecurity as well as novel initiatives like The Healthy Corner Store projects that aim to bring nutritious foods closer to people's homes. Healthy Corner Stores must meet three criteria: 1) location in an area with low access to healthy foods, 2) location in an area with high rates of diet-related disease and 3) meeting specific requirements that address access to healthy foods and leads to certification as a Healthy Corner Store. Started as a local program in Philadelphia Healthy Corner Stores have spread through the U.S. coast to coast.

Chapter 7 IT/Communication

Dr. Alibin validates the concept of information technology and communication as an essential social determinant of health in this essay. By focusing on the provision of cultural and linguistic appropriate services in healthcare and the importance of health literacy in achieving best practices health outcomes, he grounds the concept of IT/Communication as an SDH.

His chapter illustrates IT's power in improving health outcomes describing a unique program spearheaded by the March of Dimes to address reproductive services in "Maternity Care Deserts" throughout the U.S. In 2020, one in four Native American babies (26.7%) were born in areas of limited or no access to maternity care services; one in six Black babies (16.3%) were born in areas of limited or no access to maternity care services. 36% of U.S. counties are classified as maternity care deserts, statistics that signal the importance of the March of Dimes strategy (March of Dimes, 2022).

Dr. Alibin embellishes the essay with insights into the expansion of broadband technology in the United States and initiatives to improve IT access throughout the country calculated to improve health literacy and health outcomes nationwide.

Chapter 8 Education

Dr. Delos Santos cuts to the chase solidifying education as a social determinant of health in her dissertation on education in Chapter 8.

"Compared to those with a college education, Americans with less education die earlier. At age 25, U.S. adults without a high school diploma can expect to die 9 years sooner than college graduates" (Virginia Commonwealth University Center on Society and Health, 2022).

She strengthens her arguments showing education's impact on the prevalence chronic disease, multimorbidity, and functional limitations (disability).

This chapter concludes with detailed dialog pertaining to the 2023 Supreme Court ruling on affirmative action, educational opportunity, and the probability of intensified limitations on access to education for minorities (Supreme Court of the United States, 2023).

Chapter 9 Work Environments

This essay illuminates work environments as an SDH through the lens of the COVID-19 pandemic and industrial asbestos exposure, exploiting the physical and emotional consequences of each.

Dr. Lynde details in thorough discussion how COVID-19 drove burnout to such an extent that health professionals of all stripes have abandoned healthcare to pursue alternate career paths.

Taking on occupational lung disease, she focuses on asbestos related disorders including disclosure that despite known harms due to exposure, workers were misinformed regarding long-term hazards including mesothelioma. Exposure ultimately resulted in a tragic legacy of occupational diseases while simultaneously driving the push for safer working conditions and stricter safety regulations (National Cancer Institute, 2017), according to Dr. Lynde's dissertation. Due to known harms, the industrial use of asbestos is now regulated by the Environmental Protection Agency and is forbidden in most industrial applications, she concludes.

Chapter 10 Water & Sanitation

Dr. Croskey starts the chapter with the following United Nations declaration: "An adequate supply of fresh (i.e., clean potable and uncontaminated) water is essential for individual and public health, as well as being a social determinant of health" (United Nations General Assembly, 2015).

She initiates the chapter with a discussion on the many sources of water pollution – industrial and agricultural – to the extent of contamination with chemicals like arsenic and lead and substances like fertilizers, animal waste and pesticides.

Central to her essay are dissertations on the Jackson, Mississippi water crisis and the Flint, Michigan water debacle, both graphically illustrating the political features of applied systemic racism and the dire health consequences associated.

Chapter 11 Employment

Dr. Epstein tackles employment as a social determinant of health in the context of health, access to care, food security, poverty, and standard of living. She presents a cogent discussion on the concepts of living wage vs. minimum wage and the egregious fact that the minimum wage in the United States has not been increased since 2009 (Office of the Assistant Secretary for Planning and Evaluation, 2023) and as recently as March 4th 2021, the Senate voted down an amendment to increase the Federal minimum wage to $15 an hour by 2025 (Cochrane and Edmondson, 2021).

Her dialog on the 2023 United Auto Workers strike provides a lively discussion on the subject of union/non-union employment. Congruent with the discussion on living wage perspectives, her writing articulates a persuasive argument for collective bargaining as a beneficial tool for workers clamoring after improved working conditions and wages.

Chapter 12 Health Care Access

This essay centers on barriers to health access in the U.S. and international comparisons of health access and health outcomes like life expectancy, multiple chronic conditions, obesity, suicide, death rates from COVID-19, infant mortality, and maternal mortality. It draws heavily on the data compiled and analyzed by The Commonwealth Fund (Gunja, Gumas, and Williams, 2023).

Dr. Otto's discussion on politics, policies, and governance explores the right to abortion through the lens of the SCOTUS decision in *Dobbs v. Jackson Women's Health Organization* (2022), which overturned *Roe v. Wade* (1973), that granted the right to abortion. "Held: The Constitution does not confer a right to abortion; *Roe* and *Casey* are overruled; and the authority to regulate abortion is returned to the people and their elected representatives" (Supreme Court of the United States, 2022).

Chapter 13 Transportation

This essay highlights the reality of transportation as an SDH well beyond the need for transportation to get to doctor appointments and the grocery store. Dr. Pecsok unravels the U.S.

legacy of nation building based on the principles of Manifest Destiny and Eminent Domain that established unfettered construction of U.S. railroads and the Interstate highway system without regard to the human rights and civil rights of Native, African, and Mexican Americans. Laden in the conversation, Pecsok provides evidence that transportation networks propel national progress forward, albeit at the expense and to the detriment of disproportionately affected groups.

That aside, he examines the concept of transportation resilience detailing the importance of protecting infrastructure "so vital to the United States that the incapacity or destruction of such systems and assets would have a debilitating impact on security, national economic security, national public health or safety, or any combination of those matters" (AASHTO, 2017).

Chapter 14 Housing

Dr. Whitehill begins her essay on housing by examining the realities affecting people experiencing homelessness (PEH). In the 2022 ~500,000 people experienced homelessness in the U.S. . Minority groups were disproportionately affected as were males over the age of 25 years. As an SDH, she points out that homeless people have significantly higher rates of chronic disease, communicable disease, trauma, and victimization and suffer from exposure to environmental toxins, lead, rodents, pests, and molds. PEH have high rates of substance abuse, alcoholism, traumatic injuries, and homicide from gun violence, stabbings and beatings.

Homeless people live in poverty, which aligns across minority groups. In the U.S., the 2020 Census Bureau pegged the poverty rate across the U.S. at ~12%, however, American Indians & Alaskan Natives (24%), Black people (20%), and Hispanics (17%) shouldered a disproportionate share of the poverty burden. By comparison, White, not Hispanic stood at just 8% (Bureau, U.C., 2021). In summary Dr. Whitehill concludes, "The downward spiral that marks homelessness places the victims of this epidemic in a cyclical, if not perpetual swirl of exposure to infectious diseases, trauma, malnutrition, limited access to healthcare, disrupted family relationships, increased drug and alcohol use and deteriorating health due to its many manifestations."

Chapter 15 Environment

Dr. Karl Riecken tackles the environment focusing on the collision of climate change and pollution in the context of education, working conditions, food security, housing, early childhood development and healthcare access.

At conclusion, Dr. Riecken makes a strident call to action, "Climate change threatens the world order creating an urgent call to action for healthcare professionals to educate patients and the public about climate change and the environment (Tan Ngo, 2021). Our voices must be loud and clear as we advocate on local and national levels in support of public policy that embraces the devastating consequences of climate change. Healthcare professionals and major medical organizations represent trusted sources of information – duty neglected; we violate that trust." He further reminds us that the Paris Climate Agreement, 2015 leads us in that direction.

The Paris Climate Agreement

According to the National Resources Defense Council (NRDC), U.S. President Barrack Obama announced in December 2015 that the United States, along with nearly 200 other countries, had committed to the Paris Climate Agreement, an ambitious global action plan to fight climate change. Obama envisioned that the accord would leave today's children, "A world that is safer and more secure, more prosperous, and more free."

However, less than two years later, then-president Donald Trump put that future in jeopardy by announcing his plan to withdraw the United States from the accord—a step that became official on November 4, 2020—as part of a larger plan to dismantle decades of U.S. environmental policy. Fortunately, American voters also got their say in November 2020, ousting Trump and sending Joe Biden and Kamala Harris to the White House.

On his first day in office, President Biden sent a letter to the United Nations, formally signaling that the United States would rejoin the Paris Agreement. Thirty days later (as is required), on February 19, 2021, the nation was re-entered.

National Resources Defense Council (NRDC) (2021). Paris Climate Agreement: Everything You Need to Know [online] Available at:https://www.nrdc.org/stories/paris-climate-agreement-everything-you-need-know#sec-whatis

Chapter 16 Exposome & Microbiome

The dawn of the Human Genome Project completed in 2003 spawned the science of exposomics. Dr. Greco unfolds exposomics and microbiomics in this chapter. The exposome represents "the measure of all of the exposures an individual has in a lifetime and how those exposures relate to health. The exposome represents the totality of exogenous (external) and endogenous (internal) exposures from conception onwards" (Juárez, 2018).

Dr. Greco cuts the array of exposomes and complexity of exposomics into digestible bites. For example, he utilizes the ubiquitous disorder of periodontal disease (an exposure) to illustrate it's connection with cardiovascular disease, dementia, cancer, preterm birth, immune system dysregulation and rheumatoid arthritis.

Conceptually framed in exposomic terms, healthy life expectancy can be visualized as the consequence of accumulated exposures shaped by and through the social determinants of health.

Chapter 17 Obesity: The Social Determinant of Health Connection

Experiencing a lifetime in the trenches caring for children and teaching the art and science of pediatrics, Dr. Estroff rightfully claims expertise in childhood obesity. Citing the near vertical trajectory of obesity in the U.S. and around the world, this chapter exposes 21st century ultra processed foods, poverty, and stressors (violence, homelessness, racism, food insecurity and adverse childhood experiences) as prime drivers of the obesity pandemic. Dr. Estroff draws on peer reviewed research and institutional resources to validate his perspective that the neglect of the social determinants health foster a path to overweight and obesity as well as it's untoward health consequences.

Dr. Estroff holds the distinction of Clinical Professor Emeritus of Pediatrics, University of Washington.

Chapter 18 Social Determinants and Health Behaviors

Dr. Chen scrutinizes specific lifestyles and behaviors associated with substance use while dissecting the underlying social-economic, cultural, and environmental conditions propelling these behaviors. She provides an overarching analysis of smoking, alcohol and substance use in the context of the social determinants of health progressing to international comparisons of use Australia, Canada, France, Germany, Japan, the Netherlands, New Zealand, Norway, Sweden, the UK, and the United States.

In making comparisons, readers discover the alarming incidence of opioid deaths in the U.S. compared to other countries.

Chapter 19 Expressions

This just for fun essay traces the journey of writers, musicians, artists and filmmakers over the centuries who chronicled the sentinel events of their time. Commencing with the philosophers of the Enlightenment and concluding with film makers of the 20th and 21st centuries, readers develop an appreciation for the role of arts and letters in propelling social change. Links to access the creative works are provided to facilitate purchase for those interested.

Chapter 20 Epilogue

Dr. Lenhart pulls together the concepts explored throughout the text with an explanation why the United States, the richest country on the planet, fails to deliver on the promise of world class health outcomes and why increases in life expectancy over the past four decades in the U.S. lag other high-income countries by substantial margins.

References:

AASHTO (2017). *Understanding Transportation Resilience: A 2016 - 2018 Roadmap*. [online] Available at: https://transportation.org/ctssr/wp-content/uploads/sites/37/2023/01/UTR-1-book-vers-5.pdf [Accessed 1 Feb. 2024].

ACLU (2023). *Striking Down Texas Law Against Same-Sex 'Sodomy,' Supreme Court Rights Egregious Wrong of 17 Years, Signaling New Era for Gay Rights*. [online] American Civil Liberties Union. Available at: https://www.aclu.org/press-releases/striking-down-texas-law-against-same-sex-sodomy-supreme-court-rights-egregious-wrong [Accessed 1 Feb. 2024].

Bambra, C., Gibson, M., Sowden, A., Wright, K., Whitehead, M. and Petticrew, M. (2010). Tackling the wider social determinants of health and health inequalities: evidence from systematic reviews. *Journal of Epidemiology & Community Health*, [online] https://doi.org/10.1136/jech.2008.082743 [Accessed 1 Feb. 2024].

Bradshaw, D. (2008). *Determinants of Health and Their Trends*. [online] Available at: https://journals.co.za/doi/epdf/10.10520/EJC35512 [Accessed 24 Jan. 2024].

Bureau, U.C. (2021). *Income and Poverty in the United States: 2020*. [online] Census.gov. Available at: https://www.census.gov/library/publications/2021/demo/p60-273.html#:~:text=The%20official%20poverty%20rate%20in%202020%20was%2011.4 [Accessed 24 Jan. 2024].

Cochrane, E. and Edmondson, C. (2021). Minimum wage increase fails as 7 Democrats vote against the measure. *The New York Times*. [online] 5 Mar. Available at: https://www.nytimes.com/2021/03/05/us/minimum-wage-senate.html [Accessed 1 Feb. 2024].

Davidson, A. (2019). *Social Determinants of Health A Comparative Approach 2nd Ed.* Oxford University Press [Accessed 24 Jan. 2024].

Helliwell, J. and Putnam, R. (2004). The social context of well–being. *Philosophical Transactions of the Royal Society of London. Series B: Biological Sciences*, https://doi.org/10.1098/rstb.2004.1522 [Accessed 24 Jan. 2024].

Juárez, P. (2018). The Public Health Exposome. *Springer eBooks*, pp.23–61. https://doi.org/10.1007/978-3-319-89321-1_2 [Accessed 1 Feb. 2024].

March of Dimes (2022). *Healthy Moms. Strong Babies. No Where to Go: Maternity Care Deserts across the U.S.* [online] March of Dimes. Available at: https://www.marchofdimes.org/sites/default/files/2022-10/2022_Maternity_Care_Report.pdf [Accessed 1 Feb. 2024].

Marmot, M. and Wilkinson, R. (2006). *Social Determinants of Health 2nd Ed.* Oxford Press.

National Cancer Institute (2017). *Asbestos Exposure and Cancer Risk Fact Sheet*. [online] National Cancer Institute. Available at: https://www.cancer.gov/about-cancer/causes-prevention/risk/substances/asbestos/asbestos-fact-sheet [Accessed 1 Feb. 2024].

National Resources Defense Council (NRDC) (2021). Paris Climate Agreement: Everything You Need to Know [online] Available at: https://www.nrdc.org/stories/paris-climate-agreement-everything-you-need-know#sec-whatis [Accessed 27 September 2023].

Office of the Assistant Secretary for Planning and Evaluation (2023). *Poverty guidelines*. [online] ASPE. Available at: https://aspe.hhs.gov/topics/poverty-economic-mobility/poverty-guidelines [Accessed 1 Feb. 2024].

Ratcliff, K. (2017). *The Social Determinants of Health: Looking Upstream 1st Ed.* Polity.

SUPREME COURT OF THE UNITED STATES (2022). *Dobbs v. Jackson Women's Health Organization*. [online] Available at: https://www.supremecourt.gov/opinions/21pdf/19-1392_6j37.pdf [Accessed 1 Feb. 2024].

Supreme Court of the United States (2023). *Students for Fair Admissions, Inc. v. President and Fellows of Harvard College*. [online] Available at: https://www.supremecourt.gov/opinions/22pdf/20-1199_hgdj.pdf [Accessed 1 Feb. 2024].

The Commonwealth Fund (2023). *U.S. Health Care from a Global Perspective, 2022: Accelerating Spending, Worsening Outcomes*. [online] www.commonwealthfund.org. Available at: https://www.commonwealthfund.org/publications/issue-briefs/2023/jan/us-health-care-global-perspective-2022#1 [Accessed 1 Feb. 2024].

United Nations (2015). *Human right to water and sanitation | International Decade for Action 'Water for Life' 2005-2015*. [online] Available at: https://www.un.org/waterforlifedecade/human_right_to_water.shtml [Accessed 1 Feb. 2024].

Virginia Commonwealth University Center on Society and Health (2022). [online] societyhealth.vcu.edu. Available at: https://societyhealth.vcu.edu/work/the-projects/education-it-matters-more-to-health-than-ever-before.html#gsc.tab=0 [Accessed 1 Feb. 2024].

Wilkinson, R. and Marmot, M. (1998). Social determinants of health : the solid facts. *Who.int*. [online] https://iris.who.int/bitstream/handle/10665/108082/9289012870-eng.pdf?sequence=1&isAllowed=y [Accessed 24 Jan. 2024].

AUTHOR'S BIO SKETCH

James Lenhart. MD, FAAFP, MPH

Dr. Lenhart graduated from the University of New Mexico School of Medicine and took residency in Family Medicine from Brown University Affiliated Hospitals in Pawtucket/Providence, Rhode Island. In 2010 he completed a Master of Public Health degree from the University of Liverpool. He holds the distinction of academic rank of full professor from the University of North Carolina-Chapel Hill, University of Nevada, and University of Arizona.

He now serves as an Associate Program Director for the residency in Family Medicine at Community Health Care in Tacoma, Washington, a University of Washington affiliated program. In that capacity, Dr. Lenhart leads curriculum development including research and scholarship at the residency where he holds academic rank of Associate Clinical Professor.

Chapter 2

Justice as a Social Determinant of Health

Andrea Saunders, JD, Author
James Lenhart, MD, FAAFP, MPH, Editor

"Everyone has the right to an effective remedy by the competent national tribunals for acts violating the fundamental rights granted...by the constitution or by law."
- The Universal Declaration of Human Rights, Article 8, The United Nations, 1948

"Injustice anywhere is a threat to justice everywhere. We are caught in an inescapable network of mutuality, tied in a single garment of destiny. Whatever affects one directly affects all indirectly."
- Martin Luther King, Jr., Letter from Birmingham Jail, 1963

Justice as a Social Determinant of Health

Introduction

The social determinants of health (SDH) framework establishes that health outcomes are greatly, or mostly, determined by "non-medical factors" (World Health Organization, 2023). A person or population's health depends on access to tangible resources and support, such as education, nutritious food, healthcare access, safe and secure employment, a livable wage, habitable and stable housing, and committed family relationships. Clinical care replete with state-of-the-art technology and innovative therapeutics cannot effectively remedy the detrimental effects of neglected "non-medical factors." For example, poor housing conditions can "cause or exacerbate asthma, skin rashes, lead poisoning, fires, and common illnesses...While their *consequences* can be treated medically, the *causes* require robust *enforcement* of existing laws" (Law as a Social Determinant of Health, 2016) [emphasis added].

Justice is "the maintenance or administration of what is *just* especially by the impartial adjustment of conflicting claims or the assignment of merited rewards or punishments" (Merriam-Webster, 2019). To be just is to have "a basis in or conforming to fact or reason," as well as conforming to what is "morally upright or good," "merited," and "legally correct," (Merriam-

Webster, 2019). In the example of substandard housing, there may be law and policy to promote public health protections. However, a separate determinant of health is justice – fair and impartial *enforcement* of existing laws to promote that which rises to right and just. Lack of justice or *access* to justice characterizes social determinant of health neglect.

This chapter first examines justice as a tenant of medical ethics and whether distributive justice is achieved in the American healthcare system. Next, we turn to the legal system and several illustrations where health was either promoted or undermined by the administration of justice. These illustrations overlap with other SDHs, such as race, housing, education, gender, and poverty. They are offered as an introduction only. Law and justice impact virtually every facet of society and influence health outcomes in countless ways.

Fair enforcement of and remedy for one's legal claims is a human right identified in the United Nations Declaration of Human Rights (1948). When one does not have access to enforce their rights, they cannot achieve health and wellbeing. Attorney Bryan Stevenson notes, "My work with the poor and the incarcerated has persuaded me that the opposite of poverty is not wealth; the opposite of poverty is justice" (Stevenson, 2014). Throughout this chapter, we consider what circumstances led to a particular case being brought to court, whether justice was served in the outcome, and how public health was impacted as a result.

The bottom line. No matter what legal protections are legislated, justice not accessible predicts population health not served. Justice indeed is a social determinant of health.

Justice as a Social Determinant of Health

In the context of Medical Ethics

Health professionals learn through structured didactics or osmotic experiences the importance of professional behavior in the realm of patient care. Nevertheless, the tension of what is right, and in the patient's best interest, may clash with conflicts of interest. For instance, the tension to persist or terminate a treatment protocol without reasonable hope for recovery in a patient suffering from disease related intractable pain.

Beginning with Hippocrates over 2000 years ago, health professionals have been guided by ethical principles and related oaths. Over time and circumstance, medical ethics, once limited to an individual's professional conduct, expanded to "an extensive scope that includes research ethics, public health ethics, organizational ethics, and clinical ethics" in direct response to numerous "deplorable abuses of human subjects in research, medical interventions without informed consent, experimentation in concentration camps in World War II, along with salutary advances in medicine and medical technology and societal changes" (Varkey, 2021).

The ethics model proposed by Varkey includes seven separate principles that serve to steer healthcare professionals and policies:

Seven Principles of Medical Ethics

Beneficence: the obligation to act for the benefit of patients promoting altruism, well-being, and best practices care. Beneficence includes a moral obligation to protect and defend the rights of others.
Nonmaleficence: literally construed as to do no harm. "The practical application of nonmaleficence is for the physician to weigh the benefits against burdens of all interventions and treatments, to eschew those that are inappropriately burdensome, and to choose the best course of action for the patient," (Varkey, 2021).
Autonomy: the right for self-determination underpins autonomy – an individual's choice to make rational decisions and moral choices.
Informed consent: the obligation to disclose the risks and benefits of proposed therapies. This principle intertwines with autonomy and requires full disclosure, the patient's capacity to understand, comprehend, decide, and act voluntarily, and consent to the proposed action.
Truth-Telling: discloses not only the risk and benefits of proposed therapies, but the consequence of not electing for any of the proposed treatment options.
Confidentiality: without the patient's directed consent healthcare information must not be shared with others.
Justice: supports the precept of fair, appropriate, and equitable treatment for all people. In medical ethics, ***distributive justice*** is central to this doctrine.

Varkey, B. (2021). Principles of clinical ethics and their application to practice. *Medical Principles and Practice*, [online] Available at: https://doi.org/10.1159/000509119

For purposes of this treatise, the final tenet – justice – calls for specific attention. According to Varkey (2021), *social policies* dole out healthcare based on various principles and strategies. For example, resource distribution based on equal shares, or based on individual need or based on effort, contribution, or merit, or based on free-market exchanges. Taken singly or in combination, governing bodies legislate policies for the distribution of healthcare resources. In the U.S., the distribution of healthcare is the obligation of individual states. In *ethical principles* of distributive justice, healthcare is first and foremost what is fair to the patient (Varkey, 2021).

Socially progressive principles of distributive justice argue for distribution *independent* of merit, i.e., everyone deserves healthcare resources regardless of merit. Further, merit "making" should <u>not</u> begin until basic goods (housing, healthcare, education, and food) have been equally distributed to everyone (Fleischacker, 2004).

A long-time outlier in the fight against inequality, Väänänen (2020) applauds Finland's model of distributive justice. At a time when the gap between the rich and the poor is widening in most countries around the world, Finland consistently works to ensure that its poorest citizens are looked after. For example, "The country's novel 'housing first' principle ensures that, after being given the right support, rough sleepers [meaning those who are homeless and sleep on the streets] can own a home of their own, a non-traditional approach to a traditional problem" (Väänänen, 2020). In Finland, "it's about living in a country where all conceivable basic needs are met, whether that's healthcare, education, or having a job that makes you feel fulfilled" (Väänänen, 2020).

In stark contrast, distributive justice driven by free-market exchanges profoundly corrupts equal access to healthcare (and other basic needs). Profit making drives healthcare in the United States. Pharmaceutical corporations, the healthcare insurance industry, and hospital corporations maintain a tight fist on maximizing the financial bottom line. Beholden to shareholders, stock prices, and executive compensation, the cost of healthcare in the United States leads all other high-income countries yet trails substantially in health outcomes including life expectancy (The Commonwealth Fund, 2023).

Financial data gathered by Macrotrends (2024) demonstrates the staggering profit of healthcare giants in the United States. Net income reflects the bottom line after accounting for **all** revenue, income, expenses, and taxes in 2022:

- Pfizer annual net income for 2022 was $31.372B, a 42.74% increase from 2021,
- UnitedHealth Group annual net income for 2022 was $20.12B, a 16.4% increase from 2021,
- HCA Healthcare annual net income for 2022 was $5.643B, a 18.88% decline from 2021,
- Biogen annual net income for 2022 was $3.047B, a 95.8% increase from 2021,
- IQVIA Holdings annual net income for 2022 was $1.091B, a 12.94% increase from 2021 (Macrotrends, 2024).

The selected corporations are indicative of massive earnings within American health care, despite growing concerns about quality and access. Furthermore, the examples provided do not capture the largest healthcare corporations (Eli Lilly, Johnson & Johnson, Merck as examples). Pfizer appeared as a top 10 largest healthcare company based on data as of December 21, 2022 (Investopedia, 2023).

Executive compensation within the enterprise of healthcare is astonishing. It reflects high accumulation and concentration of wealth within an industry of "limited resources" ostensibly driven by world class health outcomes. The following chart documents the top 20 healthcare CEOs compensation for 2022 according to Newitt (2023).

Executive Compensation for Healthcare CEOs in the United States

Total compensation includes information disclosed in company proxy statements, including base salary, bonus, stock awards and option awards, as well as other benefits and perks.

1. Albert Bourla, PhD, Pfizer (New York City) — $30.54 million

2. Christopher Viehbacher, Biogen (Cambridge, Mass.) — $30.49 million

3. Ari Bousbib, IQVIA Holdings (Durham, N.C.) — $29.71 million

4. Marc Casper, Thermo Fisher Scientific (Waltham, Mass.) — $28.21 million

5. Franis deSouza, Illumina (San Diego) — $26.75 million

6. Richard Gonzalez, AbbVie (North Chicago, Ill.) — $25.85 million

7. Joseph Zubretsky, Molina Healthcare (Long Beach, Calif.) — $22.13 million

8. Daniel Patrick O'Day, Gilead Sciences (Foster City, Calif.) — $21.62 million

9. Robert Ford, Abbott Laboratories (Abbott Park, Ill.) — $21.45 million

10. Robert Bradway, Amgen (Thousand Oaks, Calif.) — $21.40 million

11. David Ricks, Eli Lilly and Co. (Indianapolis) — $21.40 million

12. Karen Lynch, CVS Health Corp. (Woonsocket, R.I.) — $21.32 million

13. David Cordani, The Cigna Group (Bloomfield, Conn.) — $20.97 million

14. Gail Koziara Boudreaux, Elevance Health (Indianapolis) — $20.93 million

15. Andrew Witty, UnitedHealth Group (Minnetonka, Minn.) — $20.87 million

16. Brian Tyler, PhD, McKesson Corp. (Irving, Texas) — $20.22 million

17. Rainer Blair, Danaher Corp. (Washington, D.C.) — $20.20 million

18. Giovanni Caforio, MD, Bristol-Myers Squibb Co. (Lawrence Township, N.J.) — $20.05 million

19. Stephane Bancel, Moderna (Cambridge, Mass.) — $19.36 million

20. Joseph Hogan, Align Technology (Tempe, Ariz.) — $18.68 million

Newitt, P. (2023). The 20 highest-paid Healthcare CEOs. [online] www.beckersasc.com. Available at: https://www.beckersasc.com/leadership/the-20-highest-paid-healthcare-ceos.html

Executive compensation identified above does not account for the numerous seven and eight figure salaries of downstream corporate minions in the industry. Taken in aggregate, extraordinary corporate profits and executive salaries punctuate the conviction that healthcare in the U.S. is for profit and insulting to the ethical principle of healthcare justice distributed equally.

Justice, and particularly distributive justice, play a critical role in the delivery of ethical healthcare. Distribution of healthcare resources directly implicates access to healthcare as a social determinant of health and adds a dimension of fairness and equity to patients. The figures above indicate that limited healthcare, tight resources, and disrupted allocation might be artificial, rather than inherent. Reliance on free-market distribution does not achieve best in class outcomes, but it does provide best-in-class executive compensation and corporate profit.

The U.S is the only high-income country that does not guarantee health coverage (Gunja, Gumas, and Williams, 2023); 10.1% of U.S. individuals under the age of 65 years were uninsured in 2022 at the time of the National Health Survey (Cohen, Makuc and Ezzati-Rice, 2022); U.S. life expectancy a birth is 3 years lower than the OECD average (Gunja, Gumas, and Williams, 2023). These data strongly suggests that healthcare not championed by health justice for all flies in the face of what's best for the patients, populations, and nations.

Justice as a Social Determinant of Health

Shifting from Medical Ethics to Legal Systems

We next pivot to justice as a social determinant of health in the American legal system. The following explorations show how the law has harmed or improved health, often involving other named social determinants. We will explore how justice, what is right and fair, is independent and separate from each determinant as traditionally understood ***and*** is independent and separate from overarching public health laws, policy, and governance.

These issues are infinitely complex, nuanced, and full of history. The following sections are a starting point, or introduction, for further inquiry and research. This only scratches the surface of a vast and rich social history.

Justice as a Social Determinant of Health

In the context of Race

The Supreme Court of the United States – the highest court in the land – has an egregious history in dealing with race and racial justice. The decisions of the Court establish an arbitrary hierarchy which directly implicates health, access, and basic human rights.

Prior to the Civil War, the Supreme Court explicitly "found," or decided, that enslaved persons were not people, rather the property of those who enslaved them *Dred Scott v. Sandford* (1857). "In this ruling, the U.S. Supreme Court stated that enslaved people were not citizens of the United States and, therefore, could not expect any protection from the federal government or the courts. The opinion also stated that Congress had no authority to ban slavery from a Federal territory" (National Archives, 2021). The horrifying treatment of human beings as property cannot more clearly demonstrate the role of justice and injustice on health.

Systemic racism and many violations of Black justice persist, despite the Civil War, executive actions, and Congressional legislation. In 1868, the 14th Amendment to the United States Constitution was ratified and established certain rights and protections for citizens and residences. Section 1 states:

> "All persons born or naturalized in the United States, and subject to the jurisdiction thereof, are citizens of the United States and of the State wherein they reside. No State shall make or enforce any law which shall abridge the privileges or immunities of citizens of the United States; nor shall any State deprive any person of life, liberty, or property, without due process of law; nor deny to any person within its jurisdiction the equal protection of the laws" (National Archives, 2024).

Though the 14th Amendment enshrined due process and equal protection, all levels of government continued egregious acts towards the most marginalized of society. Immediately following the Civil War and passage of the 14th Amendment, state and local government officials enacted laws enforcing racial segregation, also known as Jim Crow laws, throughout the country (Reed, 2021).

In one such Jim Crow law, Louisiana passed the Separate Car Act in 1890, legislating separate railway carriages for whites and Black people. In June 1892, Homer Plessy defied the law, was arrested, and jailed. In 1896, nearly four years after his arrest and decades after the conclusion of the Civil War and the passage of the 14th Amendment, the Supreme Court of the United States heard *Plessy v. Ferguson*. Rather than uphold what is right and just, it cemented segregation as an overarching principle of race relations in the United States and guaranteed ongoing race inequality.

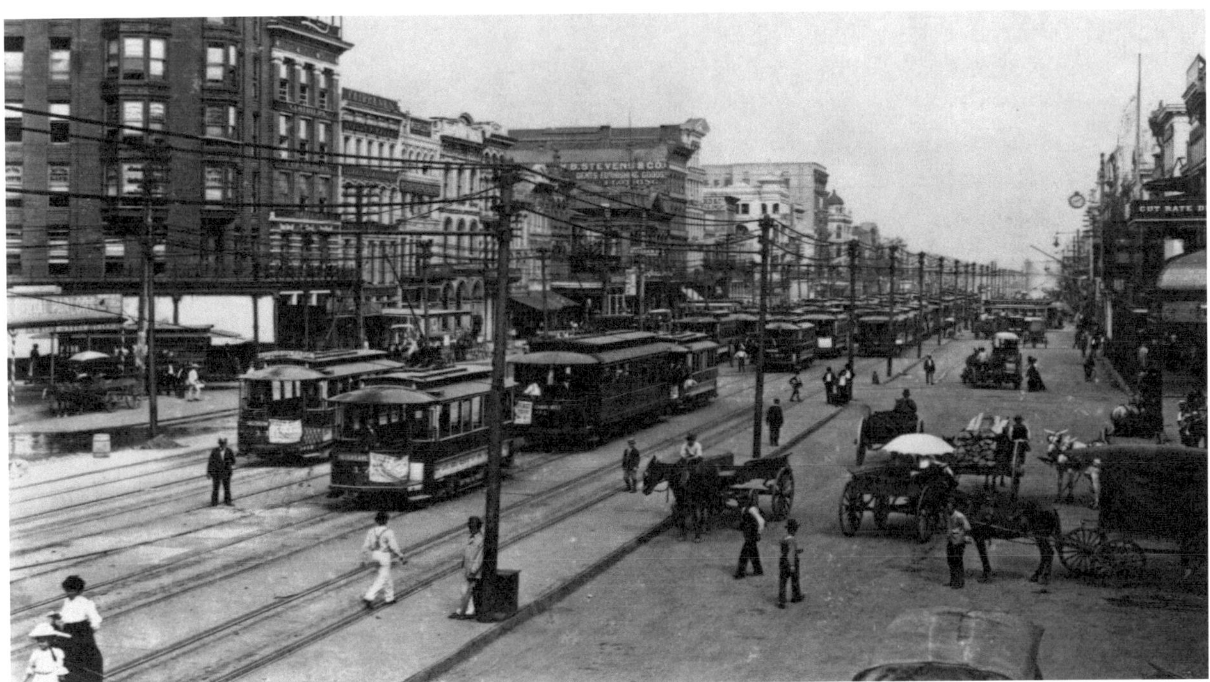

New Orleans railway carriages circa 1896.

McNamara, R. (2019). *What You Should Know About the Notorious Plessy v. Ferguson Decision.* [online] ThoughtCo. Available at: https://www.thoughtco.com/plessy-v-ferguson-1773294

Plessy v. Ferguson (1896)
Excerpts of Justice Henry Billing Brown's majority opinion

This case turns upon the constitutionality of an act of the General Assembly of the State of Louisiana, passed in 1890, providing for separate railway carriages for the white and colored races. The first section of the statute enacts "that all railway companies carrying passengers in their coaches in this State shall provide equal but separate accommodations for the white and colored races by providing two or more passenger coaches for each passenger train, or by dividing the passenger coaches by a partition so as to secure separate accommodations. No person or persons, shall be admitted to occupy seats in coaches other than the ones assigned to them on account of the race they belong to."

By the second section, it was enacted "that the officers of such passenger trains shall have power and are hereby required to assign each passenger to the coach or compartment used for the race to which such passenger belongs; any passenger insisting on going into a coach or compartment to which by race he does not belong shall be liable to a fine of twenty-five dollars, or in lieu thereof to imprisonment for a period of not more than twenty days in the parish prison.

We consider the underlying fallacy of the plaintiff's argument to consist in the assumption that the enforced separation of the two races stamps the colored race with a badge of inferiority. If this be so, it is not by reason of anything found in the act, but solely because the colored race chooses to put that construction upon it.

The argument also assumes that social prejudices may be overcome by legislation, and that equal rights cannot be secured to the negro except by an enforced commingling of the two races. We cannot accept this proposition. If the two races are to meet upon terms of social equality, it must be the result of natural affinities, a mutual appreciation of each other's merits, and a voluntary consent of individuals.

As was said by the Court of Appeals of New York in People v. Gallagher, 93 N.Y. 438, 448, "This end can neither be accomplished nor promoted by laws which conflict with the general sentiment of the community upon whom they are designed to operate. When the government, therefore, has secured to each of its citizens equal rights before the law and equal opportunities for improvement and progress, it has accomplished the end for which it was organized, and performed all of the functions respecting social advantages with which it is endowed."

Legislation is powerless to eradicate racial instincts or to abolish distinctions based upon physical differences, and the attempt to do so can only result in accentuating the difficulties of the present situation. If the civil and political rights of both races be equal, one cannot be inferior to the other civilly or politically. If one race be inferior to the other socially, the Constitution of the United States cannot put them upon the same plane.

Justia Law. (n.d.). *Plessy v. Ferguson, 163 U.S. 537 (1896).* [online] Available at: https://supreme.justia.com/cases/federal/us/163/537/#tab-opinion-1917401.

There was but one lone dissenter to the decision written by Justice John Marshall Harlan. No other Justice joined the dissenting opinion, written in opposition to the Court's ruling.

Plessy v. Ferguson (1896)
Excerpts of Justice John Marshall Harlan's dissenting opinion

Under this statute, no colored person is permitted to occupy a seat in a coach assigned to white persons, nor any white person to occupy a seat in a coach assigned to colored persons. The managers of the railroad are not allowed to exercise any discretion in the premises but are required to assign each passenger to some coach or compartment set apart for the exclusive use of his race.

If a passenger insists upon going into a coach or compartment not set apart for persons of his race, he is subject to be fined or to be imprisoned in the parish jail. The 13th amendment having been found inadequate to the protection of the rights of those who had been in slavery, it was followed by the Fourteenth Amendment, which added greatly to the dignity and glory of American citizenship and to the security of personal liberty by declaring that "all persons born or naturalized in the United States, and subject to the jurisdiction thereof, are citizens of the United States and of the State wherein they reside," and that "no State of the United States; nor shall any State deprive any person of life, liberty or property without due process of law, nor deny to any person within its jurisdiction the equal protection of the laws."

If a State can prescribe, as a rule of civil conduct, that whites and blacks shall not travel as passengers in the same railroad coach, why may it not so regulate the use of the streets of its cities and towns as to compel white citizens to keep on one side of a street and black citizens to keep on the other?

The white race deems itself to be the dominant race in this country. And so it is in prestige, in achievements, in education, in wealth and in power. So, I doubt not, it will continue to be for all time if it remains true to its great heritage and holds fast to the principles of constitutional liberty. But in view of the Constitution, in the eye of the law, there is in this country no superior, dominant, ruling class of citizens. There is no caste here. Our Constitution is color-blind, and neither knows nor tolerates classes among citizens. In respect of civil rights, all citizens are equal before the law.

The present decision, it may well be apprehended, will not only stimulate aggressions, more or less brutal and irritating, upon the admitted rights of colored citizens, but will encourage the belief that it is possible, by means of state enactments, to defeat the beneficent purposes which the people of the United States had in view when they adopted the recent amendments of the Constitution, by one of which the blacks of this country were made citizens of the United States and of the States in which they respectively reside, and whose privileges and immunities, as citizens, the States are forbidden to abridge.

I am of opinion that the statute of Louisiana is inconsistent with the personal liberty of citizens, white and black, in that State, and hostile to both the spirit and letter of the Constitution of the United States. If laws of like character should be enacted in the several States of the Union, the effect would be in the highest degree mischievous. Slavery, as an institution tolerated by law would, it is true, have disappeared from our country, but there would remain a power in the States, by sinister legislation, to interfere with the full enjoyment of the blessings of freedom to regulate civil rights, common to all citizens, upon the basis of race, and to place in a condition of legal inferiority a large body of American citizens now constituting a part of the political community called the People of the United States, for whom and by whom, through representatives, our government is administered.

Justia Law. (n.d.). *Plessy v. Ferguson, 163 U.S. 537 (1896)*. [online] Available at: https://supreme.justia.com/cases/federal/us/163/537/#tab-opinion-1917401

Plessy v. Ferguson condoned and emboldened Jim Crow laws and racial segregation in the United States, giving states and local governments Carte Blanc permission to enact similar laws throughout the land for over 58 years. "The decision, which would not be overturned until 1954 in the landmark case *Brown v. Board of Education of Topeka,* placed a seal of approval on the segregationist laws that began to spread across the country" (Reed, 2021).

Such segregationist laws limited access to all manner of public accommodations, resources, housing, and property. One method of segregation came through racially restrictive covenants against African Americans. Racially restrictive covenants refer to contractual agreements that prohibit the purchase, lease, or occupation of a piece of property by a particular group of people. Racially restrictive covenants included mutual agreements between property owners in a neighborhood not to sell to certain races and cooperation of real estate boards and neighborhood associations to enforce the restrictions.

Racially restrictive covenants became particularly common after 1926 following the U.S. Supreme Court decision, *Corrigan v. Buckley* (1926), which validated their use (The Fair Housing Center of Boston, n.d.). History confirms as well that the National Housing Act of 1934 introduced the practice of redlining, which marked off areas determined too risky to underwrite mortgage guarantees. Simultaneously, the National Association of Realtors wrote language into its code of ethics directing realtors to never introduce to a neighborhood, members of any race or nationality detrimental to property values (Evans, 2022).

In 1911, a neighborhood in St. Louis, Missouri enacted a racially restrictive covenant designed to prevent African Americans and Asian-Americans ("people of the Negro or Asian Race") from occupying property in the community. More than three decades later, in 1945, an African American family named Shelley moved into the neighborhood without being informed that the covenant existed. Another resident of the community, Louis Kraemer, brought a suit to enforce the covenant and prevent the Shelleys from moving into their house, even though he lived several blocks away (Justia Law, 2019).

Shelley v. Kraemer (1948)
Excerpts of Chief Justice Fred M. Vinson's majority opinion

These cases present for our consideration questions relating to the validity of court enforcement of private agreements, generally described as restrictive covenants, which have as their purpose the exclusion of persons of designated race or color from the ownership or occupancy of real property. Basic constitutional issues of obvious importance have been raised.

Petitioners have placed primary reliance on their contentions, first raised in the state courts, that judicial enforcement of the restrictive agreements in these cases has violated rights guaranteed to petitioners by the Fourteenth Amendment of the Federal Constitution and Acts of Congress passed pursuant to that Amendment.

Whether the equal protection clause of the Fourteenth Amendment inhibits judicial enforcement by state courts of restrictive covenants based on race or color is a question which this Court has not heretofore been called upon to consider.

It cannot be doubted that among the civil rights intended to be protected from discriminatory state action by the Fourteenth Amendment are the rights to acquire, enjoy, own and dispose of property. Equality in the enjoyment of property rights was regarded by the framers of that Amendment as an essential pre-condition to the realization of other basic civil rights and liberties which the Amendment was intended to guarantee.

We hold that in granting judicial enforcement of the restrictive agreements in these cases, the States have denied petitioners the equal protection of the laws and that, therefore, the action of the state courts cannot stand. We have noted that freedom from discrimination by the States in the enjoyment of property rights was among the basic objectives sought to be effectuated by the framers of the Fourteenth Amendment. That such discrimination has occurred in these cases is clear.

Because of the race or color of these petitioners they have been denied rights of ownership or occupancy enjoyed as a matter of course by other citizens of different race or color. The Fourteenth Amendment declares "that all persons, whether colored or white, shall stand equal before the laws of the States, and, in regard to the colored race, for whose protection the amendment was primarily designed, that no discrimination shall be made against them by law because of their color."

U.S. Supreme Court (1948). *Shelley v. Kraemer CASES ADJUDGED IN THE.* [online] Available at: https://tile.loc.gov/storage-services/service/ll/usrep/usrep334/usrep334001/usrep334001.pdf

Six Justices joined the majority opinion, three recused, none dissented.

The Court found in *Shelley v. Kraemer* (1948) that government enforcement of racially restrictive covenants was a violation of the 14th Amendment, yet the practice by private citizens and property owners was lawful. *Shelley v. Kraemer* did nothing to outlaw private racially restrictive covenants, and so discriminatory practices in housing continued. This led to the passage of the Fair Housing Act of 1968. Tragically, according to Evans (2022), "segregation was well entrenched and the old alliances that had kept the covenants in place found a way to circumvent the new system and even keep the discriminatory covenants in their deeds—even if they couldn't legally enforce them." Racial inequalities in housing, land ownership, and wealth, social determinants of health in their own right, persist today as a direct result of legal race discrimination (Evans, 2022).

Race and education collided in *Brown v. Board of Education (1954)* and the Court overturned its previous endorsement of racial segregation. "On May 17, 1954, U.S. Supreme Court Justice Earl Warren delivered the unanimous ruling in the landmark civil rights case *Brown* v. *Board of Education of Topeka, Kansas*. State-sanctioned segregation of public schools was a violation of the 14th amendment and was therefore unconstitutional.

This historic decision marked the end of the 'separate but equal' precedent set by the Supreme Court nearly 60 years earlier in *Plessy* v. *Ferguson* and served as a catalyst for the expanding civil rights movement during the decade of the 1950s" (National Archives, 2021a).

The U.S. Supreme Court delivered a unanimous opinion, joined by all Justices.

Brown v. Board of Education of Topeka (1954)
Excerpts from Justice Warren's opinion

These cases come to us from the States of Kansas, South Carolina, Virginia, and Delaware. In each of the cases, minors of the Negro race, through their legal representatives, seek the aid of the courts in obtaining admission to the public schools of their community on a nonsegregated

Brown v. Board of Education of Topeka (1954) (continued)
Excerpts from Justice Warren's opinion

basis. In each instance, they had been denied admission to schools attended by white children under laws requiring or permitting segregation according to race. This segregation was alleged to deprive the plaintiffs of the equal protection of the laws under the Fourteenth Amendment. In each of the cases federal district courts denied relief to the plaintiffs on the so-called "separate but equal" doctrine announced by this Court in Plessy v. Ferguson, 163 U. S. 537.

Today, education is perhaps the most important function of state and local governments. Compulsory school attendance laws and the great expenditures for education both demonstrate our recognition of the importance of education to our democratic society. It is required in the performance of our most basic public responsibilities, even service in the armed forces. It is the very foundation of good citizenship. Today it is a principal instrument in awakening the child to cultural values, in preparing him for later professional training, and in helping him to adjust normally to his environment. In these days, it is doubtful that any child may reasonably be expected to succeed in life if he is denied the opportunity of an education. Such an opportunity, where the state has undertaken to provide it, is a right which must be made available to all on equal terms.

We come then to the question presented: Does segregation of children in public schools solely on the basis of race, even though the physical facilities and other "tangible" factors may be equal, deprive the children of the minority group of equal educational opportunities? We believe that it does.

We conclude that in the field of public education the doctrine of "separate but equal" has no place. Separate educational facilities are inherently unequal."' Therefore, we hold that the plaintiffs and others similarly situated for whom the actions have been brought are, by reason of the segregation complained of, deprived of the equal protection of the laws guaranteed by the Fourteenth Amendment.

Of Topeka et al. No. 1. Appeal from the united states district court for the district of Kansas.*. (1954). Available at: https://tile.loc.gov/storage-services/service/ll/usrep/usrep347/usrep347483/usrep347483.pdf

There is little doubt that desegregation positively impacted health outcomes and promoted racial justice in areas beyond access to education. The Civil Rights and Voting Rights Acts of 1964 followed *Brown* "placing Congress's seal of approval on *Brown* and the project of desegregation, and [making] civil rights a national commitment of the executive and legislative branches of the federal government" setting the stage for passing the Civil Rights and Voting Rights Acts of the 1960s (Lens, 2021).

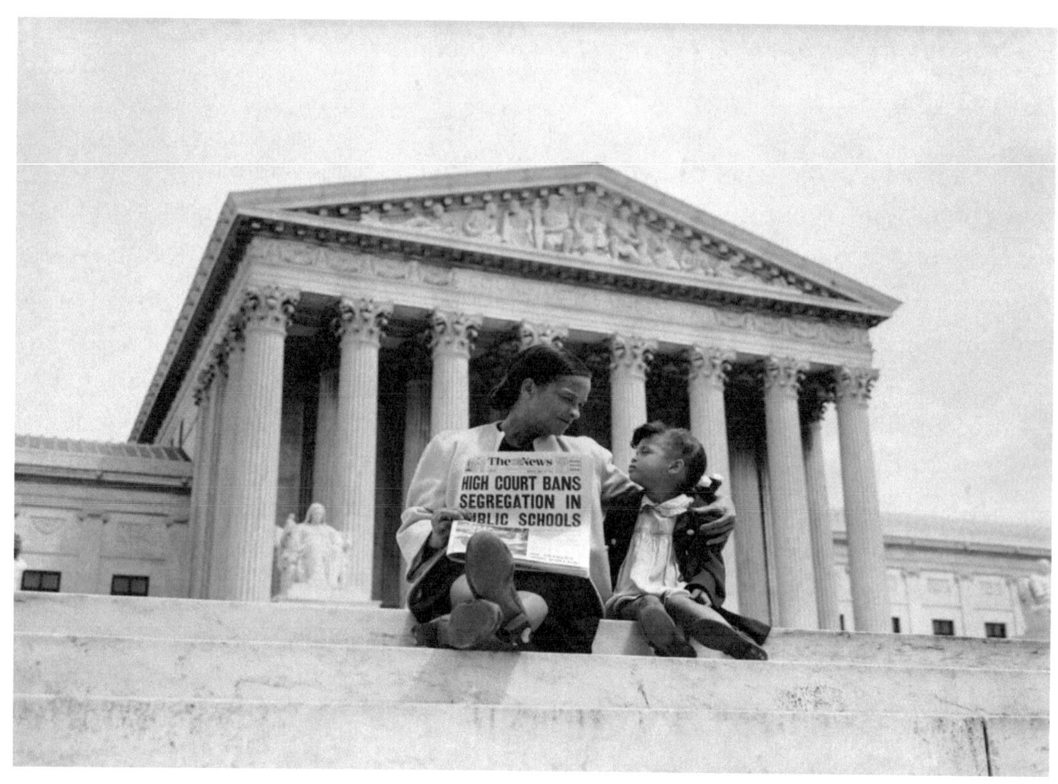

Legal Defense Fund (n.d.). *Brown v. Board of Education Case Portal*. [online] NAACP Legal Defense and Educational Fund. Available at: https://www.naacpldf.org/brown-vs-board/

Unfortunately, progress can be rolled back. Efforts to achieve desegregation have been defeated on the same grounds as *Brown v. Board of Education*, such as *Parents Involved in Community Schools v. Seattle School District No. 1* (2007), which "determined that earlier decisions for college affirmative action do not apply to public schools and that racial diversity is not a compelling government interest for public school admission. Furthermore, they held that the denial of admission to a public school because of a student's race in the interest of achieving racial diversity is unconstitutional," (Stahl, 2015).

Most recently, *Students for Fair Admissions, Inc. v. President and Fellows of Harvard College* (2023) struck down President John F. Kennedy's 1963 Affirmative Action policies that promoted racial equality in education. While *Brown v. Board of Education* remains binding law, the matter of *how* to achieve racial justice and equality is frustrated, at best. Without enforcement, there is no justice, and without justice, there cannot be consummate population health.

Justice as a Social Determinant of Health

In the context of Gender

The 14th Amendment safeguards all protected classes of people, including gender. This section will briefly focus on the Court's treatment of women within legal proceedings. In the selected case, the Court overturned a blind and discriminatory preference for men over women in court proceedings.

At issue was an Idaho state law from 1864 which required that when two parents of a deceased person apply to be the estate administrator, the court must appoint the father, not the mother. Sally Reed challenged the law when the probate court selected her ex-husband the administrator. "In a terse and unanimous opinion, the Idaho Supreme Court rejected Sally Reed's contention that the statute's preference for men over women was 'arbitrary and capricious'" and refused to grant relief under the 14th Amendment (Supreme Court Historical Society, n.d.).

However, the United States Supreme Court ruled differently, reversing the Idaho court's decision and extended 14th Amendment equal protection to gender.

When the Supreme Court handed down its opinion in *Reed v. Reed* in November of 1971, the decision made headlines across the country. More than 100 years after the passage of the 14th Amendment, the Court struck down a state law on the ground that it discriminated against women in violation of the Equal Protection Clause. Conversely, the Court declined to give as much scrutiny to gender discrimination as given to racial classifications, leaving more room for legislative deference and discretion (Supreme Court Historical Society, n.d.).

Reed v. Reed (1971)
Excerpts from Justice Burger's majority opinion

Idaho Supreme Court first dealt with the governing statutory law and held that under § 15-

Reed v. Reed (1971) (Continued)
Excerpts from Justice Burger's majority opinion

312 "a father and mother are 'equally entitled' to letters of administration," but the preference given to males by § 15-314 is "mandatory" and leaves no room for the exercise of a probate court's discretion in the appointment of administrators. Having thus definitively and authoritatively interpreted the statutory provisions involved, the Idaho Supreme Court then proceeded to examine, and reject, Sally Reed's contention that § 15-314 violates the Equal Protection Clause by giving a mandatory preference to males over females, without regard to their individual qualifications as potential estate administrators.

Sally Reed thereupon appealed for review by this Court pursuant to 28 U. S. C. § 1257 (2), and we noted probable jurisdiction. 401 U. S. 934. Having examined the record and considered the briefs and oral arguments of the parties, we have concluded that the arbitrary preference established in favor of males by § 15-314 of the Idaho Code cannot stand in the face -of the Fourteenth Amendment's command that no State deny the equal protection of the laws to any person within its jurisdiction. In such situations, § 15-314 provides that different treatment be accorded to the applicants on the basis of their sex; it thus establishes a classification subject to scrutiny under the Equal Protection Clause.

The Equal Protection Clause of that amendment does, however, deny to States the power to legislate that different treatment be accorded to persons placed by a statute into different classes on the basis of criteria wholly unrelated to the objective of that statute. A classification "must be reasonable, not arbitrary, and must rest upon some ground of difference having a fair and substantial relation to the object of the legislation, so that all persons similarly circumstanced shall be treated alike."

Regardless of their sex, persons within any one of the enumerated classes of that section are similarly situated with respect to that objective. By providing dissimilar treatment for men and women who are thus similarly situated, the challenged section violates the Equal Protection Clause.

U.S. Supreme Court (1971). *Reed v. Reed.* [online] Available at: https://tile.loc.gov/storage-services/service/ll/usrep/usrep404/usrep404071/usrep404071.pdf [Accessed 27 Dec. 2023].

Justice as a Social Determinant of Health

In the context of a Fair System of Justice

We see clearly that Constitutional protections do not necessarily guarantee just outcomes and that progress can be undone or undermined. It is important to consider *who* has access to enforce laws and rights, and *how* they do so. In the United States, a great divide between those with means and those without exists; in other words, between those with the resources to access legal professionals and those who must go at it alone. It is often said we have "two systems of justice" in the United States.

Two Supreme Court decisions sought to remedy this dichotomy. In *Miranda v. Arizona (1966),* the Supreme Court restricted the use of defendants' statements if they were not properly informed of their constitutional rights, coined "Miranda warnings." In *Gideon v. Wainwright (1963),* the Supreme Court found that indigent criminal defendants were entitled to a defense attorney, at public expense, to guarantee their constitutional rights, and established the right to legal representation.

Gideon v. Wainwright 1963 – essentials of the case

Clarence Earl Gideon was a man with an eighth-grade education who ran away from home when he was in middle school. He spent much of his early adult life as a drifter, spending time in and out of prisons for nonviolent crimes.

Gideon was charged with breaking and entering with the intent to commit a misdemeanor, which is a felony under Florida law. At trial, Gideon appeared in court without an attorney. In open court, he asked the judge to appoint counsel for him because he could not afford one. The trial judge denied Gideon's request.

At trial, Gideon represented himself – he made an opening statement to the jury, cross-examined the prosecution's witnesses, presented witnesses in his own defense, declined to testify himself, and made arguments emphasizing his innocence. Despite his efforts, the jury found Gideon guilty, and he was sentenced to five years imprisonment.

US Courts (n.d.). *Facts and Case Summary - Gideon v. Wainwright.* [online] United States Courts. Available at: https://www.uscourts.gov/educational-resources/educational-activities/facts-and-case-summary-gideon-v-wainwright

***Gideon v. Wainwright* (1963)**

Excerpts from Justice Black's majority opinion

Since 1942, when *Betts v. Brady*, 316 U. S. 455, was decided by a divided Court, the problem of a defendant's federal constitutional right to counsel in a state court has been a continuing

Gideon v. Wainwright (1963) (continued)

Excerpts from Justice Black's majority opinion

source of controversy and litigation in both state and federal courts.

The facts upon which Betts claimed that he had been unconstitutionally denied. The right to have counsel appointed to assist him are strikingly like the facts upon which Gideon here bases his federal constitutional claim. Betts was indicted for robbery in a Maryland state court. On arraignment, he told the trial judge of his lack of funds to hire a lawyer and asked the court to appoint one for him. Betts was advised that it was not the practice in that county to appoint counsel for indigent defendants except in murder and rape cases. He then pleaded not guilty, had witnesses summoned, cross-examined the State's witnesses, examined his own, and chose not to testify himself. He was found guilty by the judge, sitting without a jury, and sentenced to eight years in prison.

The Sixth Amendment provides, "In all criminal prosecutions, the accused shall enjoy the right . . . to have the Assistance of Counsel for his defense." We have construed this to mean that in federal courts counsel must be provided for defendants unable to employ counsel unless the right is competently and intelligently waived.' Betts argued that this right is extended to indigent defendants in state courts by the Fourteenth Amendment.

The fact is that in deciding as it did that "appointment of counsel is not a fundamental right, essential to a fair trial" the Court in Betts v. Brady made an abrupt break with its own well-considered precedents.

In returning, to these old precedents, sounder we believe than the new, we but restore constitutional principles established to achieve a fair system of justice.

Not only these precedents but also reason and reflection require us to recognize that in our adversary system of criminal justice, any person haled into court, who is too poor to hire a lawyer, cannot be assured a fair trial unless counsel is provided for him. This seems to us to be an obvious truth. Governments, both state and federal, quite properly spend vast sums of money to establish machinery to try defendants accused of crime. Lawyers to prosecute are everywhere deemed essential to protect the public's interest in an orderly society. Similarly, there are few defendants charged with crime, few indeed, who fail to hire the best lawyers they can get to prepare and present their defenses. That government hires lawyers to prosecute and defendants who have the money hire lawyers to defend are the strongest indications of the widespread belief that lawyers in criminal courts are necessities, not luxuries. The right of one charged with crime to counsel may not be deemed fundamental and essential to fair trials in some countries, but it is in ours.

US Courts (n.d.). *Facts and Case Summary - Gideon v. Wainwright*. [online] United States Courts. Available at: https://www.uscourts.gov/educational-resources/educational-activities/facts-and-case-summary-gideon-v-wainwright

Justice as a Social Determinant of Health

In the context of Civil Law – the Justice Gap

Both *Miranda* and *Gideon* demonstrate an understanding that most people cannot be expected to fully understand or enforce legal protections without access to legal information, advice, and representation. In contrast, there is *no* such right to counsel in civil cases. Access to legal services in cases of domestic violence or for those threatened with eviction or loss of child custody goes unmet.

Legal scholars call this ongoing disparity the "Justice Gap." While federal law established the Legal Services Corporation to address this issue (Legal Services Corporation, 1974), the overwhelming majority of people go without legal services, directly limiting the ability to seek legal remedies and obtain justice. "Every day, millions of low-income Americans grapple with civil legal problems, which often involve basic needs like safe housing, access to health care, child custody, and protection from abuse" (Legal Services Corporation, 2022). It is reported that "low-income Americans did not receive any legal help or enough legal help for 92% of the [civil legal] problems that substantially impacted them in the past year" (Legal Services Corporation, 2022). Often, the legal remedies lost to this gap are those related to basic human needs and well-established social determinants of health.

Injustice and its negative impact on health is further seen in adjudication of domestic violence, child abuse, and family law cases. The United Nations Human Rights Council argues that reform is needed to end and reverse "long-lasting harm done to individuals, families and societies" through the U.S. family court system, frequently made worse by lack of access to legal representation. "The report addresses the link between custody cases, violence against women and violence against children, with a focus on the abuse of the term 'parental alienation' and similar pseudo-concepts" (Alsalem, 2023).

Bias continues to interrupt access to a fair system of justice. A report published by Lamba Legal Black and Pink National notes the current trends of discrimination and harmful practices within the court system that undermine access to justice for LGBTQ2A communities (Frazer, et al., 2022). Further research has demonstrated ongoing bias and negative outcomes based on gender, race, and language discrimination, among other marginalized identities, within the legal system.

Just as medical ethics champion distributive justice in healthcare, social determinants of health must be promulgated with distributive justice in law, policy, and governance. Studies have identified the positive effect of access to legal professionals, for example, as a critical facet of community response to intimate partner violence (Hartley & Renner, 2018). This reflects the principles of *Gideon* and *Miranda*. Communities need access to legal professionals to secure just outcomes, as they need access to medical professionals for clinical care. Access to a fair system of justice is a critical social determinant of health.

Justice as a Social Determinant of Health

In the context of Poverty

Poverty derails access to food, housing, water and sanitation, education and health care resulting in unfavorable health outcomes – significant increases in diabetes, cardiovascular disease, obesity, hypertension, and mental health disorders to those affected. People living in poverty are subject to amplified prevalence of incarceration, infectious diseases, trauma, domestic violence, and adverse childhood experiences. Worldwide data provide compelling evidence that legislative strategies and social welfare policies to reduce and ameliorate poverty improve health outcomes and population well-being.

Vicki Lens, MSW, JD, PhD Associate Dean and Professor at the Silberman School of Social Work at Hunter College-CUNY provides a deep dive into Supreme Court decisions levied over the last 60 years that have affected poor and racial minorities (Social Justice and the Supreme Court, 2021). Lens' treatise specifically appraised the Supreme Court's "doctrinal contributions from 1953 to the present across three foundational elements of social justice on behalf of the poor and people of color: 1) the school integration cases under the Equal Protection Clause, 2) a series of cases under the Fourth Amendment which sanctioned the police tactic of stop-and-frisk, and 3) attempts to secure economic security for the poor through Constitutional decree under the Due Process and Equal Protection Clauses." Historically, social movements campaigning for civil rights, gender equality, or economic security have viewed the judiciary, and especially the Supreme Court, as a potential and essential ally according to Lens (2021).

Brown v. Board of Education, as discussed above, ended over a hundred years of segregated public school in the United States. It also marked the beginning of a new strategy for securing social justice—engaging the judiciary. Sensing that change was more likely in the courts than in Congress, the National Association for the Advancement of Colored People (NAACP) formulated a litigation strategy to overturn the legacy of Jim Crow (Lens, 2021).

Brown galvanized the Civil Rights movement. The Montgomery Bus Boycott began a year after the decision. Demonstrations and protests spread throughout the South, including in Birmingham and Selma. In 1964 the Civil Rights Act and Voting Rights Act were passed, 'placing Congress's seal of approval on *Brown* and the project of desegregation, and [making] civil rights a national commitment of the executive and legislative branches of the federal government' (Lens, 2021). Embellishing these tactics, President Lyndon Johnson launched his War on Poverty.

Strategies to promote the War included the Legal Services Program led by Edward Sparer. According to Lens (2021), Sparer laid out a scheme to create a "bill of rights" for welfare recipients that campaigned for a constitutional right for economic security, the "right to live" Sparer called it. Sparer's long-term fantasy transformed "welfare from a categorical entitlement to a universal and constitutional right" (Lens, 2021). The Supreme Court thus heard *King v. Smith* (1968), the campaign's first case.

Under the state practices challenged in *King v. Smith*, "ninety percent of the children who were cut off from aid were Black. Eighteen other states had similar rules, affecting about 500,000 children" (Lens, 2021). *King v. Smith* was part of the Center for Law and Social Policy's Southern strategy for "constitutionalizing" welfare, which focused on the South because of its deep poverty, but also, because Southern federal judges had been exposed to the use of the courts for social change through successful civil rights litigation and was a component of the Center's strategy to link poverty and civil rights together (Lens, 2021).

King v. Smith (1968)
Excerpts from Chief Justice Warren's majority opinion

Under the Aid to Families with Dependent Children Program (AFDC) established by the Social Security Act of 1935 funds are made available for a "dependent child" largely by the Federal Government. The AFDC program is one of three major categorical public assistance programs established by the Social Security Act of 1935.

Section 406 (a) of the Act defines a "dependent child" as one who has been deprived of "parental" support or care by reason of the death, continued absence, or incapacity of a "parent."

Alabama, which like all other States, participates in the AFDC program, in 1964 promulgated its "substitute father" regulation under which AFDC payments are denied to the children of a mother who "cohabits" in or outside her home with an able-bodied man, a "substitute father" being considered a non-absent parent within the federal statute.

King v. Smith (1968) (continued)

Excerpts from Chief Justice Warren's majority opinion

Between June 1964, when Alabama's substitute father regulation became effective, and January 1967, the total number of AFDC recipients in the State declined by about 20,000 persons, and the number of children recipients by about 16,000, or 22%. As applied in this case, the regulation has caused the termination of all AFDC payments to the appellees, Mrs. Sylvester Smith and her four minor children.

The AFDC program is based on a scheme of cooperative federalism. See generally Advisory Commission Report, supra, at 1-59. It is financed largely by the Federal Government, on a matching fund basis, and is administered by the States. States are not required to participate in the program, but those which desire to take advantage of the substantial federal funds available for distribution to needy children are required to submit an AFDC plan for the approval of the Secretary of Health, Education, and Welfare (HEW).

Also not involved in this case is the question of Alabama's general power to deal with conduct it regards as immoral and with the problem of illegitimacy. This appeal raises only the question whether the State may deal with these problems in the manner that it has here by flatly denying AFDC assistance to otherwise eligible dependent children.

The most recent congressional amendments to the Social Security Act further corroborate that federal public welfare policy now rests on a basis considerably more sophisticated and enlightened than the "worthy-person" concept of earlier times.

In sum, Congress has determined that immorality and illegitimacy should be dealt with through rehabilitative measures rather than measures that punish dependent children, and that protection of such children is the paramount goal of AFDC.

All responsible governmental agencies in the Nation today recognize the enormity and pervasiveness of social ills caused by poverty. The causes of and cures for poverty are currently the subject of much debate. We hold today only that Congress has made at least this one determination: that destitute children who are legally fatherless cannot be flatly denied federally funded assistance on the transparent fiction that they have a substitute father.

U.S. Supreme Court (1968). *King v. Smith.* [online] Available at: https://tile.loc.gov/storage-services/service/ll/usrep/usrep392/usrep392309/usrep392309.pdf

Related to the *King* case, *Shapiro v. Thompson* (1969) challenged residency requirements pertaining to eligibility for Aid to Families with Dependent Children Program (AFDC) based on 14th Amendment Equal Protection.

"The freedom to move from state to state unimpeded by barriers is a right most travelers within the United States take for granted. Occasionally, however, state legislatures have employed subtle methods to prevent people from entering their borders. Through the enactment of statutory restrictions burdensome to those wishing to immigrate, states may discourage the entrance of unwelcome newcomers, while avoiding the public censure which would be engendered by more blatant forms of exclusion such as barbed wire or armed guards."

In the case of *Shapiro v. Thompson*, the Court considered the constitutionality of statutes whose provisions allegedly deterred the free movement of individuals between states. At issue were the 1-year residency requirements imposed by Connecticut, the District of Columbia, and Pennsylvania as a condition for welfare eligibility. "Unlike some previous legislative attempts to burden interstate travel, the statutes under attack in Shapiro exacted no direct penalty from an indigent entering or residing in the state. Nevertheless, by denying access to public assistance for 1 year, the statutes had the effect of discouraging an indigent from leaving a state where he qualified for financial aid" (Hammarström, 1970).

Lens (2021) argues "A more enlightened view of poverty was on full display in *Goldberg v. Kelly* (1970), which mirrored the changing tenor toward poverty in the 1960s. The Court expressed sympathy for the poor, recognizing the "brutal need" of welfare recipients who were deprived of "the very means by which to live while he waits" and whose situation "becomes immediately desperate." In a stirring passage (Lens 2021), the Court also "absolved the poor for their poverty, lauding welfare as a means for promoting American values of social inclusion and equality as embodied in the Constitution," in *Goldberg v. Kelly* (1970).

Goldberg v. Kelly (1970)
Excerpts from Mr. Brennen's majority opinion

Goldberg v. Kelly (1970) (continued)

Excerpts from Mr. Brennen's majority opinion

The question for decision is whether a State that terminates public assistance payments to a particular recipient without affording him the opportunity for an evidentiary hearing prior to termination denies the recipient procedural due process in violation of the Due Process Clause of the Fourteenth Amendment. This action was brought in the District Court for the Southern District of New York by residents of New York City receiving financial aid under the federally assisted program of Aid to Families with Dependent Children (AFDC) or under New York State's general Home Relief program.1 Their complaint alleged that the New- York State and New York City officials administering these programs terminated, *or were about to terminate, such aid without prior notice and hearing, thereby denying them due process of law.

The constitutional issue to be decided, therefore, is the narrow one whether the Due Process Clause requires that the recipient be afforded an evidentiary hearing before the termination of benefits… we agree with the District Court that when welfare is discontinued, only a pre-termination evidentiary hearing provides the recipient with procedural due process.

For qualified recipients, welfare provides the means to obtain essential food, clothing, housing, and medical care.

Thus, the crucial factor in this context … is that termination of aid pending resolution of a controversy over eligibility may deprive an *eligible* recipient of the very means by which to live while he waits. Since he lacks independent resources, his situation becomes immediately desperate. His need to concentrate upon finding the means for daily subsistence, in turn, adversely affects his ability to seek redress from the welfare bureaucracy.

From its founding the Nation's basic commitment has been to foster the dignity and well-being of all persons within its borders. We have come to recognize that forces not within the control of the poor contribute to their poverty.

Welfare, by meeting the basic demands of subsistence, can help bring within the reach of the poor the same opportunities that are available to others to participate meaningfully in the life of the community. At the same time, welfare guards against the societal malaise that may flow from a widespread sense of unjustified frustration and insecurity. Public assistance, then, is not mere charity, but a means to "promote the general Welfare, and secure the Blessings of Liberty to ourselves and our Posterity."

U.S. Supreme Court (1970b). *Goldberg v. Kelly*. [online] Available at: https://tile.loc.gov/storage-services/service/ll/usrep/usrep397/usrep397254/usrep397254.pdf

The hope that the procedural rights announced in Kelly would morph into a substantive constitutional right to welfare was dashed that same term in *Dandridge v. Williams (1970).*

Dandridge involved Maryland's maximum grant regulation, which capped the amount of public assistance a family could receive based on the size of their family, leaving large families with less assistance per family member than smaller families (Lens, 2021).

The Court deferred to state officials and did not expand protections to the poor:

Dandridge v. Williams (1970)
Excerpts from Mr. Stewart's majority opinion

This case involves the validity of a method used by Maryland, in the administration of an aspect of its public welfare program, to reconcile the demands of its needy citizens with the finite resources available to meet those demands. Under this jointly financed program, a State computes the so-called "standard of need" of each eligible family unit within its borders.

Some States provide that every family shall receive grants sufficient to meet fully the determined standard of need. Other States provide that each family unit shall receive a percentage of the determined need. Still others provide grants to most families in full accord with the ascertained standard of need but impose an upper limit on the total amount of money any one family unit may receive.

Maryland, through administrative adoption of a "maximum grant regulation," has followed this last course.

The operation of the Maryland welfare system is not complex. By statute 2 the State participates in the AFDC program. It computes the standard of need for each eligible family based on the number of children in the family and the circumstances under which the family lives. In general, the standard of need increases with each additional person in the household, but the increments become proportionately smaller.

The appellees urged in the District Court that the maximum grant limitation operates to discriminate against them merely because of the size of their families, in violation of the Equal Protection Clause of the Fourteenth Amendment.

It cannot be gainsaid that the effect of the Maryland' maximum grant provision is to reduce the per capita benefits to the children in the largest families. Although the appellees argue that the younger and more recently arrived children in such families are totally deprived of aid, a more realistic view is that the lot of the entire family is diminished because of the presence of additional -children without any increase in payments.

As we have noted, the practical effect of the Maryland regulation is that all children, even in very large families, do receive some aid. We find nothing in 42 U. S. C. § 602 (a)(10) (1964 ed., Supp. IV) that requires more than this. So long as some aid is provided to all eligible families and all eligible children, the statute itself is not violated.

In the area of economics and social welfare, a State does not violate the Equal Protection Clause merely because the classifications made by its laws are imperfect. If the classification

Dandridge v. Williams (1970) (continued)
Excerpts from Mr. Stewart's majority opinion

has some "reasonable basis," it does not offend the Constitution simply because the classification "is not made with mathematical nicety or because in practice it results in some inequality."

The Constitution does not empower this Court to second-guess state officials charged with the difficult responsibility of allocating limited public welfare funds among the myriad of potential recipients.

Conflicting claims of morality and intelligence are raised by opponents and proponents of almost every measure, certainly including the one before us. But the intractable economic, social, and even philosophical problems presented by public welfare assistance programs are not the business of this Court.

U.S. Supreme Court (1970a). *Dandridge v. Williams.* [online] Available at: https://tile.loc.gov/storage-services/service/ll/usrep/usrep397/usrep397471/usrep397471.pdf

In other words, the Court in *Dandridge* refused to consider the poor as a suspect class. It readily accepted the state's rationales for the regulation, including that it helped preserve fiscal funds, functioned as an incentive for work, and a disincentive for childbearing. It helped distinguish between working families and the welfare poor, all of which played into stereotypes of the poor as lazy, promiscuous, and different than other Americans. Missing was the inclusive, empathetic, and aspirational language of Kelly that elevated rather than denigrated the poor (Lens, 2021).

In *Wyman v. James (1971),* the Court traveled full circle, taking away rather than expanding the rights of the poor. It allowed the receipt of welfare benefits contingent upon a visit and search of a recipient's home, holding that the 4th Amendment did not apply, thus treating the homes of welfare recipients different from other citizens whose homes could not be breached without a warrant. The Court also returned to the language of charity rather than entitlements, comparing the receipt of benefits to the receipt of private charity, the givers of which "rightly expects" to know how their money is being spent (Lens, 2021).

"In short, over a space of only a few years, a welfare rights campaign that began with the promise of King, Kelly and Shapiro quickly fizzled, and advocates abandoned their long-term goal of establishing a constitutional right to live.

"While the Court spoke forcibly about education as an equalizing force for Black children, it failed to address the connection between race, education, and poverty. And while the Court was willing to impose wholesale changes on the public school system, it was not willing to do the same for the public welfare system. By refusing to recognize not only a right to education but a right to live, it read the poor out of the Constitution" (Lens, 2021).

The Court's unwillingness to secure basic human rights for those living in poverty has dire health consequences in the United States. Poverty is baked into America's fabric through its years long history of white supremacy, racism, discrimination, and bias. Without the will to leverage justice as a honed instrument to fight poverty, inequities in population health will persist.

Concluding Remarks

The illustrations in this chapter cement the perspective that justice in the realm of population well-being rises to a foremost social determinant of health. Distributive justice as a principle of healthcare ethics cries for delegation of healthcare resources equally amongst the population – not based on need, contribution, merit, or social position but *to each person an equal share.* And just as medical ethics champion distributive justice in healthcare, social determinants of health must be promulgated with distributive justice in law, policy, and governance. Countries that embrace the concepts of healthcare for all and policies that ensure that all conceivable basic needs are met, boast unparalleled health outcomes compared to the U.S. on far less national wealth. The evidence is persuasive.

Further, the illustrations send an invitation for readers to explore ways that law is formed, adjudicated, and administered. Justice is more than laws and public policy as written. Justice is access to a fair, distributive, and equal system to enforce one's rights. We have not yet achieved the promise of equal justice or fully recognized the legal system's effect on social determinants of health. The examples illustrated show that nothing is set in stone. Even with forward progress, justice is fragile. As community advocates, health professionals, legal professions, and policymakers, we are called to continue striving forward to secure justice and wellbeing for all.

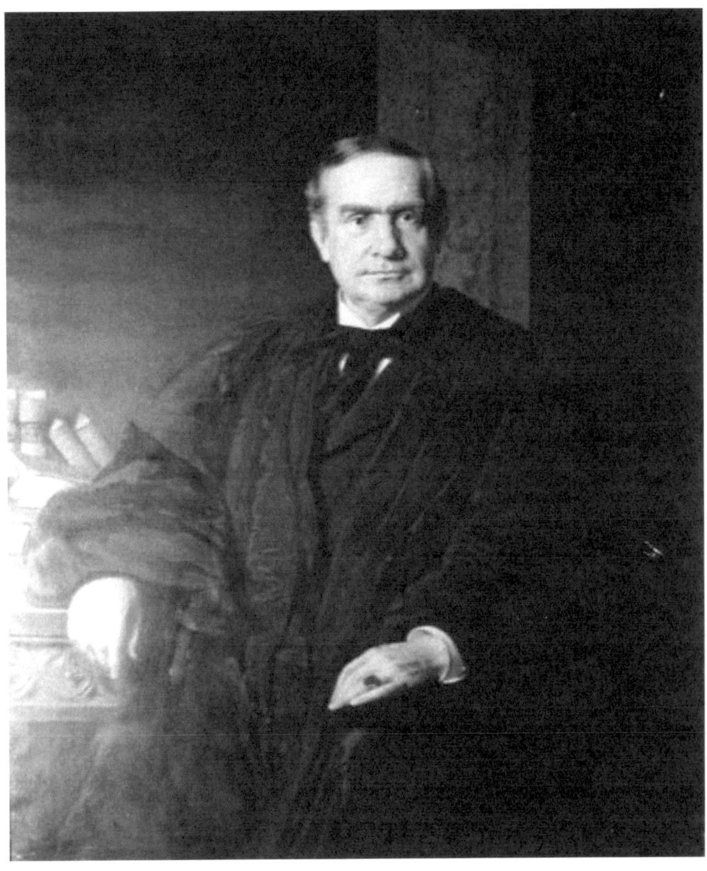

Justice Henry Billings Brown (Harvard Law) wrote the majority opinion in *Plessy v. Ferguson*

Smithsonian Institution (n.d.). *Henry Billings Brown*. [online] Smithsonian Institution. Available at: https://www.si.edu/object/npg_G966.3

Questions for Further Consideration:

1. What is meant by the "right to live" as a constitutional right? See Lens (2021) at: https://open.mitchellhamline.edu/cgi/viewcontent.cgi?article=1046&context=policypractice
2. Health care ethics articulates distributive justice as a rooted principle. How does distributive justice infer the concept of health care for all? How is access to healthcare in the United States distributed?
3. Discuss three or more ways justice meets the criteria for a social determinant of health.
4. Several measures have been enacted to ensure access to housing, yet homelessness is endemic in most cities across the U.S. Cite possible injustices leading to this crisis.

Sentinel Readings for a Deeper Dive

Lens, V. (2021). *Social Justice and the Supreme Court: Lessons from the Past. Mitchell Hamline Law Journal of Public Policy and Practice*. [online] Available at: https://open.mitchellhamline.edu/cgi/viewcontent.cgi?article=1046&context=policypractice

Law as a Social Determinant of Health (2016). *Social Determinants of Health and the Role of Law in Optimizing Health: Chapter 7*. [online] Available at: https://samples.jblearning.com/9781284162585/Chapter7.pdf

Väänänen, H. (2020). *What Makes Finland the Happiest Country In The World?* [online] Forbes. Available at: https://www.forbes.com/sites/heikkivaananen/2020/05/26/what-makes-finland-the-happiest-country-in-the-world/?sh=3ba7c23875cc

Varkey, B. (2021). Principles of clinical ethics and their application to practice. *Medical Principles and Practice*, [online] Available at: https://doi.org/10.1159/000509119

Alsalem, R. (2023). *Custody, violence against women and violence against children*. [online]. Available at: https://documents.un.org/doc/undoc/gen/g23/070/18/pdf/g2307018.pdf?token=P6e7LJoR1eyhud59uW&fe=true

References

Alsalem, R. (2023). *Custody, violence against women and violence against children*. [online]. Available at: https://documents.un.org/doc/undoc/gen/g23/070/18/pdf/g2307018.pdf?token=P6e7LJoR1eyhud59uW&fe=true [Accessed 10 January 2024].

Evans, F. (2022). *How Neighborhoods Used Restrictive Housing Covenants to Block Nonwhite Families*. [online] Available at: https://www.history.com/news/racially-restrictive-housing-covenants [Accessed 28 December 2023].

Fleischacker, S. (2004). *A Short History of Distributive Justice*. [online] *Google Books*. Harvard University Press. Available at: https://books.google.com/books?hl=en&lr=&id=NBCIh8yrNP0C&oi=fnd&pg=PR9&ots=Ybw8ZVW_1c&sig=yQW12vbcJ1MercV9L6l0A7Mj11M#v=onepage&q&f=false [Accessed 26 Dec. 2023].

Frazer, S., Saenz, R., Aleman, A. and Laderman, L. (2022). *2022 Community Survey of LGBTQ+ People and People Living with HIV's Experiences with the Criminal Legal System A Message from Black and Pink National VIII*. [online] Available at: https://static1.squarespace.com/static/62618573e937d62bddbf367d/t/646d326d98eb7343d67c91ab/1684877933977/Protected_and_Served_report.pdf [Accessed 10 Jan. 2024].

Hammarström, K. (1970). *Recent Decisions: Constitutional Law -Equal Protection - Recent Decisions: Constitutional Law -Equal Protection*. [online] Available at: https://scholarlycommons.law.case.edu/cgi/viewcontent.cgi?article=2802&context=caselrev [Accessed 28 December 2023].

Hartley, C. and Renner, L.M. (2018). Economic Self-Sufficiency among Women Who Experienced Intimate Partner Violence and Received Civil Legal Services. *Journal of Family Violence*, [online] https://doi.org/10.1007/s10896-018-9977-0 [Accessed 6 January 2024].

Investopedia.com. (2023). *10 Biggest Healthcare Companies* [online] Available at: https://www.investopedia.com/articles/markets/030916/worlds-top-10-health-care-companies-unh-mdt.asp [Accessed 28 January 2024].

Justia Law. (n.d.). *Plessy v. Ferguson, 163 U.S. 537 (1896)*. [online] Available at: https://supreme.justia.com/cases/federal/us/163/537/#tab-opinion-1917401 [Accessed 28 December 2023].

Justia Law. (2019). *Shelley v. Kraemer, 334 U.S. 1 (1948)*. [online] Available at: https://supreme.justia.com/cases/federal/us/334/1/ [Accessed 28 December 2023].

Law as a Social Determinant of Health (2016). *Social Determinants of Health and the Role of Law in Optimizing Health: Chapter 7*. [online] Available at: https://samples.jblearning.com/9781284162585/Chapter7.pdf [Accessed 8 Jan. 2024].

Legal Defense Fund (n.d.). *Brown v. Board of Education Case Portal*. [online] NAACP Legal Defense and Educational Fund. Available at: https://www.naacpldf.org/brown-vs-board/ [Accessed 28 December 2023].

Legal Services Corporation (1974). *LSC Act*. [online] LSC - Legal Services Corporation: America's Partner for Equal Justice. Available at: https://www.lsc.gov/about-lsc/laws-regulations-and-guidance/lsc-act [Accessed 6 January 2024].

Legal Services Corporation (2022). *The Report*. [online] The Justice Gap Report. Available at: https://justicegap.lsc.gov/the-report/ [Accessed 9 January 2024].

Lens, V. (2021). *Social Justice and the Supreme Court: Lessons from the Past. Mitchell Hamline Law Journal of Public Policy and Practice*. [online] Available at: https://open.mitchellhamline.edu/cgi/viewcontent.cgi?article=1046&context=policypractice [Accessed 6 January 2024].

Macrotrends.net. (2024). *Macrotrends – The Premier Research Platform for Long Term Investors.* [online] Available at: https://www.macrotrends.net/ [Accessed 28 January 2024].

Merriam-webster.com. (2019). *Definition of JUSTICE*. [online] Available at: https://www.merriam-webster.com/dictionary/justice?src=search-dict-box [Accessed 29 December 2023].

National Archives (2021a). *Brown v. Board of Education (1954)*. [online] National Archives. Available at: https://www.archives.gov/milestone-documents/brown-v-board-of-education [Accessed 8 January 2024].

National Archives (2021b). *Dred Scott v. Sandford (1857)*. [online] National Archives. Available at: https://www.archives.gov/milestone-documents/dred-scott-v-sandford [Accessed 8 January 2024].

National Archives (2024). *14th Amendment to the U.S. Constitution: Civil Rights (1868).* [online] National Archives. Available at: https://www.archives.gov/milestone-documents/14th-amendment#:~:text=No%20State%20shall%20make%20or,equal%20protection%20of%20the%20laws [Accessed 28 January 2024].

Newitt, P. (2023). *The 20 highest-paid Healthcare CEOs*. [online] Available at: https://www.beckersasc.com/leadership/the-20-highest-paid-healthcare-ceos.html [Accessed 26 Dec. 2023].

Reed, R. (2021). *Plessy v. Ferguson at 125*. [online] Harvard Law School. Available at: 26 https://hls.harvard.edu/today/plessy-v-ferguson-at-125/ [Accessed 26 December 2023].

Stevenson, B. (2014). *Just Mercy: A Story of Justice and Redemption*. New York: Spiegel & Grau.

Smithsonian Institution (n.d.). *Henry Billings Brown*. [online] Smithsonian Institution. Available at: https://www.si.edu/object/npg_G966.3 [Accessed 3 Feb. 2024].

Supreme Court Historical Society. (n.d.). *Supreme Court Decisions & Women's Rights: Breaking New Ground - Reed v. Reed | SCHS Classroom Resources*. [online] Available at: https://supremecourthistory.org/classroom-resources-teachers-students/decisions-womens-rights-reed-v-reed/ [Accessed 29 December 2023].

The Fair Housing Center of Boston (n.d.). *1920s–1948: Racially Restrictive Covenants*. [online] www.bostonfairhousing.org. Available at: https://www.bostonfairhousing.org/timeline/1920s1948-Restrictive-Covenants.html#:~:text=Racially%20restrictive%20covenants%20refer%20to [Accessed 27 December 2023].

U.S. Supreme Court (1948). *Shelley v. Kraemer CASES ADJUDGED IN THE*. [online] Available at: https://tile.loc.gov/storage-services/service/ll/usrep/usrep334/usrep334001/usrep334001.pdf [Accessed 9 January 2024].

U.S. Supreme Court (1954). *Brown v. Board of Education of Topeka et al. No. 1. Appeal from the united states district court for the district of Kansas.* * [online] Available at: https://tile.loc.gov/storage-services/service/ll/usrep/usrep347/usrep347483/usrep347483.pdf [Accessed 27 December 2023].

U.S. Supreme Court (1963). *Gideon v. Wainwright* . [online] Available at: https://tile.loc.gov/storage-services/service/ll/usrep/usrep372/usrep372335/usrep372335.pdf [Accessed 27 Dec. 2023].

U.S. Supreme Court (1968). *King v. Smith*. [online] Available at: https://tile.loc.gov/storage-services/service/ll/usrep/usrep392/usrep392309/usrep392309.pdf [Accessed 9 January 2024].

U.S. Supreme Court (1970a). *Dandridge v. Williams*. [online] Available at: https://tile.loc.gov/storage-services/service/ll/usrep/usrep397/usrep397471/usrep397471.pdf [Accessed 9 January 2024].

U.S. Supreme Court (1970b). *Goldberg v. Kelly*. [online] Available at: https://tile.loc.gov/storage-services/service/ll/usrep/usrep397/usrep397254/usrep397254.pdf [Accessed 9 January 2024]

U.S. Supreme Court (1971). *Reed v. Reed*. [online] Available at: https://tile.loc.gov/storage-services/service/ll/usrep/usrep404/usrep404071/usrep404071.pdf [Accessed 27 Dec. 2023].

US Courts (n.d.). *Facts and Case Summary - Gideon v. Wainwright.* [online] United States Courts. Available at: https://www.uscourts.gov/educational-resources/educational-activities/facts-and-case-summary-gideon-v-wainwright [Accessed 6 January 2024].

Väänänen, H. (2020). *What Makes Finland The Happiest Country In The World?* [online] Forbes. Available at: https://www.forbes.com/sites/heikkivaananen/2020/05/26/what-makes-finland-the-happiest-country-in-the-world/?sh=3ba7c23875cc [Accessed 28 December 2023].

Varkey, B. (2021). Principles of clinical ethics and their application to practice. *Medical Principles and Practice*, [online] https://doi.org/10.1159/000509119 [Accessed 28 December 2023].

World Health Organization (2021). *Social determinants of health.* [online] World Health Organisation. Available at: https://www.who.int/health-topics/social-determinants-of-health [Accessed 28 December 2023].

Lexicon of Listed Terms and Agencies

- **American Civil Liberties Union (ACLU):** the nation's premier defender of the rights enshrined in the U.S. Constitution. The ACLU fights government abuse and vigorously defends individual freedoms including speech and religion, a woman's right to choose, the right to due process, and citizens' rights to privacy.

- **Legal Defense Fund:** The Legal Defense Fund (LDF) is America's premier legal organization fighting for racial justice. Using the power of law, narrative, research, and people, we defend and advance the full dignity and citizenship of Black people in America.

- **Legal Services Corporation (LSC):** LSC is the single largest funder of civil legal aid for low-income Americans in the nation. Established in 1974, LSC operates as an independent 501(c)(3) nonprofit corporation that promotes equal access to justice and provides grants for high-quality civil legal assistance to low-income Americans.

- **U.S. Supreme Court:** The Court is the highest tribunal in the Nation for all cases and controversies arising under the Constitution or the laws of the United States. It seeks to provide "Equal Justice Under the Law"

- **World Health Organization (WHO)**: The WHO is an international organization of 194 Member States. The Member States elect the Director-General, who leads the organization in achieving its global health goals.

AUTHOR'S BIO SKETCH

Andrea Saunders, JD

Andrea Saunders is a practicing civil legal aid attorney and mother. She was born and raised in Kitsap County, Washington, where her ancestors lived for several generations after immigrating from Norway. Andrea received her undergraduate degree from Western Washington University. She studied sociology, law, inequality, and became impassioned to a career in public service. She graduated from University of San Francisco School of Law and has been admitted to the bar associations of three states and three tribal courts. She has experience in civil legal aid settings spanning California, Arizona, and Washington. Andrea believes in challenging and eliminating bias, oppression, and barriers in American courts of law.

Chapter 3

Race as a Social Determinant of Health

Joe Eubanks, MA, Author
James Lenhart, MD, MPH, Editor

"Prejudice is a burden that confuses the past, threatens the future, and renders the present inaccessible." – Maya Angelou

Race as a Social Determinant of Health

Introduction

In contemporary society, racial disparities persist across various aspects of life, including healthcare and health outcomes. These disparities can be attributed, in large part, to the social determinants of health, which encompass the conditions in the environments where people are born, live, learn, work, play, worship, and age that affect a wide range of health, functioning, and quality-of-life outcomes and risks (HHS, 2020). This chapter explores the social determinants of health and the connection to racial disparities, highlighting the impact on individual and community well-being.

In the United States significant racial disparities impact healthcare access, health insurance coverage and health outcomes. To understand health disparities, one must understand the issue is not connected to a singular matter. Health disparities pertaining to race result from policy decisions made as a society including access to care, transportation, education, housing, health insurance, food security, employment, and telecommunications. According to the World Health Organization (WHO, 2023), these circumstances are shaped by the distribution of money, power, and resources at global, national, and local levels, which are themselves influenced by policy decision making. Social determinants of health neglected create well-being inequities – the unfair and avoidable differences in health status seen within and between countries (WHO, 2023). Systematic oppression fostered by racism promotes health inequities as well.

Race as a Social Determinant of Health

Historical Context – cementing the foundation for White supremacy and racism

The legacy of slavery, segregation, and discriminatory policies have shaped the experiences and opportunities of racial and ethnic minorities for over 400 years including the intergenerational impact of systemic racism on health outcomes and access to healthcare services. Despite painstaking progress, the deep-rooted history of racism in the U.S. continues to exclude people based on race and ethnicity to this day. Galea (2017) insists that history sheds light on the roots of present-day health disparities in the U.S. This is especially true in the case of American slavery, and the legacy of Black marginalization with which people of color continue to live. The most overt consequence of slavery, our country's ugly history of racism, shaped and continues to shape, our society in many ways, with direct implications for public health (Galea, 2017). Presidential authority provides astonishing insight and historical revelation, to wit.

U.S. President Thomas Jefferson promoted the belief of White superiority compared to Black Americans in the Query 14 of his *Notes on the State of Virginia* in which he stated:

> *To these objections, which are political, may be added others, which are physical and moral. The first difference which strikes us is that of colour. Whether the Black of the negro resides in the reticular membrane between the skin and scarf-skin, or in the scarf-skin itself; whether it proceeds from the colour of the blood, the colour of the bile, or from that of some other secretion, the difference is fixed in nature, and is as real as if its seat and cause were better known to us. And is this difference of no importance? Is it not the foundation of a greater or less share of beauty in the two races? Are not the fine mixtures of red and White, the expressions of every passion by greater or less suffusions of colour in the one, preferable to that eternal monotony, which reigns in the countenances, that immoveable veil of Black which covers all the emotions of the other race? Add to these, flowing hair, a more elegant symmetry of form, their own judgment in favour of the Whites, declared by their preference of them, as uniformly as is the preference of the Oranootan for the Black women over those of his own species. The circumstance of superior beauty, is thought worthy attention in the propagation of our horses, dogs, and other domestic animals; why not in that of man?* (Jefferson, 1781-1782)
>
> University of Virginia Library, (2005). Thomas Jefferson, notes on the state of Virginia, query 14, 1781-1782 (excerpt). Jefferson, Query 14. https://mason.gmu.edu/~zschrag/hist120spring05/jeffersonquery14.htm
>
> - Thomas Jefferson, 1781-182

President Jefferson acknowledged his fear that emancipation threatened whiteness when describing his opposition to race mixture. He explained in Query 14, that there was an innate difference between Black Americans and White Americans using medical terms to explain these differences and the inferiority of Black Americans. According to Villarosa (2019), Jefferson promoted his theories in *Notes on the State of Virginia* articulating how medicine and science proved them. Myths about physical racial differences were used to justify slavery — and are still believed by doctors today (Villarosa, 2019).

In the nineteenth century, physicians and health professionals used slavery to advance the practice of medicine through human experimentation and torture. Notably, Dr. Samuel A. Cartwright advanced in-depth research on racial science during the emancipation era of American slavery. In his article, *Diseases and Peculiarities of the Negro Race*, Cartwright discussed the newly discovered "Drapetomania" a disease that causes slaves to run away.

> *DRAPETOMANIA, OR THE DISEASE-CAUSING NEGROES TO RUN AWAY.*
>
> *It is unknown to our medical authorities, although its diagnostic symptom, the absconding from service, is well known to our planters and overseers...*
> *In noticing a disease not heretofore classed among the long list of maladies that man is subject to, it was necessary to have a new term to express it. The cause in the most of cases, that induces the negro to run away from service, is as much a disease of the mind as any other species of mental alienation, and much more curable, as a general rule. With the advantages of proper medical advice, strictly followed, this troublesome practice that many negroes have of running away, can be almost entirely prevented, although the slaves be located on the borders of a free state, within a stone's throw of the abolitionists.*
>
> - Dr. Samuel Cartwright, 1851
>
> Cartwright, S. (2019). Africans in America/part 4/"diseases and peculiarities." *PBS* [online] Available at: https://www.pbs.org/wgbh/aia/part4/4h3106t.html [Accessed 18 July 2023].

Cartwright's creative, if not prolific writing gave way to other novel diagnoses. For example, he coined the condition of Dysaesthesia Aethiopica, "a disease-causing rascality" in Black people free and enslaved.

DYSAESTHESIA AETHIOPICA

Dysaesthesia Aethiopica is a disease peculiar to negroes, affecting both mind and body in a manner as well expressed by dysaesthesia, the name I have given it, as could be by a single term. There is both mind and sensibility, but both seem to be difficult to reach by impressions from without. There is a partial insensibility of the skin, and so great a hebetude of the intellectual faculties, as to be like a person half asleep, that is with difficulty aroused and kept awake. It differs from every other species of mental disease, as it is accompanied with physical signs or lesions of the body discoverable to the medical observer, which are always present and sufficient to account for the symptoms. It is much more prevalent among free negroes living in clusters by themselves, than among slaves on our plantations, and attacks only such slaves as live like free negroes in regard to diet, drinks, exercise, etc. It is not my purpose to treat of the complaint as it prevails among free negroes, nearly all of whom are more or less afflicted with it, that have not got some White person to direct and to take care of them. To narrate its symptoms and effects among them would be to write a history of the ruins and dilapidation of Hayti, and every spot of earth they have ever had uncontrolled possession over for any length of time. I propose only to describe its symptoms among slaves.

From the careless movements of the individuals affected with the complaint, they are apt to do much mischief, which appears as if intentional, but is mostly owing to the stupidness of mind and insensibility of the nerves induced by the disease. Thus, they break, waste and destroy everything they handle, --abuse horses and cattle, --tear, burn or rend their own clothing, and, paying no attention to the rights of property, steal others, to replace what they have destroyed. They wander about at night and keep in a half nodding sleep during the day. They slight their work, --cut up corn, cane, cotton or tobacco when hoeing it, as if for pure mischief. They raise disturbances with their overseers and fellow servants without cause or motive and seem to be insensible to pain when subjected to punishment. The fact of the existence of such a complaint, making man like an automaton or senseless machine, having the above or similar symptoms, can be clearly established by the most direct and positive testimony. That it should have escaped the attention of the medical profession, can only be accounted for because its attention has not been sufficiently directed to the maladies of the negro race. Otherwise, a complaint of so common an occurrence on badly governed plantations, and so universal among free negroes, or those who are not governed at all,--a disease radicated in physical lesions and having its peculiar and well-marked symptoms and its curative indications, would not have escaped the notice of the profession. The northern physicians and people have noticed the symptoms, but not the disease from which they spring. They ignorantly attribute the symptoms to the debasing influence of slavery on the mind without considering that those who have never been in slavery, or their fathers before them, are the most afflicted, and the latest from the slaveholding South the least. The disease is the natural offspring of negro liberty--the liberty to be idle, to wallow in filth, and to indulge in improper food and drinks.

- Dr. Samuel Cartwright, 1851

Cartwright, S. (2019). Africans in America/part 4/"diseases and peculiarities." *PBS* [online] Available at: https://www.pbs.org/wgbh/aia/part4/4h3106t.html [Accessed 18 July 2023].

Promulgations by southern physicians including Dr. Cartwright illustrate the extraordinary dehumanization of Black people. "Over the centuries, the two most persistent physiological myths — that Black people were impervious to pain and had weak lungs that could be strengthened through hard work — wormed their way into scientific consensus and remain rooted in modern-day medical education and practice" (Villarosa, 2019). Cartwright's research created a legacy in which his work was an inspiration to others and had a profound impact on American history, American industry, and our American society to this day (Villarosa, 2019).

Cartwright did not stand alone. According to Shaban (2014), in 1864 Benjamin Apthorp Gould launched a massive study to quantify the bodies of Union soldiers. Gould authored a 613-page report declaring that soldiers classified as "White" had higher lung capacity than those labeled "Full Blacks" or "Mulattoes." Gould's study relied on a spirometer like the devices previously used by plantation physicians to show that Black slaves had weaker lungs than White citizens. And he did not control for height, age or the recognition of living and working conditions amongst study subjects (Shaban, 2014).

Although mistaken, flawed studies like these supported the belief that Black Americans were inferior and not suitable to live amongst White Americans. Many White Americans during this era used medical and health research to create bias about Black and brown health. Thomas Jefferson's treatise *Notes on the State of Virginia*, as early as 1781 promoted theories on the dysfunction of the "pulmonary apparatus" of Black people. Lungs were used as a marker of difference, "a sign that Black bodies were fit for the field and little else." Forced labor was seen as a way to "vitalize the blood" of flawed Black physiology. By this logic, "slavery kept Black bodies alive" (Shaban, 2014).

Following the end of the Civil War, the U.S. Congress ratified the so-called Reconstruction Amendments to the U.S. Constitution. The 13th Amendment (ratified 1865) abolished slavery. The 14th Amendment (ratified 1868) ensured all people equal protection under the laws. The 15th Amendment (ratified 1870) gave *male* African Americans the right to vote. Despite these constitutional protections, based on the opinions of learned people that propagated discriminatory attitudes regarding people of color, states throughout the South held the Amendments in contempt and forged their own brand of reconstruction in defiance of the protections awarded. Hence, the birth of the Jim Crow South.

Jim Crow: a symbol for racial segregation

Jim Crow segregation was a way of life that combined a system of anti-Black laws and race-prejudiced cultural practices. The term "Jim Crow" is often used as a synonym for racial segregation, particularly in the American South. The Jim Crow South was the era during which local and state laws enforced the legal segregation of White and Black citizens from the 1870s into the 1960s. In the Jim Crow South, it was illegal for Black Americans to ride in the front of public buses, eat at a "Whites only" restaurant, or attend "White" public schools.

There was also a subtler, social dimension to Jim Crow, which required that African Americans demonstrate subservience and inferiority to Whites at all times. Most Southern Whites interpreted any claim to pride or equality by African Americans as an affront.

From the late 1800s, the name Jim Crow came to signify the social and legal segregation of Black Americans from White. After the Civil War and Reconstruction, Whites disenfranchised Black men (by the poll tax, literacy test, and more), often relegated Black workers to low-paying jobs, and poorly funded public schools for Black children. In this way, Whites in the Jim Crow South crafted a bitter web of political, economic, and social barriers to full and equal citizenship for their fellow Black citizens.

In 1896, the Supreme Court of the United States declared Jim Crow segregation legal in the ***Plessy v. Ferguson*** decision. The Court ruled that "separate but equal" accommodations for African Americans were permitted under the Constitution.

Khan Academy, 2023. *Jim Crow* [online] Available at:https://www.khanacademy.org/humanities/us-history/the-gilded-age/south-after-civil-war/a/jim-crow [Accessed 27 July 2023].

Frederick Hoffman (1865-1946) who served as a statistician at the Prudential Life Insurance Company perpetuated prevailing data to assert Black Americans lacked fitness for freedom. Hoffman claimed that "Negroes died because they were inferior, and they were inferior because they died. It is not in the conditions of life, but in the race traits and tendencies that we find the causes of excessive mortality" (Wolff, 2006). Hoffman's perspectives and credibility affected insurance eligibility and created a format for insurance redlining, according to Wolff (2006).

> In May 1896, Frederick L. Hoffman, a statistician at the Prudential Life Insurance Company, published a 330-page article in the prestigious *Publications of the American Economic Association* intended to prove—with statistic al reliability—that the American Negro was uninsurable. *Race Traits and Tendencies of the American Negro* was a compilation of statistics, eugenic theory, observation, and speculation, solicited by the Prudential in response to a wave of state legislation banning discrimination against African Americans.
>
> Wolff, M. 2002. The Myth of The Actuary: Life Insurance and Frederick L. Hoffman's "Race Traits and Tendencies of The American Negro." *Public Health Reports* [online] Available at: https://www.ncbi.nlm.nih.gov/pmc/articles/PMC1497788/ [Accessed 20 July 2023].

Hoffman's influence spread beyond insurance company enterprise. His data mobilized other factions of American industry to support and embrace White supremacy. "Prudential and Hoffman aimed to turn the racial fantasy of the extinction hypothesis into hard scientific numbers that could be deployed for both short- and long-term ends. In the short term, they helped stop the progress of anti-discrimination legislation. The implicit long-term goal was maintenance of the racial status quo. More than proving the uninsurability of the American Negro, Hoffman's publication demonstrated the social and economic power of statistical methods, and the ease with which they could be mobilized to buttress the interests and practices of private industry and White supremacy" (Wolff, 2006).

In American history, the discourse of science and medicine has been used to inflict harm on people of color. According to Lee (2022), when the bubonic plague hit Honolulu and San Francisco at the turn of the 20th century, officials in those cities quickly did what they had been doing for decades – they villainized residents of Chinese descent. Public health officials scapegoated Chinese immigrants in San Francisco, and local government officials shut down Chinatown to prevent any food or people in and out of the area, trapping 25,000 to 35,000 residents and denying most the ability to work (Lee, 2022).

The ongoing history of racial oppression in our society creates an unsafe environment for people of color regarding their health and well-being. These violations represent a long, deep-rooted history and epitomize the darkest days in our nation's history. Shirley Chisholm (1970), who became the first woman and African American to run for the U.S. Presidency wrote, "Racism is so universal in this country, so widespread, and deep-seated, that it is invisible because it is so normal." Her statement highlights that race must be viewed as a social determinant of health due to its detrimental effects on so many.

An in-depth discussion of the history racism in America exceeds the scope and purpose of this chapter, but its roots extend wide and deep and encompass our history for over 400 years. Suffice it to say heinous crimes and inhumane treatment of humans clutter the journey at the behest of White supremacy and leaves an indelible legacy that provides the foundation for race as a social determinant of health. The Indian Removal Act supplies yet another astonishing example.

The Indian Removal Act 1830

On March 28, 1830, the U.S. Congress passed, and President Andrew Jackson signed the Indian Removal Act, which launched the forced relocation of thousands of Native Americans from their ancestral homelands in Georgia, Florida, North Carolina, Tennessee, Alabama, Mississippi, and Arkansas to the "Indian Territory" in what is now Oklahoma (National Geographic, 2023).

Indian removal freed more than 25 million acres of fertile, lucrative farmland to White settlers and plantation owners who utilized slave labor to clear the land, plant and harvest profitable crops like cotton, tobacco, and hemp for export to England, France, and other European destinations (National Geographic, 2023 and McNamara, 2019a). "King" Cotton and the slave labor strategy that fueled it proved central to the southern states drive to secede from the Union and embrace slavery (McNamara, 2019a).

Pushed and pulled by the U.S. Army, estimates support that thousands of Native Americans died of disease, starvation, and exposure to extreme weather on the forced journeys, hence the commemoration of the incidents as the Trail of Tears (**Figure 1.** National Geographic, 2023).

Figure 1.

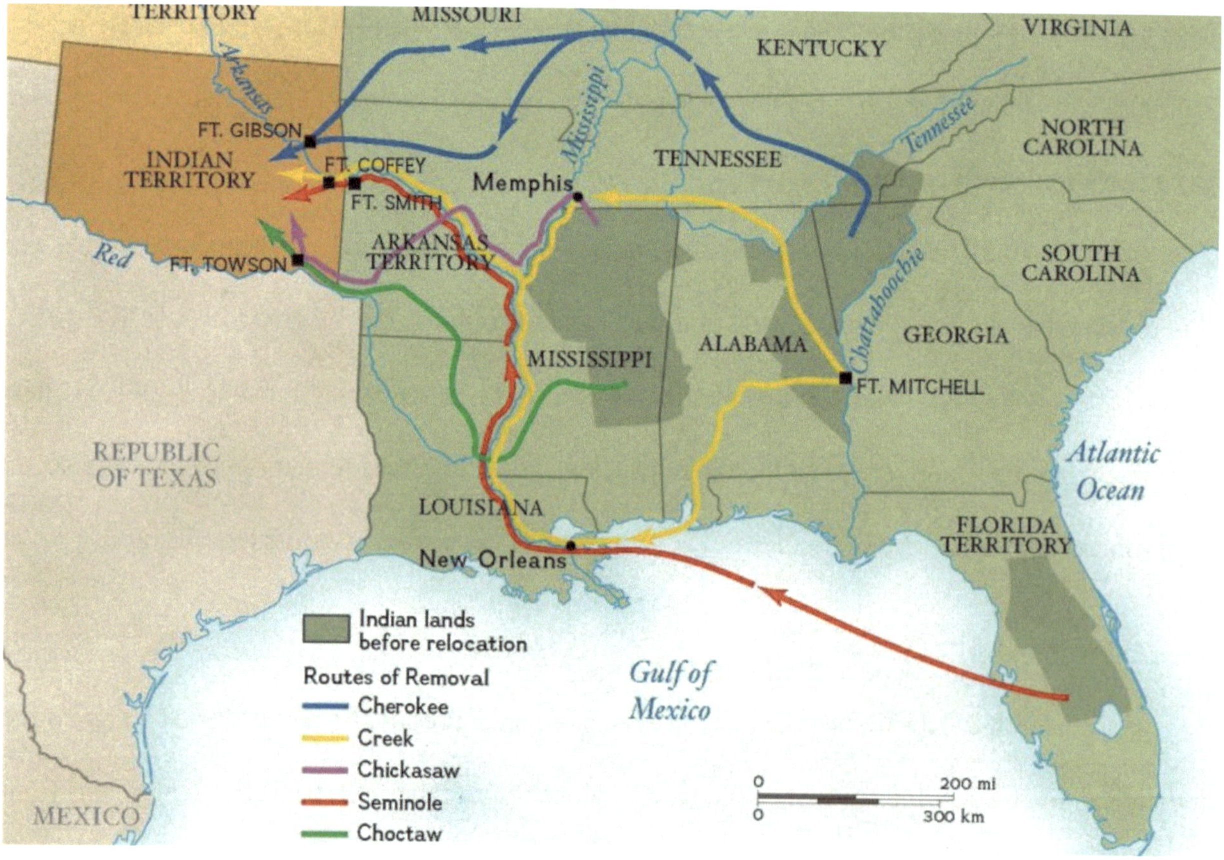

National Geographic, 2023. May 28, 1830, CE: Indian Removal Act. *National Geographic* [online] Available at: https://education.nationalgeographic.org/resource/indian-removal-act/ [Accessed 19 August 2023].

The treatment of America's Indigenous people confluent before, during and beyond the Civil War stands as another incomprehensible stain on the American ideals of democracy. History shows that Abraham Lincoln extended his presidential powers to endorse Native American injustices, while simultaneously serving as the Great Emancipator to African Americans.

> As America's 16th president, Abraham Lincoln left a towering legacy. His deep belief in the founding principles of American democracy—that every human deserved liberty and the opportunity for self-determination—compelled him to free enslaved Americans. But when it came to the nation's Indigenous peoples, who were collectively struggling for their lives, lands, and cultural survival, he fell short of applying those cherished American ideals.
>
> That meant making and breaking treaties, confiscating ancestral lands, forcing removal, pushing cultural assimilation—and, at times, turning a blind eye to acts of genocide committed by the military on the western frontier.
>
> Among the bitterest pills served to Native peoples during his administration: Lincoln signed laws that gave away millions of acres of tribal land to support White westward expansion, and he approved the hanging of 38 Dakota Sioux warriors, the largest mass execution in U.S. history.
>
> History, (n.a.) 2023. Abraham Lincoln's Uneasy Relationship with Native Americans. [online] available at: https://www.history.com/news/abraham-lincoln-native-americans

***Systematic Oppression**:*

In the context of Family Life, Well Being and Opportunity

Disparities in wealth accumulation and assets, lead to differential access to well-being resources and opportunities for optimal health. The social determinants of health reflect on the quality of life and the ability to sustain our loved ones. Racism constitutes a significant barrier to living a long and healthy life. According to Hill (2023), the COVID-19 pandemic worsened longstanding racial disparities in life expectancy and mortality within the US. 2021 provisional data show life expectancy for Black people at 70.8 years and 76.4 years for Whites.

Paradies, et al., (2015) define racism as organized systems within societies that cause avoidable and unfair inequalities in power, resources, capacities, and opportunities across racial or ethnic groups and that racism can manifest through beliefs, stereotypes, prejudices, or discrimination. Life expectancy data suggests that racial identity may mean that the health for people of color is forgotten, ignored, or even set aside.

According to Paradies, et al., (2015) racism impacts health, life expectancy and healthy life expectancy through recognized pathways:

1. reduced access to employment, housing, and education.
2. increased exposure to health risks (e.g., avoidable contact with police, environmental toxins, occupational hazards).
3. adverse cognitive/emotional experiences and associated psychopathology.
4. cumulative effects of chronic stress on mental and physical health (allostatic load).
5. diminished participation in healthy behaviors (e.g., sleep, recreation, and exercise).
6. increased engagement in unhealthy behaviors (e.g., overeating, alcohol consumption, tobacco use, substance use) either directly as stress coping, or indirectly, via reduced self-regulation.
7. physical injury due to racially motivated violence.

Data from the U.S. Census Bureau (2022) and the WorldAtlas (2017) shine important light on U.S. population and life expectancy. As to life expectancy in the U.S., Missouri, Georgia, South Carolina, District of Columbia, Tennessee, Kentucky, Arkansas, Oklahoma, Louisiana, Alabama, West Virginia, and Mississippi rank 40th through 51st respectively. States with high infant mortality are clustered in Arkansas, Louisiana, Mississippi, Alabama, West Virginia, South Carolina, and North Carolina (CDC, 2022). Likewise, maternal mortality ranks highest in Arkansas, Mississippi, Tennessee, Alabama, Louisiana, Kentucky, Georgia, and South Carolina (World Population Review, 2023). U.S. Census Bureau (2022) data reveals Black/African American populations are concentrated in the southeastern United States (**Figure 2**).

Figure 2.

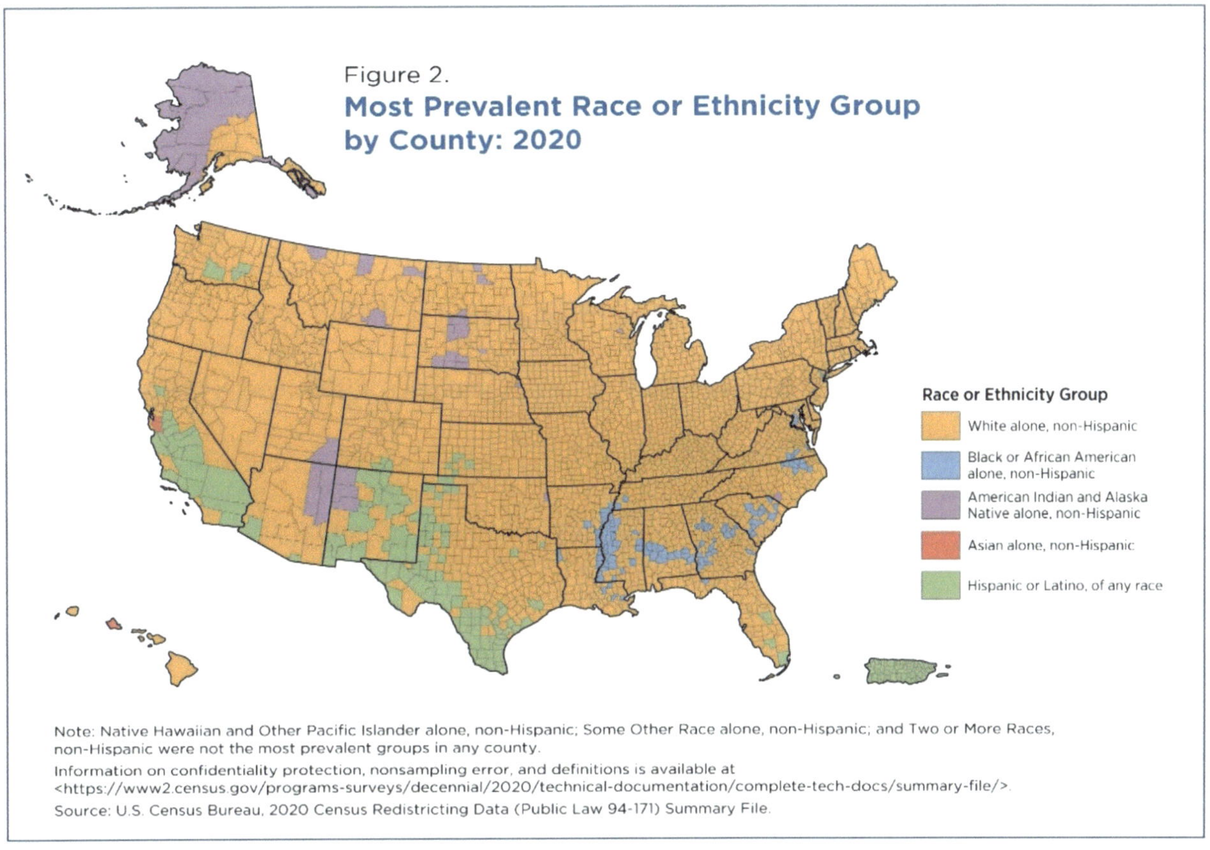

United States Census Bureau, 2022. *2020 U.S. Population More Racially and Ethnically Diverse than Measured in 2010* [online] Available at: https://www.census.gov/library/stories/2021/08/2020-united-states-population-more-racially-ethnically-diverse-than-2010.html [Accessed 29 July 2023].

Systematic Oppression

"Oppression is the inhibition of a group through a vast network of everyday practices, attitudes, assumptions, behaviors, and institutional rules," Young (1990).

Redlining

Concentrated poverty and limited access to quality housing contribute to adverse health outcomes (overcrowding, food insecurity, and personal safety) as examples. The complex story of housing discrimination takes its roots from methods that prevent communities of color from achieving affluence. Wealth (life absent from poverty) constitutes, among others, the rationale for race as a social determinant of health. "One of the biggest factors driving these disparities is housing. A home is the most valuable thing people own. And buying a nicer home in a nicer neighborhood has always been the easiest way to climb up the socioeconomic ladder," (Illing, 2020). America's cities and towns tell a clear but troubling story of home ownership and race. And this story is called redlining, "an illegal practice in which lenders avoid providing credit services to individuals living in communities of color because of the race, color or national origin of the residents in those communities," (Department of Justice, 2021).

Redlining (**Figure 3**) perpetuates a system in which communities across the United States are left behind without the financial infrastructure to build sustainable communities and access to essential services. "Historical redlining is linked to increased risk of diabetes, hypertension, and early mortality due to heart disease with evidence suggesting it impacts health through suppressing economic opportunity and human capital, or the knowledge, skills, and value one contributes to society," (Egede, 2023).

Figure 3.

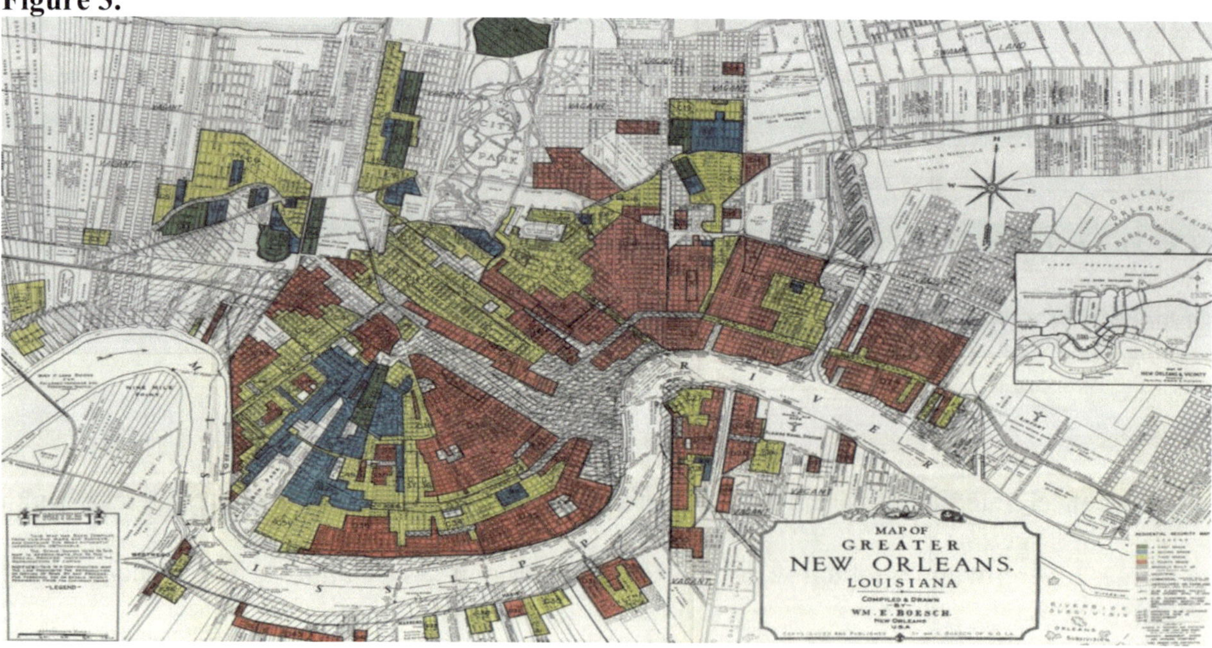

Figure 3 (above): Redline maps of New Orleans from the 1930s show Lakefront and City Park neighborhoods in green, while Central City, downtown and Garden District neighborhoods are red. Redlined areas later became primed for outside development through gentrification — from 2000 to 2016, African American populations in the Irish Channel dropped from 75 percent of the area to 27 percent.
Woodward (2021) How "redlining Shaped New Orleans [online] Available at: https://bit.ly/3QUSveQ [Accessed 19 July 2023].

According to Woodward (2021), in the early 20th century Black New Orleanians largely relied on housing without the support of commercial loans, at a significant disadvantage compared to White homeowners — and the private market also supported discriminatory policies, with the National Association of Real Estate Boards warning its members in 1924 not to integrate neighborhoods with "members of any race or nationality ... whose presence will clearly be detrimental to property values in that neighborhood." (Woodward, 2021).

Communities left behind and without access to safe drinking water provide stark examples of redlining's detriments to communities of color. Costley (2022), cites the legacy of racial zoning, segregation, and legalized redlining leading to the isolation, separation, and sequestration of racial minorities into communities with diminished tax bases, resulting in circular consequences for the built environment, including infrastructure (water, sewer/sanitation, roads, and utilities).

Poignant examples supporting Costley's research point to the minority-majority cities across America including Jackson, MS, Flint and Detroit, MI, which typify communities struggling to supply healthy drinking water to residents.

"Adequate housing is a critical determinant of health" (Martens, 2014). Redlining's influence extends beyond physical health. The psychological toll of living in disinvested neighborhoods and facing constant barriers to social mobility fosters chronic stress, mental health disorders, and reduced social cohesion. Moreover, the disruption of community networks and the intergenerational trauma perpetuated by redlining delivers lasting impacts on individuals and families, which undermines overall well-being and opportunities for upward mobility.

Systematic Oppression

Health Insurance Coverage

Disproportionate rates of uninsurance and underinsurance among racial and ethnic minority populations challenge the prospect for health equity. "Since the Jim Crow era (1875–1968), racism has implicitly and explicitly been an integral part of the U.S. government's structuring and financing of the health care system" (Yearby et al., 2022). Limited access to affordable healthcare services and preventive care impacts health outcomes, creates health disparities and promotes denigration of quality of life for disenfranchised minorities.

Structural racism in modern U.S. health care policy continues to limit the availability of health insurance for diverse groups. According to Yearby et al., (2022), the Supreme Court's decision in *National Federation of Independent Business v. Sebelius* made Medicaid expansion *optional* for the states, leading to a policy debate among certain states—primarily found in the South—about whether to expand Medicaid access. Predictably, this reinforced racial hierarchy and resulted in inequities in coverage. This is especially evident in southern states with large numbers of Black and Latino residents (Yearby, 2022).

Health insurance makes accessibility to quality and equitable health care possible. Prior to implementation of the Affordable Care Act (ACA), one in three Hispanic Americans and one in five Black Americans were uninsured leaving these minority groups without access to care. This compares to about one in eight White Americans (Young, 2022).

Race centered, exclusionary methods promote systems of grueling oppression ripping through the American Dream and extracting a heavy toll for communities of color and for society. "Racial health disparities, estimated to cost the United States $175 billion in lost life years and $135 billion per year in excess health care costs and untapped productivity, persist because of the failure to address their root cause: structural racism," (Yearby, 2020). These cost measures underscore the rationale for resources to combat racial health disparities. According to the U.S. Department of Labor, (n.d.) "the Civil Rights Act of 1964 formally outlawed discrimination based on race, color, religion, sex, and national origin" yet underrepresented minorities continue to be left behind.

Race as a Barrier to Equitable Health Care

Bias

Stemming from the works of Cartwright and Gould during the Civil War era, bias in access to care has long created challenges for people of color pertaining to the level of care they receive. According to the National Institutes of Health (2022), bias consists of attitudes, behaviors, and actions that are prejudiced in favor of or against one person or group compared to another. "A 2016 University of Virginia survey of 92 persons without medical training and 222 White medical students and residents published in The Proceedings of the National Academy of Sciences (Table 1) showed that half of them endorsed at least one myth about physiological differences between Black people and White people, including that Black people's nerve endings are less sensitive than White peoples" (Villarosa, 2019).

Percentage of White participants endorsing beliefs about biological differences between Black people and Whites comparing those with no medical training and those with medical training (medical students & medical residents)

Item	Study 1	Study 2			
	No medical training ($n = 92$)	First years ($n = 63$)	Second years ($n = 72$)	Third years ($n = 59$)	Residents ($n = 28$)
Black people age more slowly than Whites	23	21	28	12	14
Blacks' nerve endings are less sensitive than Whites'	20	8	14	0	4
Black people's blood coagulates more quickly than Whites'	39	29	17	3	4

Item	Study 1 No medical training ($n = 92$)	Study 2 First years ($n = 63$)	Second years ($n = 72$)	Third years ($n = 59$)	Residents ($n = 28$)
Whites have larger brains than Blacks	12	2	1	0	0
Whites are less susceptible to heart disease than Blacks*	43	63	83	66	50
Blacks are less likely to contract spinal cord diseases*	42	46	67	56	57
Whites have a better sense of hearing compared with Blacks	10	3	7	0	0
Blacks' skin is thicker than Whites'	58	40	42	22	25
Blacks have denser, stronger bones than Whites*	39	25	78	41	29
Blacks have a more sensitive sense of smell than Whites	20	10	18	3	7
Whites have a more efficient respiratory system than Blacks	16	8	3	2	4
Black couples are significantly more fertile than White couples	17	10	15	2	7
Whites are less likely to have a stroke than Blacks*	29	49	63	44	46
Blacks are better at detecting movement than Whites	18	14	15	5	11
Blacks have stronger immune systems than Whites	14	21	15	3	4
False beliefs composite (11 items), mean (SD)	22.43 (22.93)	14.86 (19.5)	15.91 (19.34)	4.78 (9.89)	7.14 (14.50)
Range	0–100	0–81.82	0–90.91	0–54.55	0–63.64
Combined mean (SD) (medical sample only)			11.55 (17.38)		

*Items that are factual or true.

Hoffman, K. et al., (2016). Racial bias in pain assessment and treatment recommendations, and false beliefs about biological differences between Blacks and Whites. *Proceedings of the National Academy of Sciences of the United States of America* [online] Available at: https://www.pnas.org/doi/full/10.1073/pnas.1516047113 [Accessed 20 July 2023].

According to the University of Virginia authors, this study reveals that a substantial number of White laypeople as well as medical students and residents hold false beliefs about biological differences between Black people and Whites and shows that these beliefs predict racial bias in pain perception and treatment recommendations. Taken together, this research shows that false beliefs about biological differences between Black people and Whites shapes the way Black people are perceived and treated – and the association with racial disparities, pain assessment, and treatment recommendations (Hoffman, et al., 2016). Biases promote the persistence of disparities for Black and Brown Americans. "It turns out assumptions about what it means to be Black—in terms of social status and hardship—may be behind the bias" (Silverstein, 2013). In other words, "Whites are more likely than Blacks to be prescribed adequate pain medications for equivalent ailments" (Somashekhar, 2016).

Bias is an issue that raises the call for building and nurturing supportive relationships with underrepresented and marginalized individuals or groups (allyship) in the practice of medicine. The bias disconnect allows scientists, doctors, and other medical providers — and those training to fill their positions in the future — to ignore their own complicity in health care inequality and gloss over the internalized racism and both conscious and unconscious bias that drive them to go against their very oath to do no harm" (Villarosa, 2019).

Race as a Barrier to Equitable Education

Educational Attainment

Race directly connects with the chances to reach equitable education. "School districts that predominantly serve students of color received $23 *billion* less in funding than mostly White school districts in the United States in 2016, despite serving the same number of students" (Mervosh, 2019). Consequently, students from mostly Black districts not receiving the same level of financial support as their more privileged counterparts, confront disproportionate barriers to educational attainment not attributable to ability, motivation, or disregard.

Schools in socioeconomically disadvantaged areas lack essential resources, such as experienced teachers, up-to-date curriculum materials, and extracurricular activities. "Because schools rely heavily on local taxes, drawing borders around small, wealthy communities benefits the few to the detriment of the many" (EdBuild, 2016). This system of redlining creates disparity in resources that hinder students' educational development and limit their potential for academic success. This in turn affects future financial opportunities and overall well-being. According to Demos (2015), racial disparities permeate the educational system from pre-kindergarten through completion of post-baccalaureate programs, and inequalities at each level reflect earlier disparities and contribute to those that follow. Education, in a sense, creates a 'wealth feedback loop' as the educational level of parents significantly predicts the level of education completed by their children (Demos, 2015).

Educational attainment is a major factor to enhance an individual's health. "Health disparities grew hand in hand with the socio-economic inequalities. Although the average health of the US population improved over the past decades, the gains went to the most educated groups. Inequalities in health and mortality increased steadily, to a point where we now see an unprecedented pattern: health and longevity are deteriorating among those with less education (Zajacova, 2018).

Race as a Barrier to Equitable Education

Affirmative Action

The term "affirmative action" first appeared in a 1963 executive order, signed by President John F. Kennedy, establishing the Committee on Equal Employment Opportunities to be chaired by Vice President Lyndon B. Johnson. Conceived by the committee's special counsel, Hobart Taylor, Jr., the phrase originally connoted aggressive, forward-looking efforts to combat racism, as in "by affirmative action the elimination of discrimination" (Mandery, 2023).

Over the past fifty years, affirmative action created an equal playing field and reduced barriers to educational success for diverse groups including people of color. On June 29, 2023, "The Supreme Court rejected affirmative action at colleges and universities around the nation, declaring that the race-conscious admissions programs at Harvard and the University of North

Carolina were unlawful and sharply curtailing a policy that had long been a pillar of higher education" (Liptak, 2023).

According to Maye (2023) "race-blind admissions processes will further exacerbate existing inequalities and undermine the recognition of the unique challenges that Black, Hispanic, and Native American students encounter throughout the admissions process. By disregarding the significance of race, these approaches risk a wider divide between equal opportunity and communities of color" (Maye, 2023). Bero (2023) summarizes the contradictory nature of the Court's opinion, professing that contrary to widely held belief, affirmative action is not just a "get in free" card for Black post-secondary students. Historically marginalized groups – women, people with disabilities, religious, cultural, and other disregarded groups have all benefited from Affirmative Action and now, circumstances beyond their control may exclude them from these institutions (Bero, 2023).

I believe in affirmative action!
AGGIES
DIVERSITY MATTERS
FFIRMATIVE ACTION!
VERYONE BENEFITS
INCLUDING
ASIAN
AMERICANS

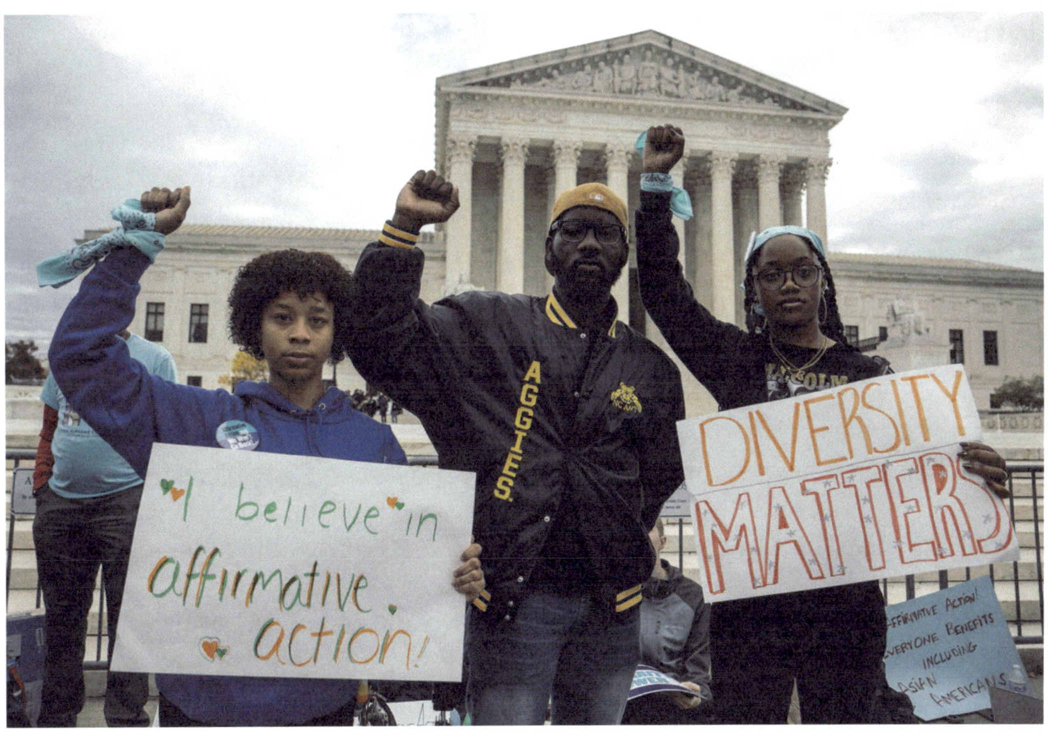

Mandery, E. (2023). How White people stole affirmative action - and ensured its demise. *POLITICO* [online] Available at: https://www.politico.com/news/magazine/2023/06/16/supreme-court-affirmative-action-college-00101963 [Accessed 20 July 2023].

The Supreme Court (SCOTUS) ruling signals major implications for the next generation of Black and Brown providers in healthcare. "Universities have warned that getting rid of affirmative action would significantly impact the diversity of their student bodies, with Harvard arguing in court briefs that taking race out of its admissions process would reduce enrollment of Black students at the school from 14% to 6% of its student body, and Hispanic enrollment from 14% to 9%." (Durkee, 2023).

The educational impact of the ruling extends to the health professions workforce. Forget data before 2023, the disparities in the workforce are severe. "Underrepresented groups including Black, Hispanic and Native American individuals, make up roughly 34% of the U.S. population, but only 19% are registered nurses, 12% are physicians, 11% are pharmacists, and 10% are dentists – a stark underrepresentation of the population it serves" (Albala, 2023).

In the context of healthcare, a diverse workforce is better equipped to understand and respond to the needs of diverse patient populations. Research consistently shows that patients who receive care from healthcare providers of similar backgrounds experience better health outcomes. Affirmative action policies facilitate the recruitment and retention of individuals from marginalized communities, leading to a more culturally competent healthcare workforce (Albala, 2023).

According to the Association of American Medical Colleges (2023) among active physicians, 56.2% identified as White, 17.1% identified as Asian, 5.8% identified as Hispanic, and 5.0% identified as Black or African American (AAMC, 2023). Prevailing opinion declares that the SCOTUS Affirmative Action ruling 2023 will worsen the racial disparities of the healthcare workforce.

Diversity in the healthcare workforce creates a tool that alleviates the healthcare disparities that impact communities of color. The end of Affirmative Action predicts major consequences on the well-being of future generations especially as we look to address health disparities.

Figure 18. Percentage of all active physicians by race/ethnicity, 2018.

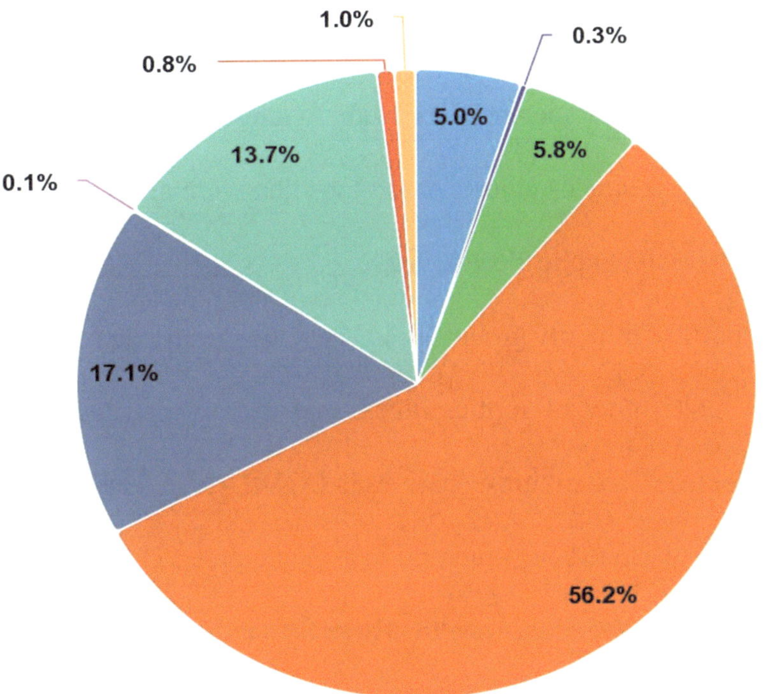

Click on legend item below to add or remove a section from the report.

- American Indian or Alaska Native (2,570)
- Asian (157,025)
- Black or African American (45,534)
- Hispanic (53,526)
- Multiple Race, Non-Hispanic (8,932)
- Native Hawaiian or Other Pacific Islander (941)
- Other (7,571)
- Unknown (126,144)
- White (516,304)

Note: Figure 18 shows the percentage of active physicians by race and ethnicity as of July 1, 2019.

Source: Race and ethnicity are obtained from a variety of sources including DBS, ERAS, APP, MCAT, SMDEP, GQ, MSQ, PMQ, FACULTY, GME, STUDENT with priority given to the most recent self-reported source

AAMC, 2023. Diversity in Medicine: Facts and Figures 2019. [online] Available at: https://www.aamc.org/data-reports/workforce/data/figure-18-percentage-all-active-physicians-race/ethnicity-2018 [Accessed 5 August 2023].

Race as a Barrier to Employment Opportunities

Job Safety, Wages and Benefits

Throughout the pandemic, Black and Hispanic people bore the brunt of higher rates of viral transmission, morbidity, and mortality across the U.S. On analysis, researchers found little evidence to suggest that these differences in outcomes were biological. On the contrary, they resulted due to longstanding and pervasive structural inequalities, systemic racism, and health inequities within the United States that increased exposure to the virus within ethnic and minority groups – during the pandemic, people of color worked jobs that were more deleterious to health than their White counterparts (UIC Public Health, 2021).

When infected, ethnic and minority groups faced barriers to accessing testing and treatment with the consequence of higher rates of serious illness and death (UIC Public Health, 2021). According to UIC Public Health, "the striking disparities in COVID-19-related outcomes for Black and Hispanic people reflect and exacerbate structural racism and persistent underlying social and economic inequities that influence individual health. These factors include, but are not limited to, disparities in income, education, health insurance and access to medical care, access to food, job characteristics, and living conditions" (UIC Public Health, 2021).

Hispanic Americans face challenges when it comes to access to health care and medical treatment. Overall, Hispanic adults are less likely than other Americans to have health insurance and to receive preventative medical care. Language and cultural barriers, as well as factors such as higher levels of poverty, particularly among recent Hispanic immigrants, push the social and economic dynamics that contribute to disparate health outcomes for Hispanic Americans. The COVID-19 pandemic is a stark illustration of health disparities: Hispanic Americans were far more likely than White Americans to be hospitalized or die because of the coronavirus (Pew Research Center, 2022).

The Pew Research Center (2022) surveyed Hispanic people for their beliefs about factors leading to worse health outcomes. Respondents declared working in jobs with a risk for health problems as the major factor (53%) with access to quality care (48%), and language, communication, and cultural barriers (44%) highly contributory.

Figure 4.

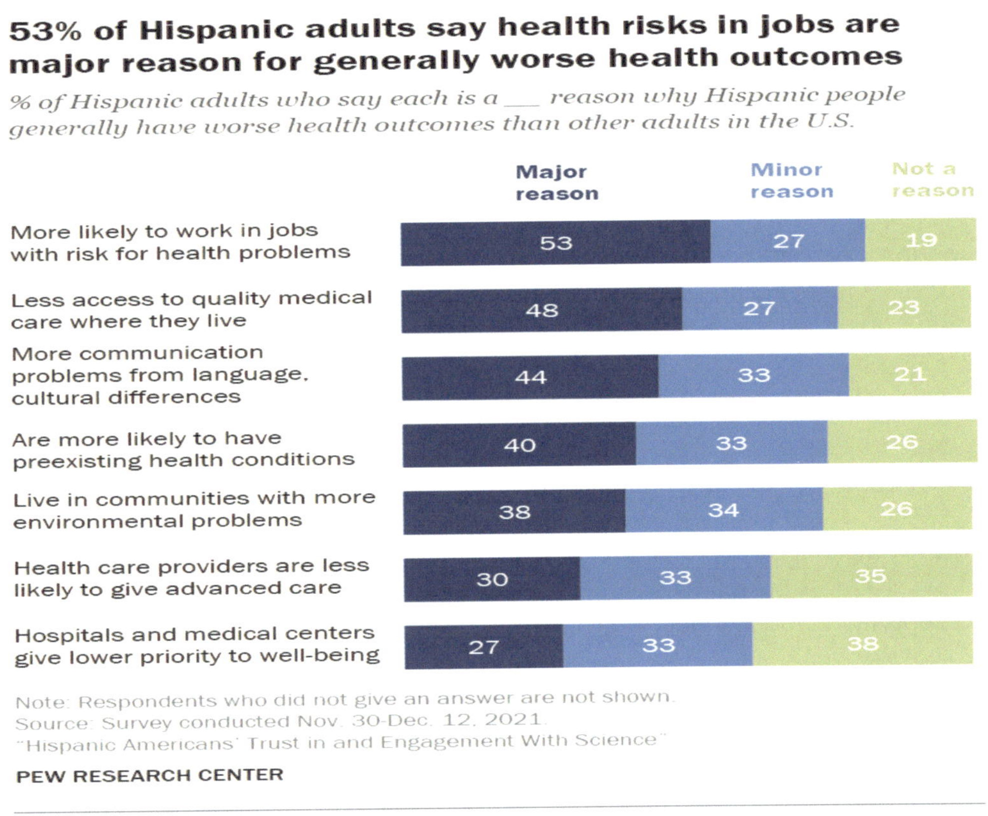

Figure 4: 53% of Hispanic Americans say that working jobs that put them at risk for health problems is a major reason for health disparities.

Funk, C. and Lopez, M. (2022). 2. Hispanic Americans' experiences with Health Care. Pew Research Center Science & Society. https://www.pewresearch.org/science/2022/06/14/hispanic-americans-experiences-with-health-care/

Certain types of jobs, especially low-wage entry-level positions in restaurants, grocery stores, retail locations and warehouses put workers at an access to health care disadvantage. "In

2017, less than a third of workers who worked at or below their state's minimum wage had an offer of health coverage through their employer" (Antonisse, 2018).

Employment disparities cut across color and gender. According to Kochhar (2023) "Looking across racial and ethnic groups, a wide gulf separates the earnings of Black and Hispanic women from the earnings of White men. In 2022, Black women earned 70% as much as White men and Hispanic women earned only 65% as much. The ratio for White women stood at 83%, about the same as the earnings gap overall, while Asian women were closer to parity with White men, making 93% as much" (Kochhar, 2023).

Race as a Barrier to Employment Opportunities

Occupational Segregation and Poverty

Occupational segregation supplies another illustration of racial disparities. It occurs when one demographic group is overrepresented or underrepresented in job categories (Zhavoronkova, et al., 2022). Occupational segregation perpetuates all forms of disparities by limiting access to higher-paying and higher-status jobs for marginalized communities. A University of Minnesota study supports occupational segregation as a driver of health inequities in Black and White workforces, supplying evidence that workforce desegregation reduces workers' health inequities and improves overall population health (Center for American Progress, 2022).

Citing Dixon (2021) and the Low Country Digital Initiative (2022), Zhavoronkova contends that race-based occupational segregation has its roots in slavery. At the time of emancipation in 1865, approximately two-thirds of enslaved people had been forced to work on farms while others worked in domestic settings. After slavery was abolished, legislation and lack of access to other employment opportunities often left Black workers no choice but to continue working in agricultural or domestic roles; in South Carolina, for example, Black residents could only work as a farmer or a servant unless they received a license from a judge (Zhavoronkova, 2022).

Individuals from racial and ethnic minority groups find themselves confined to lower-paying and low-status occupations. The struggle to move up the ladder is even tougher with, "occupational segregation as a targeted effort to relegate Black people and women to lower-paying jobs through rigid legal policy and social structures" (Whitaker, 2023).

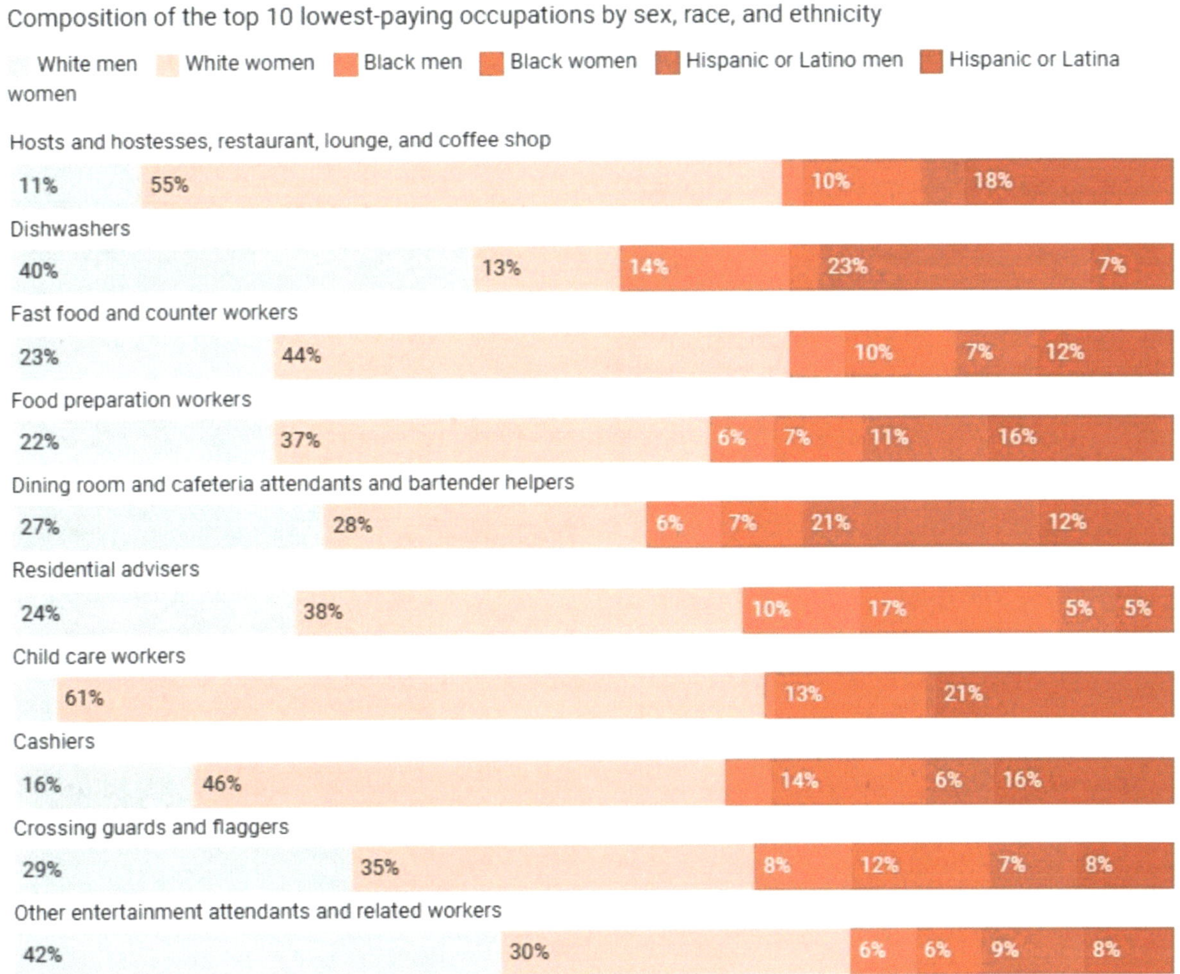

Center for American Progress. (2022). *Occupational Segregation in America.* [online] Available at: https://www.americanprogress.org/article/occupational-segregation-in- [Accessed 27 Aug. 2023].

Compare the above illustrated gender-race disadvantage with the advantage White men enjoy when it comes to high paying jobs.

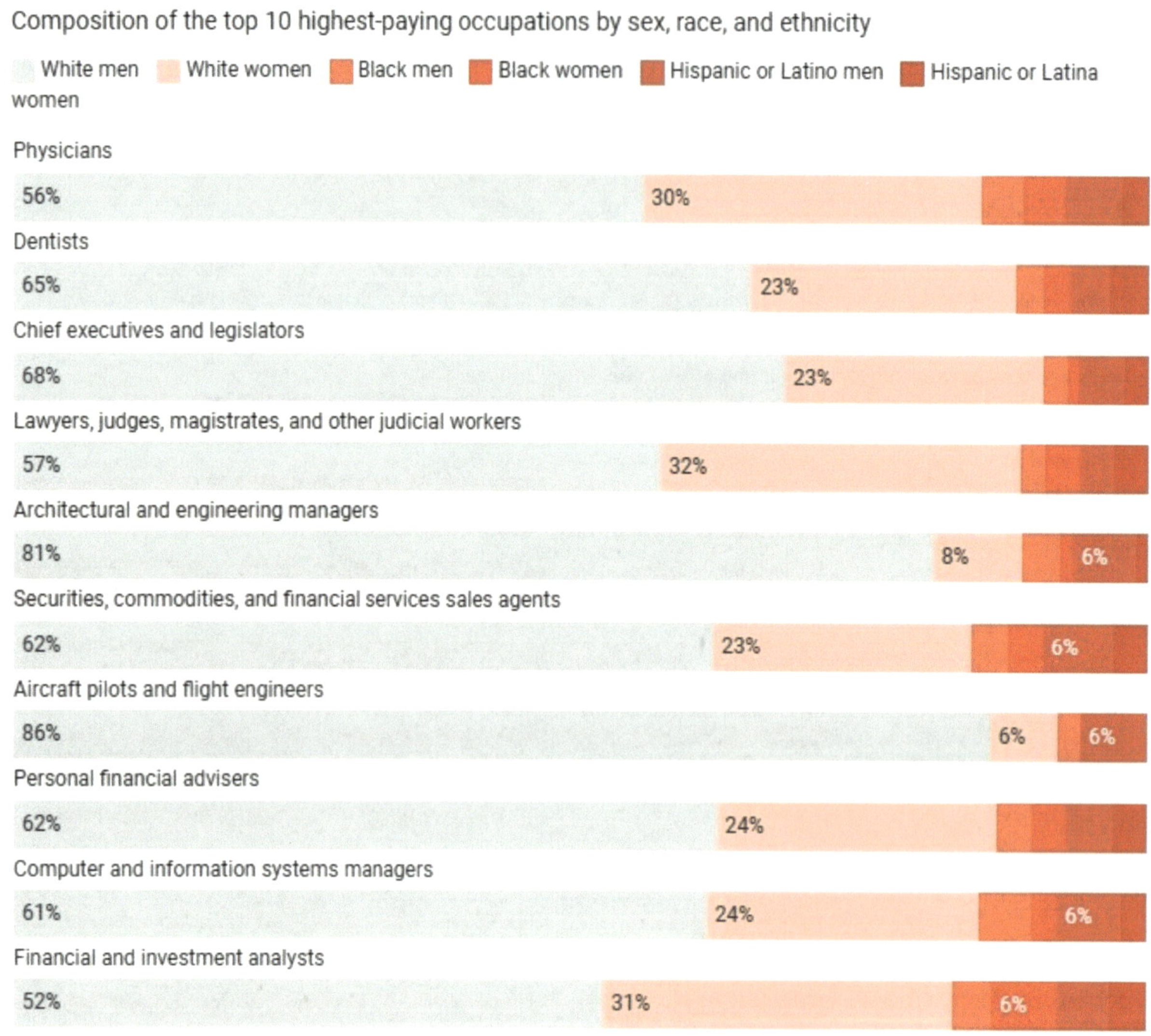

Center for American Progress. (2022). *Occupational Segregation in America.* [online] Available at: https://www.americanprogress.org/article/occupational-segregation-in- [Accessed 27 Aug. 2023].

Limited job security and low-wage work compound health disparities among marginalized populations. "As a result of structural racism in employment and wages, minority women live in poverty and have limited access to health care even after the implementation of the Affordable Care Act because they do not have health insurance from their jobs, or they cannot afford to pay for health care" (Yearby, 2022).

When taken in totality, people without job security and gainful employment live in and are stuck in poverty. Poverty, amongst all other social determinants of health, opens a flood of severe limitations in access to healthcare, housing, transportation, education, food security, employment safety, IT/communication, and legal systems.

> "A second evil which plagues the modern world is that of poverty. Like a monstrous octopus, it projects its nagging, prehensile tentacles in lands and villages all over the world. Almost two-thirds of the peoples of the world go to bed hungry at night. They are undernourished, ill-housed, and shabbily clad. Many of them have no houses or beds to sleep in. Their only beds are the sidewalks of the cities and the dusty roads of the villages. Most of these poverty-stricken children of God have never seen a physician or a dentist."
> - Dr. Martin Luther King, Nobel Peace Prize address, 1964
>
> Szabo, K. (nd.) 9 Powerful Martin Luther King Jr. Quotes on Eradicating Poverty. *Food for the Hungry* [online] Available at: https://www.fh.org/blog/mlk-ending-poverty/ [Accessed 6 August 2023].

Built Environment

According to the Environmental Protection Agency (EPA) built environment touches all aspects of our lives, encompassing the buildings we live in, the distribution systems that provide us with water and electricity, and the roads, bridges, and transportation systems we use to get from place to place. It can be described as the man-made or modified structures that provide people with living, working, and recreational spaces (EPA, 2023).

Neighborhood and Built Environment

Access to healthy food options – food security

Brusher (2022) maintains that access to good, nutritious food is essential to our ability to survive and thrive as human beings, but this right is not afforded to all Americans. Whereas Sevilla

(2021) utilizes the term "food desert" to describe low-income communities—often communities of color—where access to healthy and affordable food is limited or where there are no grocery stores.

Food insecurity affects the health and well-being of all Americans, but the problem permeates communities of color. A 2011-2017 National Health Interview Survey found that non-Hispanic Black individuals had the highest percentage of food insecurity followed by Hispanics, with lower proportions of other minorities and non-Hispanic Whites reporting food insecurity (Walker, 2021).

Neighborhood and Built Environment

Environmental Pollution

In the United States, people of color breathe more particulate air pollution on average, a finding that holds across income levels and regions of the U.S., according to a study by researchers at the EPA-funded Center for Air, Climate, and Energy Solutions (2021). The findings expand a body of evidence showing that African Americans, Hispanics, Asians, and other people of color are disproportionately exposed to a regulated air pollutant called fine particulate matter, according to the EPA (2021). Racial-ethnic minorities in the United States are exposed to disproportionately elevated levels of ambient fine particulate air pollution ($PM_{2.5}$), the largest environmental cause of human mortality according to a study in Science Advances (Tessum, 2021).

For many communities of color environmental toxins come from clear sources. "If you go to communities of color across this country and ask them, 'What's the source of the environmental problems?' they point to: the highway, the chemical plants, the refineries, the legacy pollution left over from decades ago, in the houses, air, water, and playgrounds" (Hiroko, 2021). The Environmental Integrity Project, a nonprofit group founded by former officials from the EPA released findings of separate investigation that found 13 refineries across the United States released elevated levels of benzene, another harmful pollutant, into mostly minority and lower-income neighborhoods in 2020 (EPA, 2021).

Neighborhood and Built Environment

Housing & Homelessness

According to WHO, household crowding is a condition where the number of occupants succeeds the capacity of the dwelling space available whether measured as rooms, bedrooms or floor area resulting in adverse physical and mental health outcomes. Crowding relates to the conditions of the dwelling as well as the space it provides. For example, people may crowd into rooms in their home to avoid cold or uninhabitable parts of the dwelling or to save on heating and ventilating costs.

Studies report a direct association between crowding and adverse health outcomes such as infectious disease and mental health troubles. Researchers connect crowding to poor educational attainment as well. Worldwide, crowding is marker of poverty and social deprivation. Tuberculosis, influenza, and gastroenteritis thrive in crowded living situations. Crowding promotes psychological distress, alcohol abuse, depression, and sleep disorders (WHO, 2018).

Poverty begats overcrowding. According to Austin (2013), residential segregation and ongoing poverty leaves African Americans in the least desirable housing in the lowest-resourced communities in America. In addition to higher poverty rates, Black people suffer from concentrated poverty. Half (45 percent) of poor Black children live in neighborhoods with concentrated poverty, but only a tenth (12 percent) of poor White children live in similar neighborhoods. Children in neighborhoods with concentrated poverty experience more social and behavioral problems, have lower educational test scores, and are more likely to drop out of school (Austin, 2013). **Figure 5.**

Figure 5.

Nearly half of poor black children live in neighborhoods with concentrated poverty
Percent of poor children living in areas of concentrated poverty, by race/ethnicity, 2006–2010 average

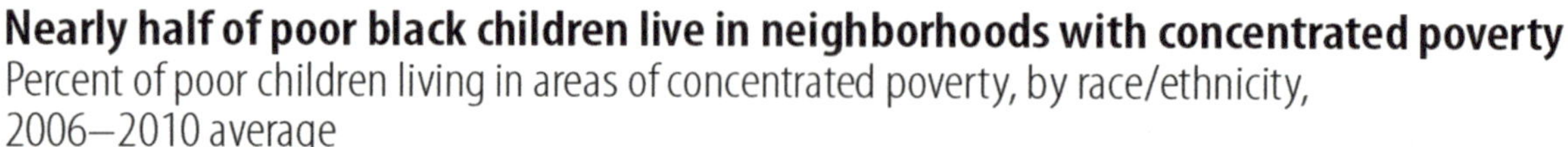

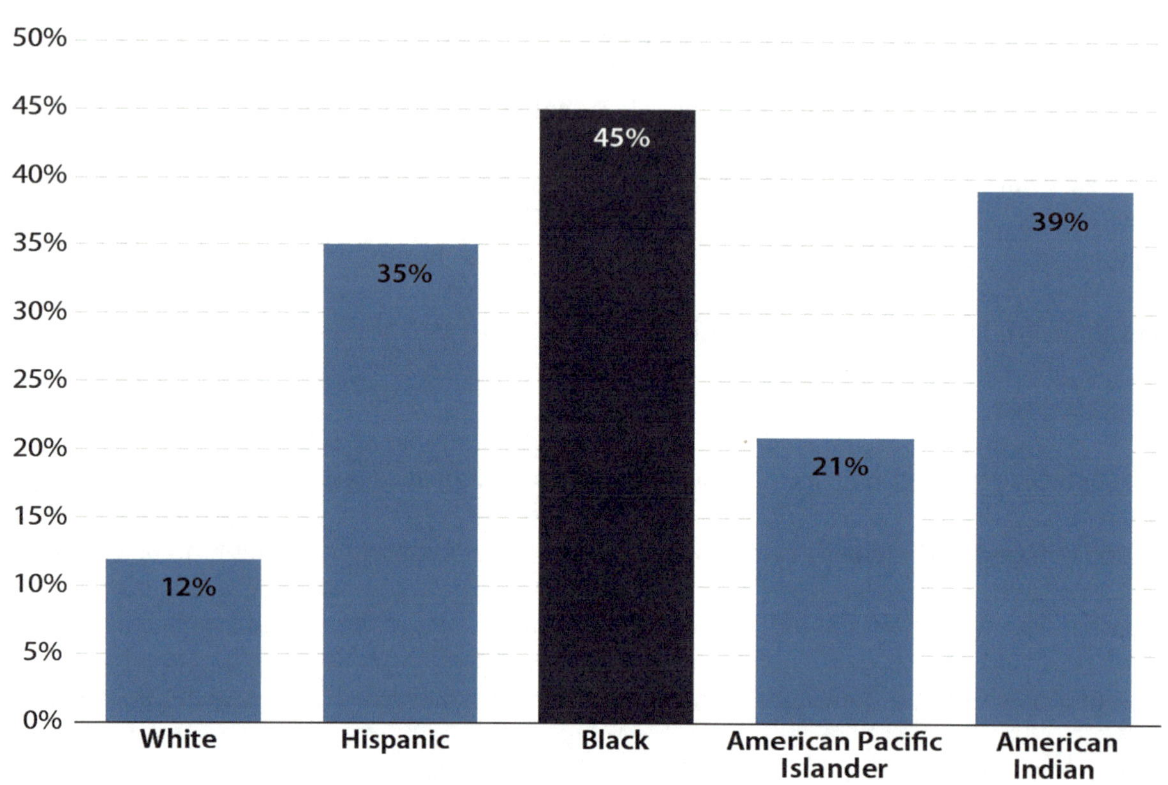

Note: "Concentrated poverty" is defined as a census tract with a poverty rate of 30 percent or higher.
Source: Kids Count (2012)

ECONOMIC POLICY INSTITUTE

Austin, A. (2013). African Americans are still concentrated in neighborhoods with high poverty and still lack full access to decent housing. Economic Policy Institute [online] Available at: https://www.epi.org/publication/african-americans-concentrated-neighborhoods/ [Accessed 6 August 2023].

Inglis (2015) links poor mental health status, reduction in coping strategies, increased risk of childhood injuries, exposure to respiratory issues, infectious diseases, and poor school performance to household overcrowding.

Researchers at the University of California San Francisco found that the epidemic of homelessness in the state of California results from the availability of affordable housing coupled with the limited economic means of persons seeking housing after displacement from their former residence also known as gentrification (Demas, 2023).

Neighborhood and Built Environment

Safe Neighborhoods

Our communities embody the spirit and lifeline of culture, customs, well-being, and health. Safety sits central to well-being; unsafe neighborhoods negatively impact health. Race plays a part in this challenge. "Gun violence alone reduces the life expectancy of Black Americans by four years. And yet, the U.S. ignores the external, systemic factors driving inequality and violence in Black neighborhoods" (Brady, 2019). According to the Centers for Disease Control (2018), homicide ranks in the top 10 for the leading causes of death for Black and Hispanic men, at 4.5% and 2.2% percent respectively, but homicides did not crack the top 10 for leading causes of death for White men during the same period of analysis (CDC, 2022). **Figures 6, 7 & 8.**

Figure 6.

Hispanic, Males All ages

Leading Causes of Death, United States, Males, 2016, Hispanic, all ages		
Rank	**Disease**	**Percent**
1	Heart Disease	20.2%
2	Cancer	19.4%
3	Unintentional Injuries	11.3%
4	Stroke	4.7%
5	Diabetes	4.5%
6	Chronic Liver Disease & Cirrhosis	4.1%
7	Suicide	3.1%
8	Chronic Lower Respiratory Disease	2.6%
9	Alzheimer's Disease	2.3%
10	Homicide	2.2%

Centers for Disease Control and Prevention (2022a). Leading causes of death – males – Hispanic – United States, 2018. *Centers for Disease Control and Prevention*. [online] Available at: https://www.cdc.gov/minorityhealth/lcod/men/2018/hispanic/index.htm [Accessed 23 July 2023].

Figure 7.

Non-Hispanic Black, Male, All ages

Leading Causes of Death, United States, Non-Hispanic Black Males, 2018, all ages		
Rank	**Disease**	**Percent**
1	Heart Disease	24.1%
2	Cancer	19.7%
3	Alzheimer's Disease	7.9%
4	Stroke	5.0%
5	Homicide	4.5%
6	Diabetes	4.4%
7	Chronic Lower Respiratory Disease	3.3%
8	Kidney Disease	2.7%
9	Septicemia	1.7%
10	Hypertension	1.7%

Centers for Disease Control and Prevention (2022b) Leading causes of death - males - non-Hispanic, Black-United States, 2018. *Centers for Disease Control and Prevention.* [online] Available at: https://www.cdc.gov/minorityhealth/lcod/men/2018/nonhispanic-Black/index.htm [Accessed 23 July 2023]

Figure 8.

Non-Hispanic White, Male, All ages

Leading Causes of Death, United States, Non-Hispanic White Males, 2018, all ages		
Rank	**Disease**	**Percent**
1	Heart Disease	24.8%
2	Cancer	22.2%
3	Unintentional Injuries	6.9%
4	Chronic Lower Respiratory Disease	5.8%
5	Stroke	4.1%
6	Diabetes	2.9%
7	Alzheimer's Disease	2.9%
8	Suicide	2.7%
9	Influenza & Pneumonia	2.0%
10	Chronic Liver Disease & Cirrhosis	1.7%

Centers for Disease Control and Prevention. (2022c). Leading causes of death - males - non-Hispanic, White-United States, 2018. *Centers for Disease Control and Prevention.* [online] Available at: https://www.cdc.gov/minorityhealth/lcod/men/2018/nonhispanic-White/index.htm [Accessed 23 July 2023].

Neighborhood safety illustrates race as a social determinant of health. According to Brady (2019) the same cities that experience disproportionate gun homicide — Detroit, Baltimore, Philadelphia, New Orleans, Newark, St. Louis, Chicago — all have large, segregated Black communities with a history of disinvestment. This segregation and disinvestment didn't happen by nature, but by design (Brady, 2019). "Research shows that well after slavery ended, de-industrialization, discriminatory housing practices known as red-lining, and White flight from neighborhoods as Black families migrated north pushed large numbers of Black people into poverty, perpetuating economic inequalities between White and Black people" (Hinton, 2018).

AM I NEXT?
WHO AM I KIDDING?
I'M BLACK.
OF COURSE
I'M NEXT

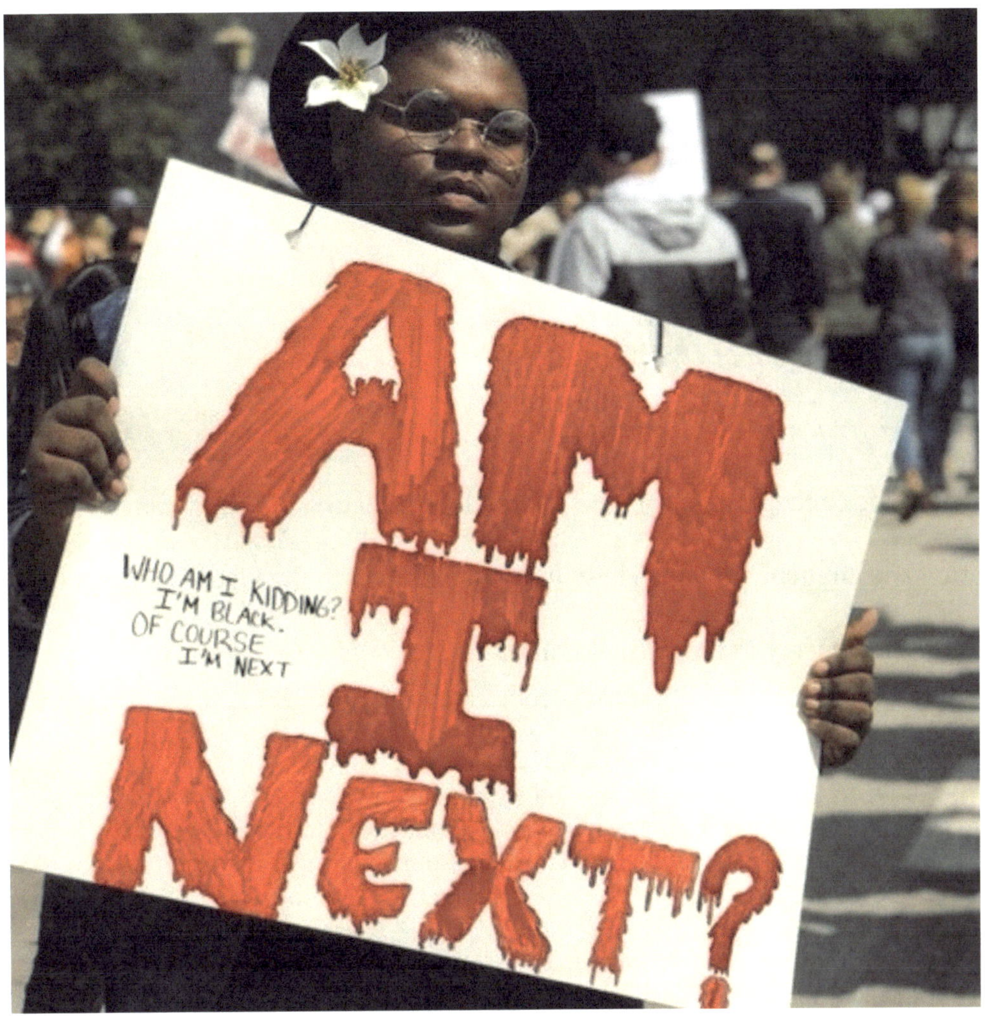

Brady (2019). Gun Violence is a Racial Justice Issue *Brady* [online] Available at: https://www.bradyunited.org/issue/gun-violence-is-a-racial-justice-issue [Accessed 23 July 2023].

The criminal justice system represents a unique element of race intertwined with health and well-being. People with mental illness are overrepresented in the criminal justice system. "What's troubling is that even though people of color are more likely to be involved in the criminal justice system, there is evidence that they are less likely to be identified as having a mental health problem" (Pope, 2019). Phrased analytically, the criminal justice system identifies people of color as criminals, marginalizing or disregarding mental health as a factor played out in their behavior.

Addressing gun violence in our society is a vital step to ensuring the livelihood of millions of Americans. "Black communities have disproportionately shouldered our nation's gun violence epidemic for decades and will continue to do so unless we take concerted, community-driven steps to address this public health crisis. It is imperative—from an equity perspective, a moral perspective, and a human perspective—that we support these communities in reducing gun violence" (Nguyen, 2023).

Race as a Social Determinant of Health

Politics, policies, governance, and the law

Two idealistic concepts underpin the foundation for nation building in the United States – manifest destiny and eminent domain. These two principles form the historical basis for systemic racism and White supremacy as it persists to this day.

Manifest Destiny

Manifest Destiny, a phrase coined in 1845, is the idea that the United States is destined – by God, its advocates believed – to expand its dominion and spread democracy and capitalism across the entire North American continent. The philosophy drove 19th-century U.S. territorial expansion and was used to *justify the forced removal of Native Americans* and other groups from their homes. The rapid expansion of the United States *intensified the issue of slavery* as new states were added to the Union.

Economically, manifest destiny justified further colonization of southern states by increasing production of cotton, tobacco, and hemp for exportation back to England and other European domains.

History.com Editors, (2019) Manifest Destiny. *History* [online] Available at: https://www.history.com/topics/19th-century/manifest-destiny#section_3

Eminent Domain

Eminent domain refers to the power of the government to take *private property* and convert it into *public use*, referred to as a *taking*. The Fifth Amendment provides that the government may only exercise this power if they provide just compensation to the property owners. A taking may be the actual seizure of property by the government, or the taking may be in the form of a regulatory taking, which occurs when the government restricts a person's use of their property to the point of it constituting a taking.

Eminent Domain (continued)
Courts broadly interpret the Fifth Amendment to allow the government to seize property if doing so will increase the general public welfare. In *Kelo v. City of New London, 545 U.S. 469 (2005)*, the Supreme Court allowed a taking when the government used eminent domain to seize private property to facilitate a private development. The Court considered the taking to be a public use because the community would enjoy the furthering of economic development. In this case, the *Kelo* court determined that a governmental claim of eminent domain is justified if the seizure is rationally related to a conceivable public purpose.

LII Legal Information Institute (2023) Eminent Domain *Cornell Law School* [online] Available at: https://www.law.cornell.edu/wex/eminent_domain

Race as a Social Determinant of Health

Justice bent.

The U.S. Supreme Court, presidents of the United States and various institutional and governing bodies throughout the Nation's history have embraced the concepts of manifest destiny and eminent domain legitimizing White supremacy to marginalize, disenfranchise, and oppress minorities for a broad array of contrived benefits. Here are just a few:

Supreme Court of the United States (SCOTUS)

Dred Scott v. Sandford (1857)
In this ruling, the U.S. Supreme Court stated that enslaved people were not citizens of the United States and, therefore, could not expect any protection from the federal government or the courts. The opinion also stated that Congress had no authority to ban slavery from a federal territory.

National Archives, (2022). Dred Scott v. Sandford (1857) *National Archives* [online] Available at: https://www.archives.gov/milestone-documents/dred-scott-v-sandford

The Civil Rights Cases of 1883
In the Civil Rights Cases of 1883, the United States Supreme Court ruled that the Civil Rights Act of 1875, which had prohibited racial discrimination in hotels, trains, and other public places, was unconstitutional.
In an 8 -1 decision, the court ruled that the 13th and 14th amendments to the Constitution did not give Congress the power to regulate the affairs of private individuals and businesses

Longley, R. (2022). About the civil Rights Cases of 1883. *ThoughtCo.* [online] Available at: https://www.thoughtco.com/1883-civil-rights-cases-4134310

Plessy v. Ferguson (1896) *Landmark 1896 Supreme Court Case Legitimized Jim Crow Laws*
The 1896 landmark Supreme Court decision *Plessy v. Ferguson* established that the policy of "separate but equal" was legal and *states could pass laws requiring segregation of the races*. By declaring that Jim Crow laws were constitutional, the nation's highest court created an atmosphere of legalized

Plessy v. Ferguson (1896) continued
discrimination that endured for nearly six decades. Segregation became common in public facilities including railroad cars, restaurants, hotels, theaters, and even restrooms and drinking fountains.

McNamara, R. (2019b) Plessy v. Ferguson *ThoughtCo.* [online} Available at: https://www.thoughtco.com/plessy-v-ferguson-1773294

Dobbs v. Jackson Women's Health organization (2022)
Dobbs v. Jackson Women's Health Organization is the 2022 Supreme Court case that reversed *Roe v. Wade* and *Planned Parenthood of Southeastern Pennsylvania v. Casey*, the decisions that originally asserted the fundamental right to an abortion prior to the viability of the fetus. *Dobbs v. Jackson* states that the Constitution does not confer a right to abortion; and, the authority to regulate abortion is "returned to the people and their elected representatives."
Dobbs disproportionately impacts people of color, the impoverished and victims of sexual assault.

Newton, C. (2022). *Dobbs v. Jackson Women's Health Organization (2022).* [online] LII / Legal Information Institute. Available at: https://www.law.cornell.edu/wex/dobbs_v._jackson_women%27s_health_organization_%282022%29

Students for Fair Admissions v. President and Fellows of Harvard College (2023)
On June 29, 2023, the U.S. Supreme Court announced its ruling in Students for Fair Admissions, Inc. v. President and Fellows of Harvard College and Students for Fair Admissions, Inc. v. University of North Carolina et al., holding that the use of race in admissions policies applied by the University of North Carolina and Harvard College violates the Equal Protection Clause of the Fourteenth Amendment and Title VI of the Civil Rights Act of 1964. This decision, which directly addressed only the universities' admissions programs, restricts approaches that institutions of higher education have been using for decades to provide students the educational benefits that derive from diverse and vibrant campus communities.

Clarke, K. and Lhamon, C. (2023) *U.S. Department of Justice* [online] Available at: https://www.justice.gov/d9/2023-08/post-sffa_cover_letter_final_508.pdf

Presidents of the United States

Thomas Jefferson (1801-1809)
President Jefferson emerged as the preeminent American authority on Black inferiority. His racist ideas ("The Blacks...are inferior to the Whites in the endowments both of body and mind") in his perennially best-selling *Notes on the State of Virginia* (1787) were impactful. His *Notes* were useful for powerful Americans rationalizing slavery after the American Revolution. In his book, Jefferson also offered the most popular race relations solution of the 19th century: the freeing, "civilizing," and colonizing of all Blacks back to "barbaric" Africa.

Andrew Jackson (1829-1837)
Jackson stepped into the U.S. presidency as a wealthy Tennessee enslaver and military general who founded and spearheaded the Democratic Party. Jacksonian Democrats, as historians call them, amassed a winning coalition of southern enslavers, White working people, and recent European immigrants who regularly rioted against abolitionists, Indigenous and Black communities, and civil rights activists before and after the Civil War.
His Indian removal policies were the most devastating of all on the lives of Native Americans (and African Americans). Beginning with the Indian Removal Act of 1830, President Jackson forced several Native Americans nations to relocate from their ancestral homelands in the Southeastern United States

Andrew Jackson (1829-1837) continued

to areas west of the Mississippi River – all to make way for those enslaved Africans being forcibly hauled into the Deep South to clear, sow and harvest lucrative crops. President Jackson helped forge this trail of Native American tears out of the Deep South, and a trail of African tears into the Deep South.

Andrew Johnson (1865-1869)

When President Johnson issued his Reconstruction proclamations on May 29, 1865, he deflated the high hopes of civil rights activists. President Johnson offered amnesty, property rights, and voting rights to all but the highest Confederate officials (most of whom he pardoned a year later). He eventually ordered the return of land to pardoned Confederates, null and voided those wartime orders that granted Blacks forty acres and a mule and removed many of the Black troops from the South.

President Johnson vetoed the Freedmen's Bureau Bill and Civil Rights Bill of 1866, compelling Congress to pass them over his veto. President Johnson also opposed the 14th and 15th Amendments to the U.S. constitution, and in 1868 became the first American president to be impeached by the House of Representatives.

Woodrow Wilson (1913-1921)

President Wilson oversaw the re-segregation of the federal government. Black federal workers were fired, and those that remained faced separate and unequal workspaces, lunchrooms, and bathrooms. He refused to appoint Black ambassadors to Haiti and the Dominican Republic, as was custom. President Wilson unapologetically backed what he called the "great Ku Klux Klan," and championed the Klan's violent disenfranchisement of southern African Americans in the late 19th century.

Calvin Coolidge (1923-1929)

President Coolidge signed the most racist and ethnocentric immigration act in history, an act championed by Republican eugenicists and Democratic Klansmen. The Immigration Act of 1924 was co-authored by Washington Congressman Albert Johnson, well-schooled in theories of "yellow peril" that rationalized discrimination against west coast Asians for decades. The bipartisan measure further restricted immigration from southern and eastern Europe, severely restricted African immigrants, and banned the immigrations of Arabs and Asians. "America must be kept American," President Coolidge had said during his first annual message to Congress in 1923.

Franklin Delano Roosevelt (1933-1945)

President Roosevelt's executive order in 1942 that rounded up and forced more than 100,000 Japanese Americans into prisons during World War II is the most racist executive order in American history. That he spared German and Italian Americans from the military prisons signals his racist perspectives related to persons of color.

The job benefits in Roosevelt's New Deal, like minimum wage, social security, unemployment insurance, and unionizing rights did not extend to Blacks. Farmers and domestics – southern Blacks' primary vocations – were excluded from the New Deal; and federal relief was locally administered, satisfying southern segregationists.

Northern segregationists were also satisfied by the housing discrimination in New Deal initiatives, like coding Black neighborhoods as unsuitable for the new mortgages. As such, Black communities remained buried in the Great Depression long after the 1930s while these New Deal policies (combined with the GI Bill) exploded the size of the White middle class.

Dwight D. Eisenhower (1953-1961)

When NAACP lawyers persuaded the U.S. Supreme Court to rule Jim Crow as unconstitutional in 1954, President Eisenhower did not endorse *Brown v. Board of Education* and dragged his feat to enforce it. At a White House dinner, the year before, President Eisenhower told Chief Justice Earl Warren he could

Dwight D. Eisenhower (1953-1961) continued
understand why White southerners wanted to make sure "their sweet little girls [are not] required to sit in school alongside some big Black buck."
During those critical years after the 1954 *Brown* decision, the former five-star World War II general did not wage war against segregation.

George Walker Bush (2001-2009)
President Bush's No Child Left Behind Act (NCLBA) in 2003 increased the stranglehold of standardized testing on America's children – tests antiracists have long argued were racist. NCLBA encouraged funding mechanisms that decreased (or did not increase) funding to schools when students were struggling or not making improvements on tests, thus privately leaving the neediest students of color behind.
President Bush's Federal Emergency Management Agency (FEMA) publicly left thousands of stranded Black residents behind after Hurricane Katrina hit on August 29, 2005. Federal officials made excuses for their delays, quickening the death spiral in New Orleans.

Kendi, I. (2017) The 11 Most Racist U.S. Presidents. *HUFFPOST* [online] Available at: https://www.huffpost.com/entry/would-a-president-trump-m_b_10135836

Legislative Acts

The Indian Removal Act 1830
On March 28, 1830, the U.S. Congress passed, and President Andrew Jackson signed and enforced the Indian Removal Act – despite Chief Justice John Marshall's Supreme Court ruling in Worcester v. Georgia [1832] that Native American lands were sovereign – launching the forced relocation of thousands of Native Americans - Cherokee, Creek, Chickasaw, Seminole and Choctaw - from their ancestral homelands in Georgia, Florida, North Carolina, Tennessee, Alabama, Mississippi, and Arkansas to the "Indian Territory" in what is now Oklahoma.

National Geographic (2023). Indian Removal Act. *National Geographic* [online] Available at: https://education.nationalgeographic.org/resource/indian-removal-act/ [Accessed 19 August 2023].

The Compromise of 1877
By the 1870s, support was waning for the racially egalitarian policies of Reconstruction, a series of laws (14th and 15th Amendments) put in place after the Civil War to protect the rights of African Americans, especially in the South. Following emancipation, many southern Whites resorted to intimidation and violence to keep Black people from voting and to restore White supremacy in the region.
The Compromise of 1877 was an informal agreement between southern Democrats and allies of Republican Rutherford Hayes to settle the result of the 1876 presidential election.
Immediately after the presidential election of 1876, it became clear that the outcome of the race hinged on disputed returns from Florida, Louisiana, and South Carolina—the only three states in the South with Reconstruction-era Republican governments still in power. Allies of the Republican Party candidate Rutherford Hayes met in secret with moderate southern Democrats in order to negotiate acceptance of Hayes' election. The Democrats agreed not to block Hayes' victory on the condition that Republicans withdraw all federal troops from the South, thus consolidating Democratic control over the region.
The Compromise of 1877 effectively ended the Reconstruction era. Southern Democrats' promises to protect the civil and political rights of Black people were not kept, and the end of federal interference in southern affairs led to widespread disenfranchisement of Black voters.

The Compromise of 1877 (continued)
From the late 1870s onward, southern legislatures passed a series of laws requiring the separation of Whites from "persons of color" on public transportation, in schools, parks, restaurants, theaters and other locations (Jim Crow laws).

History (2023). Compromise of 1877. *A&E Television Networks* [online] Available at: https://www.history.com/topics/us-presidents/compromise-of-1877

The Nelson Act 1905
In 1905 Congress passed the Nelson Act which established a separate system of education for Alaska Natives, giving the Bureau of Indian Affairs (BIA) exclusive control over Alaska Native education until well after Alaska Statehood. The Interior Department made contracts with various missionary associations, giving them authority over education in Alaska. These associations developed a network of Native village schools, which were notorious for prohibiting the speaking of Native languages. During this period children were also being sent out of State to boarding schools, including the notorious *Carlisle School*.

University of Alaska Fairbanks, (n.d.). Early Education and Effects of the Nelson Act (1905) [online] Available at: https://www.uaf.edu/tribal/academics/112/unit-2/earlyeducationandeffectsofthenelsonact1905.php [Accessed 26 August 2023].

Carlisle School 1879
Opened in 1879 in Pennsylvania, the Carlisle Indian Industrial School was the first government-run boarding school for Native Americans. Civil War veteran Lt. Col. Richard Henry Pratt spearheaded the effort to create an off reservation boarding school with the goal of forced assimilation.
Students were forced to cut their hair, change their names, stop speaking their Native languages, convert to Christianity, and endure harsh discipline including corporal punishment and solitary confinement. This approach was used by hundreds of other Native American boarding schools, some operated by the government and many more operated by churches.
Pratt, like many others at that time, believed that the only hope for Native American survival was to shed all native culture and customs and assimilate fully into White American culture. His common refrain was "Kill the Indian, Save the Man."
Carlisle closed in 1918, but its legacy and that of the many boarding schools modeled after it continues to impact Native American families today. From the generational impact of trauma to the loss of cultural identity, many Natives today still feel the pain of Carlisle.

Carlisle Indian School Project (2020) *Past* [online] Available at: https://carlisleindianschoolproject.com/past/ [Accessed 26 August 2023].

Interracial Marriage 1661 - 1967
In 1661 Virginia passed legislation prohibiting interracial marriage and later passed a law that prohibited ministers from marrying racially mixed couples.
In 1691, Virginia required that any White woman who bore a mulatto child pay a fine or face indentured servitude for five years for herself and thirty years for her child.
Over the years, regulations outlawing interracial marriage became commonplace to the extent that in 1924 a Virginia law was passed that prohibited Whites from marrying anyone with "a single drop of Negro blood".
Virginia was not unique; marriage between Whites and Black people was by this time illegal in thirty-eight states.
Loving v. Commonwealth of Virginia 1967
Virginians Perry Loving and his wife Mildred Jeter were arrested and sentenced to prison in 1958 stemming from their interracial marriage. At the trial, the Virginia judge gave the Lovings a choice: they

Interracial Marriage 1661 - 1967 (continued)
could spend one year in jail or move to another state. In his opinion, the judge said: *"Almighty God created the races, White, Black, yellow, malay and red, and he placed them on separate continents. And but for the interference with his arrangement there would be no cause for such marriages. The fact that he separated the races shows that he did not intend for the races to mix."*
The Lovings appealed their case, which eventually made it to the U.S. Supreme Court. Ultimately, the Court found the laws against interracial marriage unconstitutional. Chief Justice Earl Warren wrote the Court's decision: "Under our Constitution, the freedom to marry or not marry a person of another race resides with the individual and cannot be infringed upon by the State." With that decision, all the remaining anti-miscegenation laws in the country were null and void.

Jim Crow Museum (n.d.). *Laws that Banned Mixed Marriages - 2010 - Question of the Month - Jim Crow Museum.* [online] Available at: https://jimcrowmuseum.ferris.edu/question/2010/may.htm

The National Housing Act of 1934
The National Housing Act of 1934 intended to strengthen the residential real estate market and promote homeownership. A cornerstone of FDR's New Deal, the act established the Federal Housing Administration (FHA) which, by creating a federally guaranteed mortgage insurance program, allowed banks to issue lower-cost loans and make them more accessible to more people.

Hayes, A. and Brock, T. 2022 National Housing Act; Overview, Impact, Criticisms, *Investopedia* [online] Available at: https://www.investopedia.com/terms/n/national-housing-act.asp

The FHA was tasked with insuring "economically sound" loans, as part of an overhaul of the system of residential mortgage finance that had been decimated by the Depression. The FHA began redlining at the very beginning of its operations in 1934, as FHA staff concluded that no loan could be economically sound if the property was located in a neighborhood that was or could become populated by Black people, as property values might decline over the life of the 15- to 20-year loans they were attempting to standardize. For example, the FHA's 1938 Underwriting Manual emphasized the negative impact of "infiltration of inharmonious racial groups" on credit risk.

Federal Reserve History (2023). *Redlining | Federal Reserve History.* [online] www.federalreservehistory.org. Available at: https://www.federalreservehistory.org/essays/redlining.

Conclusion:

Understanding the social determinants of health and their relationship to racial disparities is crucial for addressing health inequities. Efforts to promote health equity require a comprehensive approach that addresses structural racism, improves healthcare access and quality, and tackles socioeconomic and environmental factors that contribute to racial health disparities. By dismantling systemic barriers and promoting equitable policies, societies can move toward a future where health outcomes are no longer determined by race, ethnicity, or color of skin.

Questions for Further Consideration:

1. How can healthcare organizations increase racial diversity to better address the social determinants of health?
2. Considering the 2023 SCOTUS decision on Affirmative Action, what measures can be taken to increase racial diversity in education at the college and university level?
3. What policy and legislative recommendations could create bridges to enhance racial equity in healthcare and remove barriers regarding access to care?
4. How can data collection be improved to better understand the social determinants of health and race, and inform targeted interventions?

Sentinel Readings for a Deeper Dive

Allen, B.J. (2011). *Difference matters: communicating social identity*. Long Grove, Ill.: Waveland Press.

Kingsford, Abigail N., Angela N. Gist-Mackey, and Angie E. Pastorek. "Welfare recipients communicated pathways to resilience during stigma and material hardship in the heartland of America." Journal of Applied Communication Research 50, no. 4 (2022): 363-381

EdBuild (2016). *EdBuild | 23 Billion*. [online] Edbuild.org. Available at: https://edbuild.org/content/23-billion

Hahn, R.A., Truman, B.I. and Williams, D.R. (2018). Civil rights as determinants of public health and racial and ethnic health equity: Health care, education, employment, and housing in the United States. *SSM - Population Health*, 4, pp.17–24. doi:https://doi.org/10.1016/j.ssmph.2017.10.006

Thomas, S.B. and Casper, E. (2019). The Burdens of Race and History on Black People's Health 400 Years After Jamestown. *American Journal of Public Health*, [online] 109(10), pp.1346–1347. doi:https://doi.org/10.2105/ajph.2019.305290

Williams, D.R., Lawrence, J.A. and Davis, B.A. (2019). Racism and Health: Evidence and Needed Research. *Annual Review of Public Health*, [online] 40(1), pp.105–125. doi:https://doi.org/10.1146/annurev-publhealth-040218-043750

References

AAMC. (n.d.). *Figure 18. Percentage of all active physicians by race/ethnicity, 2018*. [online] Available at: https://www.aamc.org/data-reports/workforce/data/figure-18-percentage-all-active-physicians-race/ethnicity-2018 [Accessed 5 August 2023].

Albala, B.B. (n.d.). *In an Era of No Affirmative Action: The Right Reasons for Diversifying the Health Workforce*. [online] Forbes. Available at: https://www.forbes.com/sites/bernadettebodenalbala/2023/07/07/in-an-era-of-no-affirmative-action-the-right-reasons-for-diversifying-the-health-workforce/?sh=e2aeb401d50b. [Accessed 27 Aug. 2023].

Antonisse, L. and Garfield, R. (2018). *The Relationship Between Work and Health: Findings from a Literature Review*. [online] The Henry J. Kaiser Family Foundation. Available at: https://www.kff.org/medicaid/issue-brief/the-relationship-between-work-and-health-findings-from-a-literature-review/ [Accessed 20 July 2023].

Austin, A. (2013). *African Americans are still concentrated in neighborhoods with high poverty and still lack full access to decent housing*. [online] Economic Policy Institute. Available at: https://www.epi.org/publication/african-americans-concentrated-neighborhoods/. [Accessed 6 August 2023].

Bero, T. (2023). Affirmative action is over in the United States, but only for Black people. *The Guardian*. [online] 30 Jun. Available at: https://www.theguardian.com/commentisfree/2023/jun/30/affirmative-action-over-only-Black-people. [Accessed 21 July 2023].

Brady. (2019). *Gun Violence is a Racial Justice Issue*. [online] Available at: https://www.bradyunited.org/issue/gun-violence-is-a-racial-justice-issue. [Accessed 23 July 2023].

Carlisle Indian School Project (2020). *Carlisle Indian School Project | Richard Henry Pratt Carlisle Indian School*. [online] Carlisle Indian School Project. Available at: https://carlisleindianschoolproject.com/past/. [Accessed 26 August 2023].

Cartwright, S. (2019). *Africans in America/Part 4/ 'Diseases and Peculiarities'*. [online] Pbs.org. Available at: https://www.pbs.org/wgbh/aia/part4/4h3106t.html. [Accessed 18 July 2023].

Centers for Disease Control and Prevention (2022a). *From the CDC-Leading Causes of Death-Males all races and origins 2018*. [online] Centers for Disease Control and Prevention. Available at: https://www.cdc.gov/minorityhealth/lcod/men/2018/hispanic/index.htm [Accessed 21 July 21023].

Centers for Disease Control and Prevention (2022b). *From the CDC-Leading Causes of Death-Males all races and origins 2018*. [online] Centers for Disease Control and Prevention. Available at: https://www.cdc.gov/minorityhealth/lcod/men/2018/nonhispanic-Black/index.htm [Accessed 21 July 21023].

Centers for Disease Control and Prevention (2022c). *From the CDC-Leading Causes of Death-Males all races and origins 2018*. [online] Centers for Disease Control and Prevention. Available at: https://www.cdc.gov/minorityhealth/lcod/men/2018/nonhispanic-White/index.htm [Accessed 21 July 21023].

Center for American Progress. (2022). *Occupational Segregation in America*. [online] Available at: https://www.americanprogress.org/article/occupational-segregation-in- [Accessed 22 July 2023].

Centers for Disease Control and Prevention (2019). *Stats of the states - infant mortality*. [online] cdc.gov. Available at: https://www.cdc.gov/nchs/pressroom/sosmap/infant_mortality_rates/infant_mortality.htm. [Accessed 29 July 2022].

Costley, D. and Pettus, E. (2022). Decades of systemic racism seen as root of Jackson Mississippi Water Crisis. *PBS* [online] Available at: https://www.pbs.org/newshour/nation/decades-of-systemic-racism-seen-as-root-of-jackson-mississippi-water-crisis [Accessed 21 July 2023].

Demos. (n.d.). *Less Debt, More Equity: Lowering Student Debt While Closing the Black-White Wealth Gap*. [online] Available at: https://www.demos.org/research/less-debt-more-equity-lowering-student-debt-while-closing-Black-White-wealth-gap. [Accessed 21 July 2023].

Department of Justice (2021). *Justice Department Announces New Initiative to Combat Redlining*. [online] Available at: https://www.justice.gov/opa/pr/justice-department-announces-new-initiative-combat-redlining. [Accessed 21 July 2023].

Dixon, R. (2021). *Testimony of Rebecca Dixon National Employment Law Project from Excluded to Essential: Tracing the Racist Exclusion of Farmworkers, Domestic Workers, and Tipped Workers from the Fair Labor Standards Act Hearing before the U.S. House of Representatives Education and Labor Committee, Workforce Protections Subcommittee From Excluded to Essential: Tracing the Racist Exclusion of Farmworkers, Domestic Workers, and Tipped Workers from the Fair Labor Standards Act*. [online] Available at: https://s27147.pcdn.co/wp-content/uploads/NELP-Testimony-FLSA-May-2021.pdf. [Accessed 6 August 2023].

Durkee, A. (2023). *Supreme Court Gets Rid of Affirmative Action in College Admissions*. [online] Forbes. Available at: https://www.forbes.com/sites/alisondurkee/2023/06/29/supreme-court-gets-rid-of-affirmative-action-in-college-admissions/?sh=5cf20f2857ad [Accessed 21 July 2023].

EdBuild (2016). *EdBuild | 23 Billion.* [online] Edbuild.org. Available at: https://edbuild.org/content/23-billion [Accessed 21 July 2023].

Egede, L.E., Walker, R.J., Campbell, J.A., Linde, S., Hawks, L.C. and Burgess, K.M. (2023). Modern Day Consequences of Historic Redlining: Finding a Path Forward. *Journal of General Internal Medicine*. doi:https://doi.org/10.1007/s11606-023-08051-4. [Accessed 19 July 2023].

EPA (2021). *Study Finds Exposure to Air Pollution Higher for People of Color Regardless of Region or Income.* [online] www.epa.gov. Available at: https://www.epa.gov/sciencematters/study-finds-exposure-air-pollution-higher-people-color-regardless-region-or-income [Accessed 21 July 2023].

EPA (2023). Basic Information about the Built Environment. www.epa.gov. [online] Available at: https://www.epa.gov/smm/basic-information-about-built-environment [Accessed 21 July 2023].

Federal Reserve History (2023). *Redlining | Federal Reserve History*. [online] www.federalreservehistory.org. Available at: https://www.federalreservehistory.org/essays/redlining. [Accessed 26 august 2023]

Funk, C. and Lopez, M. (2022). *Hispanic Americans' experiences with health care*. [online] Pew Research Center Science & Society. Available at: https://www.pewresearch.org/science/2022/06/14/hispanic-americans-experiences-with-health-care/. [Accessed 21 July 2023].

Hayes, A. and Brock, T. (2022) National Housing Act; Overview, Impact, Criticisms, *Investopedia* [online] Available at: https://www.investopedia.com/terms/n/national-housing-act.asp [Accessed 26 August 2023].

Hill, L and Artiga, S. (2023). *What is Driving Widening Racial Disparities in Life Expectancy?* [online] KFF. Available at: https://www.kff.org/racial-equity-and-health-policy/issue-brief/what-is-driving-widening-racial-disparities-in-life-expectancy/. [Accessed 29 July 2023].

Hinton, E., Henderson, L. and Reed, C. (2018). *For the Record an Unjust Burden: The Disparate Treatment of Black Americans in the Criminal Justice System.* [online] Available at: https://www.vera.org/downloads/publications/for-the-record-unjust-burden-racial-disparities.pdf. [Accessed 23 July 2023].

History (2023). *Compromise of 1877.* HISTORY. [online] Available at: https://www.history.com/topics/us-presidents/compromise-of-1877. [Accessed 20 August 2023].

History, (n.a.) 2023. Abraham Lincoln's Uneasy Relationship with Native Americans. [online] available at: https://www.history.com/news/abraham-lincoln-native-americans [Accessed 7 August 2023].

History.com. Editors (2019). *Manifest Destiny - Definition, Facts & Significance*. HISTORY. [online] Available at: https://www.history.com/topics/19th-century/manifest-destiny#section_3. [Accessed 20 August 2023].

Hoffman, K., Trawalter, S., Axt, J. and Oliver, M. (2016). Racial Bias in Pain Assessment and Treatment recommendations, and False Beliefs about Biological Differences between Blacks and Whites. *Proceedings of the National Academy of Sciences*, [online] Available at: https://www.pnas.org/doi/full/10.1073/pnas.1516047113 [Accessed 20 July 2023].

HHS (2020). *Social determinants of health*. [online] Healthy People 2030. Available at: https://health.gov/healthypeople/priority-areas/social-determinants-health [Accessed 18 July 2023].

Illing, S. (2019). *The Sordid History of Housing Discrimination in America*. [online] Vox. Available at: https://www.vox.com/identities/2019/12/4/20953282/racism-housing-discrimination-keeanga-yamahtta-taylor. [Accessed 19 July 2023].

Inglis, D.J. (2015). Crowding as a Possible Factor for Health Outcomes in Children. *American Journal of Public Health*, [online] Available at: https://ajph.aphapublications.org/doi/full/10.2105/AJPH.2014.302458 [Accessed 22 July 2023].

Jim Crow Museum (n.d.). *Laws that Banned Mixed Marriages - 2010 - Question of the Month - Jim Crow Museum*. [online] Available at: https://jimcrowmuseum.ferris.edu/question/2010/may.htm. [Accessed 26 August 2023].

Kendi, I. (2017). *The 11 Most Racist U.S. Presidents*. [online] HuffPost. Available at: https://www.huffpost.com/entry/would-a-president-trump-m_b_10135836. [Accessed 21 August 2023].

Kochhar, R. (2023). *The Enduring Grip of the Gender Pay Gap*. [online] Pew Research Center. Available at: https://www.pewresearch.org/social-trends/2023/03/01/the-enduring-grip-of-the-gender-pay-gap/
[Accessed 22 July 2023].

Lee, M. (2022). *When Chinese Americans Were Scapegoated for Bubonic Plague*. [online] HISTORY. Available at: https://www.history.com/news/bubonic-plague-honolulu-fire-san-francisco. [Accessed 20 July 2023].

LII Legal Information Institute, (2022) Dobbs v. Jackson Women's Health organization (2022) *Cornell Law School* [online] Available at: https://www.law.cornell.edu/wex/dobbs_v._jackson_women%27s_health_organization_%282022%29 [Accessed 20 August 2023].

LII Legal Information Institute (2023) Eminent Domain *Cornell Law School* [online] Available at: https://www.law.cornell.edu/wex/eminent_domain [Accessed 20 August 2023].

Liptak, A. (2023). Supreme Court Rejects Affirmative Action Programs at Harvard and U.N.C. *The New York Times*. [online] 29 Jun. Available at: https://www.nytimes.com/2023/06/29/us/politics/supreme-court-admissions-affirmative-action-harvard-unc.html. [Accessed 22 July 2023].

Longley, R. (2022). About the Civil Rights Cases of 1883. *ThoughtCo.* [online] Available at: https://www.thoughtco.com/1883-civil-rights-cases-4134310 [Accessed 20 August 2023].

Low Country Digital Initiative (2022) *After Slavery: Educator Resources: 8. South Carolina's 'Black Code'* [online] Available at; https://ldhi.library.cofc.edu/exhibits/show/after_slavery_educator/unit_three_documents/document_eight [Accessed 6 August 2023].

Mandery, E. (2023). How White people stole affirmative action - and ensured its demise. *POLITICO* [online] Available at: https://www.politico.com/news/magazine/2023/06/16/supreme-court-affirmative-action-college-00101963 [Accessed 20 July 2023].

Maye, A. (2023). *The Supreme Court's ban on affirmative action means colleges will struggle to meet goals of diversity and equal opportunity*. Economic Policy Institute [online] Available at: https://www.epi.org/blog/the-supreme-courts-ban-on-affirmative-action-means-colleges-will-struggle-to-meet-goals-of-diversity-and-equal-opportunity/. [Accessed 20 July 2023].

McNamara, R. (2019a). King Cotton and the Economy of the Old South. *ThoughtCo.* [online] Available at: https://www.thoughtco.com/king-cotton-1773328 [Accessed 19 August 2023].

McNamara, R. (2019b). Plessy v. Ferguson *ThoughtCo.* [online} Available at: https://www.thoughtco.com/plessy-v-ferguson-1773294 [Accessed 20 August 2023].

Mervosh, S. (2019). How much wealthier are White school districts than non-White ones? $23 billion, report says. *The New York Times*. [online] 27 Feb. Available at: https://www.nytimes.com/2019/02/27/education/school-districts-funding-White-minorities.html. [Accessed 21 July 2023].

National Archives (2022). *Dred Scott v. Sandford (1857)*. [online] National Archives. Available at: https://www.archives.gov/milestone-documents/dred-scott-v-sandford. [Accessed 20 August 2023].

National Geographic Society (2023). *May 28, 1830, CE: Indian Removal Act | National Geographic Society*. [online] education.nationalgeographic.org. Available at: https://education.nationalgeographic.org/resource/indian-removal-act/. [Accessed 20 August 2023].

National Institutes of Health (2022). Implicit Bias [online] Available at https://diversity.nih.gov/sociocultural-factors/implicit-bias [Accessed 21 July 2023].

Newton, C. (2022). *Dobbs v. Jackson Women's Health Organization (2022)*. [online] LII / Legal Information Institute. Available at: https://www.law.cornell.edu/wex/dobbs_v._jackson_women%27s_health_organization_%282022%29. [Accessed 20 August 2023].

Nguyen, A. and Drane, K. (2023). Gun violence in Black Communities *Giffords Law Center* [online] Available at: https://giffords.org/lawcenter/memo/gun-violence-in-Black-communities/ [Accessed 23 July 2023].

Paradies, Y., Ben, J., Denson, N., Elias, A., Priest, N., Pieterse, A., Gupta, A., Kelaher, M. and Gee, G. (2015). Racism as a Determinant of Health: A Systematic Review and Meta-Analysis. *PLOS ONE*, [online] 10(9), pp.1–48. doi:https://doi.org/10.1371/journal.pone.0138511. [Accessed 19 July 2023].

Pope, L. (2019). *Racial Disparities in Mental Health and Criminal Justice | NAMI: National Alliance on Mental Illness*. [online] Nami.org. Available at: https://www.nami.org/Blogs/NAMI-Blog/July-2019/Racial-Disparities-in-Mental-Health-and-Criminal-Justice. [Accessed 23 July 2023].

Sevilla, N. (2021). *Food Apartheid: Racialized Access to Healthy Affordable Food*. [online] www.nrdc.org. Available at: https://www.nrdc.org/bio/nina-sevilla/food-apartheid-racialized-access-healthy-affordable-food. [Accessed 20 July 2023].

Shaban, H. (2014). *How Racism Creeps Into Medicine.* [online] The Atlantic. Available at: https://www.theatlantic.com/health/archive/2014/08/how-racism-creeps-into-medicine/378618/. [Accessed 19 July 2023].

Silverstein, J. (2013). *Why White People Don't Feel Black People's Pain.* [online] Slate Magazine. Available at: https://slate.com/technology/2013/06/racial-empathy-gap-people-dont-perceive-pain-in-other-races.html. [Accessed 21 July 2023].

Somashekhar, S. (2016). The disturbing reason some African American patients may be undertreated for pain. *The Washington Post.* [online] 4 Apr. Available at: https://www.washingtonpost.com/news/to-your-health/wp/2016/04/04/do-Blacks-feel-less-pain-than-Whites-their-doctors-may-think-so/. [Accessed 21 July 2023].

Szabo, K. (2017) *9 Powerful Martin Luther King Jr. Quotes on Eradicating Poverty.* Food for the Hungry [online] Available at: https://www.fh.org/blog/mlk-ending-poverty/ [Accessed 6 August 2023]

Tessum, C., Paolella, D., Chambliss, S., Apte, J., Hill, J. and Marshall, J. (2021). PM2.5 polluters disproportionately and systemically affect people of color in the United States. *Science Advances*, [online] 7(18), p.eabf4491. doi:https://doi.org/10.1126/sciadv.abf4491 [Accessed 21 July 21023].

UIC Public Health (2021). *Black, Hispanic Americans are Overrepresented in Essential Jobs | School of Public Health | University of Illinois at Chicago.* [online] Available at: https://publichealth.uic.edu/news-stories/Black-hispanic-americans-are-overrepresented-in-essential-jobs/. [Accessed 21 July 2023].

University of Alaska Fairbanks (n.d.). *Early Education and Effects of the Nelson Act (1905) | Tribal Governance.* [online] Available at: https://www.uaf.edu/tribal/academics/112/unit-2/earlyeducationandeffectsofthenelsonact1905.php [Accessed 27 Aug. 2023].

University of Virginia Library, (2005). Thomas Jefferson, notes on the state of Virginia, query 14, 1781-1782 (excerpt). Jefferson, Query 14. https://mason.gmu.edu/~zschrag/hist120spring05/jeffersonquery14.htm [Accessed 20 July 2023].

U.S. Census Bureau (2022). *2020 U.S. Population More Racially and Ethnically Diverse Than Measured in 2010.* [online] The United States Census Bureau. Available at: https://www.census.gov/library/stories/2021/08/2020-united-states-population-more-racially-ethnically-diverse-than-2010.html [Accessed 29 July 2023].

U.S. Department of Labor (n.d.). *Legal Highlight: The Civil Rights Act of 1964*. [online] www.dol.gov. Available at: https://www.dol.gov/agencies/oasam/civil-rights-center/statutes/civil-rights-act-of-1964#:~:text=In%201964%2C%20Congress%20passed%20Public [Accessed 18 July 2023].

Villarosa, L. (2019). How False Beliefs in Physical Racial Difference Still Live in Medicine Today. *The New York Times*. [online] 14 Aug. Available at: https://www.nytimes.com/interactive/2019/08/14/magazine/racial-differences-doctors.html. [Accessed 21 July 21023].

Walker, R.J., Garacci, E., Dawson, A.Z., Williams, J.S., Ozieh, M. and Egede, L.E. (2021). Trends in Food Insecurity in the United States from 2011–2017: Disparities by Age, Sex, Race/Ethnicity, and Income. *Population Health Management*, 24(4). Available at: https://www.liebertpub.com/doi/10.1089/pop.2020.0123 [Accessed 21 July 2023].

Whitaker, P. (2023). *Occupational Segregation as a Driver of Racial Health Disparities among Black Women*. [online] Race, Racism and the Law. Available at: https://racism.org/articles/basic-needs/health-and-health-care/health-status/89-disparities-in-health-status/11349-occupational-segregation [Accessed 27 Aug. 2023].

WHO (2023). *Taking action on the social determinants of health*. [online] Available at: https://www.who.int/westernpacific/activities/taking-action-on-the-social-determinants-of-health [Accessed 19 July 2023].

Wolff, M.J. (2006). The Myth of The Actuary: Life Insurance and Frederick L. Hoffman's Race Traits and Tendencies Of The American Negro. *Public Health Reports*, [online] 121(1), pp.84–91. Available at: https://www.ncbi.nlm.nih.gov/pmc/articles/PMC1497788/. [Accessed 20 July 2023].

Woodward, A. (2021). *How 'redlining' shaped New Orleans neighborhoods — is it too late to be fixed?* [online] NOLA.com. Available at: https://www.nola.com/gambit/news/how-redlining-shaped-new-orleans-neighborhoods-is-it-too-late-to-be-fixed/article_215014ce-0c15-5917-b773-8d1d2fdaa655.html. [Accessed 19 July 2023].

World Health Organization (2018). *Household crowding*. [online] *www.ncbi.nlm.nih.gov*. World Health Organization. Available at: https://www.ncbi.nlm.nih.gov/books/NBK535289/. [Accessed 6 August 2023].

World Population Review (2023). *Maternal Mortality Rate by State 2020*. [online] worldpopulationreview.com. Available at: https://worldpopulationreview.com/state-rankings/maternal-mortality-rate-by-state [Accessed 29 July 2023].

WorldAtlas (2017). *US States by Life Expectancy*. [online] Available at: https://www.worldatlas.com/articles/us-states-by-life-expectancy.html. [Accessed 29 July 2023].

Yearby, R. (2020). Structural Racism: The Root Cause of the Social Determinants of Health. *Bill of Health Examining the Intersection of Health Law, Biotechnology, and Bioethics* [online] Available at: https://blog.petrieflom.law.harvard.edu/2020/09/22/structural-racism-social-determinant-of-health/ [Accessed 17 July 2023].

Yearby, R., Clark, B., and Figueroa, J. (2022). Structural Racism in Historical and Modern US Health Care Policy. *Health Affairs*, [online] 41(2), pp.187–194. doi:https://doi.org/10.1377/hlthaff.2021.01466 [Accessed 17 July 2023].

Young, C. (2020). *There are clear, race-based inequalities in health insurance and health outcomes*. [online] Brookings. Available at: https://www.brookings.edu/blog/usc-brookings-schaeffer-on-health-policy/2020/02/19/there-are-clear-race-based-inequalities-in-health-insurance-and-health-outcomes/ [Accessed 17 July 2023].

Young, I.M. (1990). *Justice and the Politics of Difference*. Princeton: Princeton University Press.

Zajacova, A. and Lawrence, E.M. (2018). The Relationship Between Education and Health: Reducing Disparities Through a Contextual Approach. *Annual Review of Public Health*, [online] 39(1), pp.273–289. doi:https://doi.org/10.1146/annurev-publhealth-031816-044628 [Accessed 17 July 2023].

Zhavoronkova, M., Khattar, R., and Brady, M. (2022). Occupational Segregation in America. *Center for American Progress* [online] Available at: https://www.americanprogress.org/article/occupational-segregation-in-america/ [Accessed 22 July 2023].

Lexicon of Listed Terms and Agencies

- **American Slavery** was a situation or practice in which people were entrapped and exploited in the United States.

- **Civil Rights Act of 1964** is a comprehensive legislation intended to end discrimination based on race, color, religion or national origin.

- **Centers for Disease Control and Prevention (CDC)** is an agency of the Department of Health and Human Services responsible for the prevention and control of disease and for health promotion and education.

- **Department of Justice** is a federal executive division responsible for law enforcement and allied programs and services.

- **Department of Labor** is a federal executive division responsible for enforcing labor statutes and promoting the general welfare of U.S. wage earners.

- **Deindustrialization** refers to the reduction or destruction of a nation's or region's industrial capacity.

- **Entry Level** refers to being at the lowest level of a hierarchy.

- **Environmental Protection Agency (EPA)** is an independent agency in the executive branch charged with controlling and abating environmental pollution.

- **Jim Crow** Jim Crow segregation was a way of life that combined a system of anti-Black laws and race-prejudiced cultural practices. The term "Jim Crow" is often used as a synonym for racial segregation, particularly in the American South.

- **Patient Protection and Affordable Care Act** aims to provide health care coverage to all Americans and prevent escalation of health care costs.

- **Segregation** is the separation or isolation of a race, class, or ethnic group by enforced or voluntary residence in a restricted area, by barriers to social intercourse, by separate educational facilities, or by other discriminatory means.

AUTHOR'S BIO SKETCH

Joe Eubanks, MA

Joe Eubanks was born and raised in New Orleans, Louisiana. Joe noticed a need for social reform at an early age after seeing the widespread hardship created due to Hurricane Katrina. He received his undergraduate degree in political science from the University of Mississippi. There, he developed an intense interest in changing political narratives around Black poverty. His passion for public service and policy, helped him organize against Confederate flag displays at the University of Mississippi. He received his master's degree in Leadership, Diversity and Inclusion from the University of Kansas, with a focus on disability justice. An avid runner, Joe runs in long-distance marathons and lives by the quote from his favorite athlete Muhammad Ali, "Don't Count the Days, Make the Days Count."

Chapter 4

Gender as a Social Determinant of Health

Joshua Monson, MD, Author
James Lenhart, MD, MPH, Editor

"You never completely have your rights, one person, until you have all have your rights."
- Marsha P. Johnson, prominent gay rights activist in New York City 1960 - 1970s.

Gender as a Social Determinant of Health

While often related to sex, which refers to biological characteristics typically attributed to male or female, gender comprises numerous characteristics that affect how a person interacts with society. These characteristics include appearance, behavior and societal expectations for profession, parenting, education, and hobbies. Characteristics of gender are often assigned to traditional ideas of men and women. The designation of a dress as a feminine article of clothing, despite having no distinct biological function nor purpose, characterizes one example of a gender norm. Historically, gender has played a significant role in individuals' access to healthcare rooted in a differential power dynamic. As described by the World Health Organization (WHO), "Gender is hierarchical and produces inequalities that intersect with other social and economic inequalities" (WHO, 2019).

The high rate of violence against girls and women world-wide manifests this power differential. The World Health Organization (WHO, 2021) reports that ~ 30% of women experience violence from an intimate partner or sexual violence from a non-partner during their lifetime. Exposure to violence is related to negative mental health outcomes and results in PTSD, depression, substance abuse, suicidal ideation, and suicidal behaviors (Coker et. Al., 2002). The act of violence itself carries significant risk for lasting harm and a substantial portion of murders perpetrated against women (~38%) are performed by an intimate partner (WHO, 2021).

On a global scale, women experience inequity in the domains of food insecurity, poverty, education, nutrition, and participation in governance which leads to negative effects on several factors that contribute to overall well-being (WHO, 2021). These effects often compound with other social determinants including race and socioeconomic status.

Consider some of the following facts reported by UN Women (2018):

- *As of September 2017, women held just 23.7% of parliamentary seats globally.*
- *Globally, women and girls are over-represented among the poor: 330 million women and girls live on less than US $1.90 a day.*
- *In 18 countries across the world, husbands can legally prevent their wives from working.*
- *49 countries lack laws protecting women from domestic violence.*
- *More than 50% of urban women in developing countries live in conditions where they lack at least one of the following: access to clean water, improved sanitation facilities, durable housing, or sufficient living area.*
- *While men are more likely to be killed on the battlefield, women are disproportionately subjected to sexual violence and abducted, tortured and forced to leave their homes during times of war.*

UN Women (2018). *Turning Promises into Action: Gender Equality in the 2030 Agenda for Sustainable Development.* [online] Available at: https://www.unwomen.org/sites/default/files/Headquarters/Attachments/Sections/Library/Publications/2018/SDG-report-Fact-sheet-Europe-and-Northern-America-en.pdf?la=en&vs=3554.

The "Motherhood Penalty" and "Fatherhood Bonus" exemplify the disparate respect afforded men and women in the workforce and results in significant economic repercussions for women. Women with children comprise a significant fraction of workers in America, with up to 71% of mothers continuing to work despite responsibility for children in the home. In fact, mothers are the sole or primary source of income for their family in up to 41% of households (AAUW, n.d.). Despite this, mothers are often hired at lower rates than men and women without children offered lower starting salaries. In contrast, men who become fathers often see an increase in their salary. Both effects have a relationship which scales off the number of children, decreasing salary for women and increasing compensation for men respectively (Yu and Hara, 2021).

Figure 1.

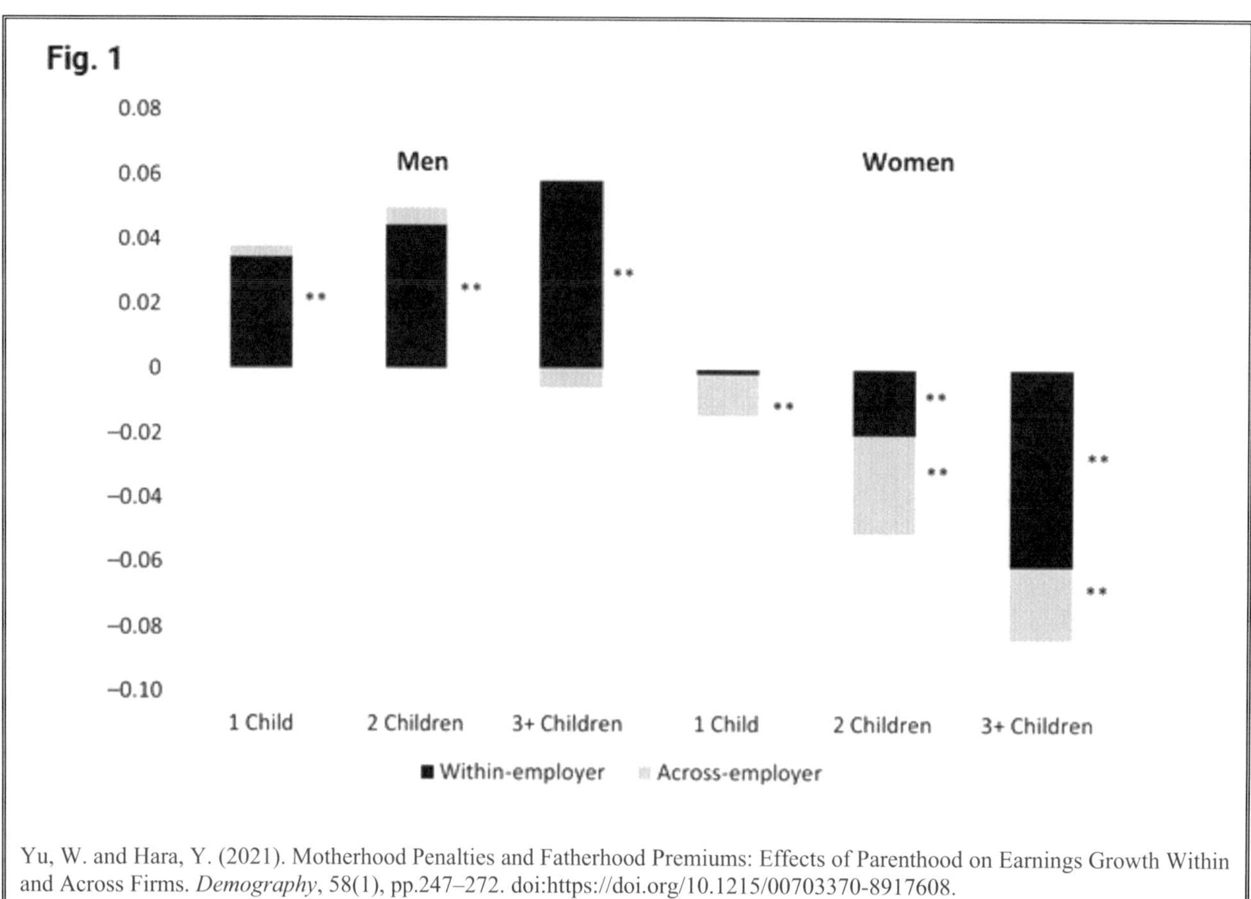

Yu, W. and Hara, Y. (2021). Motherhood Penalties and Fatherhood Premiums: Effects of Parenthood on Earnings Growth Within and Across Firms. *Demography*, 58(1), pp.247–272. doi:https://doi.org/10.1215/00703370-8917608.

Figure 1 shows that the Fatherhood Bonus is most prominent within the same employer for men, but the Motherhood Penalty applies both within and across employers for women. This suggests the event of becoming a father offers a bonus for men who stay with their same employer while women find reduced salary regardless for whom they work. Theory proposes a multifactorial rationale behind this inequity stemming from societal stereotypes of how men and women *should* behave. For example, if a woman talks about her children at work, she can be seen as a "distracted" employee, while a man discussing his children may be viewed as a "caring" father (Zalis, 2019).

Gender as a Social Determinant of Health

In the context of physical and emotional well-being

Perception of behavior based on gender bias affects treatment of patients in the healthcare system. In the United States, chronic pain presents one of the most prevalent conditions affecting individuals' daily life with about 1 in 5 Americans reporting pain daily or almost daily (Yong, 2021). Chronic pain profoundly effects quality of life and negatively affects mental health, finances, and interpersonal relationships (McCarberg et al., 2008).

In a systematic review of pain research and management, investigators found that men were often described as "stoic" and women tagged as "sensitive to pain." These labels left women feeling dismissed or judged when seeking care for their pain and men describing pain as threatening to their masculinity (Samulowitz et al., 2018). Traditional phrases such as "man up" when a young boy complains of pain or other sources of discomfort suggest the stereotypical root of such expressions. Some words even have their etymology rooted in gendered stereotypes. Hysteria stems from the Latin word for uterus to describe a "neurotic condition peculiar to women" (Etymonline, 2021).

Social pressure encourages men to ignore or endure physical and emotional pain, with negative effects on health. While mental health disorders such as anxiety and depression commonly overwhelm men and women, men are much less likely to seek psychiatric treatment, which may explain the sobering fact that men die by suicide four times more commonly than women (Mental Health America, 2020).

Foss (2022) describes the concept of toxic masculinity as the internalization of the traditional interpretation of masculinity with focus on aggression, power, emotional suppression, and dominance to the detriment of one's own health or the freedom of another. This definition does not insinuate that masculinity is inherently harmful. Rather, issues arise when traditional interpretation of masculinity leads to rigidity in expression and suppression of individuality causing dissonance in thoughts and behaviors. For example, internalizing the phrase "boys don't cry," can lead to avoidance of mental health services which in turn contributes to the higher risk of suicide and substance abuse (Chatmon, 2020).

Household income provides an example of how toxic masculinity leads to upheaval in relationships that diverge from historical standards. The power differentiating term "Wearing the pants in the family," refers to the primary breadwinner for a family and stems from a time when, traditionally, only men wore pants. Men not fitting within this conventional prototype often suffer increased stress. According to Syrda (2019), research demonstrates that men experience increased psychological stress as their wives' salary contribute an increasing proportion of the household income past 40% and reaches its peak at complete economic dependence. Subsequently, divorce rates rise as wives' salary increases, showing the negative interpersonal effect income parity has on marriage (Syrda, 2019). In one study, "while women's income was protective against intimate partner violence (IPV), women who contributed more financially than their partners had greater IPV risk. Poverty and tensions over men's inability to provide appear as potentially important drivers of this association" (Abramsky, 2019).

Women finally received the right to vote in the United States of America in 1920 with the passage of the 19th amendment and, despite progress in equity over the last century, not all women have been afforded equal rights or protections and face uncertainty in the recent ebb and flow of American policy (England, Levine and Mishel, 2020).

Transgender Americans (individuals whose gender identities differ from their sex assigned at birth) were not granted protected access to healthcare that aligns with their identity until 2016 when the Office of Civil Rights and the Department of Health and Human Services determined that section 1557 of the Affordable Care Act included gender identity in its prohibitions of discrimination based on sex (Gonzales & McKay, 2017).

President Trump reversed this policy in 2020, however, Federal Judge Frederic Block of the US District Court in Brooklyn blocked Trump's reversal and it was reinstated under the Biden administration in 2021 (Lewis et al., 2021). Translated, in 5 years transgender Americans saw their rights expanded, rescinded, and then reinstated. Such a sequence of events exposes the fragility of civil rights and access to healthcare in the U.S.

Even when transgender Americans are provided access to healthcare, they still face bias and discrimination that has far-reaching implications for their overall health and well-being. In a survey of trans individuals, 41% reported experiencing discrimination in the setting of healthcare, employment, and/or housing, all which constitute determinants of health. Comparable results have been found in studies of major cities including San Francisco, Chicago, and Philadelphia (Bradford et al., 2013). Persistent exposure to discrimination and stress leads to staggering rates of depression and suicidal ideation up to rates of 80%, particularly among transgender youth (Austin, et al., 2022). These rates decline significantly when transgender individuals receive gender-affirming and congruent care demonstrating the importance of providing appropriate services (Mann, Campbell, and Nguyen, 2022).

Gender as a Social Determinant of Health

In the context of Diversity, Equity, and Inclusion

While sexuality is distinct from, and not necessarily connected to gender, the LGBTQ+ community includes both sexual and gender identities that do not conform to heteronormative definitions connected by a shared history of discrimination and hardship. From the history of same-sex relationships in Greek mythology to the "Two-Spirit" identity of many Indigenous cultures, evidence of alternative sexual and gender identities appears throughout history, yet the catalyst for the modern LGBTQ+ movement is attributed to the rebellion at Stonewall Inn by LGBTQ+ patrons in 1969.

The Birth of Pride

Through most of the twentieth century, and certainly prior to, US courts punished same sex behavior as criminal offenses in every state other than Illinois (History.com, 2017). Public displays, such as holding hands or kissing, led to jail-time and legal prosecution. In New York City, this led to mafia management of the establishments where LGBTQ+ individuals would gather without fear of being reported for illegal behavior to law enforcement. Nevertheless, police frequently buttonholed locations like the Stonewall Inn.

During a police raid on June 28th, 1969, the Stonewall Inn patrons fought back against state-sponsored brutality in a monumental act of rebellion. While the exact spark that ignited the rebellion remains shrouded in mythos, protests and demonstrations continued for the next six days as thousands took to the streets surrounding Stonewall. Word of the events at Stonewall traveled throughout the LGBTQ+ community and energized the movement to promote equal rights. To commemorate the anniversary of the Stonewall Uprising on June 28, 1970, thousands of protestors marched in New York City as the first Pride demonstration. This tradition continues to manifest worldwide during the June Pride month (The Library of Congress, 2015).

The Library of Congress. (2015). *Today in History - June 28.* [online] Available at: https://www.loc.gov/item/today-in-history/june-28/

Despite inroads made for equal recognition under the law in many countries, 76 nations worldwide still outlaw consensual same-sex relationships with the death penalty applying in at least 5 (United Nations, 2015). Even in jurisdictions with more progressive policies like the United

States, up to 16% of LGBTQ+ individuals report discrimination during healthcare encounters and, as a result, are less likely to seek medical care (Casey et al., 2019).

Medicine's history of pathologizing the queer community and ignoring issues attributed to "deviant" behavior runs long and deep. For example, homosexuality was not removed as a disease diagnosis from the Diagnostic and Statistical Manual of the American Psychiatric Association until 1973 (Drescher, 2015). The United States AIDS Epidemic first began in 1981 labeled as a diagnosis of opportunistic infections in young, gay males in Los Angeles. For a decade-and-a-half fear, anger, and loss characterized huge proportions of the Gay community in urban centers decimated by HIV and AIDS (CDC, 2023; Rosenfeld, 2018). Who could blame them? HIV/AIDS misperceptions abounded, the media regularly pronounced there was never to be a vaccine, loved ones lay dying in hospital wards and physicians were handcuffed with little more than symptoms-based therapy to combat it. This crisis occurred in the context of a sluggish national response under Raegan-era policy intended to reduce public spending on those whom society deemed "immoral" (Brier, 2009; Rosenfeld, 2018). The effects of the epidemic on survivors are still not fully appreciated, with many suffering from depression and complex grief (Ingram, Jones, and Smith, 2016).

The US Supreme Court ruled so-called sodomy laws unconstitutional in *Lawrence vs. Texas* in 2003 (Gilkis, 2018) paving the way for universal freedom to have consensual, intimate experiences with members of the same sex. According to Shern, Blanch and Steverman (2014), this complex relationship with the legal system, medicine, and society at large potentiates toxic stress and detrimental effects on both physical and mental health.

The following highlighted paragraphs expand on the nuances of the Supreme Court decision.

Lawrence vs. Texas *June 26, 2003*

In an historic decision with wide-ranging implications, the U.S. Supreme Court today struck down a Texas law that makes some kinds of sexual intimacy a crime, but only for gay people. The decision overrules the court's 1986 decision in *Bowers v. Hardwick,* which was widely condemned for treating gay people as second-class citizens. It was hailed by the American Civil Liberties Union (n.d.) as a major milestone in the fight for constitutional rights.

"This decision will affect virtually every important legal and social question involving lesbians and gay men," said James Esseks, Litigation Director of the ACLU's Lesbian and Gay Rights Project. "For years, whenever we have sought equality, we've been answered both in courts of law and in the court of public opinion with the claim that we are not entitled to equality because our love makes us criminals. That argument – which has been a serious block to progress — is now a dead letter." Esseks added, "from now on, cases and political debates about employment, custody and the treatment of same-sex couples should be about merit, not about who you love."

In sweeping language, the Court said the Constitution protects the right of gay people to form intimate relationships and "retain their dignity as free persons." Gay people, the Court said, have the same right to "define one's concept of existence, of meaning, or the universe, and of the mystery of human life," that heterosexuals do. The Bowers decision, the Court said, "demeans the lives of homosexual persons."

Since 1986, lower courts have relied on Bowers v. Hardwick to take away or limit custody to gay parents and to uphold firing or refusing to hire gay people. Bowers has frequently been invoked in legislative debates as a reason not to protect gay people from discrimination.

"With this decision, the Court has finally recognized that we are part of the American family. Now it's time for the rest of society to do the same," Esseks said. "Our civil rights laws need to make the workplace fair, our schools safe, and to give basic respect to the relationships at the core of our lives–with our partners and our children. By acknowledging that we are not criminals, this decision will make it far easier for us to get society to change."

ACLU (2023). *Striking Down Texas Law Against Same-Sex "Sodomy," Supreme Court Rights Egregious Wrong of 17 Years, Signaling New Era for Gay Rights* [online] Available at: https://www.aclu.org/press-releases/striking-down-texas-law-against-same-sex-sodomy-supreme-court-rights-egregious-wrong [Accessed 25 June 2023].

Gender as a Social Determinant of Health

Policy, Politics and Governance

The political landscape for women and members of the LGBTQ+ community ebbs and flows in a dynamic of constant flux often with disastrous, if not unintended consequences. According to a complaint filed by the Texas Medical Association (TMA), due to the June 24, 2022 decision by the United States Supreme Court to break from federal precedent to protect access to abortion set by *Roe V. Wade*, some pregnant women have been denied healthcare, even when appropriate (Dallas News, 2022). The Texas Medical Board received a letter from the TMA describing examples of doctors refusing treatment for certain medical and pregnancy related conditions out of fear of prosecution if a court were to decide the patient's life was not in "enough danger" to warrant intervention. This included the report of a physician being told to wait to treat an ectopic pregnancy until it ruptured, posing serious risk of harm to the pregnant woman including death. Further illustrating the diversity, equity, and inclusion (DEI) conundrum, state legislators introduced over 500 anti-LGBTQ+ laws in the first six months of 2023 alone, most of them targeting transgender Americans. Many of these bills restrict access to gender affirming care posing significant risk of harm to individuals that are affected (Fields, 2023).

Internationally, women in Afghanistan saw the progress made for their equality stripped away after the Taliban recaptured control of the country in 2021. Since then, access to healthcare, education, transportation, and employment opportunities has been severely limited for Afghan women with many describing feelings of hopelessness and despair (Human Rights Watch, 2022).

Given the circumstances nationally and internationally illustrated in this essay, an obligation to support DEI in the broad context of human rights and human health represents health professions call to action on every level. Support for the work of the National Association for Equity, Diversity and Inclusion and the American Association for Access Equity and Diversity on a national level as well as the World Health Organization and United Nations internationally, promotes limitation of the adverse effects of gender and sexual discrimination and advances the hope of healthcare for all toward fulfilment.

Gender Terms

Sex refers to a person's biological status and is typically assigned at birth, usually based on external anatomy. Sex is typically categorized as male, female, or intersex.

Gender is often defined as a social construct of norms, behaviors and roles that varies between societies and over time. Gender is often categorized as male, female, or nonbinary.

Gender identity is one's own internal sense of self and their gender, whether that is man, woman, neither or both. Unlike gender expression, gender identity is not outwardly visible to others. For most people, gender identity aligns with the sex assigned at birth, the American Psychological Association notes. For transgender people, gender identity differs in varying degrees from the sex assigned at birth.

Gender expression is how a person presents gender outwardly, through behavior, clothing, voice, or other perceived characteristics. Society identifies these cues as masculine or feminine, although what is considered masculine or feminine changes over time and varies by culture.

Wamsley, L. (2021) *A Guide to Gender Terms* NPR: Pride Month [online] Available at: https://www.npr.org/2021/06/02/996319297/gender-identity-pronouns-expression-guide-lgbtq [Accessed 17 August 2023].

Questions for Further Consideration:

1. How does the gender bias in STEM fields affect the gender wage gap and subsequent access to high-paying professions?
2. How does gender bias affect patients' trust and willingness to follow medical advice?
3. What effects will state-wide bans on gender affirming care, particularly for transgender youth, have on transgender individuals?
4. What effects will the repeal of *Roe v. Wade* have on women's access to other domains of healthcare? For example, will pregnant women be unable to receive important medical care such as treatment for systemic infections, seizures, cholecystitis, or appendicitis due to clinician fear of harming the fetus?

Sentinel Readings for a Deeper Dive

History.com Editors (2017). *Stonewall Riots*. [online] HISTORY. Available at: https://www.history.com/topics/gay-rights/the-stonewall-riots

Human Rights Watch (2022). Afghanistan: Taliban Deprive Women of Livelihoods, Identity. Human Rights Watch. [online] Available at: https://www.hrw.org/news/2022/01/18/afghanistan-taliban-deprive-women-livelihoods-identity

UN Women (2018). *Turning Promises into Action: Gender Equality in the 2030 Agenda for Sustainable Development*. [online] Available at: https://www.unwomen.org/sites/default/files/Headquarters/Attachments/Sections/Library/Publications/2018/SDG-report-Fact-sheet-Europe-and-Northern-America-en.pdf?la=en&vs=3554

World Health Organization (2021). *Violence against women*. World Health Organization. [online] Available at: https://www.who.int/news-room/fact-sheets/detail/violence-against-women

References

AAUW (n.d.). *The motherhood penalty*. AAUW : Empowering Women since 1881. [online] Available at: https://www.aauw.org/issues/equity/motherhood/ [Accessed Feb - June 2023].

Abramsky, T., Lees, S., Stöckl, H., Harvey, S., Kapinga, I., Ranganathan, M., Mshana, G. and Kapiga, S. (2019). Women's income and risk of intimate partner violence: secondary findings from the MAISHA cluster randomised trial in North-Western Tanzania, *BMC Public Health* [online] Available at: https://bmcpublichealth.biomedcentral.com/articles/10.1186/s12889-019-7454-1 [Accessed June 25, 2013].

ACLU (2003). *Striking Down Texas Law Against Same-Sex "Sodomy," Supreme Court Rights Egregious Wrong of 17 Years, Signaling New Era for Gay Rights* [online] Available at: https://www.aclu.org/press-releases/striking-down-texas-law-against-same-sex-sodomy-supreme-court-rights-egregious-wrong [Accessed 25 June 2023].

American Civil Liberties Union. (n.d.). *Update on the Status of Sodomy Laws*. [online] Available at: https://www.aclu.org/other/update-status-sodomy-laws#:~:text=Sodomy%20laws%20generally%20prohibit%20oral [Accesses Feb. - June 2023].

Austin, A., Craig, S., D'Souza, S. and McInroy, L. (2020). Suicidality Among Transgender Youth: Elucidating the Role of Interpersonal Risk Factors. *Journal of Interpersonal Violence*, [online] Available at: https://journals.sagepub.com/doi/abs/10.1177/0886260520915554?journalCode=jiva [Accessed Feb. - June 2023].

Bradford, J., Reisner, S., Honnold, J. and Xavier, J. (2013) Experiences of Transgender-Related Discrimination and Implications for Health: Results from the Virginia Transgender Health Initiative Study. *American Journal of Public Health*, [online] Available at: https://www.ncbi.nlm.nih.gov/pmc/articles/PMC3780721 [Accesses Feb. - June 2023].

Brier, J. (2009) Infectious Ideas: U.S. Political Responses to the AIDS Crisis. [online] *Google Books. Univ of North Carolina Press*. Available at: https://books.google.co.uk/books?hl=en&lr=&id=ZxV8CpKfhI0C&oi=fnd&pg=PR7&ots=eMvNkvt-dH&sig=Sow51phrvSKs-WA2DYXuCxiPWic#v=onepage&q&f=false. [Accesses Feb. - June 2023].

Casey, L., Reisner, S., Findling, M., Blendon, R., Benson, J., Sayde, J. and Miller, C. (2019). Discrimination in the United States: Experiences of lesbian, gay, bisexual, transgender, and queer Americans. *Health Services Research*, [online] Available at: https://www.ncbi.nlm.nih.gov/pmc/articles/PMC6864400 [Accessed Feb. - Mar. 2023].

CDC (2023). HIV and AIDS Timeline. *National Prevention Information Network* [online] Available at: https://npin.cdc.gov/pages/hiv-and-aids-timeline. [Accessed Feb. - Mar. 2023].

Chatmon, B. (2020) Males and Mental Health Stigma. *American Journal of Men's Health*, [online] Available at: https://www.ncbi.nlm.nih.gov/pmc/articles/PMC7444121/ [Accessed Feb. - Mar. 2023].

Coker, A. et al. (2002) Social Support Protects against the Negative Effects of Partner Violence on Mental Health. *Journal of Women's Health & Gender-Based Medicine*, [online] Available at: https://pubmed.ncbi.nlm.nih.gov/12165164/ [Accessed Feb. - Mar. 2023].

Dallas News, (2022) *Texas hospitals fearing abortion law delay pregnant women's care, medical association says*. [online] Available at: https://www.dallasnews.com/news/politics/2022/07/14/texas-hospitals-fearing-abortion-law-delay-pregnant-womens-care-medical-association-says/ [Accessed 29 Nov. 2022].

Drescher, J. (2015) Out of DSM: Depathologizing homosexuality. *Behavioral Sciences*, 5(4), pp.565–575. [online] Available at: https://www.ncbi.nlm.nih.gov/pmc/articles/PMC4695779/ [Accesses Feb. - June 2023].

England, P., Levine, A. and Mishel, E. (2020) Progress toward gender equality in the United States has slowed or stalled. *Proceedings of the National Academy of Sciences*, [online] https://www.pnas.org/doi/10.1073/pnas.1918891117 [Accessed Feb. - Mar. 2023].

Etymonline (2021) *Origin and meaning of hysterical by Online Etymology Dictionary*. [online] Available at: https://www.etymonline.com/word/hysterical. [Accessed Feb. - June 2023].

Fields, A. (2023) Human Rights Campaign: Pride is More than a Parade. *Human Rights Campaign* [online] Available at: https://www.hrc.org/press-releases/human-rights-campaign-pride-is-more-than-a-parade. [Accessed Feb - Mar. 2023].

Foss, K. (2022) *What is Toxic Masculinity and How it Impacts Mental Health*. Anxiety & Depression Association of America [online] Available at: https://adaa.org/learn-from-us/from-the-experts/blog-posts/consumer/what-toxic-masculinity-and-how-it-impacts-mental [Accessed Feb. - June 2023].

Gilkis, K. (2018) *Lawrence v. Texas*. LII / Legal Information Institute. [online] Available at: https://www.law.cornell.edu/wex/lawrence_v._texas. [Accessed Feb. - June 2023].

Gonzales, G. and McKay, T. (2017) What an Emerging Trump Administration Means for Lesbian, Gay, Bisexual, and Transgender Health. *Health Equity*, [online] Available at: https://www.ncbi.nlm.nih.gov/pmc/articles/PMC6071884/ [Accessed Feb. - June 2023].

History.com Editors (2017) *Stonewall Riots*. [online] HISTORY. Available at: https://www.history.com/topics/gay-rights/the-stonewall-riots [Accessed Feb. - June 2023].

Human Rights Watch (2022) Afghanistan: Taliban Deprive Women of Livelihoods, Identity. *Human Rights Watch* [online] Available at: https://www.hrw.org/news/2022/01/18/afghanistan-taliban-deprive-women-livelihoods-identity [Accessed Feb. - June 2023].

Ingram, K., Jones, D., and Smith N. (2001) Adjustment among People who have Experienced Aids-Related Multiple Loss: The Role of Unsupportive Social Interactions, Social Support, and Coping. *OMEGA - Journal of Death and Dying* [online] Available at: https://journals.sagepub.com/doi/abs/10.2190/TV1J-543L-M020-B93V [Accessed Feb. - June 2023].

Lewis, C., et al. (2021) Federal Government Eliminates Health Care Protections for Transgender Americans. *The Commonwealth Fund* [online] Available at: https://www.commonwealthfund.org/blog/2018/federal-protections-health-care-risk-transgender-americans. [Accessed Feb. - June 2023].

Library of Congress, (2015). *Today in History - June 28*. [online] Available at: https://www.loc.gov/item/today-in-history/june-28/. [Accessed Feb. - June 2023].

Mann, S., Campbell, T. and Nguyen, D. (2022) Access to Gender-Affirming Care and Transgender Mental Health: Evidence from Medicaid Coverage. *SSRN* [online] Available at: https://papers.ssrn.com/sol3/papers.cfm?abstract_id=4164673 [Accessed Feb. - June 2023].

McCarberg, B., Nicholson, B., Todd, K., Palmer, T. and Penles, L. (2008). The Impact of Pain on Quality of Life and the Unmet Needs of Pain Management: Results from Pain Sufferers and Physicians Participating in an Internet Survey. *American Journal of Therapeutics*, [online] Available at: https://pubmed.ncbi.nlm.nih.gov/18645331 [Accessed Feb. – Mar. 2023].

Mental Health America (2020) Infographic: Mental Health for Men *Mental Health America.* [online] Available at: https://www.mhanational.org/infographic-mental-health-men. [Accessed Feb. - Mar. 2023].

Rosenfeld, D. (2018) The AIDS epidemic's lasting impact on gay men. *The British Academy.* [online] Available at: https://www.thebritishacademy.ac.uk/blog/aids-epidemic-lasting-impact-gay-men/. [Accessed Feb. – Mar. 2023].

Samulowitz, A., Gremyr, I., Eriksson, E. and Hensing, G. (2018). 'Brave Men' and 'Emotional Women': A Theory-Guided Literature Review on Gender Bias in Health Care and Gendered Norms towards Patients with Chronic Pain. *Pain Research and Management.* [online] Available at: https://www.hindawi.com/journals/prm/2018/6358624/. [Accessed Feb. - June 2023].

Shern, D., Blanch, A. and Steverman, S. (2014). Impact of Toxic Stress on Individuals and Communities: A Review of the Literature. *Mental Health America* [online] Available at: https://www.mhanational.org/sites/default/files/Impact%20of%20Toxic%20Stress%20on%20Individuals%20and%20Communities-A%20Review%20of%20the%20Literature.pdf. [Accessed Feb. - June 2023].

Syrda, J. (2019) Spousal Relative Income and Male Psychological Distress. *Personality and Social Psychology Bulletin*, [online] https://doi.org/10.1177/0146167219883611. [Accessed Feb. - June 2023].

UN Women (2018) *Turning Promises into Action: Gender Equality in the 2030 Agenda for Sustainable Development*. [online] Available at: https://www.unwomen.org/sites/default/files/Headquarters/Attachments/Sections/Library/Publications/2018/SDG-report-Fact-sheet-Europe-and-Northern-America-en.pdf?la=en&vs=3554. [Accessed Feb. - June 2023].

United Nations Human Rights (2015) Ending violence and discrimination against lesbian, gay, bisexual, transgender and intersex people. *UNODC* [online] Available at: https://cdn.who.int/media/docs/default-source/documents/gender/joint_lgbti_statement_eng.pdf?sfvrsn=fad54fc7_3. [Accessed Feb. - June 2023].

Wamsley, L. (2021) *A Guide to Gender Terms* NPR: Pride Month [online] Available at: https://www.npr.org/2021/06/02/996319297/gender-identity-pronouns-expression-guide-lgbtq [Accessed June 26 2023]

WHO (2019) *Gender and health*. World Health Organization. [online] Available at: https://www.who.int/health-topics/gender#tab=tab_1. [Accessed Feb. - June 2023].

WHO (2021) *Violence against women*. World Health Organization. [online] Available at: https://www.who.int/news-room/fact-sheets/detail/violence-against-women [Accessed Feb. - June 2023].

Yong, R., Mullins, P. and Bhattacharyya, N. (2021) The prevalence of chronic pain among adults in the United States. *Pain*, [online] Available at: https://pubmed.ncbi.nlm.nih.gov/33990113/ [Accessed Feb. - June 2023].

Yu, W. and Hara, Y. (2021) Motherhood Penalties and Fatherhood Premiums: Effects of Parenthood on Earnings Growth Within and Across Firms. *Demography*, [online] Available at: https://pubmed.ncbi.nlm.nih.gov/33834238/ [Accessed Feb. - June 2023].

Zalis, S. (2019) The Motherhood Penalty: Why We're Losing Our Best Talent to Caregiving. Forbes [online] Available at: https://www.forbes.com/sites/shelleyzalis/2019/02/22/the-motherhood-penalty-why-were-losing-our-best-talent-to-caregiving/?sh=bc1627a46e5c [Accessed Mar. - June 2023].

Lexicon of Listed Terms and Agencies

- **UN Women** is a branch of the UN that focuses on monitoring and improving gender inequality worldwide. https://www.unwomen.org/

- **The World Health Organization** (WHO) is an international organization that seeks to improve and provide healthcare on a global level. https://www.who.int/

- **The Library of Congress** is a governmental agency that stores vast amounts of historical information and includes numerous articles of the origin of the LGTBQ+ movement and Pride in the United States. https://www.loc.gov/lgbt-pride-month/

- **The Human Rights Campaign** is an organization based in the United States that works to provide advocacy for LGBTQ+ individuals. https://www.hrc.org/

AUTHOR'S BIO SKETCH

Joshua Monson, MD

Joshua Monson grew up in the small rural town Littlerock, Washington just outside of Olympia. He studied Neuroscience at the University of Minnesota before moving on to medical school at the University of Washington where he locked into the field of Family Medicine. He received residency training at Community Health Care, a Federally Qualified Health Center in Tacoma that provides services to many of the underserved populations in Pierce County. As a family physician, he has a passion for LGBTQIA+ health and working with historically marginalized groups. He has two cats and a wonderful partner who also works in the healthcare field.

Chapter 5

Poverty as a Social Determinant of Health

Jessica Skelton, DO, Author
Cliff Moeckelmann, MD, Editor

"Overcoming poverty is not a gesture of charity. It is an act of justice. It is the protection of a fundamental human right, the right to dignity and a decent life. While poverty persists, there is no true freedom."
- Nelson Mandela

Poverty as a Social Determinant of Health

This chapter explores the detrimental impact of poverty on health and well-being. It aims to undertake a sweeping examination of poverty, exposing the myriad ways income shapes overall health. It places particular emphasis on the correlation between poverty and life expectancy as well as quality of life. Furthermore, the essay conducts an exploration of the distinctive challenges faced by children in poverty, a demographic constituting the majority within impoverished populations. Within this context, it casts a spotlight on the heightened risks for chronic and infectious diseases associated with impoverishment. The overarching conclusion suggests potential solutions to mitigate poverty's escalated health risks, thereby contributing to a more nuanced and comprehensive understanding of the intricate interplay between poverty and health.

Poverty as a Social Determinant of Health

In the context of Life Expectancy

An analysis of 1.4 billion U.S. tax records revealed a substantial and thought-provoking disparity: men who fall within the highest one percent of income earners exhibit an average lifespan that is notably extended by 14 years when compared to their counterparts residing in the lowest one percent income bracket. A parallel observation revealed a discernible discrepancy of 10 years greater life expectancy for women in upper income levels (Chetty et al., 2016). **Figure 1.**

Figure 1. Disparities in life expectancy associated with varying income levels

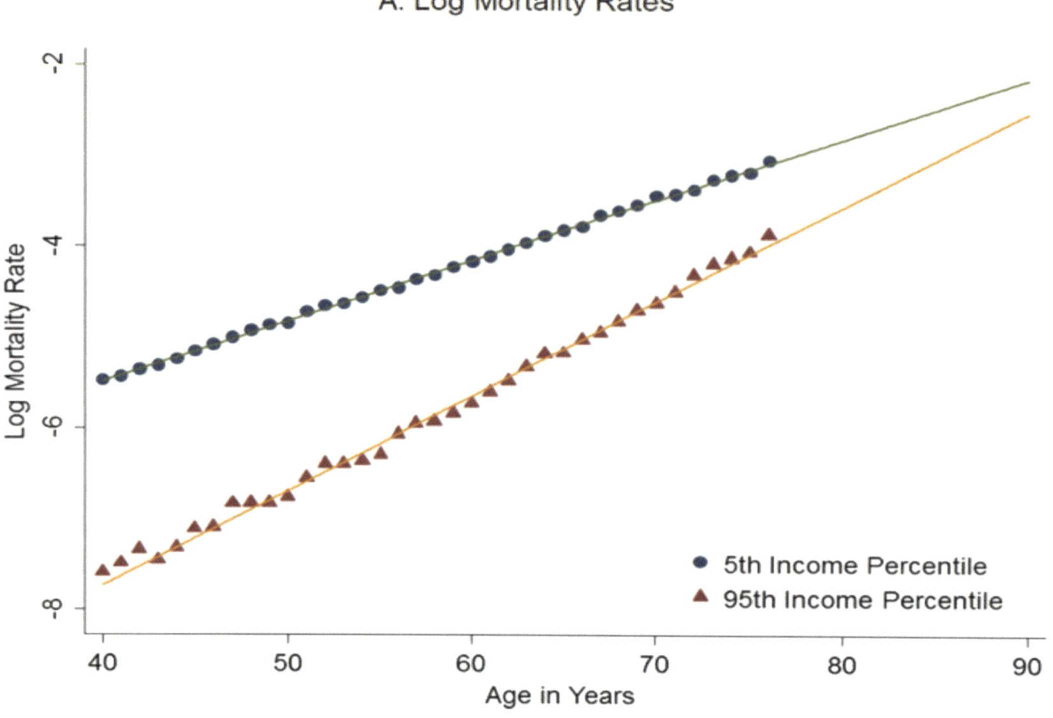

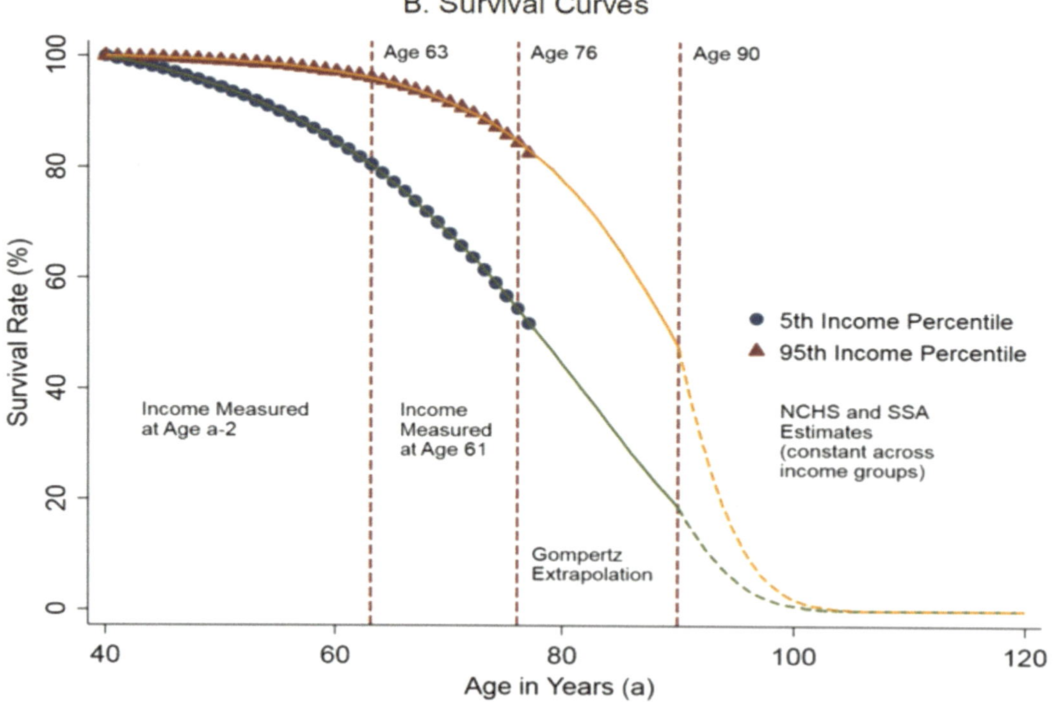

Chetty, R., Stepner, M., Abraham, S., Lin, S., Scuderi, B., Turner, N., Bergeron, A. and Cutler, D. (2016). The Association between Income and Life Expectancy in the United States, 2001-2014. *JAMA*, [online] Available at https://doi.org/10.1001/jama.2016.4226

The significance of this discovery lies in the intriguing revelation that life expectancy is intricately linked to financial status, a notion that takes on added weight in the context of a developed nation with abundant resources and opportunities.

This pattern persists not only at the individual level but also extends to national metrics. According to the Organization for Economic Co-operation and Development (OECD, 2017), there exists a direct correlation between country GDP and life expectancy at birth, with higher GDP levels associated with longer life expectancies. **Figure 2.**

Figure 2. Life Expectancy at birth and country GDP per capita, 2015

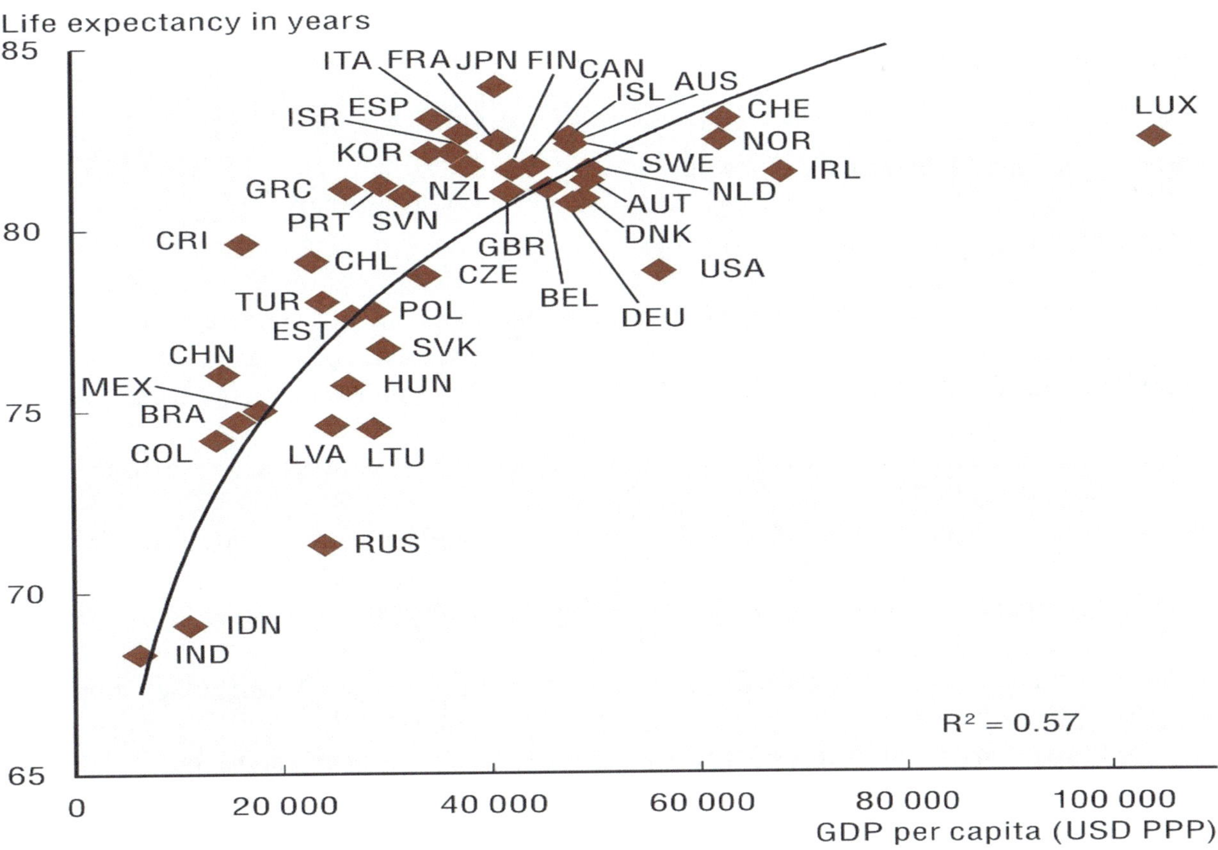

Source: OECD Health Statistics 2017.

OECD (2017a). *Health at a Glance 2017: OECD Indicators.* [online] *OECD iLibrary*. Paris: Organisation for Economic Co-operation and Development. Available at: https://www.oecd-ilibrary.org/docserver/health_glance-2017-en.pdf [Accessed 27 Nov. 2023].

Distribution of income within countries influences this relationship. For instance, in countries like the United States, life expectancy is lower than anticipated partially due to unequal distribution of GDP. In contrast, Spain exhibits the opposite trend, boasting a higher life expectancy than expected for its GDP, due to more equitable allocation of income among its population. These findings underscore the significance of economic equality within a population, emphasizing its crucial role in shaping life expectancy outcomes (OECD, 2017b). According to Woolf, et al., (2013) the so-called U.S. health disadvantage can be explained in part due to income inequality, "although the income of Americans is higher on average than in other countries, the United States also has higher levels of poverty (especially child poverty) and income inequality and lower rates of social mobility."

Poverty as a Social Determinant of Health

In the context of Quality of Life

A detrimental interconnection exists between illness and poverty, forming a vicious cycle. Diminished health results in missed days of work, translating to a reduction in income, thereby exacerbating the challenges of poverty. This deeper descent into impoverished circumstances, in turn, contributes to more unfavorable health outcomes. A comprehensive study involving over 1,500 cancer patients in New York brought to light a noteworthy imbalance: those without employment reported lower functional well-being at a rate 1.4 times higher than their employed or retired counterparts (Lui et al., 2022). The repercussions of poverty extend beyond influencing health outcomes and lifespan, as they are intricately correlated with a diminished quality of life (QOL).

Individuals in the lowest income bracket in the United States experience the lowest quality of life. The U.S. Department of Health and Human Services' Healthy People Initiative, conducted every decade since 1980, examines diverse factors influencing quality of life with the aim of enhancing the well-being of Americans. Residents of impoverished communities have reduced access to resources that are needed to support healthy QOL, such as stable housing, healthy foods, and safe neighborhoods. Poverty limits access to educational and employment opportunities, which further contributes to income inequality and perpetuates the cyclical effects of low income (Healthy People 2030, 2020).

Healthy People 2030: Poverty

Across the lifespan, residents of impoverished communities are at increased risk for mental illness, chronic disease, higher mortality, and lower life expectancy. Children make up the largest age group of those experiencing poverty. Childhood poverty is associated with developmental delays, toxic stress, chronic illness, and nutritional deficits. Individuals who experience childhood poverty are more likely to experience poverty into adulthood, which contributes to generational cycles of poverty.

In addition to the lasting effects of childhood poverty, adults living in poverty are at a higher risk of adverse health effects from obesity, smoking, substance use, and chronic stress. Finally, older adults with lower incomes experience higher rates of disability and mortality. One study found that men and women in the top 1 percent of income were expected to live 14.6 and 10.1 years longer respectively than men and women in the bottom 1 percent.

Unmet social needs, environmental factors, and barriers to accessing health care contribute to worse health outcomes for people with lower incomes. For example, people with limited finances have more difficulty obtaining health insurance and paying for expensive procedures and medications. Neighborhood factors, such as limited access to healthy foods and higher instances of violence, affect health by influencing health behaviors and stress.

Healthy People 2030 (2020). *Poverty - Healthy People 2030.* [online] health.gov. Available at: https://health.gov/healthypeople/priority-areas/social-determinants-health/literature-summaries/poverty

Assessing 26 different metrics, including medical insurance, air quality, and infant deaths, the Healthy People Initiative establishes target goals for improvement in heath. Researchers found a significant statistical difference between income classes, with individuals in the lowest incomes being half as likely to achieve the target goals when compared to those in the highest income brackets (Healthy People 2030, 2020).

Poverty as a Social Determinant of Health

In the context of Disease Prevalence and Health Behaviors

Nunes, et al., (2022) studied the prevalence of *anxiety disorder* in a cohort of over 2,500 adults utilizing the General Anxiety Disorder-7 Questionnaire (GAD-7). The GAD-7 is a validated screening tool used to measure and follow-up patients diagnosed with generalized anxiety disorder in primary care settings. Higher GAD-7 scores were associated with female sex, unemployment, low socioeconomic status (SES), annual income less than $25,000, and less than or equal to 12 years of education. The authors concluded that "clinicians and provider organizations need to consider both the physical manifestations of the disorder and their patients' *social determinants of health* when considering treatment pathways and designing interventions."

To understand what contributes to the disparities in *high infant mortality* rates between the United States and other developed countries, research conducted by Mohamoud, Kirby, and Ehrenthal (2021) revealed that infant mortality is associated with poverty. Investigators correlated birth/infant death files for 2012 - 2015 utilizing U.S. poverty estimates and county urban-rural classifications. Term infant deaths were classified as sudden unexpected death in infancy (SUDI) aka sudden infant death syndrome, congenital malformations, perinatal conditions, and all other causes. "The relative risk of term infant deaths because of SUDI was 1.6 (95% CI, 1.5-1.8) times higher in medium-poverty counties and 2.3 (95% CI, 1.2-2.5) times higher in high-poverty counties than in low-poverty counties."

According to Finer and Zolna (2016), *unintended pregnancies* in the United States most commonly affect impoverished women and girls, especially those cohabiting, while teenagers living 100% below the poverty line experience the highest prevalence of unintended pregnancies. In Canada, research conducted by the Canadian government disclosed that 68% of families led by teenage mothers depended on social assistance as their primary income source (Hovdestad, et al., 2015). In aggregate, these data suggest that women of little or low income are 1) particularly vulnerable to unintended pregnancies, 2) subjected to the consequences of high infant mortality and 3) mired in circumstances perpetuating vulnerability to ongoing cycles of poverty for them and their children.

"*Childhood neglect* accounts for over three-quarters of confirmed cases of child maltreatment in the United States—far more than physical or sexual abuse—but it continues to receive less attention from practitioners, researchers, and the media," according to the U.S. Department of Health and Human Services (2012). Risk factors for childhood neglect include poverty, lack of social support, single parent households, domestic violence, unemployment or low socioeconomic status, young maternal age, mental illness, and substance abuse. Young children are particularly in harm's way.

The consequences of neglect include alterations in:

- Health and physical development
- Intellectual and cognitive development
- Emotional and psychological development and
- Social and behavioral development (Department of Health and Human Services, 2012).

Not surprisingly, poverty and adverse childhood experiences correlate hand in hand (Centers for Disease Control and Prevention, 2020a). In contemporary nomenclature, recognizing adverse childhood experiences or ACEs assist health professionals in tackling the consequences of childhood neglect. For example, research reveals that adults with ACEs scores of four or more compared to adults with ACEs scores of zero are approximately twice as likely to confront premature death and have a twofold increased risk of developing *cardiovascular disease* (Godoy, et al., 2020).

Among other harmful behaviors, *smoking* enhances the risks for cardiovascular disease. The prevalence of tobacco use among impoverished populations is substantial and accounts in part for the increased incidence of *cardiovascular disease* among people in poverty. Garrett, et al., (2019) researched tobacco use and poverty. Prevalence overall was 41.1% among men with incomes below the federal poverty level and 23.7% among men with incomes at or above the poverty level. Prevalence was 32.5% among women with incomes below the federal poverty level and 18.3% among those with incomes at or above the poverty level.

Tobacco companies have historically been cognizant of the socioeconomic status of their customer base. In 1994, the Merit cigarette brand distributed 7,000 advertising blankets to a New York homeless shelter. Tobacco companies extended their efforts to distribute samples of their cigarettes, with Lorillard tobacco company providing 100 sample packs each to mental health associations, soup kitchens, and homeless shelters one month in 1990 (Apollonio & Malone, 2005). Similar contributions were consistently recorded over a decade, spanning from 1983 to 1993. Although nefarious marketing practices have been curtailed over the last several years, tobacco companies continue consumer directed advertising schemes in convenience stores and similar commercial outlets.

Elevated smoking rates rank as a significant factor in the decline of quality of life amongst impoverished populations. According to the CDC, "For every person who dies because of smoking, at least 30 people live with a serious smoking-related illness." Smoking is associated with an increased risk of conditions such as lung cancer, chronic obstructive pulmonary disease (COPD), cardiovascular disease, and stroke (Centers for Disease Control and Prevention, 2020b).

Research reveals that no threshold of smoking avoids the associated risks. A robust systematic review and meta-analysis of 141 cohort studies examining the relative risk of cardiovascular disease concluded that even smoking a single cigarette per day carried significant increase in cardiovascular disease. "Smoking only about one cigarette per day carries a risk of developing coronary heart disease and stroke much greater than expected: around half that for people who smoke 20 per day. No safe level of smoking exists for cardiovascular disease. Smokers should aim to quit instead of cutting down to significantly reduce their risk of these two common major disorders," Hackshaw, et al., (2018).

The intensified susceptibility of individuals in poverty to chronic diseases goes beyond smoking. Utilizing Behavioral Risk Factor Surveillance System to study chronic disease disparities by economic status and metropolitan classification found that the prevalence of *hypertension*, *arthritis*, and *poor health* in the poorest counties was 9%, 13%, and 15% higher, respectively, than in the most affluent counties (Shaw et al., 2016).

Obesity disproportionally affects low-income individuals. According to (Bentley, Ormerod and Ruck, 2018), a 2015 study revealed that in states where the median income was less than $45,000, 35% of the population were obese, compared to states where the median income exceeded $65,000, less than 25% of population were obese. The proportion of obese individuals in industrialized nations correlates inversely with median household income and has been described as the "poverty-obesity paradox" according to Hruschka and Han (2017). In the simplest view, obesity in developed economies is a result of over-abundance of inexpensive food calories combined with decreases in daily physical activity in the industrialized world and its built environment (Mattson et al., 2014).

This observation is likely linked to limited *access to nutritious food* and reduced opportunities for physical activity. Approximately 6.1 percent of the U.S. population resides in a food desert where the nearest supermarket is 1 to 10 miles away making access to affordable, nutritious foods challenging (Rhone, A. 2022). The correlation between poverty and *decreased minutes of weekly exercise* is well-documented. For example, a Colorado survey investigating factors influencing reduced exercise in children found that common responses from parents included a lack of affordable exercise options and concerns about the safety of the environment for physical activity (Finkelstein, Peterson, and Schottenfeld, 2017).

The repercussions of impoverished living extend well beyond those already discussed – increased prevalence of chronic disease, anxiety, infant mortality, unintended pregnancies, childhood neglect, cardiovascular disease, tobacco use, obesity, reductions in exercise, and access to nutritious foods. They encompass as well significant concerns for *personal safety, access to quality education, and infectious diseases*. Individuals residing in poverty were more than twice as likely to become victims of violent crime compared to those with higher incomes (Harrell et al., 2014). *Intimate partner violence* is most frequently experienced by those of low SES (Rosenberg, Benson, and Blasdell, 2023). Furthermore, quality education in low-income areas falls short of that in high-income areas. Those in the top 10% of income levels outperform the bottom 10% by 1 standard deviation on standardized testing (Hanushek, et al., 2022). The reasons for this educational disparity are multifactorial, with school funding from property taxes undeniably playing a role. For example, higher-income neighborhoods, characterized by more expensive houses, lead to increased funding through property taxation in their respective school districts.

Figure 3. Tuberculosis incidence compared to individuals living on $2 daily

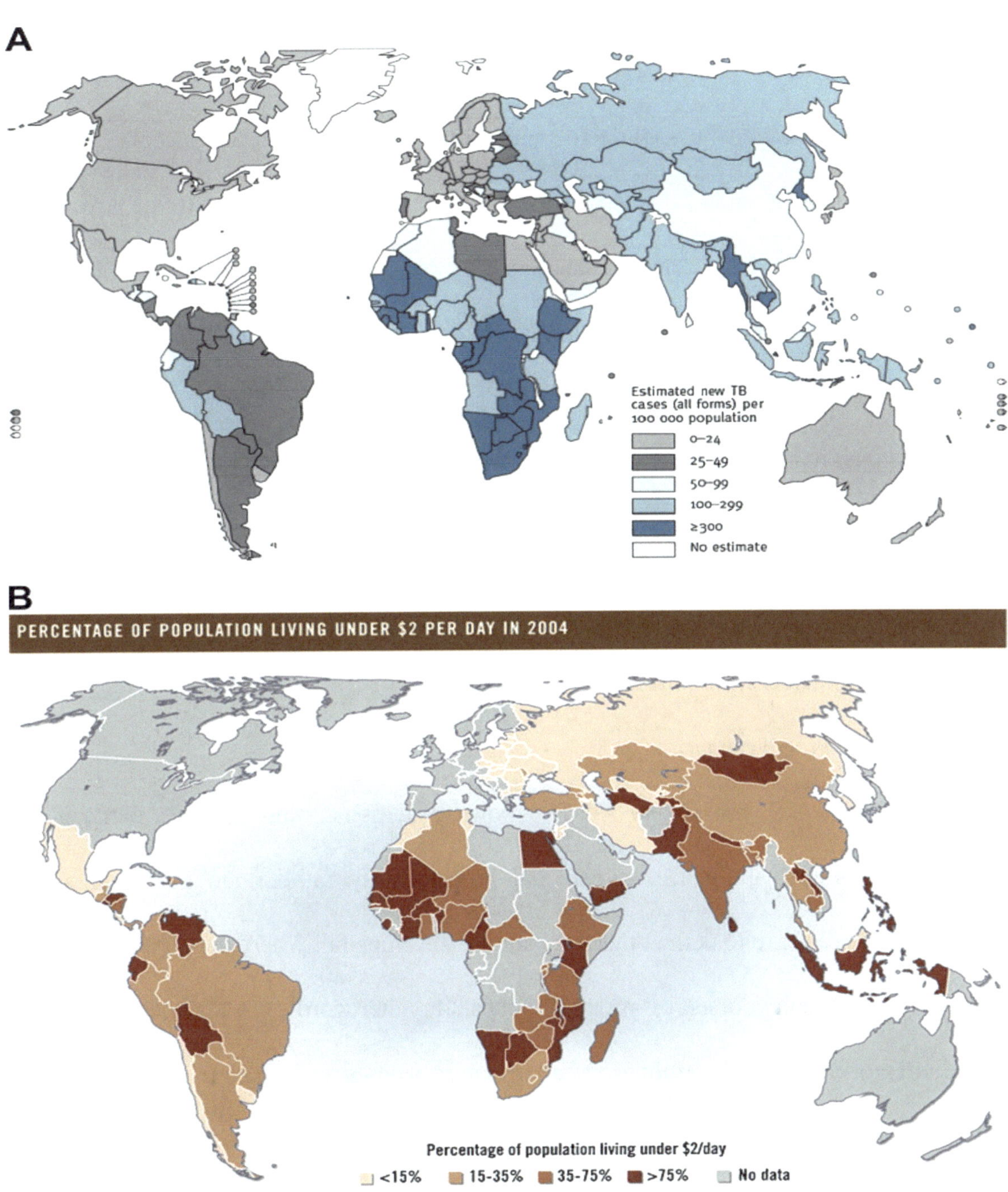

Alsan, M., Westerhaus, M., Herce, M., Nakashima, K. and Farmer, P.E. (2011). Poverty, Global Health, and Infectious Disease: Lessons from Haiti and Rwanda. Infectious Disease Clinics of North America [online] Available at: https://doi.org/10.1016/j.idc.2011.05.004

Figure 3 juxtaposes income and rates of tuberculosis worldwide and illustrates the impact of poverty on the incidence of tuberculosis. The World Bank defines extreme poverty as living on less than $2.15 per day. Tuberculosis (TB) is a bacterial infection spread by the inhalation of respiratory droplets emitted by an infected individual through coughing, sneezing, screaming, yelling, and singing. Untreated TB often results in death. Persons living in extreme poverty and in crowded conditions with limitations on sleeping quarters, water, sanitation, and access to health care are highly vulnerable to the acquisition of this life-threatening respiratory disease as demonstrated (Alsan et al., 2011)

The United States witnessed analogous trends during the COVID-19 pandemic, as counties with the lowest median income displayed higher rates of incidence and subsequent fatalities from corona virus infection (Jung et al., 2021).

Poverty as a Social Determinant of Health

Politics, policies, and governance

Historically, U.S. lawmakers sidestep poverty demonstrating distaste to meaningfully address it and viewing indigence as personal responsibility rather than the assignment of government – it's easier to look the other way and let the chips fall where they may. Conservative rhetoric proclaims, "pull yourself by your bootstraps." In other words, get a grip, improve your lot through hard work and self-determination rather than relying on assistance from others.

This essay, and the many others throughout this treatise, spell out an ugly truth. When it comes to health and well-being for most individuals in the United States the chips are falling.

According to the Organization for Economic Co-Operation and Development (OECD 2015) "The gap between rich and poor keeps widening. Growth, if any, has disproportionally benefited higher income groups while lower income households have been left behind. This longrun increase in income inequality not only raises social and political concerns, but also economic ones. It tends to drag down GDP growth, due to the rising distance of the lower 40% from the rest of society. Lower income people have been prevented from realising their human capital potential, which is bad for the economy as a whole."

Countries characterized by *lower levels of income inequality* consistently achieve higher well-being scores, according to OECD (2022). On the other hand, in healthcare systems that fail to prioritize universal affordability, vulnerable populations with low socioeconomic status find themselves at increased susceptibility to adverse health outcomes (Zieff et al., 2020). According to the U.S. Census Bureau, the percentage of Americans with health insurance coverage for all or part of the year in 2020 was 91.4% leaving 28 million individuals without insurance coverage (Bureau, U.C., 2021).

Figure 4. Income Inequality by Country

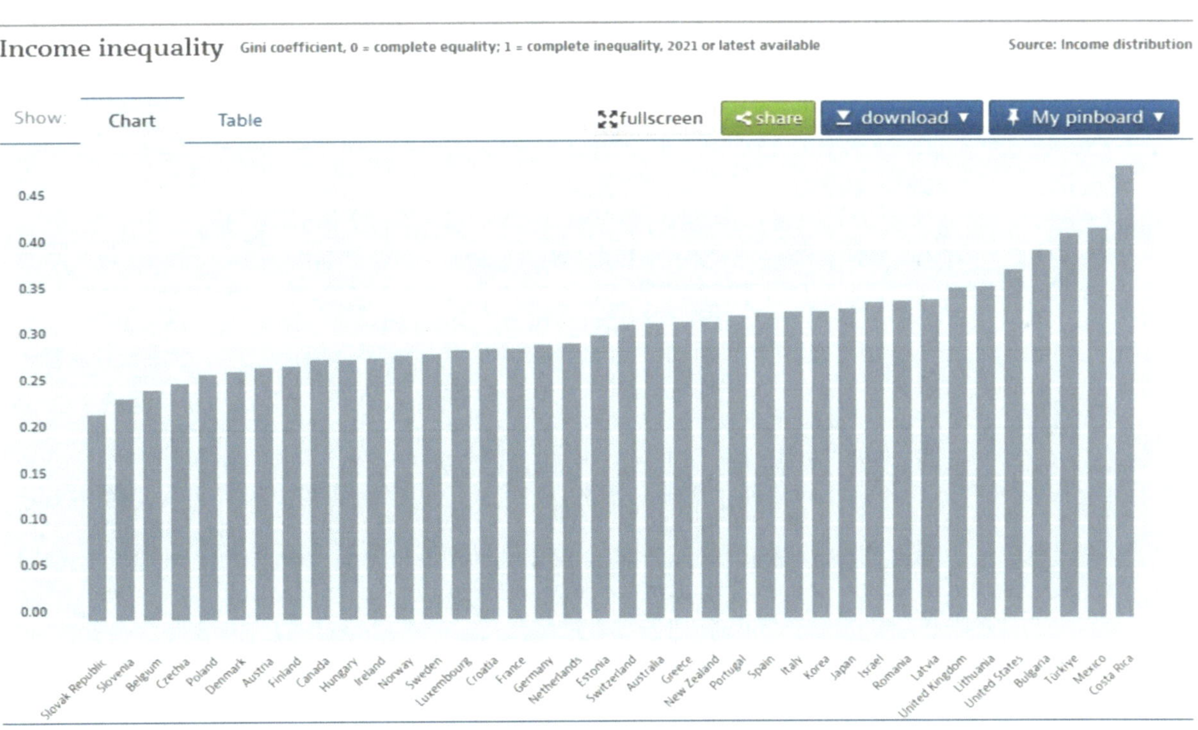

OECD (2022). *Inequality - Income inequality - OECD Data.* [online] OECD. Available at: https://data.oecd.org/inequality/income-inequality.htm#indicator-chart

Figure 4 illustrates the variation of income inequality among Organization for Economic Co-operation and Development (OECD) countries. Notably, Finland exhibits low-income inequality, while the United States displays high-income inequality. In international happiness surveys, Finland ranks first in happiness, now six years running, based on income equality, high social support, healthy life expectancy, freedom to make life choices, generosity, and low levels of corruption (Dorling, 2023). Out of 153 countries analyzed, Denmark, Switzerland, Iceland, Norway, Netherlands, Sweden, New Zealand, Austria, and Luxembourg round out the top ten – Canada 11th, the United States 18th, Hungary 53rd, Japan 62nd, Russia 73rd and Afghanistan 153rd (Helliwell, et al., 2020). In 2021, life expectancy in Finland rose to 81.2 years; in the United States it fell to 76.4 years (OECD, 2017b).

What Makes Finland the Happiest Country in the World? - Opinion

Finland has been a long-time outlier in the fight against inequality. At a time when the gap between the rich and the poor is widening in most countries around the world, Finland has consistently worked to ensure that its poorest citizens are looked after. The fight against inequality is one that many countries continually struggle with, but Finland is one that has made a point to stay the course and keep it atop the priority list.

There is a Finnish philosophy that is said to underpin everything that it means to be Finnish - 'sisu'. While it's nearly impossible to translate 'sisu' into English, the closest translation would be something similar to 'strength of will' or 'stoic perseverance'. Finland embodies this principle in countless ways, such as with its successful approach to ending homelessness. The country's novel 'housing first' principle ensures that, after being given the right support, rough sleepers can own a home of their own, a non-traditional approach to a traditional problem.

The happiness of the Finnish people stems not only from its substantial number of welfare policies, its intrinsic affinity for mutual trust and equality but also from freedom. The mindset that one can only be free and independent if everyone is equally free and independent drives the country's policymaking and underpins what it means to be Finnish.

For many, it's about living in a country where all conceivable basic needs are met, whether that's healthcare, education, or having a job that makes you feel fulfilled. The overarching theme is that Finland remains ahead of the curve in so many facets of life. For now, Finland is ranking top, but the hope is that the example Finland is setting helps other countries to better care for their people. The fact that the country continues to pioneer social and economic welfare, education and working best-practice is something of which other countries should take note when looking at improving the happiness and well-being of their people.

Väänänen, H. (2020). *What Makes Finland the Happiest Country in The World?* [online] Forbes. Available at: https://www.forbes.com/sites/heikkivaananen/2020/05/26/what-makes-finland-the-happiest-country-in-the-world/?sh=3ba7c23875cc [Accessed 21 Dec. 2023].

The data, illustrations, descriptions and opinions presented in this essay and others throughout this book, provide evidence for a health and well-being crisis in the United States. As life expectancy, health outcomes, well-being and happiness in the U.S. tumble behind other high-income countries, we wonder why. Nordic countries provide ample evidence that programs and attitudes that endorse social support promote population health and well-being. According to Healthy People 2030 (2020), various safety net strategies like Earned Income Tax Credit, Child Tax Credit, Medicaid, and Supplemental Nutrition Assistance Program serve to ameliorate poverty in the U.S. But for the country boasting the world's highest GDP, it is clearly too little too late. Social progressives might conclude, "You can't pull yourself up by your bootstraps if you are unable to afford them."

Questions for Further Consideration:

1. Universal Healthcare provides a potential solution to close the gaps in health outcomes between high- and low-income individuals. Name barriers to initiating this in the U.S.
2. If it were adopted in the United States, should individuals migrated illegally have access to Universal Healthcare?
3. What would be the consequences of a long-term commitment to provide everyone enough money to meet their basic needs?
4. How do systemic factors contribute to the cycle of poverty and poor health outcomes, and what strategies can break this cycle?

Sentinel Readings for a Deeper Dive

Universal Basic Income: Short-Term Results from a Long-Term Experiment in Kenya *. [online] Available at: https://basicincome.org/wp-content/uploads/2023/12/Give-Directly-Kenya-report-2-years.pdf

Health-Related Quality of Life and Well-Being. CDC [online] Available at: https://www.cdc.gov/nchs/data/hpdata2020/HP2020MCR-C18-HRQOL-WB.pdf

Billions left behind on the path to universal health coverage. WHO [online] Available at: https://www.who.int/news/item/18-09-2023-billions-left-behind-on-the-path-to-universal-health-coverage#:~:text=In%202021%2C%20about%204.5%20billion,of%20the%20COVID%2D19%20pandemic.

Tracking Universal Health Coverage 2023 global report. WHO [online] Available at: https://iris.who.int/bitstream/handle/10665/374059/9789240080379-eng.pdf?sequence=1

Universal Healthcare in the United States of America: A healthy debate. MDPI. [online] Available at: https://www.mdpi.com/1648-9144/56/11/580

References

Alsan, M., Westerhaus, M., Herce, M., Nakashima, K. and Farmer, P. (2011). Poverty, Global Health, and Infectious Disease: Lessons from Haiti and Rwanda. *Infectious Disease Clinics of North America* https://doi.org/10.1016/j.idc.2011.05.004 [Accessed 29 November 2023].

Apollonio, D. and Malone, R. (2005). Marketing to the marginalised: Tobacco Industry Targeting of the Homeless and Mentally Ill. *Tobacco Control*, [online] Available at: https://tobaccocontrol.bmj.com/content/14/6/409 [Accessed 20 Dec. 2023].

Banerjee, A., Faye, M., Krueger, A., Niehaus, P., Suri, T., Amuku, C., Asman, S., Chandra, S., Chilakapati, P., Fleischman, G., Jain, P., Kioko, E., Lezcano, T., Mwangi, B., Narayanan, A., Robertson, S., Mit, Princeton, G. and Mit (2023). *Universal Basic Income: Short-Term Results from a Long-Term Experiment in Kenya* *. [online] Available at: https://basicincome.org/wp-content/uploads/2023/12/Give-Directly-Kenya-report-2-years.pdf [Accessed 21 Dec. 2023].

Bentley, R., Ormerod, P. and Ruck, D. (2018). Recent Origin and Evolution of obesity-income Correlation across the United States. *Palgrave Communications* [online] https://www.nature.com/articles/s41599-018-0201-x [Accessed 28 November 2023].

Bureau, U.C. (2021). *Health Insurance Coverage in the United States: 2020.* [online] Census.gov. Available at: https://www.census.gov/library/publications/2021/demo/p60-274.html#:~:text=Highlights%201%20In%202020%2C%208.6%20percent%20of%20people%2C [Accessed 19 December 2023].

Centers for Disease Control and Prevention. (2020a). *Adverse childhood experiences (ACES).* [online] Available at: https://www.cdc.gov/violenceprevention/aces/riskprotectivefactors.html [Accessed 19 December 2023].

Centers for Disease Control and Prevention. (2020b). *Health Effects.* [online] Available at: https://www.cdc.gov/tobacco/basic_information/health_effects/index.htm [Accessed 28 November 2023].

Chetty, R., Stepner, M., Abraham, S., Lin, S., Scuderi, B., Turner, N., Bergeron, A. and Cutler, D. (2016). The Association between Income and Life Expectancy in the United States, 2001-2014. *JAMA*, [online] Available at: https://jamanetwork.com/journals/jama/article-abstract/2513561 [Accessed 27 December 2023].

Dorling, D. (2023). *Why Finland is the happiest country in the world – an expert explains.* [online] The Conversation. [online] Available at: https://theconversation.com/why-finland-is-the-happiest-country-in-the-world-an-expert-explains-203016 [Accessed 21 December 2023].

Finer, L. and Zolna, M. (2016). Declines in Unintended Pregnancy in the United States, 2008–2011. *New England Journal of Medicine*, [online] Available at: https://doi.org/10.1056/nejmsa1506575 [Accessed 28 November 2023].

Finkelstein, D., Petersen, D. and Schottenfeld, L. (2017). Promoting Children's Physical Activity in Low-Income Communities in Colorado: What Are the Barriers and Opportunities? *Preventing Chronic Disease*, [online] https://www.cdc.gov/pcd/issues/2017/17_0111.htm [Accessed 28 November 2023].

Garrett, B., Martell, B., Caraballo, R. and King, B. (2019). Socioeconomic Differences in Cigarette Smoking Among Sociodemographic Groups. *Preventing Chronic Disease* [online] Available at: https://www.cdc.gov/pcd/issues/2019/18_0553.htm [Accessed 22 December 2023].

Godoy, L., Frankfurter, C., Cooper, M., Lay, C., Maunder, R. and Farkouh, M. (2021). Association of Adverse Childhood Experiences with Cardiovascular Disease Later in Life: A Review. *JAMA Cardiology*, [online] Available at: https://doi.org/10.1001/jamacardio.2020.6050 [Accessed 27 November 2023].

Hackshaw, A., Morris, J., Boniface, S., Tang, J. and Milenković, D. (2018). Low Cigarette Consumption and Risk of Coronary Heart Disease and stroke: meta-analysis of 141 Cohort Studies in 55 Study Reports. *BMJ*, [online] Available at: https://www.bmj.com/content/360/bmj.j5855 [Accessed 28 November 2023].

Hanushek, E., Peterson, P., Talpey, L. and Woessmann, L. (2019). *The Achievement Gap Fails to Close: Half Century of Testing Shows Persistent Divide between Haves and have-nots - Education next*. Education Next. [online] Available at: https://www.educationnext.org/achievement-gap-fails-close-half-century-testing-shows-persistent-divide/ [Accessed 19 December 2023].

Harrell, E., Langton, L., Statisticians, M., Berzofsky, P., Couzens, L. and Smiley-Mcdonald, H. (2014). *Special Report Household Poverty and Nonfatal Violent Victimization, 2008-2012.* [online] Available at: https://bjs.ojp.gov/content/pub/pdf/hpnvv0812.pdf [Accessed 29 November 2023].

Healthy People 2030 (2020). *Poverty - Healthy People 2030.* [online] Available at: https://health.gov/healthypeople/priority-areas/social-determinants-health/literature-summaries/poverty [Accessed 27 November 2023].

Helliwell, J., Layard, R., Sachs, J., De, J.-E., Associate, N., Aknin, L., Huang, H. and Wang, S. (2020). *World Happiness Report 2020.* [online] Available at: https://happiness-report.s3.amazonaws.com/2020/WHR20.pdf [Accessed 21 December 2023].

Hovdestad, W., Shields, M., Williams, G. and Tonmyr, L. (2015). Vulnerability within families headed by teen and young adult mothers investigated by child welfare services in Canada. *Health Promotion and Chronic Disease Prevention in Canada* [online] Available at: https://doi.org/10.24095/hpcdp.35.8/9.06 [Accessed 28 November 2023].

Hruschka, D. and Han, S. (2017). Anti-fat discrimination in marriage more clearly explains the poverty–obesity paradox. *Behavioral and Brain Sciences* https://doi.org/10.1017/s0140525x1600145x [Accessed 28 November 2023].

Jung, J., Manley, J. and Shrestha, V. (2021). Coronavirus infections and deaths by poverty status: The effects of social distancing. *Journal of Economic Behavior & Organization* https://doi.org/10.1016/j.jebo.2020.12.019 [Accessed 29 November 2023].

Lui, F., Finik, J., Leng, J. and Gany, F. (2022). Social Determinants and Health-related Quality of Life in a Sample of diverse, Low Socioeconomic Status Cancer Patients. *Psycho-Oncology*, online [Available at]: https://onlinelibrary.wiley.com/doi/10.1002/pon.6006 [Accessed 27 November 2023].

Mattson, M., Allison, D., Fontana, L., Harvie, M., Longo, V., Malaisse, W., Mosley, M., Notterpek, L., Ravussin, E., Scheer, F., Seyfried, T., Varady, K.A. and Panda, S. (2014). Meal Frequency and Timing in Health and Disease. *Proceedings of the National Academy of Sciences*, [online] Available at: https://www.pnas.org/doi/full/10.1073/pnas.1413965111 [Accessed 28 November 2023].

Mohamoud, Y., Kirby, R. and Ehrenthal, D. (2021). County Poverty, Urban–Rural Classification, and the Causes of Term Infant Death. *Public Health Reports*, [online] Available at: https://doi.org/10.1177/0033354921999169 [Accessed 28 November 2023].

Nunes, J., Carroll, M., Mahaffey, K., Califf, R., Doraiswamy, P., Short, S., Shah, S., Swope, S., Williams, D., Hernandez, A. and Hong, D. (2022). General Anxiety Disorder-7 Questionnaire as a marker of low socioeconomic status and inequity. *Journal of Affective Disorders*, [online] Available at: doi: https://doi.org/10.1016/j.jad.2022.08.085 [Accessed 27 November 2023].

OECD (2015). *In It Together: Why Less Inequality Benefits All*. OECD {online] Available at: https://doi.org/10.1787/9789264235120-en [Accessed 29 November 2023].

OECD (2017a). *Health at a Glance 2017: OECD Indicators*. [online] *OECD iLibrary*. Paris: Organisation for Economic Co-operation and Development. [online] Available at: https://www.oecd-ilibrary.org/docserver/health_glance-2017-en.pdf [Accessed 18 Dec. 2023].

OECD (2017b). *Health status - Life expectancy at birth - OECD Data*. [online] the OECD. Available at: https://data.oecd.org/healthstat/life-expectancy-at-birth.htm [Accessed 30 November 2023].

OECD (2022). *Inequality - Income inequality - OECD Data*. [online] OECD. [online] Available at: https://data.oecd.org/inequality/income-inequality.htm#indicator-chart [Accessed 30 November 2023].

Rhone, A. (2022). *USDA ERS - Documentation*. [online] Available at: https://www.ers.usda.gov/data-products/food-access-research-atlas/documentation/ [Accessed 28 November 2023].

Rosenberg, O., Benson, B. and Blasdell, R. (2023). Socioeconomic Status/Poverty and Domestic Violence. *Springer eBooks* [online] Available at: https://doi.org/10.1007/978-3-030-85493-5_1574-1 [Accessed 19 December 2023].

Shaw, K., Theis, K., Self-Brown, S., Roblin, D. and Barker, L. (2016). Chronic Disease Disparities by County Economic Status and Metropolitan Classification, Behavioral Risk Factor Surveillance System, 2013. *Preventing Chronic Disease*, [online] Available at: https://www.cdc.gov/pcd/issues/2016/16_0088.htm [Accessed 28 November 2023].

U.S. Department of Health and Human Services (2012). *BULLETIN FOR PROFESSIONALS*. [online] Available at: https://www.1001kritiekedagen.nl/wp-content/uploads/2021/07/An-overview-of-child-neglect.pdf [Accessed 19 Dec. 2023].

Väänänen, H. (2020). *What Makes Finland the Happiest Country in The World?* [online] Forbes. Available at: https://www.forbes.com/sites/heikkivaananen/2020/05/26/what-makes-finland-the-happiest-country-in-the-world/?sh=3ba7c23875cc [Accessed 21 Dec. 2023].

Woolf, S., Braveman, P., Christiansen, K., Crimmins, E., Diez Roux, A., Jamison, D., Mackenbach, J., McQueen, D., Palloni, A., Preston, S. and Aron, L. (2013). *COMMITTEE ON POPULATION*. [online] *The National Academies*. Available at: https://nap.nationalacademies.org/resource/13497/dbasse_080620.pdf [Accessed 19 Dec. 2023].

Zieff, G., Kerr, Z., Moore, J. and Stoner, L. (2020). Universal healthcare in the United States of America: A healthy debate. *Medicina*, [online] https://doi.org/10.3390/medicina56110580 {Accessed 30 November 2023].

Lexicon of Listed Terms and Agencies

- **ACEs:** A medical questionnaire used to screen for adverse childhood experiences.
- **CDC:** CDC is the nation's leading science-based, data-driven, service organization that protects the public's health.
- **Functional well-being (FWB):** Ability for individual to conduct tasks of daily living including social roles.
- **GAD-7:** A validated medical questionnaire used to screen for generalized anxiety disorder.
- **GDP:** Gross domestic product or the total value of the economies products and services.
- **OECD:** The Organisation for Economic Co-operation and Development (OECD) is an international organisation that works to build better policies for better lives. Our goal is to shape policies that foster prosperity, equality, opportunity and well-being for all.
- **Socioeconomic status (SES):** The collective resources that an individual has. It is often measured as a combination of education, occupation, and income.

AUTHOR'S BIO SKETCH

Jessica Skelton, DO

Dr. Skelton is a comprehensive family medicine physician driven by a profound commitment to enhance the well-being of underserved communities. Having personally faced the challenges of poverty as a young single parent to a disabled child, she brings a unique perspective to her medical practice. Dr. Skelton earned her bachelor's degree in biology with a minor in chemistry from Washington State University and completed her medical education at A.T. Still University in Missouri. She remains dedicated to serving the community by continuing her work at the Community Health Care residency program in Tacoma, Washington. Outside of her medical endeavors, she finds joy in engaging with her four children through games, experimenting with new culinary creations, and expressing her creativity through art and crafts.

Chapter 6

Food Security as a Social Determinant of Health

Kathryn Annand, MD, Author
James Lenhart, MD, FAAFP, MPH, Editor

"Everyone has the right to a standard of living adequate for the health and well-being of himself and of his family, including food, clothing, housing and medical care and necessary social services, and the right to security in the event of unemployment, sickness, disability, widowhood, old age or other lack of livelihood in circumstances beyond his control."

- The Universal Declaration of Human Rights, Article 25 1. The United Nations,1948

Food Security as a Social Determinant of Health

Marmot and Wilkinson (2003) echoed the sentiment of the Universal Declaration of Human rights when they stated, "a good diet and adequate food supply are central for promoting health and wellbeing." Despite widespread acknowledgement that access to nutritious food is fundamental for good health, the Food and Agriculture Organization of the United Nations (FAO) estimates that healthy diets are unaffordable for almost 3.1 billion people around the world (FAO, 2022). In 2020 the United States Department of Agriculture (USDA) found that 10.5% of the U.S. population did not have enough money to purchase an adequate amount of food for all members of their family at some point in the year (USDA, 2022a). A 2017 study estimated that within the United States, 54.4 million individuals or 17.7% of the population had limited access to a supermarket or grocery store, thus restricting their ability to buy and consume affordable, nutritious food (Rhone et al., 2017).

These data illustrate the harsh reality of food insecurity in the United States and throughout the world. Many factors contribute to individual ability or inability to access nutritious foods. This chapter highlights the interplay between geographic and socioeconomic inequalities and how politics, policies and governance aim to improve access to food in the United States.

Food Security as a Social Determinant of Health

In the context of Food Security

The USDA measures food security in the United States through the Current Population Survey Food Security supplement (CPS-FSS).

The USDA food security survey is an annual supplement to the CPS-FSS, a nationally representative survey conducted by the Census Bureau, which measures the extent and severity of food insecurity in U.S. households. The survey uses a three-stage design with screeners and different modules for households with and without children. The survey also collects data on food spending, use of federal and community food assistance programs, and food defense measures. The survey results are analyzed by USDA's Economic Research Service and are used to inform USDA's food and nutrition assistance programs. Food security is measured at the household level in three categories: food secure, low food security and very low food security. Each category is measured by a total count and as a percentage of the total population. Categories and measurements are broken down further based on the following demographic characteristics: household composition, race/ethnicity, metro/nonmetro area of residence, and geographic region.

The food security scale includes questions about households and their ability to purchase enough food and balanced meals, questions about adult meals and their size, frequency skipped, weight lost, days gone without eating, questions about children's meals, including diversity, balanced meals, size of meals, skipped meals and hunger. Questions are also asked about the use of public aid and supplemental food assistance.

The food security scale is eighteen items that measure insecurity. A score of 0-2 means a house is food secure, from 3-7 shows low food security, and 8-18 means very low food security. The scale and the data also report the frequency with which each item is experienced.

US Department of Agriculture, Economic Research Service (2016). Food Security in the United States [online] Available at: https://data.nal.usda.gov/dataset/food-security-united-states-0

The USDA defines food *security* as "access by all people [in a household] at all times to have enough food for an active, healthy life" and food *insecurity* as "a household-level economic and social condition of limited or uncertain access to adequate food" as assessed by their annual CPS-FSS (USDA, 2022b). According to the USDA, the defining characteristics of very low food security is that – at times during the year – food intake of household members is reduced, and normal eating patterns disrupted because the household lacks money and other recourses for food (USDA, 2022a).

In 2020 approximately 89.5% of U.S households were classified as food secure for the entire duration of the year. The remaining 10.5% of the population – about 13.8 million households – were food insecure at some time throughout the year **Figure 1** (Coleman-Jenson, 2021).

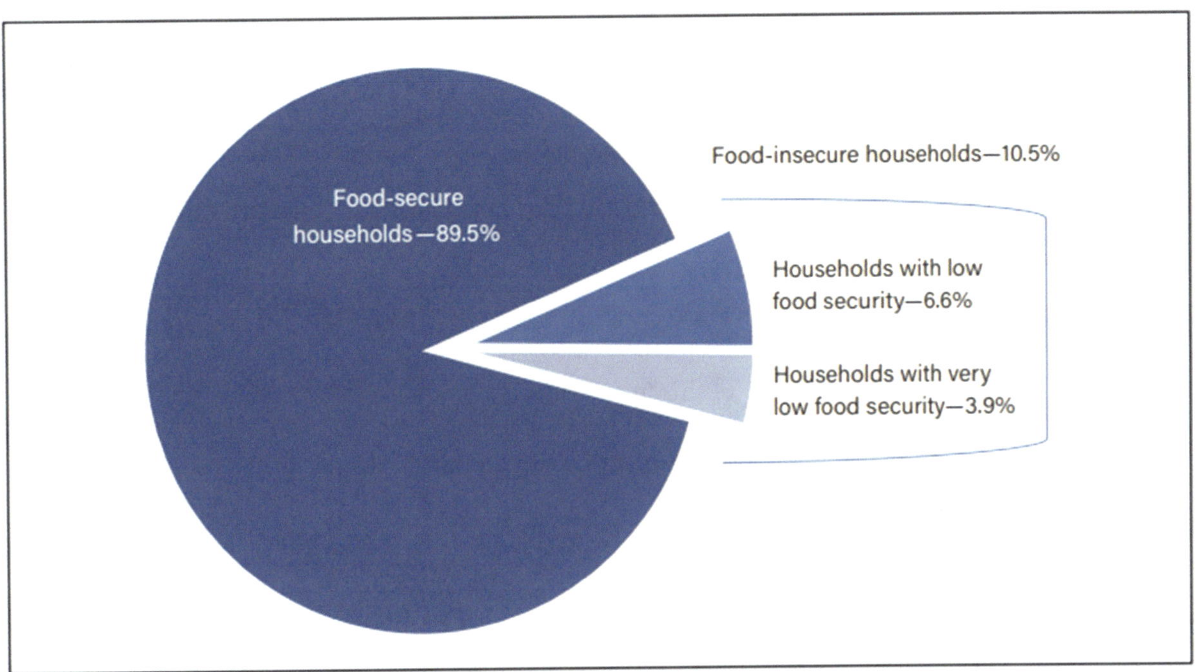

Figure 1: U.S. Households by food security status, 2020.
Coleman-Jensen, A., Gregory, C. and Singh, A. (2021). Household Food Security in the United States in 2020. *SSRN Electronic Journal*, [online] Available at: https://www.ers.usda.gov/webdocs/publications/102076/err-298.pdf

According to Coleman-Jensen, food insecurity impacts both dietary quantity and dietary quality with food insecure households, spending less on food, buying fewer calories overall and having lower quality food purchases than food secure households (Coleman-Jenson, 2021).

Lee et al. (2012) frame food insecurity in an alternative light, "the cycle of having enough food followed by a food shortage has been documented among food-insecure households and is thought to play a direct role in nutritional compromise, the accumulation of visceral fat, and weight gain." Beyond contributing to the development of chronic illness, food insecurity negatively affects the ability to manage chronic disease. For example, Lee et al. (2012) cites studies that show associations between food insecurity, poor diabetic management, difficulty following diabetic diets and decreased confidence in the ability to manage diabetic diets.

The CDC maintains that individuals without adequate access to nutritious food, either seek out energy-dense, nutrient poor (EDNP) foods or they go without any food (CDC, 2020). Both options have their associated negative consequences. Extended periods without food intake results in undernutrition or micronutrient related malnutrition (WHO, 2021). The World Health Organization (WHO) defines undernutrition as wasting (low weight for height), stunting (low height for age), underweight (low weight for age) and deficiencies in vitamins and minerals.

Children run particular risk for these conditions due to high metabolic demands. The WHO estimated in 2010 that 115 million children worldwide were underweight, fifty-five million children had low weight for height and 171 million children under the age of five years had stunted growth (WHO, 2014). Childhood malnutrition ranks as the underlying cause of death in approximately 35% of all deaths among children under the age of five with more than two million children dying each year because of undernutrition (WHO, 2014).

The US Department of Agriculture (USDA) calculates that the demand for food will rise 70 to 100 percent worldwide by 2050 (U.S. Department of Agriculture, 2009). The Centers for Disease Control (CDC) postulates that climate change will threaten food production and quality globally. According to the CDC, the collision of rising demand for food and climate alterations in food production portends increased food insecurity worldwide secondary to rising food prices, increased cost of raw materials, a shortage of key foods for populations living in isolated geographic regions, and changes in the nutritional profile of foods secondary to elevated atmospheric carbon dioxide (Centers for Disease Control and Prevention, 2019).

Food insecurity and the lack of access to affordable nutritious food are associated with increased risk for multiple chronic health conditions such as diabetes, obesity, heart disease, mental health disorders and other chronic diseases (NIMHH, 2023). Household food insecurity, defined as a form of economic struggle that includes the lack of access to enough food for an active and healthy life, is associated with negative physical and mental health outcomes in children and adults such as poor child development, increased hospitalizations, anemia, asthma, suicidal ideation, depression and anxiety, diabetes, and chronic disease (Chilton, 2017).

National Institute on Minority Health and Health Disparities (2023). Food Accessibility, Insecurity and Health Outcomes. [online] Available at: https://www.nimhd.nih.gov/resources/understanding-health-disparities/food-accessibility-insecurity-and-health-outcomes.html

Chilton, et al. (2017). The Intergenerational Circumstances of Household food Insecurity and Adversity. Journal of Hunger & Environmental Nutrition. [online] Available at: https://www.ncbi.nlm.nih.gov/pmc/articles/PMC5399810 [Accessed 22 July 2023].

Food Security as a Social Determinant of Health

In the context of Nutritional Value and Health

In 2022 the WHO estimated that non-communicable diseases (NCDs) kill forty-one million people each year, accounting for 74% of deaths globally. NCDs, also known as chronic diseases, include but are not limited to cardiovascular disease, chronic respiratory disease, and diabetes. These conditions often result from a combination of genetic, physiological, environmental, and behavioral factors. Diet works as a modifiable behavioral risk factor that contributes to NCDs. For example, adhering to nutritious foods not containing high volume added sugar or elevated levels of sodium reduces the incidence of NCDs (WHO, 2022).

The USDA publication *Dietary Guidelines for Americans (DGA)* supplies advice on what foods to eat and drink to meet nutrient needs, promote health and help prevent chronic disease. Revised and re-released every five years, the DGA advocates limitations on foods and beverages high in added sugars, saturated fat, and sodium as well as alcoholic beverages (DGA, 2020).

The *Dietary Guidelines for Americans* recommended limits include:

1. Added sugars – less than 10 percent of calories per day starting at age 2. Avoiding foods and beverages with added sugars for those younger than age 2.
2. Saturated fat – less than 10 percent of calories per day starting at age 2.
3. Sodium – less than 2,300 milligrams or less per day for children younger than age 14.

In addition to limiting sugars, sodium, and saturated fats, the DGA recommends incorporating fruits and vegetables into diets as these foods are nutrient-dense (high in nutrients, low in calories) and minimally processed. According to the DGA, adults should consume 1.5-2 cup-equivalents of fruits and 2-3 cup-equivalents of vegetables each day in addition to other nutrient-dense foods like whole grains, dairy products, and lean protein with the goal of 85% of calories each day coming from these nutrient rich foods (Dietary Guidelines for Americans, 2020).

Although the dietary patterns of citizens in the United States have improved, most Americans do not meet the dietary recommendations established by the USDA, according to Rehm et al. (2016). Utilizing 2019 Behavioral Risk Factor Surveillance System (BRFSS) data, Lee et al. (2022) studied the demographics of nutrient patterns in the US. Their research concluded that only 12.5% and 10.0% of adults met fruit and vegetable intake recommendations, respectively. Consuming the recommended intake of fruit was highest among Hispanic adults (16.4%) and lowest among males (10.1%). Consuming the recommended intake of vegetables was highest among adults over the age of 51 (12.5%) and lowest (6.8%) among adults with poverty level income (Lee et al. 2022).

Consumption of energy-dense, nutrient-poor foods harms the health of U.S. residents. To illustrate, the CDC estimates that Americans consume over 3400 mg of sodium daily, well over the recommended 2300 mg or less. Over 70% of this sodium comes from energy-dense, nutrient-poor packaged and processed foods (CDC, 2022). Sodium contributes to elevated blood pressure (hypertension) which increases the risk for heart attack and stroke.

Consumption of energy-dense, nutrient-poor foods leads to obesity, a problem within the United States and globally. The CDC estimates that obesity confronts 42% of US adults at health care costs of $173 billion dollars annually (CDC, 2022). The prevalence of obesity varies between groups with non-Hispanic Black adults the most affected with a rate of 49.9% and non-Hispanic Asian adults the least affected with a rate of 16.1% (CDC, 2021). In 2016 the World Medical Association (WMA) declared obesity as one of the single most important health issues facing the world in the twenty first century, affecting all countries, socio-economic groups and representing a serious drain on health care resources (WMA, 2019). Obesity affects children as well as adults; the CDC estimates that 20% of people ages 2 through 19 have obesity (CDC, 2021).

The National Institute of Diabetes and Digestive and Kidney Diseases asserts that obesity increases risks for Type 2 diabetes, high blood pressure, heart disease, stroke, sleep apnea, metabolic syndrome, fatty liver disease, osteoarthritis gall bladder disease, kidney damage, complications of pregnancy and depression (NIDDK, 2019).

National Institute of Diabetes and Digestive and Kidney Disease (2019). *Health Risks of Overweight & Obesity* [online] Available at: https://www.niddk.nih.gov/health-information/weight-management/adult-overweight-obesity/health-risks [Accessed 23 July 2023].

Food Security as a Social Determinant of Health

In the context of geographic and socioeconomic inequalities - International

On a global scale, the World Health Organization (WHO) estimates that 45% of deaths among children under the age of five are linked to some form of undernutrition. These deaths disproportionately affect children living in low- and middle-income countries (WHO, 2021). Even when malnutrition is not severe enough to lead to death, it fosters untoward impact on development. Low height for age in combination with nutrient deficiencies such as low iron and iodine levels prevent an estimated two hundred million children from reaching their full development potential (WHO, 2014).

National and international conflict significantly impacts food security. In 2018, the United Nations Security Council, in conjunction with the World Food Programme (WFP) acknowledged the link between hunger and war. “Food insecurity inevitably worsens when fighting drives large numbers of people from their homes, their land and their jobs” (WFP, 2018).

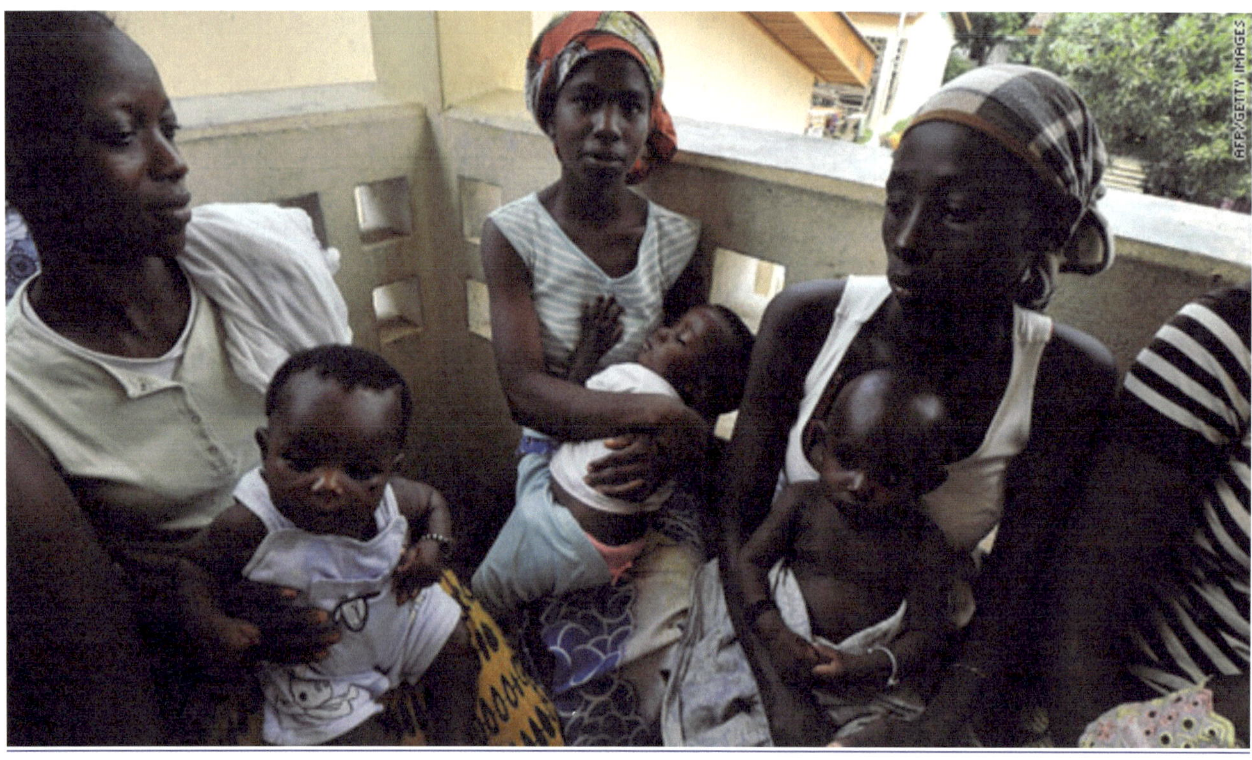

Families fleeing fighting and unrest in Abidjan rest at a shelter for internally displaced people, near Anyama on the south-eastern coast of Africa. War and famine ravaged the area in 2011. CNN News, 2011. [online] Available at: http://www.cnn.com/2011/WORLD/africa/03/26/ivory.coast.obama/index.html

Of the 800 million individuals chronically food insecure in the world, approximately 490 million (~61%) live in countries affected by war. Indeed, most children classified with stunted growth live in countries with major conflicts (Beasley, 2018). Husain (2017) showed that elevated levels of *undernourishment contribute to the occurrence and intensity of armed conflict* illustrating the complex interplay of food insecurity and war.

> ***How Russia's War on Ukraine Is Worsening Global Starvation***
>
> Moscow blocks most shipments from Ukraine, one of the world's largest wheat producers, and its attacks on the country's energy grid also disrupt the flow of food.
>
> An enduring global food crisis has become one of the farthest-reaching consequences of Russia's war, contributing to widespread starvation, poverty, and premature deaths.
>
> The United States and allies are struggling to reduce the damage. American officials are organizing efforts to help Ukrainian farmers get food out of their country through rail and road networks that connect to Eastern Europe and on barges traveling up the Danube River.
>
> But as deep winter sets in and Russia presses assaults on Ukraine's infrastructure, the crisis is worsening. Food shortages are already worsened by a drought in the Horn of Africa and unusually harsh weather in other parts of the world.
>
> The United Nations World Food Program estimates that more than 345 million people are suffering from or at risk of acute food insecurity, more than double the number from 2019.
>
> Wong, E. and Swanson, A., 2023. How Russia's War on Ukraine Is Worsening Global Starvation. *New York Times,* [online] Available at: https://www.nytimes.com/2023/01/02/us/politics/russia-ukraine-food-crisis.html [Accessed 26 July 2023].

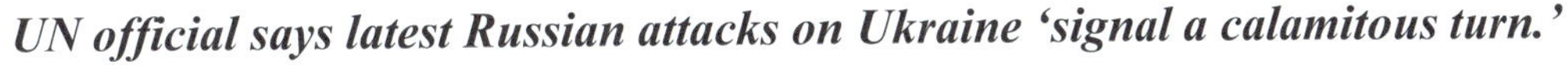

UN official says latest Russian attacks on Ukraine 'signal a calamitous turn.'

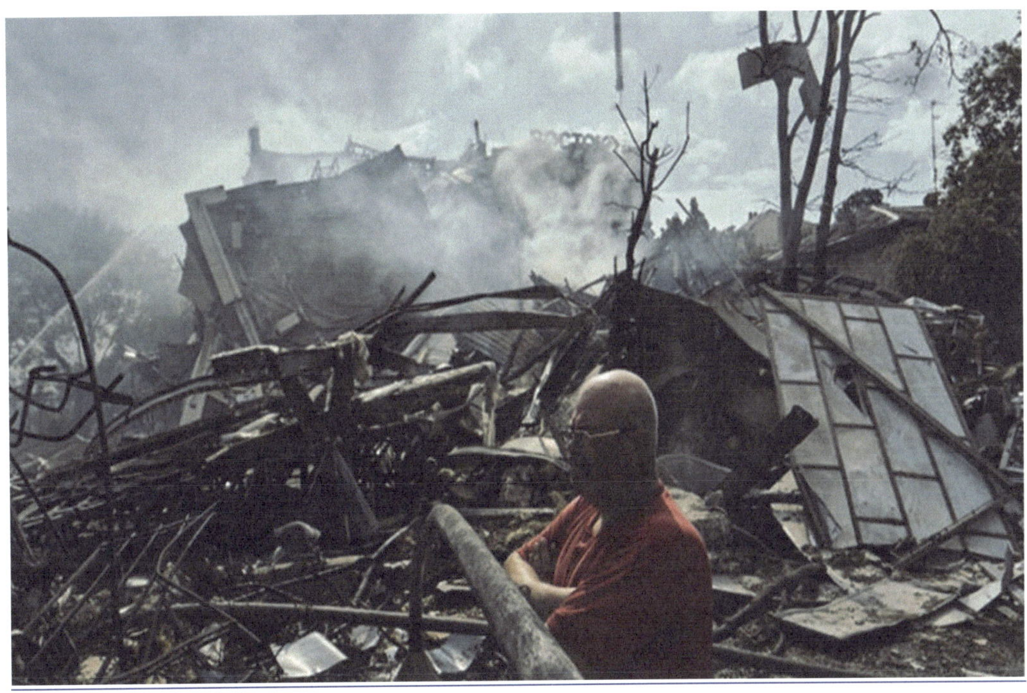

Looking over the devastation in Odessa, Ukraine *The Hill*, 26 July 2023. Available at: https://www.yahoo.com/news/un-official-says-latest-russian-233118394.html [Accessed 27 July 2023].

July 26, 2023
The Hill

UN official says latest Russian attacks on Ukraine 'signal a calamitous turn.'

A top United Nations official on Wednesday called recent attacks by Russia on the city of Odesa and other southern Ukrainian port areas "the latest casualties in this senseless, brutal war." Speaking to the U.N. Security Council in a briefing on Ukraine, Mohamed Khaled Khiari, an assistant secretary-general, called for such attacks to end "immediately" and suggested they "signal a calamitous turn" in the war.

"These attacks targeting Ukraine's grain export facilities, similarly to all attacks against civilians and civilian infrastructure, are unacceptable and must stop immediately," Khiari said in prepared remarks. "I must emphasize that attacks against civilians and civilian infrastructure may constitute a violation of international humanitarian law."

Khiari pointed to a Russian attack Sunday that damaged a historic cathedral in Odesa, which followed multiple nights of attacks targeting the city and other southern ports in Ukraine. "We have now seen disturbing reports of further Russian strikes against port infrastructure, including grain storage facilities, in Reni and Izmail ports on the Danube River – a key route for shipment of Ukrainian grain, not far from Ukraine's borders with Moldova and Romania," Khiari said.

"Deliberately targeting infrastructure that facilitates the export of food to the rest of the world could be life-threatening to millions of people who need access to affordable food," he added. Russia last week pulled out of a wartime deal negotiated by the United Nations. that allowed for Ukraine to export grain to countries in Asia, Africa and the Middle East, a move widely condemned by the West.

"In the wake of Russia's withdrawal from the Black Sea Initiative, these latest attacks signal a calamitous turn for Ukrainians and the world," Khiari said Wednesday.

Suter, T. (2023). UN official says latest Russian attacks on Ukraine 'signal a calamitous turn.' *The Hill* [online] Available at: https://www.yahoo.com/news/un-official-says-latest-russian-233118394.html

Food as a Social Determinant of Health

In the context of geographic and socioeconomic inequalities – U.S. National

Data from the U.S. Department of Agriculture, Economic Research Service (2021) exposes the strong association between food insecurity and income, race, household size, marital status, and geographic location. To wit in the United States rates of food insecurity in 2020 were statistically significantly higher than the national average (10.5%) for the following groups:

- All households with children (14.8%)
- Households with children under age 6 (15.3%)
- Households with children headed by a single woman (27.7%) or a single man (16.3%)
- Households with Black, non-Hispanic (21.7%) and Hispanic (17.2%) household reference persons
- Households with incomes below 185 percent of the poverty threshold (28.6%)
- Households within the principal cities of metropolitan areas (12.7%) and nonmetropolitan (rural) areas (11.6%) when compared with suburbs and other metropolitan areas outside principal cities lines
- Food insecurity is lowest in the Northeast (9.3%), below the national average in the Midwest (9.5%) and West (9.5%), *significantly higher* than the U.S. average in the South (12.3%) (Coleman-Jensen, et al, 2021).

Transportation barriers and increased physical distance to sources of nutritious food impede the ability to adhere to a nutritious diet. Low-Income, Low-Supermarket-Access tracts (LILA), sometimes referred to as food deserts, are "neighborhoods or regions in the United States that have limited access to stores that offer a wide variety of healthy food items" according to Rhone et al. (2017). Research shows that the number of LILA increased from 2010 to 2015, despite a higher number of total groceries stores in 2015 than 2010. Rhone et al. (2017) propose that this increase is due to a lack of access to a vehicle for families that are considered low-income.

Food Security as a Social Determinant of Health

In the context of politics, policies, and governance

The United State government strives to improve food security and nutrition in two primary ways: 1) subsidization of food costs at a household level and 2) increasing access to healthy foods.

Subsidization:

Subsidization of food costs has been provided to individuals through the U.S. Department of Agriculture (USDA) since 1939 when the first food stamp program was implemented. The Supplemental Nutrition Assistance Program (SNAP) supplied benefits to 35.7 million people living in eighteen million households in the U.S. in 2019. According to the USDA (2023), SNAP provides food benefits to low-income families to supplement their grocery budget so they can afford the nutritious foods essential to health and well-being. SNAP reduces poverty and food insecurity while stimulating economic growth (USDA, 2023).

Families with earned income may be eligible for SNAP benefits, but at a lower subsidy. Unfortunately, according to Golan, et al., (2008), households not receiving maximum SNAP benefits buy more nutrient poor, energy dense foods to meet perceived nutritional needs.

Another form of food subsidization in the United States comes through the Special Supplemental Nutrition Program for Women, Infants and Children (WIC), which supplies supplemental foods and nutrition education for low-income, pregnant, breastfeeding, and non-breastfeeding mothers, infants, and children up to age 5 who meet criteria for nutritional risk. WIC launched in 1974 and has been "one of the most successful federally funded nutrition programs in the United States" (USDA, 2013). Studies show that WIC plays a key role in improving birth outcomes, increasing consumption of key nutrients resulting in improved growth in children (USDA, 2013). Despite these beneficial outcomes, the USDA argues for increased participation in WIC to address health disparities in the United States that result from food insecurity and poor nutrition. Only 70% of eligible individuals nationwide take part in this highly beneficial and successful program (USDA, 2013).

Increasing access to healthy foods

The CDC promotes strategies to increase access to healthy foods in several ways. On the community level, many programs show success in bringing higher volumes of nutritious foods to more people. The Healthy Corner Store Initiative epitomizes one such project. Piloted in Philadelphia in 2004, this program identified corner stores in lower-income communities within Philadelphia that met three criteria: 1) low access to healthy foods, 2) high rates of diet-related disease and 3) certification as a Healthy Corner Store by meeting specific goals and requirements.

The introduction of four or more new healthy food products, positive impact on local business profits, and continuing customer demand for healthier foods attests to the success of the Healthy Corner Store Initiative (Healthy Corner Store Initiative, 2014). The spread of concepts nationally to other cities like Providence, Rhode Island, Los Angeles, California and Louisville, Kentucky further cements the strategies to increase access to nutritious foods. Consequently, The National Healthy Corner Stores Network (HCSN) supports ongoing efforts to increase the availability and sales of healthy, affordable foods through small-scale stores in underserved communities (Healthy Food Access, n.d.).

Fruit and vegetable voucher programs exemplify another way communities work to increase the consumption of healthy foods among their neighborhoods. The fruit and vegetable prescription program in the Navajo Nation is an example of this intervention. The program, implemented in 2015, targeted the most vulnerable members of the Navajo Nation – children under the age of six and pregnant women – and enrolled them in an investigation. In addition to receiving prescriptions for fruits and vegetables, participants in the study attended monthly education sessions over a 6-month period designed to set goals for healthier lifestyles. Following implementation of this intervention, participants increased their consumption of fruits and vegetables by 48% (Sundberg et al., 2020).

Food Security as a Social Determinant of Health

Summary

As declared by the United Nation Universal Declaration of Human Rights (1948), access to sufficient food that is nutritious and healthy is a human right and a crucial aspect of good health. In the current global landscape where highly processed, nutrient-poor foods are inexpensive and widely available, it is important to equip people with resources that enable them to make healthy choices about their diet. Policies that make nutritious food affordable and available have been shown to improve health outcomes in the United States. The reduction of global conflict helps developing countries build the infrastructure necessary to provide a steady supply of food to their citizens. Investing in programs that enable individuals to make significant changes to their diet is not only in the best interest of countries, but necessary if we are collectively going to change the current trajectory of health across the world.

Questions for Further Consideration:

1. What role should the U.S. Government play in promoting food choices?
2. Beyond education, what can healthcare providers do to promote healthy food choices?
3. How do differences in governing bodies around the world impact the quality of food available to people?
4. The poverty as a social determinant of health plays significantly in food insecurity. What policies are in place in the U.S. to mitigate poverty. What do countries like Finland and Norway do to ensure basic needs are met for everyone?

Sentinel Readings for a Deeper Dive

Food and Agriculture Organization of the United Nations. *The State of Food Security and Nutrition in the World, 2022* [online] Available at: https://www.fao.org/3/cc0639en/online/cc0639en.html

Liu, C.H. and Liu, H. (2016). Concerns and Structural Barriers Associated with WIC Participation among WIC-Eligible Women. *Public Health Nursing.* [online] Available at: https://onlinelibrary.wiley.com/doi/10.1111/phn.12259

Yeh, M.-C., et al, 2008. Understanding barriers and facilitators of fruit and vegetable consumption among a diverse multi-ethnic population in the USA, *Health Promotion International* [online] Available at: https://academic.oup.com/heapro/article/23/1/42/555897

References

Beasley, D. (2018). Fact sheet Hunger & Conflict. *WFP* [online] Available at: https://docs.wfp.org/api/documents/WFP-0000099172/download/ [Accessed 18 Jul. 2023].

Ben Hassen, T. and El Bilali, H. (2022). Impacts of the Russia-Ukraine War on Global Food Security: Towards More Sustainable and Resilient Food Systems? *Foods,* [online] Available at: https://www.mdpi.com/2304-8158/11/15/2301 [Accessed 19 July 2023].

CDC (2020). *Healthy Food Environments: Improving Access to Healthier foods*. [online] Available at: https://www.cdc.gov/nutrition/healthy-food-environments/improving-access-to-healthier-food.html [Accessed 14 July 2023].

CDC (2021). *Adult Obesity Facts*. [online] [online] Available at: https://www.cdc.gov/obesity/data/adult.html [Accessed 18 July 2023].

CDC (2022). *Poor Nutrition.* [online] Available at: https://www.cdc.gov/chronicdisease/resources/publications/factsheets/nutrition.htm#:~:text=The%20Harmful%20Effects%20of%20Poor%20Nutrition&text=In%20the%20United%20States%2C%2020 [Accessed 15 July 2023].

Centers for Disease Control and Prevention (2019). *Climate Change and Public Health - Health Effects - Food Security*. [online] Available at: https://www.cdc.gov/climateandhealth/effects/food_security.htm [Accessed 14 July 2023].

Chilton, M., Knowles, M. and Bloom, S. (2017). The Intergenerational Circumstances of Household food Insecurity and Adversity. *Journal of Hunger & Environmental Nutrition.* [online] Available at: https://www.ncbi.nlm.nih.gov/pmc/articles/PMC5399810 [Accessed 22 July 2023].

Coleman-Jensen, A., Gregory, C. and Singh, A. (2021). Household Food Security in the United States in 2020. *SSRN Electronic Journal*, [online] Available at: https://www.ers.usda.gov/webdocs/publications/102076/err-298.pdf [Accessed 13 July 2023].

Dietary Guide for Americans (2020). *Dietary Guidelines for Americans, 2020-2025* [online] Available at: www.dietaryguidelines.gov [Accessed 17 July 2023].

FAO (2022). Agriculture Organization of the United Nations, 2022. *The State of Food Security and Nutrition in the World, 2022* [online] Available at: https://www.fao.org/3/cc0639en/online/cc0639en.html [Accessed 16 July 2023].

Golan, E., Stewart, H. Kuchler, F. and Dong, D. (2008). Can Low-Income Americans Afford a Healthy diet? *USDA-ERS.* [online] Available at: https://www.ers.usda.gov/amber-waves/2008/november/can-low-income-americans-afford-a-healthy-diet [Accessed 15 July 2023].

Healthy Corner Store Initiative (2014). Available at: https://thefoodtrust.org/wp-content/uploads/2022/07/healthy-corner-store-overview.original.pdf [Accessed 18 July 2023].

Healthy Food Access (n.d.) *Corner Stores.* [online] Available at: https://www.healthyfoodaccess.org/launch-a-business-models-corner-stores [Accessed 25 July 2023].

Husain, A. (2017). At the Root of the Exodus: Food Security, Conflict, and International Migration. *World Food Programme* [online] www.wfp.org. Available at: https://executiveboard.wfp.org/document_download/WFP-0000039350 [Accessed 13 July 2023].

Lee, J., Gundersen, C., Cook, J., Laraia, B. and Johnson, M. (2012). Food Insecurity and Health across the Lifespan. *Advances in Nutrition*, [online] Available at: https://academic.oup.com/advances/article/3/5/744/4591599 [Accessed 17 July 2023].

Lee, S., Moore, L., Park, S., Harris, D., and Blanck, H. (2022). Adults Meeting Fruit and Vegetable Intake Recommendations — United States, 2019. *MMWR. Morbidity and Mortality Weekly Report*, [online] Available at: https://www.cdc.gov/mmwr/volumes/71/wr/mm7101a1.htm [Accessed 14 July 2023].

Marmot, M. and Wilkinson, R. (2003). *Social determinants of health: the solid facts, 2nd ed* Copenhagen: Center for Urban Health, World Health Organization.

National Institute of Diabetes and Digestive and Kidney Disease (2019). *Health Risks of Overweight & Obesity* [online] Available at: https://www.niddk.nih.gov/health-information/weight-management/adult-overweight-obesity/health-risks [Accessed 23 July 2023].

National Institute on Minority Health and Health Disparities (2023). *Food Accessibility, Insecurity and Health Outcomes.* [online] Available at: https://www.nimhd.nih.gov/resources/understanding-health-disparities/food-accessibility-insecurity-and-health-outcomes.html [Accessed 22 July 2023].

Rehm, C., Peñalvo, J., Afshin, A. and Mozaffarian, D. (2016). Dietary Intake Among US Adults, 1999-2012. *JAMA* [online] Available at: https://jamanetwork.com/journals/jama/fullarticle/2529628 [Accessed 13 July 2023.

Rhone, A., Ploeg, M., Dicken, C., Williams, R. and Breneman, V. (2017) Low-Income and Low-Supermarket-Access Census Tracts, 2010-2015. *USDA ERS* [online] Available at: https://www.ers.usda.gov/publications/pub-details/?pubid=82100 [Accessed 12 July 2023].

Sundberg, M., Warren, A., VanWassenhove-Paetzold, J., George, C., Carroll, D., Becenti, L., Martinez, A., Jones, B., Bachman-Carter, K., Begay, M., Wilmot, T., Sandoval-Soland, H., MacKenzie, O., Hamilton, L., Tsosie, M., Bradburn, C., Ellis, E., Malone, J., Pon, J. and Fitch, A. (2020). Implementation of the Navajo fruit and vegetable prescription programme to improve access to healthy foods in a rural food desert. *Public Health Nutrition* [online] Available at: https://www.cambridge.org/core/journals/public-health-nutrition/article/implementation-of-the-navajo-fruit-and-vegetable-prescription-programme-to-improve-access-to-healthy-foods-in-a-rural-food-desert/854A789167B4F4A86CBB4CAC4FE8FDE3 [Accessed 19 July 2023].

Suter, T. (2023). UN official says latest Russian attacks on Ukraine 'signal a calamitous turn.' *The Hill* [online] Available at: https://www.yahoo.com/news/un-official-says-latest-russian-233118394.html [Accessed 27 July 2023].

US DEPARTMENT OF AGRICULTURE (2009). *Food Security* [online] Available at: https://www.usda.gov/topics/food-and-nutrition/food-security [Accessed 19 July 2023]

US Department of Agriculture, Economic Research Service (2016). *Food Security in the United States* [online] Available at: https://data.nal.usda.gov/dataset/food-security-united-states-0 [Accessed 22 July 2023].

USDA (2013). *About WIC- How WIC Helps | Food and Nutrition Service*. [online] Available at: https://www.fns.usda.gov/wic/about-wic-how-wic-helps [Accessed 18 July 2023].

USDA (2022a) *Definitions of Food Security* US Department of Agriculture, Economic Research Service [online] Available at: https://www.ers.usda.gov/topics/food-nutrition-assistance/food-security-in-the-u-s/definitions-of-food-security/#characteristics [Accessed 13 July 2023].

USDA (2022b) *Interactive Charts and Highlights* US Department of Agriculture, Economic Research Service [online] Available at: https://www.ers.usda.gov/topics/food-nutrition-assistance/food-security-in-the-u-s/interactive-charts-and-highlights/#trends [Accessed 13 July 2023].

WMA (2019). *World Medical Association Statement on Free Sugar Consumption and Sugar-sweetened Beverages.* [online] Available at: https://www.wma.net/policy-tags/nutrition/ [Accessed 17 July 2023].

Wong, E. and Swanson, A., 2023. How Russia's War on Ukraine Is Worsening Global Starvation. *New York Times.* [online] Available at: https://www.nytimes.com/2023/01/02/us/politics/russia-ukraine-food-crisis.html [Accessed 26 July 2023].

WFP (2018). *Fact Sheet Hunger and Conflict* World Food Programme. [online] Available at: https://docs.wfp.org/api/documents/WFP-0000099172/download/ [Accessed 13 July 2023].

WHO (2014). *Comprehensive implementation plan on maternal, infant and young child nutrition* World Health Organization [online] Available at: https://www.who.int/publications/i/item/WHO-NMH-NHD-14.1 [Accessed 18 July 2023].

WHO (2021). *Malnutrition* World Health Organization [online] Available at: https://www.who.int/health-topics/malnutrition#tab=tab_1 [Accessed 18 July 2023].

WHO (2022). *Noncommunicable Diseases* World Health Organization [online] Available at: https://www.who.int/news-room/fact-sheets/detail/noncommunicable-diseases [Accessed 15 July 2023].

Lexicon of Listed Terms and Agencies

- **The Centers for Disease Control and Prevention** (CDC) is an American governing body that operates under the Department of Health and Human Services to supply information that protects the nation against dangerous health threats.

- **The Food and Agricultural Organization of the United Nations** (FAO) is a specialized agency of the United Nations that leads international efforts to defeat hunger.

- **The Food Programme** (WFP) is a global organization that works to bring life-saving relief in emergencies and use food assistance to build peace, stability, and prosperity for the people of the world. They work with both national agencies and international agencies such as the United Nations, to conduct their goals.

- **The World Health Organization** (WHO) is a United Nations agency that aims to promote health, keep the world safe and serve the vulnerable.

- **The States Department of Agriculture** (USDA) is an American governing body responsible for supplying leadership on food, agriculture, natural resources, rural development, nutrition, and related issues.

AUTHOR'S BIO SKETCH

Kathryn Annand, MD

Kathryn Annand grew up in New Hampshire before earning her undergraduate degree in neuroscience from Furman University in Greenville, South Carolina. She completed medical school at New York Medical College in Westchester New York and is currently completing her residency at University of Washington affiliated Community Health Care in Tacoma, Washington. Outside of work she enjoys traveling, experiencing new foods and wines, exploring the outdoors and spending time with friends and family.

Chapter 7

Information Technology and Communication as Social Determinants of Health

Eloy Alibin, MD, Author
Carri Jo Timmer, DO, Editor

"The number one benefit of information technology is that it empowers people to do what they want to do. It lets people be creative. It lets people be productive. It lets people learn things they didn't think they could learn before, and so in a sense it is all about potential."
-Steve Ballmer, Microsoft CEO, 2000-2014

Information Technology and Communication as Social Determinants of Health

According to the World Health Organization (WHO), "the social determinants of health (SDH) are the non-medical factors that influence health outcomes. They are the conditions in which people are born, grow, work, live, and age, and the wider set of forces and systems shaping the conditions of daily life. These forces and systems include economic policies and systems, development agendas, social norms, social policies, and political systems" (World Health Organization, n.d.). Although not routinely cited as a social determinant of health, this chapter endorses information technology and communication as an essential SDH due to its impact on health and quality of life by increasing access to care, improving health literacy, shrinking communication barriers, and reducing health disparities.

Federal Communications Commission (FCC, 2022) research supports this assertion. After accounting for confounding factors such as rurality, education, and income, research demonstrates the significant correlation between increasing broadband access and improving health outcomes – especially notable differences between digitally connected communities from isolated ones. For example, the least connected counties throughout the U.S. had higher chronic disease prevalence like diabetes by as much as 41%, obesity by as much as 25%, and preventable hospitalizations 1.5 times greater compared to connected counties (FCC, 2022).

Information Technology and Communication as Social Determinants of Health

In the context of National Access to IT

According to the National Telecommunications and Information Administration, internet access provides a gateway to education, health care, jobs, and entertainment – an essential ingredient in modern societies. Despite this, as of 2022 one in five U.S. households (24 million) were not connected to the internet (NTIA, n.d.). While a majority – 58% of the 24 million offline households express no interest or need to be connected, there is also a substantial proportion who say they can't afford home Internet service (18%). Regardless of their stated reasons for non-use, offline households have significantly lower incomes than their online counterparts (NTIA, n.d.).

Figure 1. Illustrates factors for household non-internet use.

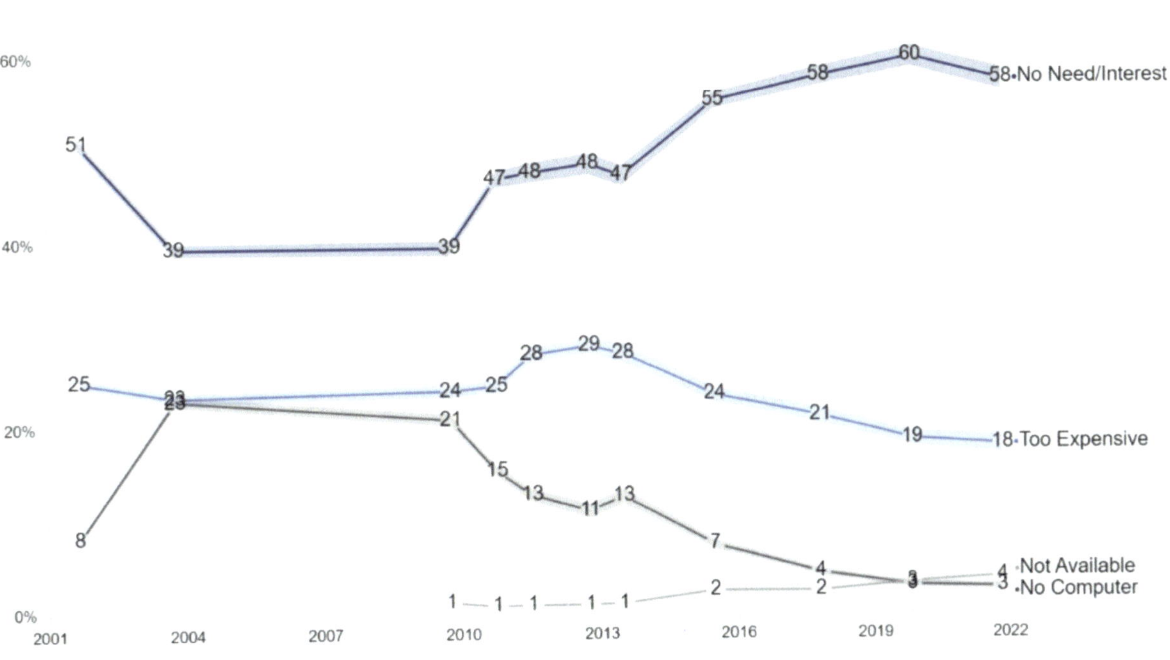

NTID (n.d.). *Switched Off: Why Are One in Five U.S. Households Not Online? | National Telecommunications and Information Administration* (no date) *www.ntia.gov*. [online] Available at: https://www.ntia.gov/blog/2022/switched-why-are-one-five-us-households-not-online

Households that cited "too expensive" as their barrier online access were more likely to have school-age children at home and identify as racial and ethnic minorities than those who were not interested in getting internet services (NTID, n.d.).

Citing the analysis, the National Telecommunications and Information Administration recommends multiple strategies to stimulate greater adoption of the internet, including subsidy programs such as the Affordable Connectivity Program (ACP), the Digital Equity Act, and other initiatives that increase digital skills, equip people with suitable devices, and ensure important online services are accessible to all (NTIA, n.d.).

As a component of the Bipartisan Infrastructure Law, crafted by Congress and signed into law by President Biden, Democrats, Republicans, and Independents collaborated to create the *Affordable Connectivity Program* (ACP) that provides eligible households $30 per month off their internet bills. ACP-eligible households receive a one-time discount of up to $100 to purchase a laptop, desktop computer, or tablet from participating providers in addition (FACT SHEET, 2022).

To deliver maximum cost savings to families, the Biden-Harris Administration secured commitments from twenty leading internet providers to offer ACP-eligible households a high-speed internet plan for no more than $30 per month. Eligible families who pair their ACP benefit with one of these plans can receive high-speed internet at no cost (Get Internet, n.d.).

Information Technology and Communication as Social Determinants of Health

In the context of Health Equity

The U.S. Department of Health and Human Services (HHS) promotes culturally and linguistically appropriate services (CLAS) to improve the quality of healthcare provided to all individuals. The provision of CLAS reduces health disparities with the goal of improving health equity – "CLAS is about respect and responsiveness: respect for the whole individual and responsiveness to the individual's health needs and preferences" (U.S. Department of Health & Human Services, 2019).

According to the HHS (2019), health inequities abound. Effectively implemented, CLAS provides a strategy to reduce and even eliminate health inequities. Services tailored to an individual's culture and language preferences give healthcare professionals a tool to bring about positive health outcomes for diverse populations.

Philosophically imagined, the provision of health services that are respectful of, and responsive to the health beliefs, practices and needs of diverse populations provide the opportunity to close gaps in population health outcomes. Further elaborating, the HSS argues "the pursuit of health equity must remain at the forefront of our efforts; we must always remember that dignity and quality of care are rights of all and not the privilege of a few" (U.S. Department of Health & Human Services, 2019).

Delivering on the promise of culturally and linguistically appropriate services requires significant and persistent organizational leadership that promote CLAS and health equity through policies and practices that allocate necessary resources to recruit, promote, and support a workforce responsive to CLAS. To sustain these services, administrative leadership and organizational workforce must provide the resources and opportunity to engage in continuous training to maintain the esprit de corps that deliver best practices CLAS services (U.S. Department of Health & Human Services, 2019).

Considering the complexities of organizational integration of CLAS, *The Commonwealth Fund* authors Goode, Dunne, and Bronheim (2006) offer this counterpoint. "Cultural and linguistic competence are widely recognized as fundamental aspects of quality in health care and mental health care—particularly for diverse patient populations—and as essential strategies for reducing disparities by improving access, utilization, and quality of care. However, it is not clear if evidence exists to support the assertion that cultural and linguistic competence improve health outcomes and well-being. Advocates of culturally and linguistically competent care state that the costs of providing such care are offset by potential benefits, but, again, there is limited evidence to support this assertion." The author's full report assesses the evidence for the impact and benefits of cultural and linguistic competence in health care and mental health care: *The Evidence Base for Cultural and Linguistic Competency in Health Care* (2006).

Despite the conclusions of the author's scholarly analysis, the provision of care that is free of bias, readily accessible, liberally uses interpretive services and respects cultural nuances, intuitively speaks to holistic, humanistic patient centered care.

Information Technology and Communications as Social Determinants of Health

In the context of Health Literacy

Health literacy is a complex phenomenon that involves individuals, families, communities, healthcare providers and systems. The concept of health literacy encompasses the materials, environments, technology, and challenges specifically associated with disease management, disease prevention and health promotion (Health Literacy, 2021).

The U.S. Department of Health and Human Services (HHS) identified two dimensions of health literacy in the Healthy People 2030 – personal health literacy and organizational health literacy.

- *Personal health literacy* is the degree to which individuals can find, understand, and use information and services to inform health-related decisions and actions for themselves and others.

- *Organizational health literacy* is the degree to which organizations equitably enable individuals to find, understand, and use information and services to inform health-related decisions and actions for themselves and others (Health Literacy, 2021).

The critical need for health literacy, moved the U.S. Department of Health and Human Services to create a *National Action Plan to Improve Health Literacy* in 2021. The Plan seeks to engage organizations, professionals, policymakers, communities, individuals, and families in a linked, multi-sector effort to improve health literacy (U.S. Department of Health and Human Services, 2021).

National Action Plan to Improve Health Literacy

The Action Plan contains seven goals that aim to improve health literacy with strategies for achieving them:

- Develop and disseminate health and safety information that is accurate, accessible, and actionable
- Promote changes in the health care system that improve health information, communication, informed decision-making, and access to health services
- Incorporate accurate, standards-based, and developmentally appropriate health and science information and curricula in child care and education through the university level
- Support and expand local efforts to provide adult education, English language instruction, and culturally and linguistically appropriate health information services in the community
- Build partnerships, develop guidance, and change policies
- Increase basic research and the development, implementation, and evaluation of practices and interventions to improve health literacy
- Increase the dissemination and use of evidence-based health literacy practices and interventions

U.S. Department of Health and Human Services (2021) National Action Plan to Improve Health Literacy | health.gov, health.gov. [online] Available at: https://health.gov/sites/default/files/2019-09/Health_Literacy_Action_Plan.pdf

The HHS bases the Action Plan on two core principles:

1. All people have the right to health information that fosters informed decisions

2. Health services should be delivered in ways that are easy to understand and that improve health, longevity, and quality of life (U.S. Department of health and Human Services, 2021).

As designed and implemented, the Plan seeks to improve the accessibility, quality, and safety of healthcare for all; reduce healthcare costs; and improve the health and quality of life for the millions of people living in the United States (U.S. Department of Health and Human Services, 2021).

Information Technology and Communication as Social Determinants of Health

In the context of Access to Health Care for Isolated Populations

Connect2Health^{FCC} (C2HFCC) a Promising Solution to the Maternal Health Crisis

According to the *Nowhere to Go: Maternity Care Deserts Across the U.S. 2022* March of Dimes report, consistent, high-quality maternity care is essential to protect the health of all moms and babies irrespective of geographic domain. Maternity care encompasses healthcare services for women throughout all stages of pregnancy, labor, delivery, and postpartum events. With over 3.5 million births in the U.S. annually, and rising rates of maternal mortality and morbidity, a pressing need to improve maternal and birth outcomes in the U.S. confronts healthcare professionals across the nation (March of Dimes, 2022).

In 2020, approximately nine hundred women died of causes related to pregnancy in the U.S., with a 14.2 percent increase in deaths from the previous year and a 30.9 percent increase since 2018. To compound the concerns, the number of women experiencing pregnancy-related complications, or severe maternal morbidity is increasing and affecting at least 50,000 women each year (March of Dimes, 2022).

A *maternity care desert* is any county without a hospital or birth center offering obstetric care and without any obstetric providers, according to the March of Dimes. Disparities punctuate access to care, further characterizing the realm of maternity care deserts. In 2020, one in four Native American babies (26.7%) were born in areas of limited or no access to maternity care services; one in six Black babies (16.3%) were born in areas of limited or no access to care to maternity care services. 36% of U.S. counties are classified as maternity care deserts (March of Dimes, 2022).

Map 1.

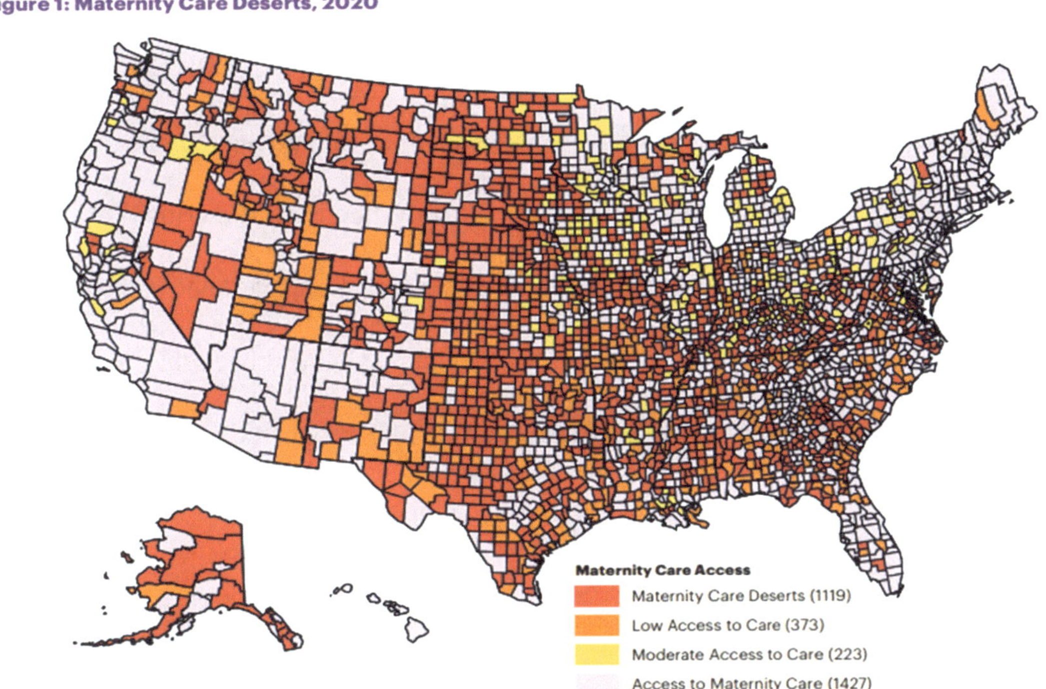

Source: U.S. Health Resources and Services Administration (HRSA), Area Health Resources Files, 2021.

March of Dimes (2022). Healthy Moms. Strong Babies. No Where to Go: Maternity Care Deserts across the U.S. (2022) [online] Available at: https://www.marchofdimes.org/sites/default/files/2022-10/2022_Maternity_Care_Report.pdf

Map 1. Graphically portrays the prevalence of *Maternity Care Deserts* and the substantial need to identify effective solutions to address the daunting challenges.

Cognizant of the urgent need to address health disparities and untoward infant and maternal health outcomes in rural and isolated communities across the United States, the U.S. Congress charged the Federal Communications Commission (FCC) to analyze the intersection of broadband, advanced information technology, and health disparities to address infant and maternal health outcomes (Connect2Health^FCC^, n.d.).

Seizing the challenge, the FCC fostered the potential role of broadband technology in addressing 1) maternal health, 2) chronic disease, and 3) opioid use. In particular, the FCC promoted the "*Data Mapping to Save Moms' Lives Act*" passed by Congress and signed into law by President Biden in 2022. The Act directed the FCC to incorporate data on maternal mortality and severe maternal morbidity into the agency's *Mapping Broadband Health in America* platform, in consultation with the Centers for Disease Control and Prevention (Connect2Health^FCC^, n.d.).

Mapping Broadband Health in America provides a novel, interactive mapping platform as developed by the Connect2Health^FCC^ task force. The platform functions as a critical resource for users to visualize, intersect and analyze broadband and health data at the national, state and county levels, providing compelling insights on opportunities and gaps (Connect2Health^FCC^, n.d.).

Addressing maternal health, the FCC discovered the following critical facts:

- The U.S. is the only developed country with increasing maternal mortality and severe maternal morbidity rates.
- Black and American Indian/Alaska Native women are two to three times more likely to die of pregnancy-related causes than white women.
- The U.S. faces an increasing prevalence of chronic diseases, worsening mental health, and substance abuse disorders among women of reproductive age and pregnant women.

- Most of these deaths and complications can be prevented. Telehealth and other broadband-enabled solutions and technologies offer exciting potential and innovations for addressing preventable deaths and improving maternal health.
- Access to maternal health care presents challenges, especially in rural areas.

Map 2. Displays locales where broadband and health coincide. The FCC utilizes these to identify those areas where broadband can be leveraged to help address the maternal health crisis. Categories are designated as: double burden, opportunity, single burden, and milestone.

Map 2.

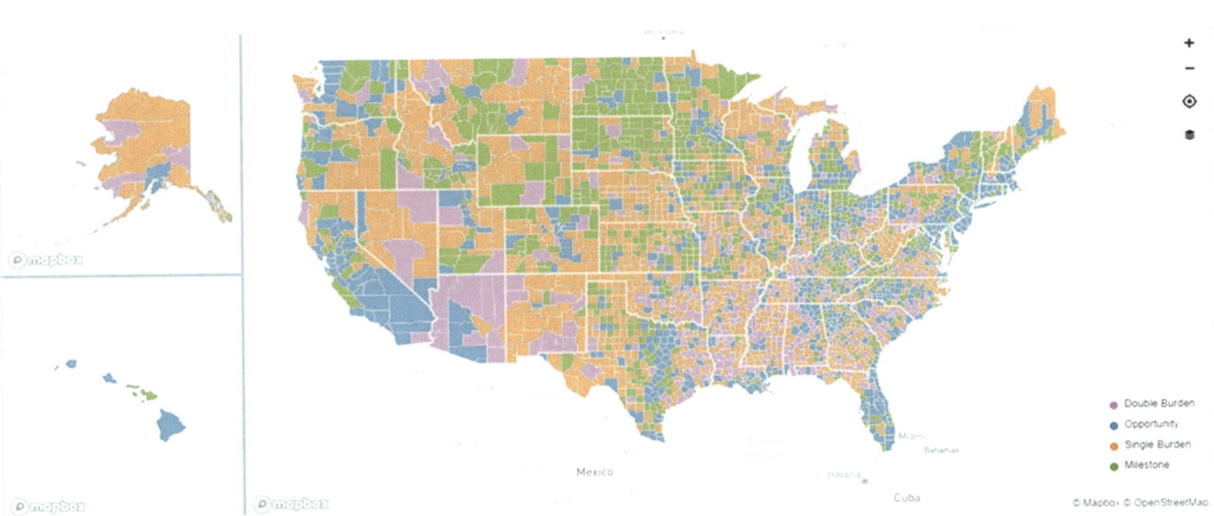

Connect2HealthFCC - Mapping Broadband Health in America (no date) www.fcc.gov. [online] Available at: https://www.fcc.gov/reports-research/maps/connect2health/background.html

County Categorization		Population Count	County Count
Double Burden		17,815,188	398
Opportunity		252,775,345	766
Single Burden		21,857,704	1,157
Milestone		35,791,286	821
Totals		**328,239,523**	**3,142**

Double burden: county or state with lower connectivity status relative to the national average and with higher health need.

Opportunity: county or state with higher connectivity status relative to the national average and with higher health need.

Single burden: county or state with lower connectivity status relative to the national average and with lower health need.

Milestone: county or state with higher connectivity status relative to the national average and with lower health need.

Given the complexity of the data and compressed time to respond to the Act, the Task Force planned and implemented a multi-phase approach (**Table 1.**).

Table 1.

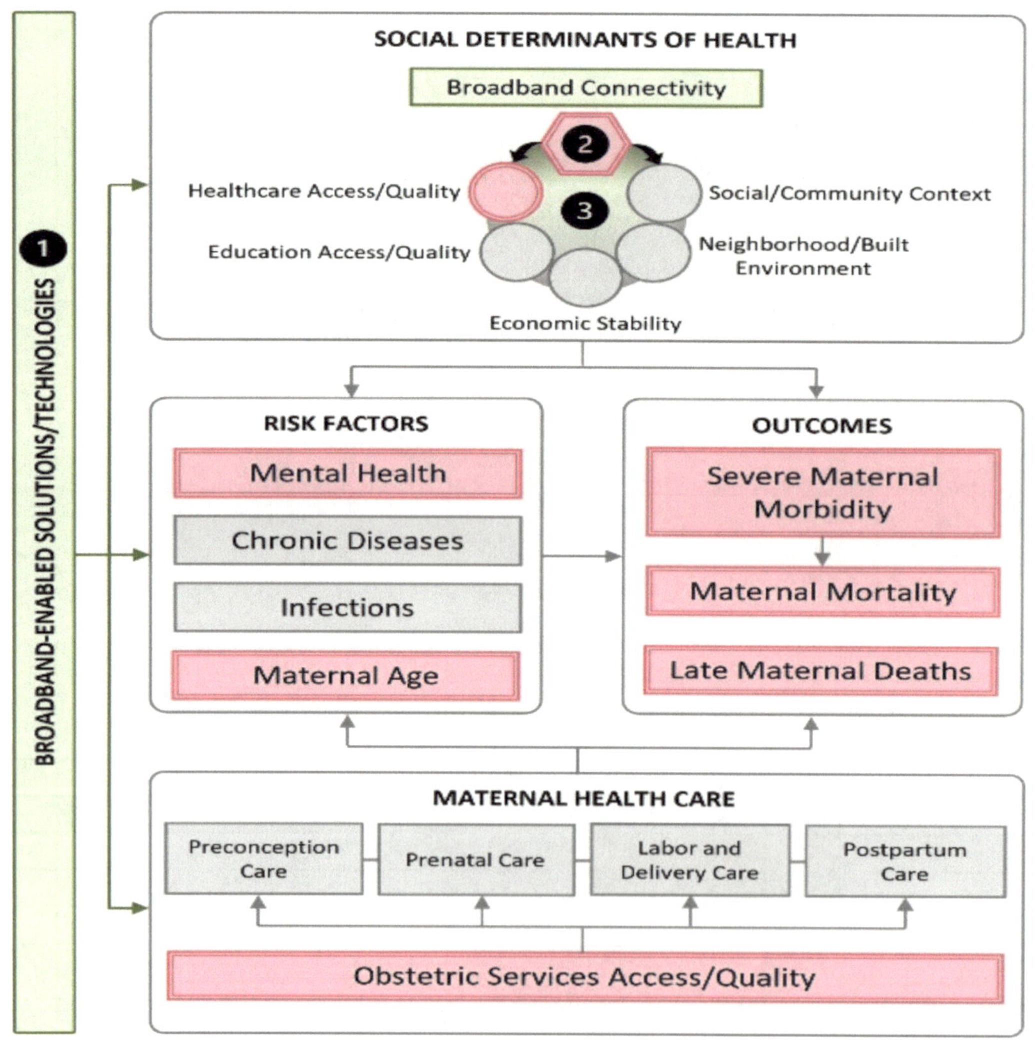

Connect2HealthFCC - Mapping Broadband Health in America (no date) *www.fcc.gov*. [online] Available at: https://www.fcc.gov/reports-research/maps/connect2health/background.html

In Phase 1, the Task Force commenced ongoing consultation with the CDC, relevant agencies within the Department of Health and Human Services, and other stakeholders to gather their input on the maternal health data and information to incorporate in the mapping platform. Based on this feedback, the Task Force developed an initial conceptual framework to guide this effort, as diagrammed in **Table 1.** above (Connect2Health^{FCC}, n.d.).

During Phase 1, the *Connect2Health* task force reviewed available literature to identify relevant risk factors and social determinants of health that influence maternal health outcomes and where broadband-enabled intervention might bridge gaps. These variables include race and ethnicity, maternal age, maternity care deserts, mental health provider shortage areas and rural geographic areas (Connect2HealthFCC, n.d.).

In the next phases of this initiative, the FCC coupled with *Connect2Health* Task Force expertise intend to incorporate additional maternal health variables and functionalities into the mapping platform, conduct important research and data analytics on the intersection of broadband connectivity to address maternal health (Connect2Health^{FCC}, n.d.). As it evolves, *Connect2Health* holds promise that advanced broadband technology can reverse maternal health outcomes in rural and isolated America.

Information Technology and Communications as Social Determinants of Health

Politics, policies, and governance

As noted above, the U.S. Congress and the Biden Administration recognize the importance of communication through internet connectivity. The Bipartisan Infrastructure Law through initiatives like the Affordable Connectivity Program and the Digital Equity Act have been passed to increase digital skills, equip people with suitable devices, and ensure that important online services are accessible to all.

Nefarious "opportunities" to disseminate false information, violate standards related to protected health information and breeches in healthcare information systems for reprehensible proposes creates the need to oversee and regulate health information technology. Listed here, some agencies granted the responsibility for that oversight:

- The Office of the National Coordinator for Health Information Technology regulates and sets standards for health information and certification of EHR (Certification of Health, n.d.).
- The *Health Information Technology for Economic and Clinical Health (HITECH) Act of 2009* grants Health and Human Services (HHS) the authority to improve the quality of healthcare by promoting health IT, EHRs, and the security and privacy of exchanging health information (HITECH, 2017).
- The *Affordable Care Act* promotes availability of health care information to uninsured low-income households amongst other important benefits promoting access to care (U.S. Department of Health & Human Services, 2022).
- The *Cures Act*, introduced in 2015, aims to promote access to health information in an accurate and convenient form, increases certification of EHR, and promotes patient communication with providers (Bonamici, 2016).

Conclusions:

As presented in this chapter, the interface of information technology and communication rise to important social determinants of health by playing a vital role in improving healthcare access, reducing health disparities, enhancing health literacy, promoting language and cultural sensitivity, and mitigating health information obstacles. Continued government finance will ensure progressive development and adoption of robust, secure health information technology for the benefit of all going forward in the future.

Questions for Further Consideration:

1. What can healthcare professionals do to deflect healthcare misinformation?
2. How do you balance freedom of speech with healthcare misinformation?
3. Should access to the internet be a human right?
4. In what ways does information technology negatively impact healthcare?

Sentinel Readings for a Deeper Dive

March of Dimes (2022). *Healthy Moms. Strong Babies. No Where to Go: Maternity Care Deserts across the U.S.* (2022) [online] Available at: *https://www.marchofdimes.org/sites/default/files/2022-10/2022_Maternity_Care_Report.pdf*

Connect2HealthFCC - Mapping Broadband Health in America (no date) *www.fcc.gov*. [online] Available at: https://www.fcc.gov/reports-research/maps/connect2health/background.html

U.S. Department of Health and Human Services (2021) *National Action Plan to Improve Health Literacy* | health.gov, health.gov. [online] Available at: https://health.gov/sites/default/files/2019-09/Health_Literacy_Action_Plan.pdf

References:

Bonamici, S. (2016). *H.R.34 - 114th Congress (2015-2016): 21st Century Cures Act.* [online] www.congress.gov. Available at: https://www.congress.gov/bill/114th-congress/house-bill/34 [Accessed 14 September 2023].

Certification of Health IT | HealthIT.gov (n.d.) *www.healthit.gov*. [online] Available at: https://www.healthit.gov/topic/certification-ehrs/certification-health-it [Accessed 14 September 2021].

Connect2HealthFCC - Mapping Broadband Health in America (no date) *www.fcc.gov*. [online] Available at: https://www.fcc.gov/reports-research/maps/connect2health/background.html [Accessed 10 October 2023].

FACT SHEET (2022): *Biden-Harris Administration's 'Internet for All' Initiative: Bringing affordable, reliable high-speed internet to everyone in America | National Telecommunications and Information Administration* (no date) *www.ntia.doc.gov*. [online] Available at: https://www.ntia.doc.gov/other-publication/2022/fact-sheet-biden-harris-administration-s-internet-all-initiative-bringing [Accessed 15 September 2023].

FCC (2022). Federal Communications Commission. *Studies and Data Analytics on Broadband and Health*. [online] Available at: https://www.fcc.gov/health/sdoh/studies-and-data-analytics [Accessed 13 September 2023].

Get Internet (n.d.). *The White House*. {online] Available at: https://www.whitehouse.gov/getinternet/?utm_source=getinternet.gov [Accessed 14 September 2023].

Goode, T., Dunne, C. and Bronheim, S. (2006) *The Evidence Base for Cultural and Linguistic Competency in Health Care | Commonwealth Fund*, *www.commonwealthfund.org*. [online] Available at: https://www.commonwealthfund.org/publications/fund-reports/2006/oct/evidence-base-cultural-and-linguistic-competency-health-care [Accessed 11 October 2023].

Health Literacy (2021). *National Institutes of Health (NIH)*. [online] Available at: https://www.nih.gov/institutes-nih/nih-office-director/office-communications-public-liaison/clear-communication/health-literacy#:~:text=Health%20literacy%20is%20a%20complex%20phenomenon%20that%20involves [Accessed 11 October 2023].

HITECH (2017). U.S. Department of Health & Human Services (2017) *HITECH Act Enforcement Interim Final Rule*, *HHS.gov*. [online] Available at: https://www.hhs.gov/hipaa/for-professionals/special-topics/hitech-act-enforcement-interim-final-rule/index.html [[Accessed 15 September 2023].

March of Dimes (2022). *Healthy Moms. Strong Babies. No Where to Go: Maternity Care Deserts across the U.S.* (2022) [online] Available at: https://www.marchofdimes.org/sites/default/files/2022-10/2022_Maternity_Care_Report.pdf [Accessed 10 October 2023].

NTID (n.d.). *Switched Off: Why Are One in Five U.S. Households Not Online? | National Telecommunications and Information Administration* (no date) *www.ntia.gov*. [online] Available at: https://www.ntia.gov/blog/2022/switched-why-are-one-five-us-households-not-online [Accessed 14 September 2023].

U.S. Department of Health & Human Services (2019) *What is CLAS? Think Cultural Health.* [online] Available at: https://thinkculturalhealth.hhs.gov/clas/what-is-clas [Accessed 10 October 2023].

U.S. Department of Health and Human Services (2021) *National Action Plan to Improve Health Literacy | health.gov, health.gov.* [online] Available at: https://health.gov/sites/default/files/2019-09/Health_Literacy_Action_Plan.pdf [Accessed 11 October 2021].

U.S. Department of Health & Human Services (2022) *About the Affordable Care Act, HHS.gov.* [online] Available at: https://www.hhs.gov/healthcare/about-the-aca/index.html [Accessed 10 October 2023].

World Health Organization (n.d.) *Social determinants of health, World Health Organization.* [online] Available at: https://www.who.int/health-topics/social-determinants-of-health#tab=tab_1 [Accessed 13 September 2023].

Lexicon of Listed Terms and Agencies

- **Affordable Care Act:** The Patient Protection and Affordable Care Act, referred to as the Affordable Care Act or "ACA" for short, is the comprehensive health care reform law enacted in March 2010. Made affordable health insurance affordable to more people, expanded Medicaid, supported methods to lower healthcare costs.

- **Federal Communications Commission (FCC):** regulates communications by radio, television, wire, satellite, and cable across the United States.

- **March of Dimes:** The **March of Dimes leads the fight for the health of all moms and babies.** We support research, lead programs, and provide education and advocacy so that every family can get the best possible start. Building on a successful 85-year legacy, we support every pregnant person.

- **National Institutes of Health (NIH)**: NIH's mission is to seek fundamental knowledge about the nature and behavior of living systems and the application of that knowledge to enhance health, lengthen life, and reduce illness and disability. The NIH provides leadership and direction to programs designed to improve the health of the Nation by conducting and supporting research.

- **National Telecommunications and Information Administration (NTIA):** a department of the executive branch responsible for advising Presidents on telecommunications an information policy issues.

- **U.S. Department of Health and Human Services (HHS):** enhances the health and well-being of all Americans, by providing effective health and human services and by fostering sound, sustained advances in the sciences underlying medicine, public health, and social services.

AUTHOR'S BIO SKETCH

Eloy Alibin, MD

Dr. Alibin originates from a rural area of the Philippines. He moved with his single parent to Honolulu, HI where he received his bachelor's degree in nursing. He completed medical school at the American University of the Caribbean and began residency in Family Medicine at University of Washington affiliated Community Health Care in Tacoma, WA in 2022. He passionately delivers health care services with a focus on the Asian and Pacific-Islander community. Eloy enjoys spending time with his family, relaxing on the beach, building gaming computers, and technology.

Chapter 8

Education as a Social Determinant of Health

Nicole Delos Santos, MD, Author
James G. Lenhart, MD, MPH, Editor

"Everyone has the right to education. Education shall be free, at least in the elementary and fundamental stages. Elementary education shall be compulsory. Technical and professional education shall be made generally available and higher education shall be equally accessible to all on the basis of merit.

Education shall be directed to the full development of the human personality and to the strengthening of respect for human rights and fundamental freedoms. It shall promote understanding, tolerance, and friendship among all nations, racial or religious groups, and shall further the activities of the United Nations for the maintenance of peace."

- The Universal Declaration of Human Rights, Article 26 The United Nations, 1948

Education as a Social Determinant of Health

Education plays a vital role as a social determinant of health. Numerous studies link education to higher health literacy, health promotion, and increased life expectancy; in addition, education contributes to the overall well-being of individuals by creating opportunities for employment and increased income potential (Office of Disease Prevention and Health Promotion, 2020).

In 2018, the United States Department of Health and Human Services released the framework of Healthy People Initiative 2030 with the aim of drilling down on the social determinants of health. In addressing education, its overarching goal aims to aid children and adolescents by increasing educational access and quality.

According to Healthy People 2030, children facing social discrimination and poverty are more likely to struggle in school, affecting their chances of graduating from high school or pursuing higher education. This in turn, reduces the ability to qualify for higher income jobs, which increases the likelihood of having chronic health conditions such as heart disease and depression as adults (Office of Disease Prevention and Health Promotion, 2020).

Education as a Social Determinant of Health

In the context of Socioeconomics, Health, and Life Expectancy

Socioeconomics

In 2007, the Centers for Disease Control and Prevention (CDC) reframed school dropout rates as a public health issue demanding attention:

> Good education predicts good health, and disparities in health and in educational achievement are linked. Despite these connections, public health professionals rarely make reducing the number of students who drop out of school a priority, although nearly one-third of all students in the United States and half of Black, Latino, and American Indian students do not graduate from high school on time.
>
> Freudenberg and Ruglis (2007). Reframing School Dropout as a Public Health Issue: Preventing Chronic Disease Centers for Disease Control and Prevention. [online] Available at: https://www.cdc.gov/pcd/issues/2007/oct/07_0063.htm [Accessed 5 May 2023].

Fast forward ten years, the American Public Health Association (APHA) declared high school dropout a public health crisis. According to the APHA (2018), 13 percent of adults 18 and older had less than a high school education in the United States, with low graduation rates disproportionately affecting people of color – Hispanic 44%, Native Americans 21%, Blacks 15%, Asian 13%, Pacific Islanders 12% and Whites 8% – centering in clusters in the Southeast (33%) and West.

According to the APHA (2018), high school dropout costs the United States more than $11 billion dollars of lost tax revenue, equating to $163,000 dollars in lost tax revenue over a lifetime for each individual dropout. More recent data reported by Lansford et al., (2016) argued that each high school dropout costs the United States economy an estimated $250,000 dollars over an individual's lifetime due to an increased reliance on welfare and Medicaid, poorer health outcomes, and increased likelihood of criminal activity.

> Lower levels of educational attainment affect health through a cascade effect, including employment, earning capacity, incarceration, and ability to secure resources that improve health. In 2016, workers with less than a high school diploma had: higher unemployment rates, annual incomes 25% lower than high school graduates, 60% lower than college graduates and higher poverty.
>
> American Public Health Association, 2018. The Dropout Crisis: A Public Health Problem and the role of School-Based Health Care. February 2018. [online] Available at: https://www.apha.org/-/media/Files/PDF/SBHC/Dropout_Crisis.ashx [Accessed May 5, 2023].

In alignment with Lansford's data, the APHA (2018) projected that by cutting U.S. high school dropout rates in half, significant annual cost savings would accrue with reductions in:

- Medicaid spending - $7.3 billion
- Heart disease - $12 billion
- Obesity - $11.9 billion
- Smoking - $8.9 billion smoking related expenditures
- Alcoholism - $6.4 billion alcoholism costs.

Although the cited research demonstrates significant adverse socioeconomic and health impacts in the United States, from a worldwide perspective, high school completion rates in the U.S. are favorable. Internationally, the Organization for Economic Cooperation and Development (OCED) reported in 2020 that the high school completion rate in the United States was higher than 28 out of the 34 other countries. **Figure 1** from the National Center for Education Statistics (NCES,

2023) website shows that high school completion rates bested the U.S. in only Canada, Slovak Republic, Poland, Lithuania, and the Czech Republic in 2020.

Figure 1.

Percentage of the population 25 to 64 years old who had completed high school, by Organization for Economic Cooperation and Development (OECD) country: 2020 and 2021.

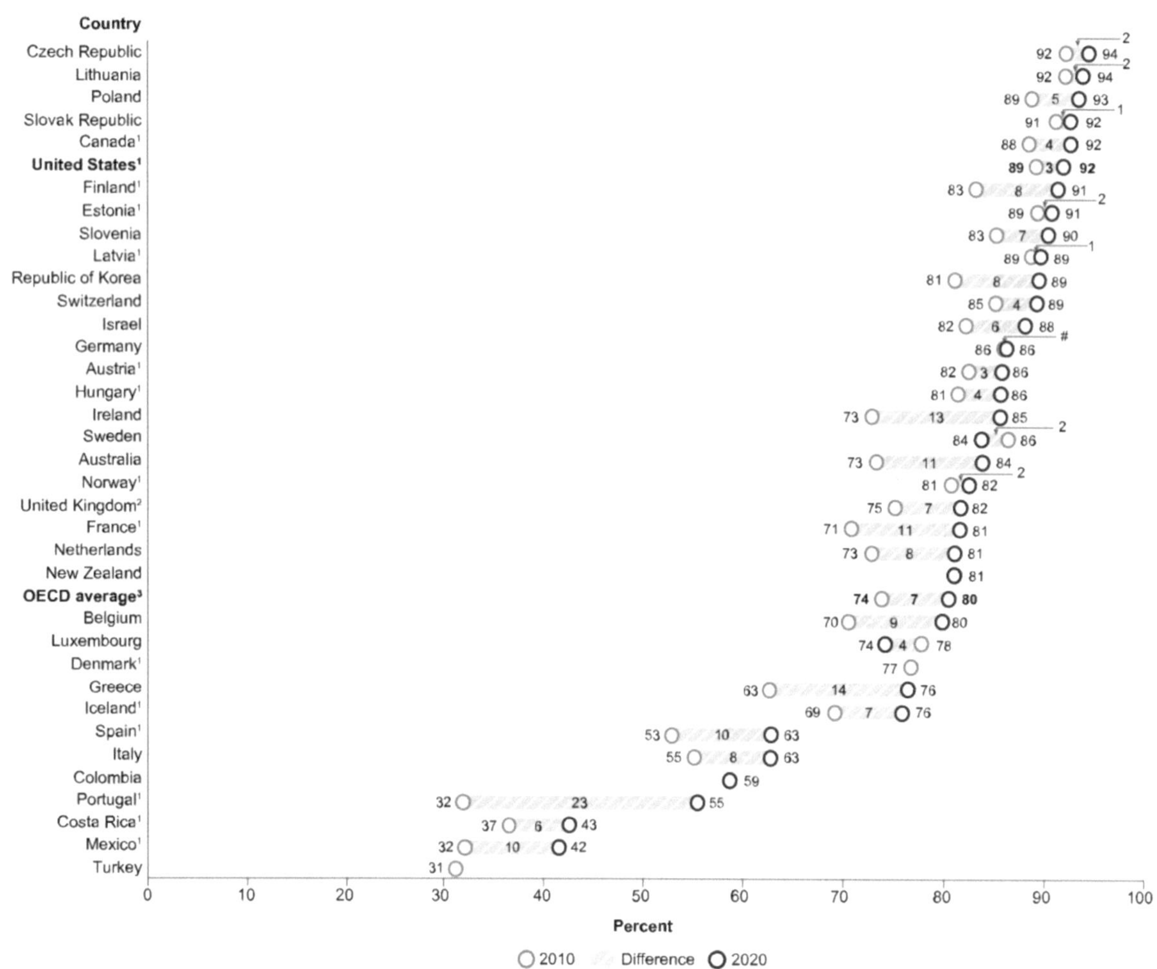

OECD, 2023. International Educational Attainment. [online] Available at: COE - International Educational Attainment

Health

According to Zajacova and Lawrence (2018), three broad theories explain the relationship between health and education. The most convincing theory, the *Fundamental Cause Theory*, states that social factors including education determine health outcomes as they lead to access in resources such as "income, safe neighborhoods, and healthier lifestyles." The second theory, the *Human Capital Theory*, emphasizes education as an investment in productivity – increased productivity results in increased knowledge, skills, reasoning, and other abilities that affect an individual's health. Finally, the third theory – the *Signaling* or *Credentialing Theory* "views earned credentials as a potent signal about one's skills and abilities and emphasizes the economic and social returns to such signals" Zajacova and Lawrence (2018).

While each theory constructs an etiology to explain the relationship of education's impact on health, taken in aggregate **Figure 2** illustrates the predicted probability of health problems based on educational attainment.

Figure 2.

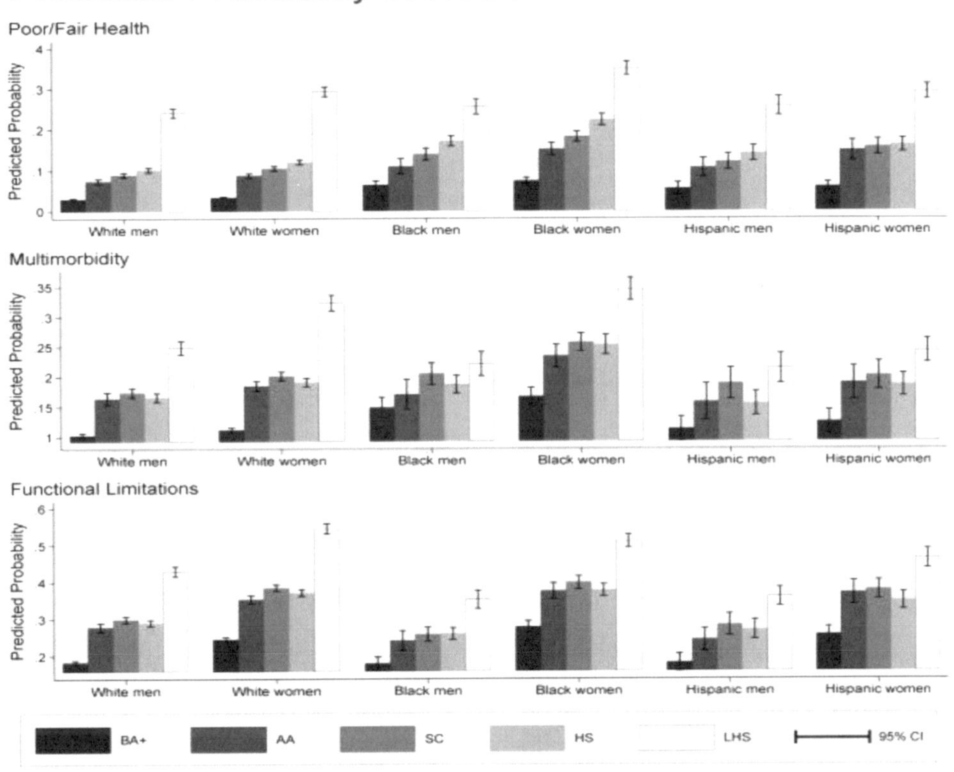

Figure 2. Zajacova, A. (2018). The Relationship Between Education and Health: Reducing Disparities Through a Contextual Approach. *Annual Review of Public Health*, [online] Available at: https://pubmed.ncbi.nlm.nih.gov/29328865/

Data from the National Interview Survey (2002-2016) of adults aged 25 - 64 years was analyzed looking at three categorical health outcomes – poor/fair health, multimorbidity, and functional limitations and their relationship with educational attainment across six different demographic groups - White men, White women, Hispanic men, Hispanic women, Black men, and Black women.

Graphically represented in **Figure 2**, BA+ represents bachelor's degree or more, AA an associate degree, SC some college, HS high school, and LHS limited high school. As illustrated, poor/fair health, multimorbidity, and functional limitations stand out as much more prevalent in those with limited high school across all demographic groups. The data reveals that women are disproportionately affected in health outcome domains across all demographic groups (health improved greater than men by increased education) and (health more adversely impacted compared to men by limited education). Visually represented, the striking contrast between BA+ and LHS across all groups astonishes and supports education as a social determinant of health (Zajacova and Lawrence, 2018).

Life Expectancy

Educational attainment directly and positively improves life expectancy. Although in 2011 U.S. mortality rates decreased substantially with life expectancies for men and women attaining just 76 years and 81 years respectively, there are significant disparities amongst population groups, including those pertaining to education attainment Hummer and Hernandez (2013). See **Figure 3**.

U.S. data for adults ages 25 to 64 shows wide variation in mortality rates by educational attainment for both white women and men. The mortality rate for white women who have not completed high school is four times higher than the rate for white women with 16 or more years of education. An even wider disparity is evident for the same categories of white men: Men with less than a high school degree have a mortality rate more than four times higher than those who have completed at least 16 years of education. Individuals who have only completed high school or some college display mortality rates in between those with the highest and lowest levels of educational attainment

Thus, each increase in educational attainment is associated with a lower mortality rate for both white women and men.

Hummer, R. et al (2013). The Effect of Educational Attainment on Adult Mortality in the United States. *Population bulletin*, [online] Available at: https://www.ncbi.nlm.nih.gov/pmc/articles/PMC4435622/#:~:text=At%20age%2025%2C%20women%20with,a%20difference%20of%2012%20years

Figure 3.

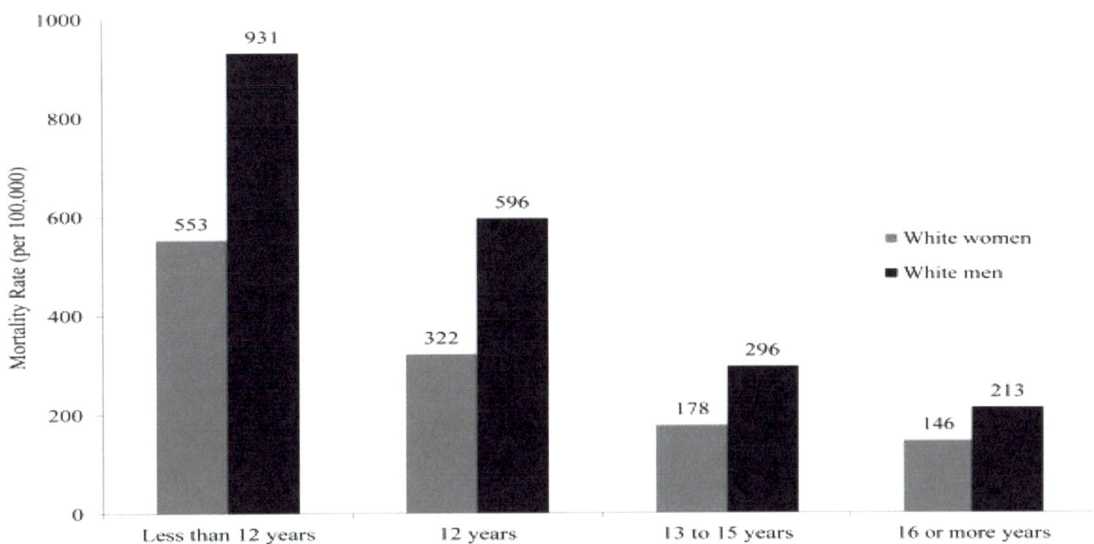

Source: Ahmedin Jemal et al., "Widening of Socioeconomic Inequalities in U.S. Death Rates, 1993-2001," *PLoS ONE*, no. 3, issue 5 (2008): 1-8.

Figure 3. Adapted from Hummer (2013) describes the inverse relationship between education and mortality rates with these differences more pronounced in males.

Hummer, R. et al (2013). The Effect of Educational Attainment on Adult Mortality in the United States. *Population bulletin*, [online] Available at: https://www.ncbi.nlm.nih.gov/pmc/articles/PMC4435622/#:~:text=At%20age%2025%2C%20women%20with,a%20difference%20of%2012%20years

Comparing these two demographic groups - White men and White women - less educated White men have substantially higher mortality rates (decreased life expectancy). Hummer and Hernandez (2013) postulated that lung cancer, respiratory diseases, accidents, and homicide account for the higher mortality rates between the two groups.

The impact of education on life expectancy amongst racial groups paints significant contrasts in outcomes. According to Hummer and Hernandez (2013), educational differences in mortality are wider among U.S. white adults than either Black or Hispanic adults. Highly educated whites have far lower mortality rates and longer life expectancies than whites with low levels of education.

Although highly educated Black and Hispanic adults also have lower mortality rates than their less-educated counterparts, compared to whites the "high education payoff" does not seem to be as strong among these minority groups (**Figure 4.**). One plausible reason is that Black people and Hispanics are more likely to attend and graduate from lower-quality high schools and colleges compared with whites and may not reap the same health and longevity benefits from their education as whites. *In addition, Black and Hispanic adults, even those with high education, encounter discrimination in various forms and contexts throughout their lives that affects their prospects for longevity.*

Hummer, R. et al (2013). The Effect of Educational Attainment on Adult Mortality in the United States. Population bulletin, [online] Available at:
https://www.ncbi.nlm.nih.gov/pmc/articles/PMC4435622/#:~:text=At%20age%2025%2C%20women%20with,a%20difference%20of%2012%20years

Figure 4.

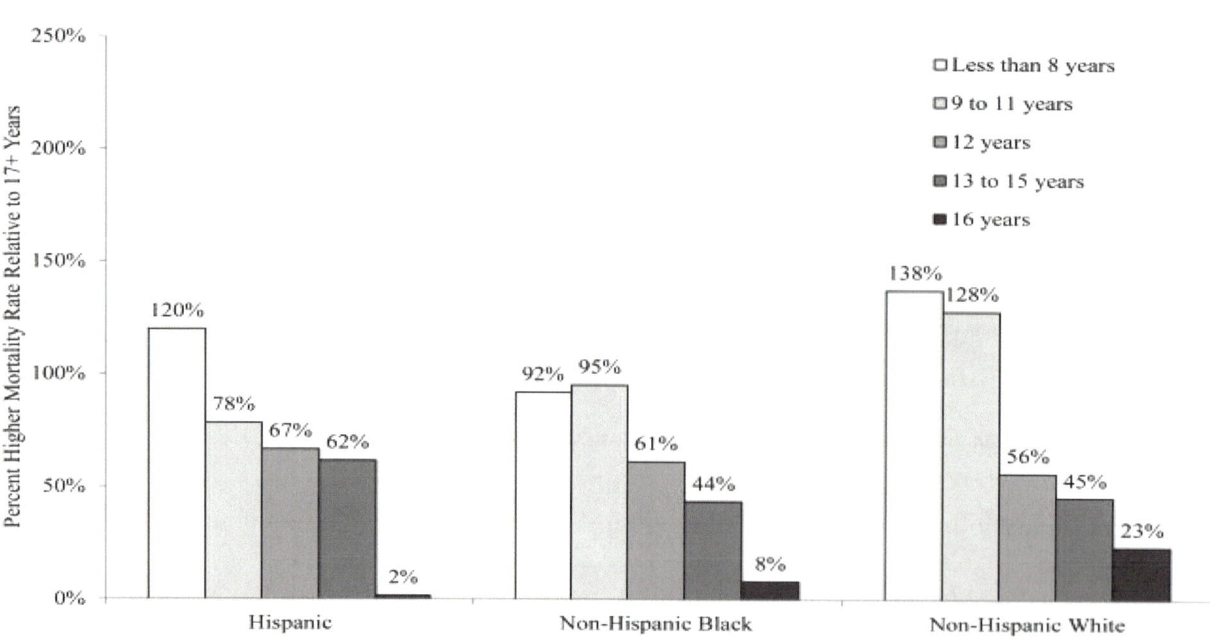

Figure 4. Adapted from Hummer (2013) shows that higher educational attainment is more beneficial in non-Hispanic whites, though the overall trend of decreased mortality rates in higher educated individuals is preserved.
https://www.ncbi.nlm.nih.gov/pmc/articles/PMC4435622/#:~:text=At%20age%2025%2C%20women%20with,a%20difference%20of%2012%20years

Roy et al. (2020) assessed the association of race/ethnicity and education on premature mortality amongst participants in a longitudinal investigation of 5114 adults recruited from 1985 to 1986 and followed for up to 29 years in the CARDIA study (1985 - 2017). Researchers balanced sex, Black and white race/ethnicity, education level (high school or less vs. greater than high school) and age. Cancer and cardiovascular disease stood out as the most common cause of mortality. Through their multivariant models, they determined that each year of lost education correlated with 1.37 less years of potential life (P=.007), while race/ethnicity were not independently associated with years of potential life lost (Roy et al., 2020).

The Virginia Commonwealth University Center on Society and Health (2022) cuts to the bottom line, *"Compared to those with a college education, Americans with less education die earlier. At age 25, U.S. adults without a high school diploma can expect to die 9 years sooner than college graduates."*

Education as a Social Determinant of Health

In the context of Employment and Income

The US Social Security Administration (2015) published relevant information on the impact of education on lifetime earnings.

> There are substantial differences in lifetime earnings by educational attainment.
> Men with bachelor's degrees earn approximately $900,000 more in median lifetime earnings than high school graduates. Women with bachelor's degrees earn $630,000 more. Men with graduate degrees earn $1.5 million more in median lifetime earnings than high school graduates. Women with graduate degrees earn $1.1 million more.
>
> Social Security Administration (2015). Education and Lifetime Earnings [online] Available at: https://www.ssa.gov/policy/docs/research-summaries/education-earnings.html

Further, the United States Bureau of Labor Statistics (2023) showed that median weekly earnings are directly correlated with level of educational attainment while unemployment rates are inversely correlated (**Figure 5**).

Figure 5.

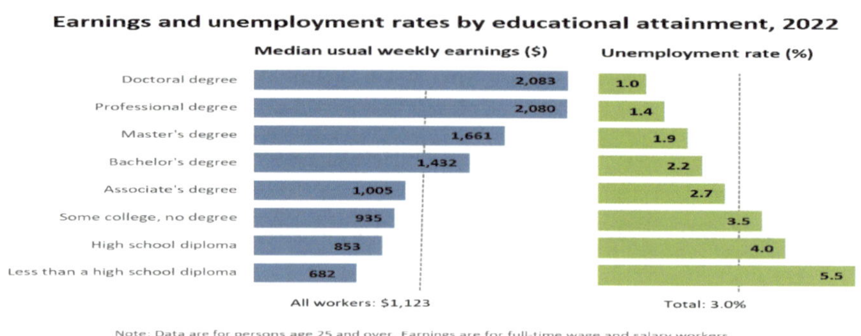

Figure 5. Adapted from the U.S. Bureau of Labor Statistics (2023), this figure demonstrates the relationship between education, median usual weekly earnings, and unemployment rates. https://www.bls.gov/emp/chart-unemployment-earnings-education.htm

The income gender gap (**Figure 6**) illustrates evidence for an ugly disparity when it comes to lifetime income demonstrating how it manifests as inequity and gender determinant of health comparing lifetime earnings of men and women.*

Figure 6.

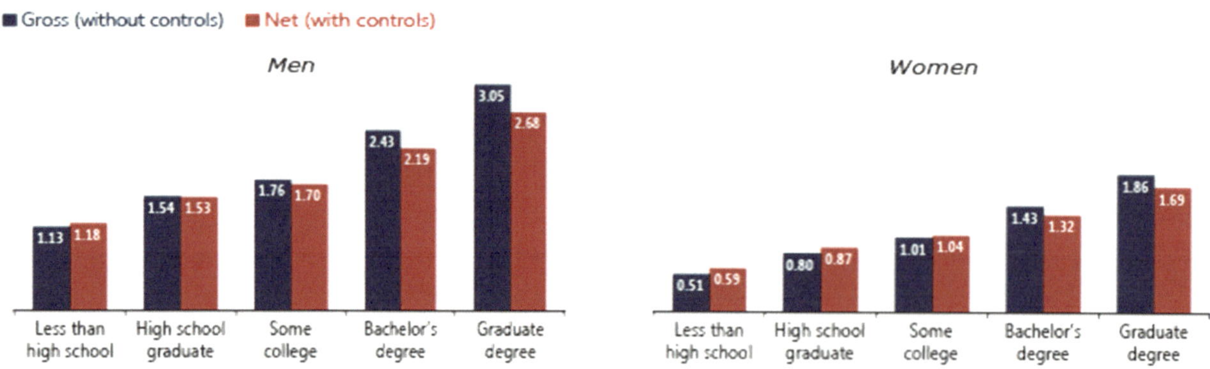

Tamborini, C. et al, (2015). Education and Lifetime Earnings in the United States. *Demography* [online] Available at: https://www.ncbi.nlm.nih.gov/pmc/articles/PMC4534330/

*Without and with controls applied/analyzed: race, marital status, geographic location, private vs. public education, college prep courses.

Politics, Policies, and Governance

Educational Attainment and Graduation Rates

According to the National Center for Education Statistics (NCES, 2021), the average adjusted cohort graduation rate in the U.S. increased from 79 percent in 2010 to 86 percent in 2018.

Figure 7, adapted from the NCES, illustrates the adjusted cohort graduation rate by state from 2018-2019.

Figure 7.

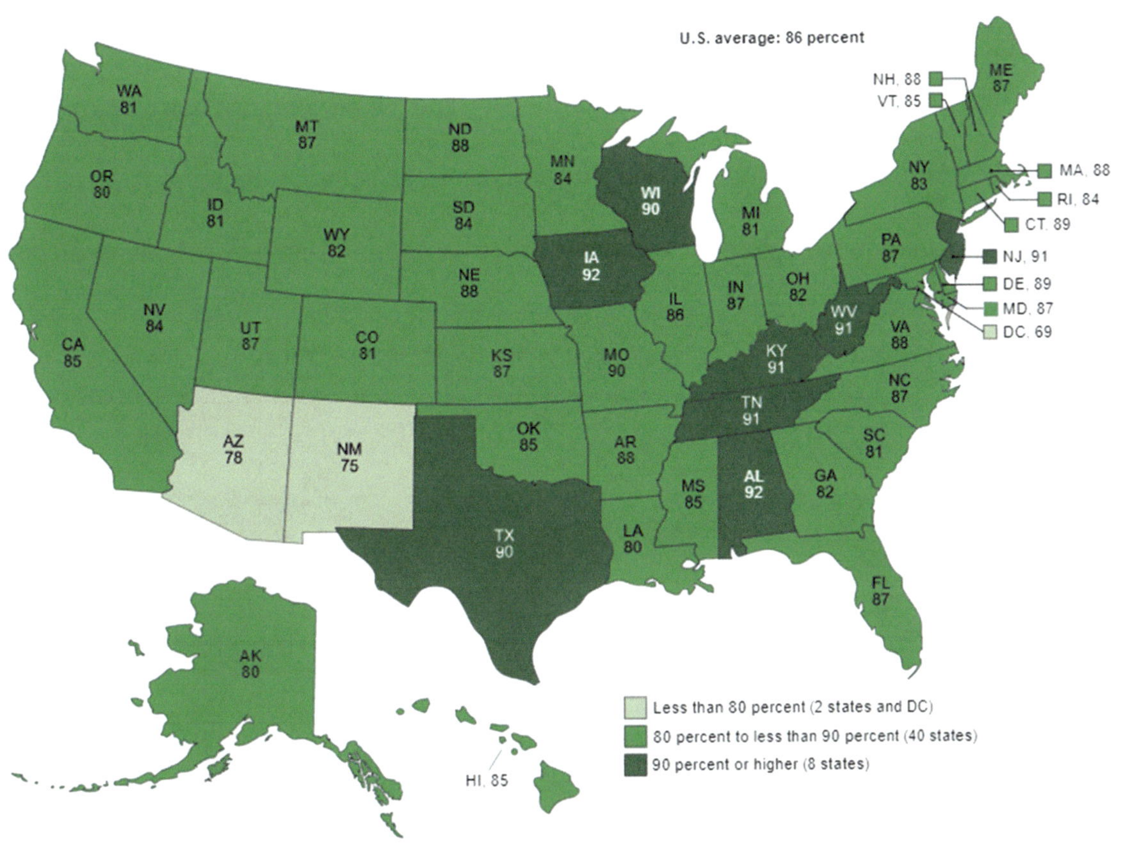

NOTE: The ACGR is the percentage of public high school freshmen who graduate with a regular diploma within 4 years of starting 9th grade. The U.S. average ACGR is for the 50 states and the District of Columbia. The graduation rates displayed above have been rounded to whole numbers. Categorizations are based on unrounded percentages. The Alabama State Department of Education has indicated that their ACGR data for some years was misstated. For more information, please see the following press release issued by the state: https://www.alsde.edu/sec/comm/News Releases/12-08-2016 Graduation Rate Review.pdf.

SOURCE: U.S. Department of Education, Office of Elementary and Secondary Education, Consolidated State Performance Report, 2018–19; and National Center for Education Statistics, EDFacts file 150, Data Group 695, and EDFacts file 151, Data Group 696, 2018–19. See *Digest of Education Statistics 2020*, table 219.46.

Figure 7. Adapted from NCES, shows the adjusted cohort graduate rate for public high school by state.
https://nces.ed.gov/programs/coe/indicator/coi/high-school-graduation-rates

Despite these encouraging gains, the Healthy People 2030 target to "increase the proportion of high school graduates in college the October after graduating" fell considerably below the 73.7% goal. Recent data from 2021 shows that only 61.8 percent of high school graduates continue to college, *a decrease from 69.1 percent* in 2018, Healthy People 2030 (2020). These statistics, coupled with the direct effect of educational attainment on health, life expectancy and income, call for research to analyze causal relationships and policy redirection on national and state levels to reverse the downward trends.

Low and Low (2019), research shows that current United States policies supporting basic education from ages 5-16 years and supporting access to post-secondary education places the United States with one of the highest rates of university and post-secondary enrollment in the world. However, despite these statistics, wide disparities exist between those able to obtain a college education, with minority children and those of low economic status less likely to do so.

Individual or Family	Neighborhood or Community	School or School System
• Low family socioeconomic status • Racial or ethnic group • Male • Special education status • Low family support for education, less opportunity for nonschool learning, few study aids and resources in the home • Low parental educational attainment • Residential mobility • Low social conformity • Low acceptance of adult authority • High levels of social isolation • Behaviors such as disruptive conduct, truancy, absenteeism, and lateness • Being held back in school • Poor academic achievement, low grades or test scores • Academic problems in early grades • Not liking school • Feelings of "not fitting in" and of not belonging • Perceptions of unfair or harsh disciplines • Feeling unsafe in school • Not engaged in school • Being suspended or expelled • Conflicts between work and school • Having to work or support family • Substance use • Pregnancy	• Living in a low-income neighborhood • Having peers with low educational aspirations • Having friends or siblings who are dropouts	• Low socioeconomic status of school population • High level of racial or ethnic segregation of students between schools in a district or within tracks or classes in a building • High proportion of students of color in school • High proportion of students enrolled in special education • Location in central city • Large school district • School safety and disciplinary policies • High-stakes testing • High student-to-teacher ratios • Academic tracking • Discrepancy between the racial or ethnic composition of students and faculty • Lack of programs and support for transition into high school for 9th and 10th graders
References: 16-20	References: 21-23	References: 16, 24-26

Table 1: Freudenberg and Ruglis (2007). Reframing School Dropout as a Public Health Issue: Preventing Chronic Disease. *Centers for Disease Control and Prevention* [online] Available at: https://www.cdc.gov/pcd/issues/2007/oct/07_0063.htm

Freudenberg and Ruglis (2007) shine light on school dropout rates and missed Healthy People 2030 targets for college enrollment following graduation. They argue that understanding reasons for dropout rates are crucial to designing policies that improve progressive educational attainment. As illustrated, multiple factors come into play – individual or family, neighborhood or community, and school or school systems **(Table 1.)**. Individual factors (left hand column) play profoundly with poverty, race, social isolation, gender, substance use, low family support for education, mental health, social isolation, and pregnancy highlighting the many family and individual explanations for school dropouts.

With such a diverse array of factors contributing to dropout, no one solution fits all; clearly, tackling the crisis demands tailor made, customized strategies that fit unique situations. According to Freudenberg and Ruglis (2007), most educational research on decreasing dropout rate focuses on interventions that alter school curriculum, improving teacher support, or changing the institutional mindset of schools. However, more attention to improving student well-being needs attention, they argue.

HEALTH INTERVENTIONS

Interventions to reduce school dropout rates seek to change individuals, families, schools, school systems, or public policies related to poverty, welfare, or employment. Most educational research has focused on evaluating interventions designed to alter the school curriculum, improve support for teachers, or change the institutional mindset in schools.

Interventions that have the potential to improve school achievement and reduce school dropout rates by improving the health of students are of particular interest to health professionals. These school-based interventions include coordinated school health programs; health clinics; mental health programs; substance abuse prevention and treatment programs; comprehensive sex education, human immunodeficiency virus infection prevention, and pregnancy prevention programs; special services for pregnant and parenting teens; violence prevention programs; and interventions to change the schools' social climate.

Freudenberg and Ruglis (2007). Reframing School Dropout as a Public Health Issue: Preventing Chronic Disease. Centers for Disease Control and Prevention [online] Available at: https://www.cdc.gov/pcd/issues/2007/oct/07_0063.htm

Based on Freudenberg's Ruglis' research the CDC makes the following policy recommendations:

CDC Policy Recommendations to Improve Educational Attainment

- Target schools and cities with the most serious dropout problems for intensive intervention.
- Develop, implement, and evaluate health interventions to improve school completion rates.
- Strengthen support for health education teachers.
- Advocate for evidence-based interventions that can improve health and reduce dropout rates.
- Put reducing high school dropout rates on the public health agenda.

Politics, Policies, and Governance

Educational Opportunity & Diversity

On June 29, 2023, the Supreme Court of the United States (2023) ruled that affirmative action policies used to increase diversity and access to educational opportunity were unconstitutional in so much as they violate the Equal Protection Clause of the 14th amendment.

The Fourteenth Amendment to the United States Constitution followed in the aftermath of the Civil War. Passed by Congress June 13, 1866, and ratified July 9, 1868, the 14th Amendment extended liberties and rights granted by the Bill of Rights to formerly enslaved people (National Archives, 2022).

14th Amendment to the U.S. constitution: Civil Rights (1868)
Section 1
All persons born or naturalized in the United States, and subject to the jurisdiction thereof, are citizens of the United States and of the State wherein they reside. No State shall make or enforce any law which shall abridge the privileges or immunities of citizens of the United States; nor shall any State deprive any person of life, liberty, or property, without due process of law; nor deny to any person within its jurisdiction the equal protection of the laws.

National Archives, 2022. *Milestone Documents. 14th Amendment to the U.S. constitution: Civil Rights (1868).* [online] Available at: https://www.archives.gov/milestone-documents/14th-amendment#:~:text=No%20State%20shall%20make%20or,Section%202

According to the American Association for Access, Equity and Diversity (AAAED, 2022), the Students for Fair Admissions (SFFA) filed a lawsuit against Harvard College in the District

Court of Massachusetts on November 17, 2014. SFFA claimed that Harvard's race conscious admissions policy was unlawful and discriminated against Asian American applicants in violation of Title VI of the Civil Rights Act of 1964.

The complaint underwent a variety of judicial rejections and appeals over the ensuing eight years when, according to the American Association for Access, Equity and Diversity (AAAED), on January 24, 2022 the Supreme court agreed to hear *SFFA v. President & Fellows of Harvard College, consolidated with SFFA v. University of North Carolina.* Unlike Harvard, UNC is a public university, which is covered by the 14th Amendment's guarantee of equal protection. In this case, the plaintiffs argued that the university's consideration of race in its undergraduate admissions process violates both Title VI and the Constitution" (AAAED, 2022).

According to their website, Students for Fair Admissions is a nonprofit membership group of more than 20,000 students, parents, and others who believe that racial classifications and preferences in college admissions are unfair, unnecessary, and unconstitutional. "Our mission is to support and participate in litigation that will restore the original principles of our nation's civil rights movement: A student's race and ethnicity should not be factors that either harm or help that student to gain admission to a competitive university" (Students for Fair Admissions, 2023a). The challenge was argued thus:

STUDENTS FOR FAIR ADMISSIONS, INC. *v.* PRESIDENT AND FELLOWS OF HARVARD COLLEGE

Argued October 31, 2022—Decided June 29, 2023

Harvard College and the University of North Carolina (UNC) are two of the oldest institutions of higher learning in the United States. Every year, tens of thousands of students apply to each school; many fewer are admitted. Both Harvard and UNC employ a highly selective admissions process to make their decisions. Admission to each school can depend on a student's grades, recommendation letters, or extracurricular involvement. It can also depend on their race. The question presented is whether the admissions systems used by Harvard College and UNC are lawful under the Equal Protection Clause of the Fourteenth Amendment.

Supreme Court of the United States (2023). Students for Fair Admission, Inc. v. President and Fellows of Harvard College [online] Available at. https://www.supremecourt.gov/opinions/22pdf/20-1199_hgdj.pdf

Chief Justice John Roberts authored the majority opinion. Justice Roberts received undergraduate and law degrees from Harvard College, graduating *magna cum laude* in 1979. President George W. Bush nominated Roberts to Chief Justice in 2005. In conclusion of his lengthy argument, Chief Justice Roberts wrote:

> For the reasons provided above, the Harvard and UNC admissions programs cannot be reconciled with the guarantees of the Equal Protection Clause. Both programs lack sufficiently focused and measurable objectives warranting the use of race, unavoidably employ race in a negative manner, involve racial stereotyping, and lack meaningful end points. We have never permitted admissions programs to work in that way, and we will not do so today.
>
> At the same time, as all parties agree, nothing in this opinion should be construed as prohibiting universities from considering an applicant's discussion of how race affected his or her life, be it through discrimination, inspiration, or otherwise. But, despite the dissent's assertion to the contrary, universities may not simply establish through application essays or other means the regime we hold unlawful today.
>
> Supreme Court of the United States (2023). Students for Fair Admission, Inc. v. President and Fellows of Harvard College [online] Available at:
> https://www.supremecourt.gov/opinions/22pdf/20-1199_hgdj.pdf

Supreme Court Associate Justice Clarence Thomas concurred with the majority opinion. According to the Supreme Court Historical Society (2023), Thomas graduated from the College of the Holy Cross in 1971 and Yale Law School in 1974. It is alleged that Thomas participated in student activism in his early years connecting with the Black Muslim and the Black Power movements and the principles of Malcolm X but disillusioned, turned away from leftist movements. He served as Assistant Secretary for Civil Rights in the United States Department of Education 1981 and on July 1, 1991, President George H. W. Bush nominated Thomas to the Supreme Court of the United States. The Senate confirmed the appointment on October 15, 1991. At the time of his appointment, he was just the second African American appointed to the U.S. Supreme Court (Supreme Court Historical Society, 2023).

According to his website, "Justice Thomas has been a vigorous defender of the First Amendment and a strong voice for Second Amendment rights. Consistent with this approach, Justice Thomas has also held that the Constitution permits no discrimination based on race, and that the Constitution leaves certain moral and social choices, such as abortion and same-sex marriage, to the States" (Justice Clarence Thomas, 2023).

His concurrence with the majority opinion is synthesized thus:

> In the 1860s, Congress proposed, and the States ratified the Thirteenth and Fourteenth Amendments. And, with the authority conferred by these Amendments, Congress passed two landmark Civil Rights Acts. Throughout the debates on each of these measures, their proponents repeatedly affirmed their view of equal citizenship and the racial equality that flows from it.
>
> In fact, they held this principle so deeply that their crowning accomplishment—the Fourteenth Amendment—ensures racial equality *with no textual reference to race whatsoever*. The history of these measures' enactment renders their motivating principle as clear as their text: All citizens of the United States, regardless of skin color, are equal before the law.
>
> Supreme Court of the United States (2023). Students for Fair Admission, Inc. v. President and Fellows of Harvard College [online] Available at:
> https://www.supremecourt.gov/opinions/22pdf/20-1199_hgdj.pdf

Associate Supreme Court Justices Sonia Sotomayor (Yale School of Law, nominated by President Barack Obama), Elena Kagan (Harvard School of Law, nominated by President Barack Obama) and Ketanji Brown Jackson (Harvard School of Law, nominated by President Joe Biden) joined in writing the dissenting opinion (Supreme Court Historical Society, 2023).

The following characterizes the basis of their dissent:

> The Equal Protection Clause of the Fourteenth Amendment enshrines a guarantee of racial equality. The Court long ago concluded that this guarantee can be enforced through race-conscious means in a society that is not, and has never been, colorblind. In Brown v. Board of Education, 347 U. S. 483 (1954), the Court recognized the constitutional necessity of racially integrated schools in light of the harm inflicted by segregation and the "importance of education to our democratic society."
>
> For 45 years, the Court extended Brown's transformative legacy to the context of higher education, allowing colleges and universities to consider race in a limited way and for the limited purpose of promoting the important benefits of racial diversity. This limited use of race has helped equalize educational opportunities for all students of every race and background and has improved racial diversity on college campuses.

Dissent (continued)

Despite the Court's unjustified exercise of power, the opinion today will serve only to highlight the Court's own impotence in the face of an America whose cries for equality resound. As has been the case before in the history of American democracy, "the arc of the moral universe" will bend toward racial justice despite the Court's efforts today to impede its progress. Martin Luther King "Our God is Marching On!" Speech (Mar. 25, 1965).

Supreme Court of the United States (2023. Students for Fair Admission, Inc. v. President and Fellows of Harvard College [online] Available at: https://www.supremecourt.gov/opinions/22pdf/20-1199_hgdj.pdf

Associate Chief Justice Ketanji Brown Jackson became the 116th Associate Justice of the Supreme Court following her nomination by President Joe Biden in 2021 and confirmation in 2022. She sits as just the 3rd African American Justice and but a handful of women Justices historically. Justice Jackson attended Harvard College for both undergraduate and law school earning Juris Doctor in 1996 (Supreme Court Historical Society, 2023). A brief portion of her articulated dissent appears as quoted below.

Gulf-sized race-based gaps exist with respect to the health, wealth, and well-being of American citizens. They were created in the distant past but have indisputably been passed down to the present day through the generations. Every moment these gaps persist is a moment in which this great country falls short of actualizing one of its foundational principles—the "self-evident" truth that all of us are created equal.

The Court has come to rest on the bottom-line conclusion that racial diversity in higher education is only worth potentially preserving insofar as it might be needed to prepare Black Americans and other underrepresented minorities for success in the bunker, not the boardroom (a particularly awkward place to land, in light of the history the majority opts to ignore). It would be deeply unfortunate if the Equal Protection Clause actually demanded this perverse, ahistorical, and counterproductive outcome. To impose this result in that Clause's name when it requires no such thing, and to thereby obstruct our collective progress toward the full realization of the Clause's promise, is truly a tragedy for us all.

Supreme Court of the United States (2023). Students for Fair Admission, Inc. v. President and Fellows of Harvard College [online] Available at:
https://www.supremecourt.gov/opinions/22pdf/20-1199_hgdj.pdf

The President and Chancellors of the University of California authored an amici curiae (https://www.law.cornell.edu/wex/amicus_curiae) on behalf of the Respondents (Harvard University and the University of North Carolina Chapel Hill). According to the brief, California's

Proposition 209 enacted in 1996, "amended California Constitution to prohibit the use of race in various settings, including university and college admissions." In the wake of Proposition 209, the proportion of students from underrepresented minority groups fell dramatically throughout the UC system" (Robinson et al., n.d.). As a result, the UC system implemented various strategies to reverse the impact of Proposition 209, which improved the student body diversity substantially.

"But recognition of that achievement is tempered by two important concerns. First, UC's diversity gains have not been shared equally among all campuses— and it is diversity at the campus level that is most relevant to students' experiences and to UC's ability to provide the educational benefits of diversity. It is on their particular campus—in classrooms, dorms, and in extracurricular activities—that students will interact with one another. Particularly at UC's most selective campuses, feelings of racial isolation persist and hinder UC's efforts to provide the educational benefits of diversity. Second, UC's student population at many of its campuses is now starkly different, demographically speaking, from the population of California high school graduates. That raises concerns that UC is not enrolling sufficient students with diverse perspectives, and that it will not be perceived as open to, and welcoming of, all students across the State—which in turn threatens its legitimacy in the eyes of citizens of California. Those two issues persist despite UC's substantial efforts since Proposition 209 to pursue the educational benefits of diversity through race-neutral programs. At the same time, UC's extensive experience with a wide range of race-neutral measures has revealed that each of these measures has limitations that prevent UC from simply increasing its reliance on each measure to further increase racial diversity" (Robinson, n.d.).

Despite the benefit of California's experience and the untoward impact of race-neutral admissions wrought by Proposition 209, the Supreme Court of the United States found for Students for Fair Admissions, Inc. in a 6-3 decision, effectively outlawing Affirmative Action in college and university admissions.

The Students for Fair Admissions now ask: "*Are universities preparing to circumvent Supreme Court decision banning affirmative action?*"

di·ver·si·ty
1: The very thing that makes the world a better place
2: The very thing that provides equal opportunity
DIVERSITY IS A NECESSITY
AFFIRM OPPORTUNITY
AFFIRM OUR FUTURE
MALDEF
#AffirmOpportunity
MY
IS
MY
STORY
#DefendDiversity

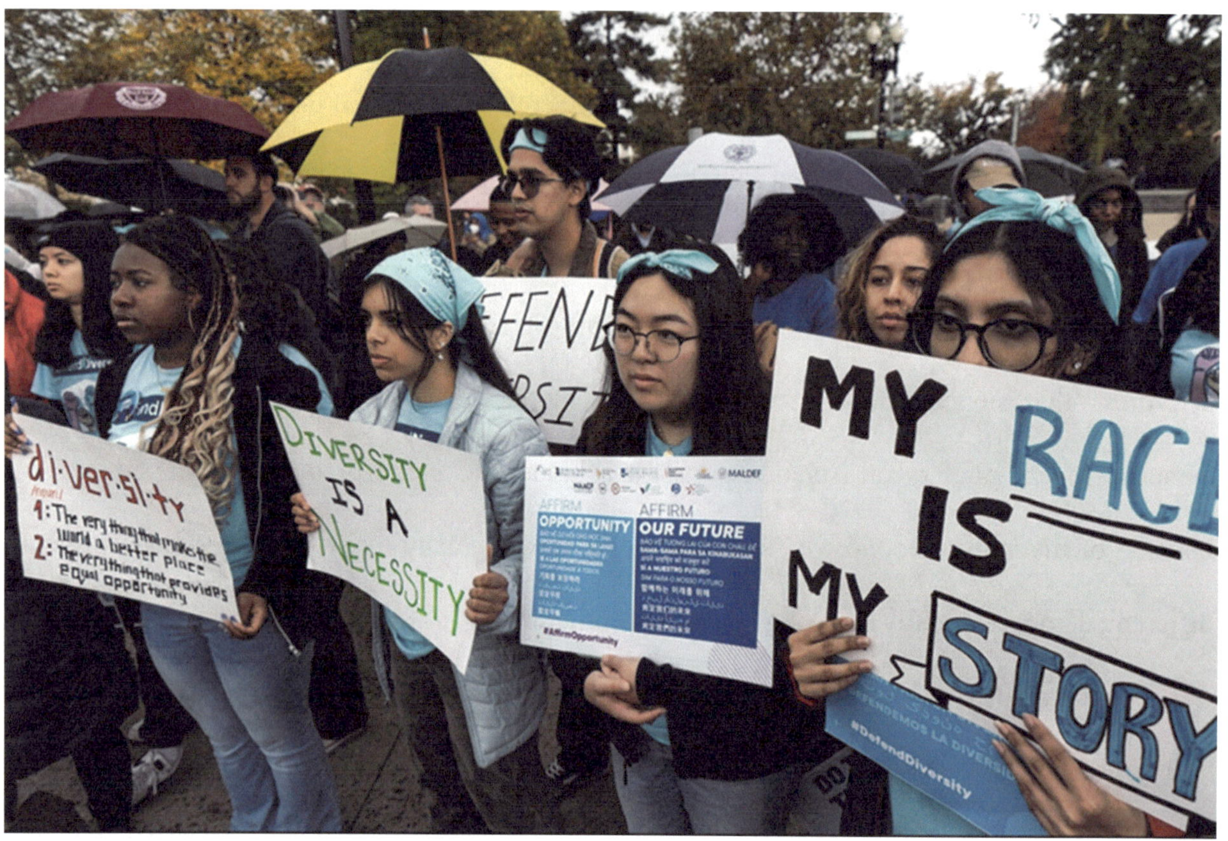

Students for Fair Admissions (2023b). *Are Universities preparing to circumvent Supreme court decision banning affirmative action?* [online] Available at: https://studentsforfairadmissions.org/are-universities-preparing-to-circumvent-supreme-court-decision-banning-affirmative-action/Asswill

Questions for Further Consideration:

1. What factors contribute to the finding that health outcomes are similar in individuals who have graduated high school and those who have had some college education (without obtaining a degree)?
2. Although high school dropout rates have steadily decreased in recent years, what factors contribute to the finding that there is a decrease in the number of high school graduates

enrolling in college as seen in the Healthy People 2030 data? What can be done to increase enrollment?

3. Of the health factors that impact high school dropout rates, teenage pregnancy leads the forefront of causes with only 40% of teenage mothers completing high school. What strategies might be employed to improve graduation rates of teenage mothers?
4. The CDC recommends several Health Interventions to reduce high school dropout. Which has been shown to be most effective?

Sentinel Readings for a Deeper Dive

Supreme Court of the United States, 2023. Students for Fair Admission, Inc. v. President and Fellows of Harvard College [online] Available at: https://www.supremecourt.gov/opinions/22pdf/20-1199_hgdj.pdf

American Public Health Association, 2018. *The Dropout Crisis: A Public Health Problem and the role of School-Based Health Care*. February 2018. [online] Available at: https://www.apha.org/-/media/Files/PDF/SBHC/Dropout_Crisis.ashx

Office of Disease Prevention and Health Promotion (2020). *Education Access and Quality - Healthy People 2030* [online] Available at: https://health.gov/healthypeople/objectives-and-data/browse-objectives/education-access-and-quality

Lansford, J., et al., (2016). A Public Health Perspective on School Dropout and Adult Outcomes: A Prospective Study of Risk and Protective Factors from Age 5 to 27 Years. *Journal of Adolescent Health* [online] Available at: https://www.ncbi.nlm.nih.gov/pmc/articles/PMC4877222/#R1

References

AAAED (2019). *History of Affirmative Action | American Association for Access Equity and Diversity - AAAED*. American Association for Access Equity and Diversity - AAAED. [online] Available at: https://www.aaaed.org/aaaed/history_of_affirmative_action.asp [Accessed 16 July 2023].

APHA (2018). The Dropout Crisis: A Public Health Problem and the role of School-Based Health Care. *American Public Health Association* [online] Available at: https://www.apha.org/-/media/Files/PDF/SBHC/Dropout_Crisis.ashx [Accessed 5 May 2023].

Freudenberg, N. and Ruglis, J. (2007). Reframing school dropout as a public health issue. *Prev Chronic Dis./Centers for Disease Control and Prevention* [online] Available at: https://www.cdc.gov/pcd/issues/2007/oct/07_0063.htm [Accessed 5 May 2023].

Hummer, R. and Hernandez, E. (2013). The Effect of Educational Attainment on Adult Mortality in the United States. *Population bulletin*, [online] Available at: https://www.ncbi.nlm.nih.gov/pmc/articles/PMC4435622/#:~:text=At%20age%2025%2C%20women%20with,a%20difference%20of%2012%20years [Accessed May – July, 2023].

Lansford, J., Dodge, K., Pettit, G. and Bates, J. (2016). A Public Health Perspective on School Dropout and Adult Outcomes: A Prospective Study of Risk and Protective Factors from Age 5 to 27 Years. *Journal of Adolescent Health* [online] Available at: https://www.ncbi.nlm.nih.gov/pmc/articles/PMC4877222/ [Accessed May – July 2023].

Low, B. and Low, D. (2019). Education and Education Policy as Social Determinants of Health. *AMA Journal of Ethics*, 8(11), pp.756–761. [online] Available at: https://journalofethics.ama-assn.org/article/education-and-education-policy-social-determinants-health/2006-11 [Accessed 5 May 2023].

National Archives (2022). *Milestone Documents. 14th Amendment to the U.S. constitution: Civil Rights (1868).* [online] Available at: https://www.archives.gov/milestone-documents/14th-amendment#:~:text=No%20State%20shall%20make%20or,Section%202 [Accessed July 16, 2023].

NCES (2021). *COE - Public High School Graduation Rates*. National Center for Education Statistics [online] Available at: https://nces.ed.gov/programs/coe/indicator/coi/high-school-graduation-rates [Accessed 5 May 2023].

NCES (2023). *COE – International Education Attainment.* National Center for Education Statistics [online] Available at: https://nces.ed.gov/programs/coe/indicator/cac/intl-ed-attainment#:~:text=The%20high%20school%20completion%20rate [Accessed May – July 2023].

Office of Disease Prevention and Health Promotion (2020). *Education Access and Quality - Healthy People 2030 | health.gov*. [online] Available at: https://health.gov/healthypeople/objectives-and-data/browse-objectives/education-access-and-quality [Accessed May - July 2023].

Robinson, C., Woodall, A., Goldstein, R., Essick, K., Yap, E., Anders, G., Verrilli, D. and Munger (n.d.). *In the Supreme Court of the United States Respondents. ON WRITS OF CERTIORARI TO THE UNITED STATES COURTS OF APPEALS FOR THE FIRST AND FOURTH CIRCUITS BRIEF FOR THE PRESIDENT AND CHANCELLORS OF THE UNIVERSITY OF CALIFORNIA AS AMICI CURIAE SUPPORTING RESPONDENTS Counsel for Amici Curiae (additional counsel on inside cover)*. [online] Available at: https://www.supremecourt.gov/DocketPDF/20/20-1199/232355/20220801134931730_20-1199%20bsac%20University%20of%20California.pdf [Accessed 15 July 2023].

Roy, B., Kiefe, C., Jacobs, D., Goff, D., Lloyd-Jones, D., Shikany, J., Reis, J., Gordon-Larsen, P. and Lewis, C. (2020). Education, Race/Ethnicity, and Causes of Premature Mortality Among Middle-Aged Adults in 4 US Urban Communities: Results From CARDIA, 1985–2017. *American Journal of Public Health*, 110(4), pp.530–536. [online] https://ajph.aphapublications.org/doi/full/10.2105/AJPH.2019.305506 [Accessed May – July, 2023].

Social Security Administration (2015). *Education and Lifetime Earnings* [online] Available at: https://www.ssa.gov/policy/docs/research-summaries/education-earnings.html [Accessed July 9, 2023].

Students for Fair Admissions (2023a). *Help Us Eliminate Race and Ethnicity from College Admissions.* [online] Available at: https://studentsforfairadmissions.org/ [Accessed 16 July 2023].

Students for Fair Admissions (2023b). *Are Universities preparing to circumvent Supreme court decision banning affirmative action?* [online] Available at: https://studentsforfairadmissions.org/are-universities-preparing-to-circumvent-supreme-court-decision-banning-affirmative-action/ [Accessed 14 July 2023].

Supreme Court Historical Society (2023). *The Current Court: Justice Clarence Thomas.* [online] Available at: https://supremecourthistory.org/supreme-court-justices/associate-justice-clarence-thomas/ [Accessed 16 July 2023].

Supreme Court of the United States (2023). Students for Fair Admission, Inc. v. President and Fellows of Harvard College [online] Available at: https://www.supremecourt.gov/opinions/22pdf/20-1199_hgdj.pdf [Accessed 12 July 2023].

Tamborini, C., Kim, C. and Sakamoto, A. (2015). Education and Lifetime Earnings in the United States. *Demography* [online] Available at: https://www.ncbi.nlm.nih.gov/pmc/articles/PMC4534330/ [Accessed 9 July 2023].

U.S. Bureau of Labor Statistics (2023). *Unemployment Rates and Earnings by Educational Attainment : U.S. Bureau of Labor Statistics*. [online] Available at: https://www.bls.gov/emp/chart-unemployment-earnings-education.htm [Accessed 9 July 2023].

Vaivada, T., Sharma, N., Das, J., Salam, R., Lassi, Z. and Bhutta, Z. (2023). Interventions for Health and Well-being in School-Aged Children and Adolescents: A Way Forward. *American Academy of Pediatrics* [online] Available at: https://publications.aap.org/pediatrics/article/149/Supplement%206/e2021053852M/186939/Interventions-for-Health-and-Well-Being-in-School?autologincheck=redirected [Accessed 7 May 2023].

Virginia Commonwealth University Center on Society and Health (2022). *Education: It Matters More to Health than Ever Before* [online] Available at: https://societyhealth.vcu.edu/work/the-projects/education-it-matters-more-to-health-than-ever-before.html#gsc.tab=0 [Accessed July 9, 2023].

Zajacova, A. and Lawrence, E. (2018). The Relationship Between Education and Health: Reducing Disparities Through a Contextual Approach. *Annual Review of Public Health*, [online] Available at: https://pubmed.ncbi.nlm.nih.gov/29328865/ [Accessed May - July 2023].

Lexicon of Listed Terms and Agencies

- **American Public Health Association**, APHA, is the publisher of the American Journal of Public Health and The *Nation's Health* newspaper. Research on public health is shared through the APHA annual meetings. APHA's mission strives to improve the health of the population and to achieve health equity.

- **National Center for Education Statistics (NCES)** is a statistical agency utilized by the United States Department of Education. Through a congressional mandate, this agency collects, analyzes, and reports statistics regarding American education.

- **The Healthy People Initiative** started as the "Healthy People: The Surgeon General's Report on Health Promotion and Disease Prevention" in 1979. Inspired by Surgeon General Julius Richmond, Healthy People set out to create 10-year objectives focusing on the nation's health and well-being. Healthy People 2030, launched in August 2020, setting out 358 core measurable objectives with an emphasis on social determinants of health, health equity and literacy.

- **The Organization for Economic Cooperation and Development**, OCED, includes 37 countries that emphasize trade and economic growth. Data is collected through this organization. Data specifically pertaining to education is reported through the NCES.

- **The Universal Declaration of Human Rights (UDHR)** represents a milestone document in the history of human rights. Drafted by representatives with different legal and cultural backgrounds from all regions of the world, the declaration was proclaimed by the United Nations General Assembly in Paris on 10 December 1948 as a common standard of achievements for all peoples and all nations. It set out, for the first time, fundamental human rights to be universally protected. The UDHR has been translated into over 500 languages. It is widely recognized as having inspired, and paved the way for, the adoption of more than 70 human rights treaties, applied today on a permanent basis at global and regional levels.

- **United States Bureau of Labor Statistics** is an agency within the United States Department of Labor that serves as part of the United States Federal Statistical System. It is a fact-finding agency for the field of labor economics and statistics.

AUTHOR'S BIO SKETCH

Nicole Delos Santos, MD

Nicole Delos Santos received the degree of Doctor of Medicine from the University of Nevada Reno in 2022. Born in Honolulu, HI she moved from her childhood home to Las Vegas, NV where she attended the University of Nevada Las Vegas receiving a Bachelor of Science in Biology. Nicole is a resident in Family Medicine at the University of Washington affiliated Community Health Care Family Residency in Tacoma, WA, a Federally Qualified Teaching Health and Patient Care Center. Dr. Delos Santos embraces a passion for working with low-income and marginalized populations who have limited access to healthcare.

Chapter 9

Work Environment as a Social Determinant of Health

Andrea Lynde, DO, Author
Stephen, Cook, MD, Editor

"A little consideration, a little thought for others, makes all the difference."
-Eeyore (from Winnie the Pooh)

"*Safety is the most basic task of all. Without a sense of safety, no growth can take place. Without safety, all energy goes to defense.*"
-Torey Hayden, special education teacher and non-fiction writer

Work Environment as a Social Determinant of Health

Introduction

Work environments profoundly influence individual well-being, making it a pivotal social determinant of health. Indicators of positive work situations encompass jobs providing physically and emotionally healthy environments, receiving a livable wage, and enjoying benefits like health insurance and paid time off. It involves prioritizing work-life balance, offering opportunities for skill growth, continuing education, advancement, and fostering positive relationships between employees and employers (Steege, et al., 2023).

Physical factors, such as air quality, personal protective equipment, ergonomic design, and safety protocols, directly affect physical health. Attention to them mitigates the potential for respiratory disorders, life threatening viral and bacterial infections, accidents, overuse syndromes, and falls. Mental health and overall quality of life are heavily influenced by job satisfaction, occupational stress levels, and work-life balance. Prolonged exposure to high-stress environments, long working hours, shift work or toxic work cultures leads to burnout and mental health disarray.

This essay takes two significant historical workplace examples – the COVID-19 pandemic and industrial exposure to asbestos – to illustrate how work environments evolve into emotional and physical health catastrophes.

Work Environment as a Social Determinant of Health

In the context of the COVID-19 Pandemic

The World Health Organization (2023) lists nine occupational hazards relating to the healthcare sector.

World Health Organization and Healthcare Risks

1. Occupational infections: tuberculosis, hepatitis B & C, HIV/AIDs, and respiratory infections (coronaviruses, influenza, RSV).
2. Exposure to hazardous chemicals: disinfecting agents, toxic medications, laboratory reagents and chemicals.
3. Exposure to radiation: ionizing and non-ionizing radiation in imaging centers, emergency departments and hospital wards.
4. Patient handling: lifting, transferring, repositioning, and moving patients without proper techniques or handling equipment.
5. Violence and harassment: incidents involving work related abuse, threats or assaults including physical, sexual, verbal, and psychological abuse and workplace harassment.
6. Psycho-social and mental health risks: lack of control over environment, shift work, time pressure, long hours, lack of support, moral injury.
7. Ambient work environment: noise, chaos, patient overcrowding, thermal discomfort.
8. Injuries: slips, trips, falls, electric shocks, fire, MVAs (ambulance, emergency vehicles).
9. Environmental hazards: inadequate sanitation, and hygiene, handling healthcare waste.

World Health Organization (2023). *Occupational Hazards in the Health Sector.* [online] www.who.int. Available at: https://www.who.int/tools/occupational-hazards-in-health-sector [Accessed 21 November 20232].

The pandemic dropped like a bomb in March 2020 leaving the entire U.S. workforce and economy dazed and confused. According to Mutikani (2020), from March 21, 2020, 26.453 million people filed claims for unemployment benefits, representing 16.2% of the labor force, leading to dire predictions of 30 million job losses during the COVID-19 pandemic and an unemployment rate at levels not seen since the Great Depression.

The chaos created by the COVID-19 pandemic exacerbated the impact of health sector occupational risks and hazards articulated by the World Health Organization (2023). The cumulative effect led to dramatic health professions burnout and for many healthcare employees who prided in their work, migration out of employment as healthcare professionals.

Burnout

In the context of the COVID-19 Pandemic

Emotional exhaustion, cynicism, and reduced personal accomplishment in the workplace define burnout. Emotional exhaustion involves the depletion of emotional and physical resources; cynicism relates to the interpersonal aspect of burnout; reduced accomplishment entails the feelings of incompetence that result from decreased productivity (Aronsson, et al., 2017). A peer reviewed meta-analysis published by Aronsson, and colleagues examined burnout concluding "while high levels of job support and workplace justice were protective for emotional exhaustion, high demands, low job control, high work load, low reward and job insecurity increased the risk for developing exhaustion" (Aronsson, et al., 2017). These negative circumstances mirror the workplace surroundings experienced by healthcare professionals – nurses, doctors, medical assistants, radiology technicians and housekeepers alike – during the COVID-19 pandemic, especially in hospital environments.

Burnout impacts both employees and employers. It translates into low motivation and job performance that metastasizes into the organizational fabric and leads to reduction in quality of services and products. Burnout promotes employee conflict that results in interruption of workflow, production schedules and reduction in manufacturing output or services (Edú-Valsania, Laguía and Moriano, 2022).

Exacerbated by the relentless demands and pressures from the healthcare industry, burnout among healthcare workers has become a critical issue. A study published in 2019 revealed that physicians in the United States have one of the highest burnout rates among all professions (Shanafelt et al., 2019). The COVID-19 pandemic further intensified this crisis as frontline workers faced unprecedented challenges and stresses. For most workers, remote work became the norm, with Zoom meetings and virtual collaboration taking precedence. Those deemed to be essential workers, such as healthcare employees, were forced to join the front lines facing a new battle not seen in over 100 years.

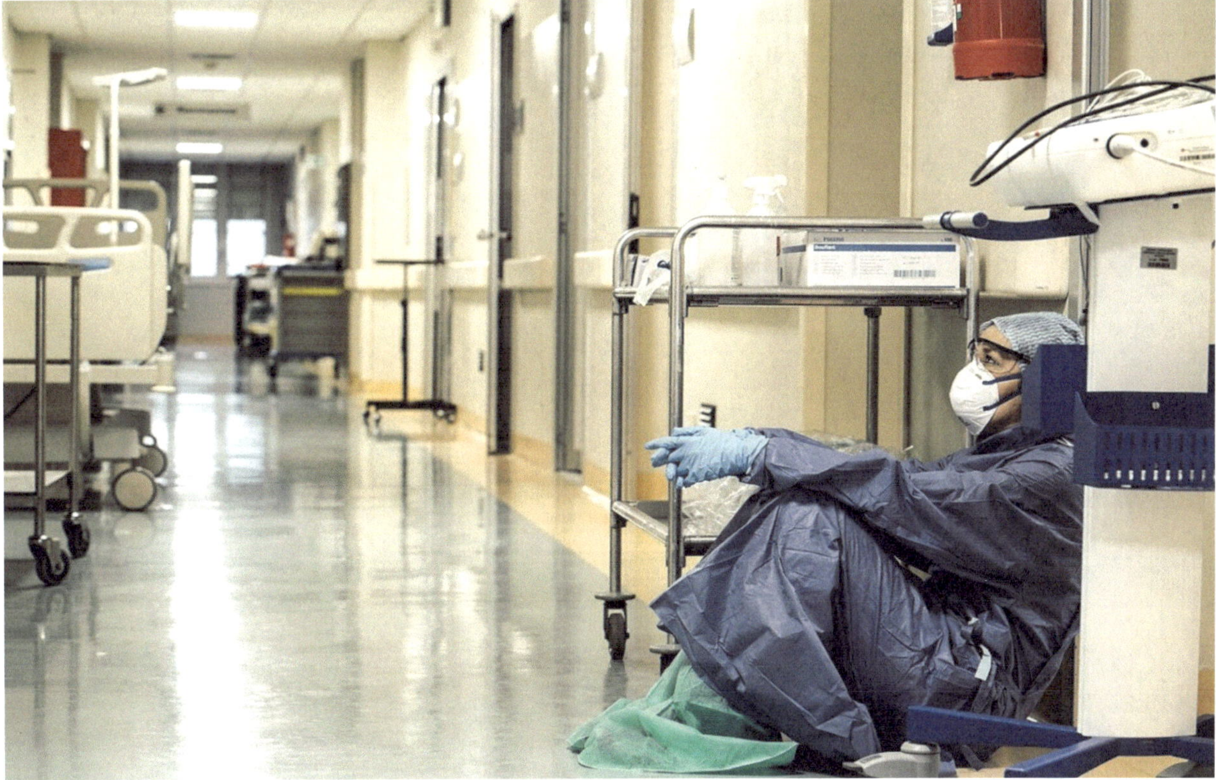

A physician sitting alone in the hospital at the end of her workday caring for COVID patients wearing the PPE required to care for these patients and maintain her own physical safety.

Hoban, R. (2022). *Within a decade, NC could be short more than 21,000 nurses.* [online] North Carolina Health News. Available at: https://www.northcarolinahealthnews.org/2022/03/02/within-a-decade-nc-could-see-nursing-shortage-of-more-than-21000/

As the pandemic progressed, it became apparent that workplace changes stemming from the COVID-19 disproportionately affected certain jobs and placed employees at increased risk of adverse effects (Armenti et al., 2023). For example, healthcare workers faced shortages of essential personal protective equipment (PPE), resorting to using garbage bags instead of isolation gowns, and employing single-use N95 masks for marathon 12-hour shifts. Nurses actively held iPads to facilitate final goodbyes with families, while refrigerated trucks were mobilized to accommodate overflowing morgues due to the overwhelming number of virus-related fatalities.

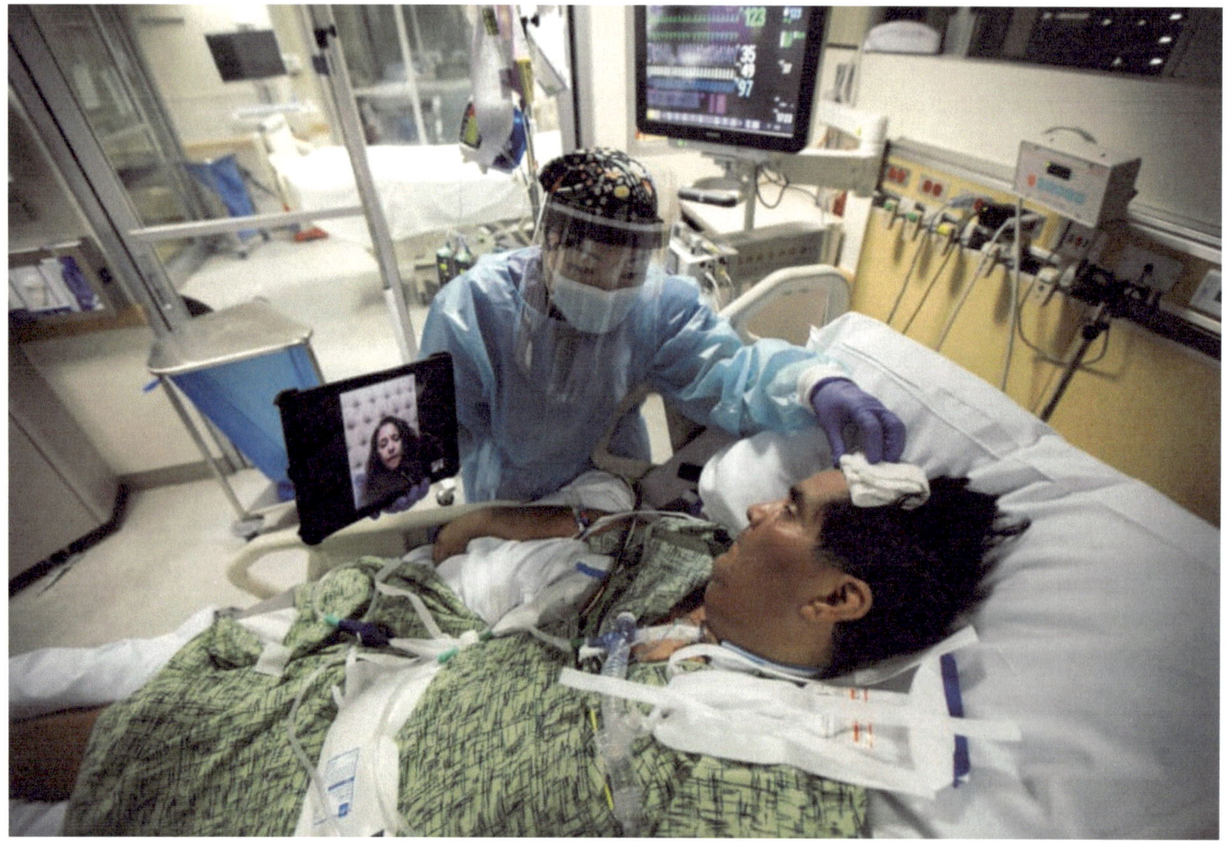

An ICU nurse holding an iPad giving her patient and his family an opportunity to see one another.

D'Couto, H. (2022). *Forcing my COVID patients to die alone is inhumane — and unnecessary*. [online] www.wbur.org. Available at: https://www.wbur.org/cognoscenti/2022/03/07/covid-patients-icu-dying-alone-helen-t-dcouto

Although posters and billboards across the nation expressed gratitude towards the "Healthcare Heroes," only those on the frontline utterly understood the day-to-day realities of battling COVID-19. A survey conducted by Mental Health America garnered responses from 1,119 healthcare workers aiming to glean insights and improve resources for those who tirelessly cared for others. The results depicted heightened levels of emotional exhaustion and psychological distress, stemming from the persistent fear of transmitting the virus to loved ones, inadequate PPE, witnessing unprecedented levels of patient suffering, and the profound challenge of not being able to deal with their own families (Mental Health America, 2021).

According to Leo, et al. (2021) frontline healthcare workers grappled with high rates of burnout, stemming from the ethical dilemmas and moral injuries resulting from the torment of making rapid life-or-death decisions in the setting of evolving care protocols.

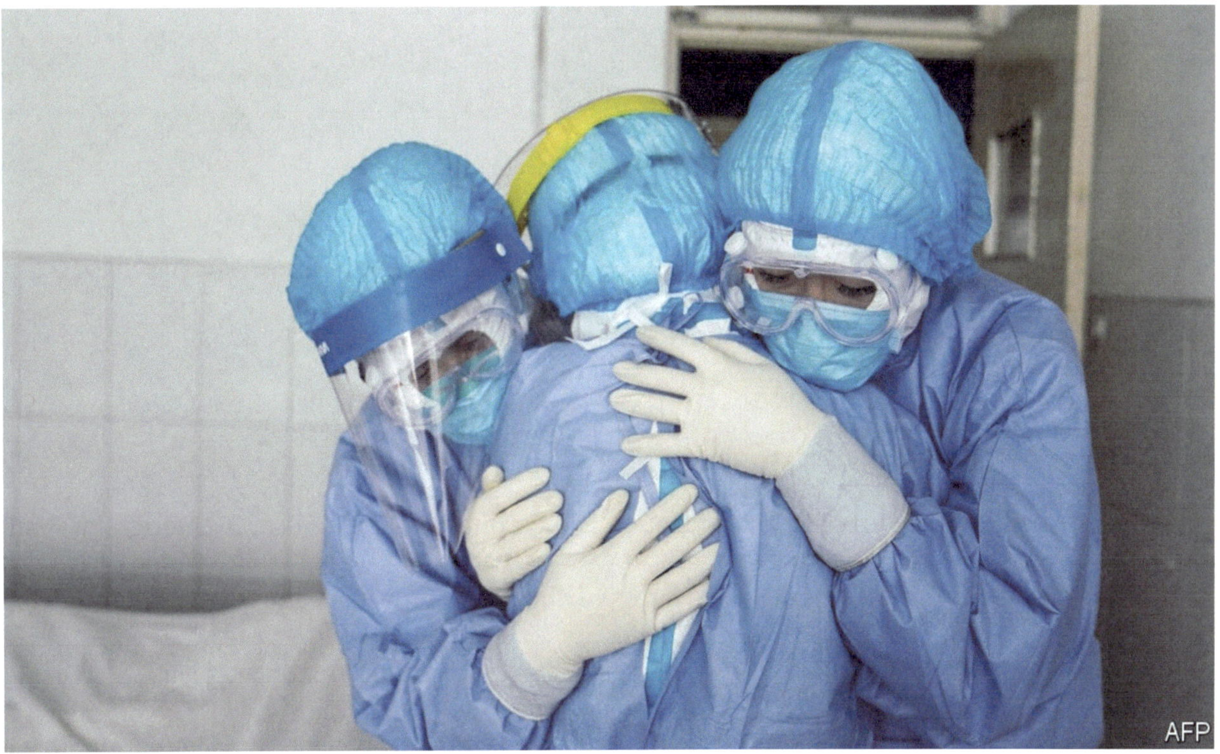

Healthcare workers embrace and provide solace to one another during the Covid-19 pandemic.

The Economist. (2020). *Health workers become unexpected targets during covid-19.* [online] Available at: https://www.economist.com/international/2020/05/11/health-workers-become-unexpected-targets-during-covid-19

Pandemic burnout directly impacted healthcare workers' psychological well-being and physical safety, contributing to elevated levels of anxiety (24.94% of employees), depression

(24.83%), and sleep disorders (44.03%). Nevertheless, many workers concealed their struggles, driven by a perceived stigma and the fear of potential repercussions on their career trajectories (Leo et al., 2021). The ripple effects extended to a 25% increase in the likelihood of alcohol abuse and a staggering 200% surge in the risk of experiencing suicidal ideation. **Figure 1.** illustrates the factors influencing workers and the subsequent outcomes with which they struggle.

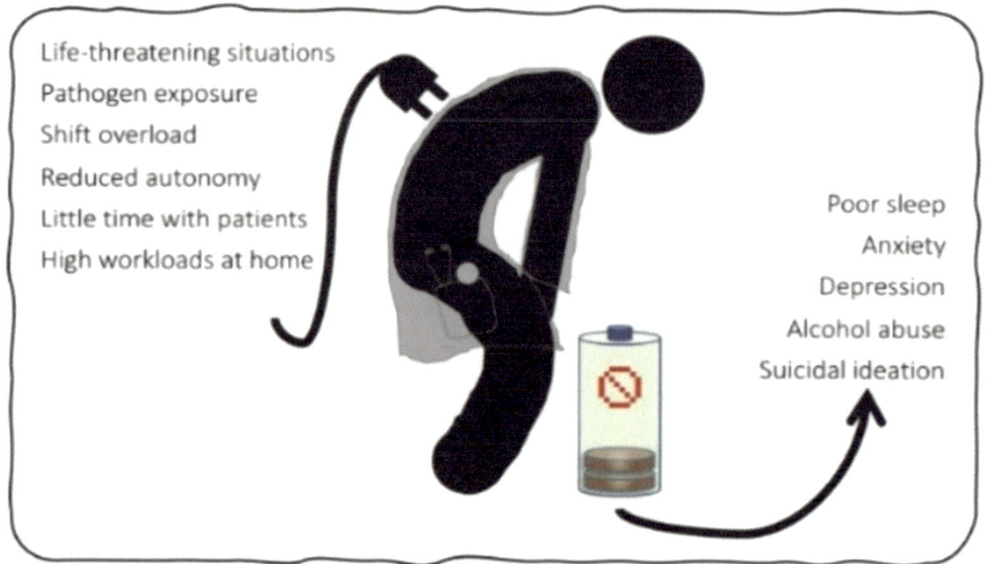

Figure 1: Summary of how several factors leads to burnout in healthcare workers

Leo, C., Sabina, S., Tumolo, M., Bodini, A., Ponzini, G., Sabato, E. and Mincarone, P. (2021). Burnout among healthcare workers in the COVID 19 era: A review of the existing literature. *Frontiers in Public Health*, [online] https://doi.org/10.3389/fpubh.2021.750529

De Hert (2020) asserts that as exhaustion and emotional depletion set in through burnout, healthcare providers exhibit diminished cognitive function and compromised decision-making abilities, resulting in medical errors, misdiagnoses, and suboptimal treatment plans. Decreased alertness and empathy hinder effective communication, leading to patients feeling marginalized, unheard, or inadequately supported. When healthcare workers leave due to burnout, it promotes increased turnover and longer patient wait times. Recognizing and addressing burnout is imperative to safeguard both the well-being of healthcare workers and the quality of care they provide to patients (De Hert, 2020).

"Never overestimate the strength of the torchbearer's arm, for even the strongest arms grow weary." A.J. Darkholme, *Rise to the Morningstar*

Burnout

In the context of Under-recognized Health Care Workers

> The COVID-19 pandemic has revealed a great irony in the labor market: workers essential to social functioning and safety are among the least valued by pay. Support workers (eg, medical assistants), direct care workers (eg, nursing assistants and personal care aides), and service workers (eg, janitors and food preparers) have long experienced wage theft and exploitation, although health care organizations would cease functioning without them. The health sector has opportunities to revisit wage hierarchies and to ensure living wages for these workers.
>
> Hallett, N. (2022). Wage Theft and Worker Exploitation in Health Care. *AMA Journal of Ethics*, [online] 24(9), pp.890–894. https://doi.org/10.1001/amajethics.2022.890

Among other important attributes, work compensated with a living wage constitutes a crucial characteristic of positive working environments. According to Hallett (2022), within healthcare labor markets, employers pay the lowest wages possible to workers considered essential. In a 2009 study, researchers found that 12% of home health aides were paid less than the minimum wage. A companion study revealed that those on a salary pay scale, were paid less than the minimum wage when accounting for total hours worked. In some instances, workers successfully take legal action resulting in just compensation for hours worked. Unfortunately, most workers lack the resources to obtain legal assistance, which sticks them in an endless cycle of long hours compensated with low wages (Hallett, 2022). This historical wage gap rolled over into the COVID-19 era and became more egregious as employees were asked to do more while simultaneously multiplying risk to health and safety. For instance, home health aides in Buffalo reported experiencing "verbal abuse, sexual harassment, bug and rodent infestations, and a lack of personal protective equipment" at their jobs. When asked about their feelings regarding their work, many expressed pride in the work itself. However, they did not view it as a long-term opportunity due to the perception that "the work was too hard, their employers too disrespectful, and the pay too low," (Hallett, 2022).

Burnout

In the context of Healthcare Workforce Shortages

The grind of the pandemic in the face of unacceptable working conditions provided the perfect storm to create yet another crisis – healthcare workforce shortages. In August 2021, having tired of low wages and offensive working conditions, more than half a million healthcare workers walked off their jobs. COVID-19 working circumstances triggered labor strikes throughout the U.S. and proliferation of labor organizations like the National Domestic Workers Alliance to provide solidarity and unified voices to address work environment issues (Hallett, 2022).

As further evidence of the pandemic's toll on healthcare workers, the Association of American Medical Colleges (AAMC) declares the U.S. faces a shortage of up to 139,000 physicians by 2033 (Heiser, 2020). Nursing workforce research projects shortages of up to 450,000 nurses by 2025 and projects that 22-32% of nurses consider leaving the profession through early retirement or departing their careers all together. And sixty-seven percent of critical care nurses contemplate leaving their vocation within the next 3 years (Martin et al., 2023).

Consider this as well. According to Spencer and Jewett (2021) more than 3,660 U.S. healthcare workers died in the first year of the pandemic – 562 nurses, 346 healthcare supports, 291 physicians, and 123 first responders. The majority were identified as people of color.

Rethinking the Healthcare Workforce

In the context of the COVID-19 Pandemic

The COVID-19 pandemic underscored the importance of actively gathering data to comprehensively grasp disease outbreaks and formulate preventive measures and disaster planning to ensure the safety and health of essential workers (Armenti et al., 2023). The pandemic emphasized the significance of establishing an equal and safe work environment for all. For nurses, however, it was not COVID-19 that rooted their desire to abandon the profession, but rather features like insufficient staffing, not feeling supported, and desire for commensurate pay (Martin et al., 2023). Employees look to administrators to actively engage and genuinely understand salient concerns through forms of collective bargaining working to develop strategies that address inequities. The expectation lies in leadership making sincere efforts to actively involve frontline essential workers by asking, listening, and acknowledging their concerns to effect constructive solutions (Shanafelt, Ripp and Trockel, 2020).

Work Environment as a Social Determinant of Health

In the context of Workplace Hazards beyond the COVID-19 Pandemic

Occupational hazards include falls and accidents, exposure to toxic chemicals and inhalation of substances known to cause lung disease.

Based on 2014 published data from the Bureau of Labor Statistics, 261,930 private industry, state and local government workers missed one or more days of work due to injuries from falls. 798 workers died from such falls. Fall injuries create a considerable financial burden: workers' compensation and medical costs associated with occupational fall incidents have been estimated at $70 billion annually in the United Sates (NIOSH, 2020).

The Occupational Safety and Health Administration (OSHA) overseas the regulation of worker exposure to chemicals to ensure workplace safety. Workers suffer more than 190,000 illnesses and 50,000 deaths annually related to chemical exposures. Workplace chemical exposures are linked to cancers, as well as other disabling and lethal disorders connected to lung, kidney, skin, heart, stomach, brain, nerve, and reproductive systems (OSHA, n.d.). Toxic chemicals include arsenic, benzene, asphalt fumes, chromium, diesel exhaust, formaldehyde, hydrogen sulfide, mercury, and methylene chloride to name a few. OSHA requires all employers with hazardous chemicals in their workplace to provide labels and safety data sheets to alert exposed workers and employee training to manage the chemicals appropriately.

According to Johns Hopkins University (2019) occupational of lung diseases are the primary cause of occupation-associated illness in U.S. based on frequency, severity, and preventability of the illnesses. They lead to functional incapacity, reduced *healthy* life-expectancy and life expectancy.

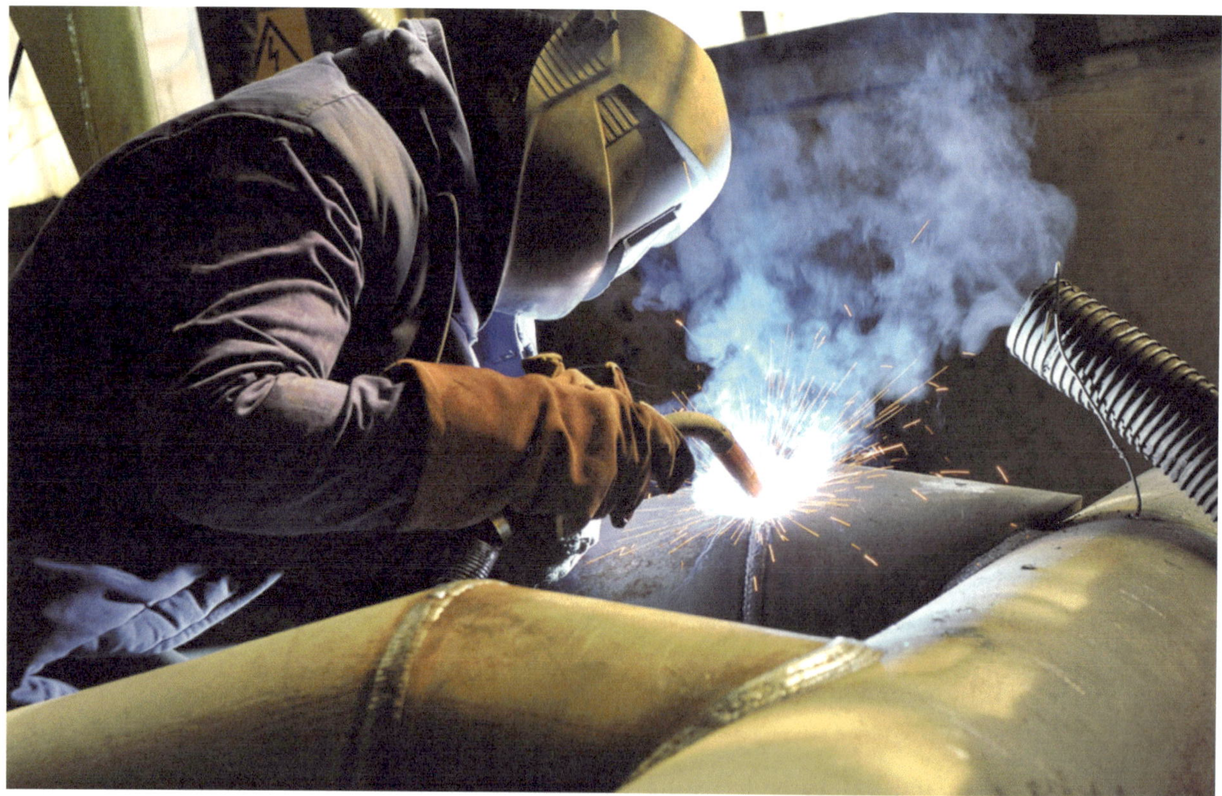

Könning, M. (2018). *Hazardous substances in welding fumes: How they affect the human body*. [online] SAFE WELDING. Available at: https://safe-welding.com/hazardous-substances-in-welding-fumes-how-they-affect-the-human-body/

Occupational Lung Disease

Repeated and long-term exposure to certain irritants on the job can lead to an array of lung diseases that may have lasting effects, including cancer, even after exposure ceases. *Occupational lung diseases are the primary cause of occupation-associated illness in the U.S. based on frequency, severity, and preventability of the illnesses.*

- Most occupational lung diseases are caused by repeated, long-term exposure, but even a severe, single exposure to a hazardous agent can damage the lungs. Persistent exposures result in chronic bronchitis, emphysema, and lung cancer.
- Occupational lung diseases are preventable.
- Smoking increases the severity of an occupational lung disease & the risk of lung cancer.

Asbestosis. Inhalation of microscopic fibers of asbestos causes asbestosis. This disease is progressive, resulting in pulmonary fibrosis; chronic exposure causes mesothelioma. An estimated 1.3 million construction and industry workers are *currently* exposed to asbestos on the job.

Coal worker's pneumoconiosis. Coal worker's pneumoconiosis is caused by inhaling coal dust. Also known as black lung disease, the condition, in severe cases, is described as pulmonary fibrosis. About 2.8 percent of coal miners have coal worker's pneumoconiosis.

Silicosis. Inhaling free crystalline silica, a dust found in the air of mines, foundries, blasting operations, and stone, clay, and glass manufacturing facilities triggers silicosis. Characterized by pulmonary fibrosis, silicosis itself can increase the risk for other lung diseases, including tuberculosis. Over one million workers per year are exposed to silica.

Byssinosis. Byssinosis is caused by dust from hemp, flax, and cotton processing. Also known as brown lung disease, the condition is chronic and exemplified by chest tightness and shortness of breath. Byssinosis affects textile workers--both former and current--and almost exclusively those who work with unprocessed cotton.

Hypersensitivity pneumonitis. Inhalation of fungus spores from moldy hay, bird droppings, and other organic dusts causes hypersensitivity pneumonitis. This disease is characterized by inflammation of alveoli, leading to pulmonary fibrosis. There are variations of hypersensitivity pneumonitis depending on the occupation, including cork worker's lung, farmer's lung, and mushroom worker's lung.

Occupational asthma. Occupational asthma is caused by inhaling certain irritants in the workplace, such as dusts, gases, fumes, and vapors. It is the most usual form of occupational lung disease and worsens pre-existing asthma. It is manifested by common asthma symptoms (such as a chronic cough, wheezing and shortness of breath). People at higher risk for occupational asthma often work in manufacturing and processing operations, farming, animal care, food processing, cotton and textile industries, and refining operations.

Johns Hopkins Medicine (2019). *Occupational Lung Diseases*. [online] Available at: https://www.hopkinsmedicine.org/health/conditions-and-diseases/occupational-lung-diseases

Work Environment as a Social Determinant of Health

In the context of Asbestos-Related Lung disease

Long before the COVID-19 pandemic, a different danger – asbestos exposure – progressively and perniciously diseased workers. The magnitude of its hazards played out for decades during the twentieth century and it was not until the 1960s that research established its link to mesothelioma. Alarms further sounded that decade when investigation proved that "the hazards of asbestos dust were not confined to heavily exposed workers in asbestos factories but extended to insulation workers, other users of products containing asbestos, and people who lived close to asbestos factories" (Bartrip, 2004).

Why Asbestos?

Asbestos is the generic term for several naturally occurring fibrous minerals. These fibers possess amazing characteristics. Uniquely among minerals, asbestos can be spun into a thread and then woven into a cloth. Clothes and soft furnishings can be manufactured from asbestos—even though it is literally a rock.

But why make such products out of a mineral except as a curiosity? The answer lies in the material's unparalleled fireproofing and insulating capabilities. However, asbestos possesses other attractive qualities: it is lightweight (an important consideration when fireproofing naval vessels), abundant, cheap to mine and process, resistant to water and acids (corrosion), durable to the point of indestructibility, electrically non-conductive, and unattractive to vermin.

Finally, it can be put to an enormous number of uses – brake linings, gaskets, insulation, fireproofing, shipbuilding, domestic products, and electrical distribution systems when blended with resins, plastics, or other materials. In many respects, therefore, asbestos is the perfect material for an industrializing and electrifying world of heat, combustion, and high-speed locomotion. Not surprisingly, it came to be viewed, for the first two thirds of the 20th century, as the "indispensable" and even the "magic" mineral.

Bartrip, P. (2004). History of asbestos related disease. *Postgraduate Medical Journal*, [online] Available at: https://doi.org/10.1136/pmj.2003.012526

Although the industrial health hazards associated with asbestos exposure emerged in the early 20th century and evidence for toxicity mounted over the next 50 years, applications of the "indispensable mineral" proliferated resulting in manufacturing consumption of over 700,000 tons in 1957 and 1967 (Bartrip, 2004).

Table 1 Raw asbestos consumption in the USA, 1917–77 (10 year intervals)

Year	Consumption (short tons)
1917	135338
1927	226365
1937	316263
1947	616194
1957	723492
1967	720583
1977	671543

US Department of Commerce. *Bureau of Mines Mineral Yearbook*. Consumption peaked at 882 908 tons in 1973. The vast bulk of American consumption (some 96% in 1956) consisted of chrysotile (white asbestos).

Bartrip, P. (2004). History of asbestos related disease. *Postgraduate Medical Journal*, [online] Available at: https://doi.org/10.1136/pmj.2003.012526

Asbestos - a group of naturally occurring minerals known for their versatility and durability.

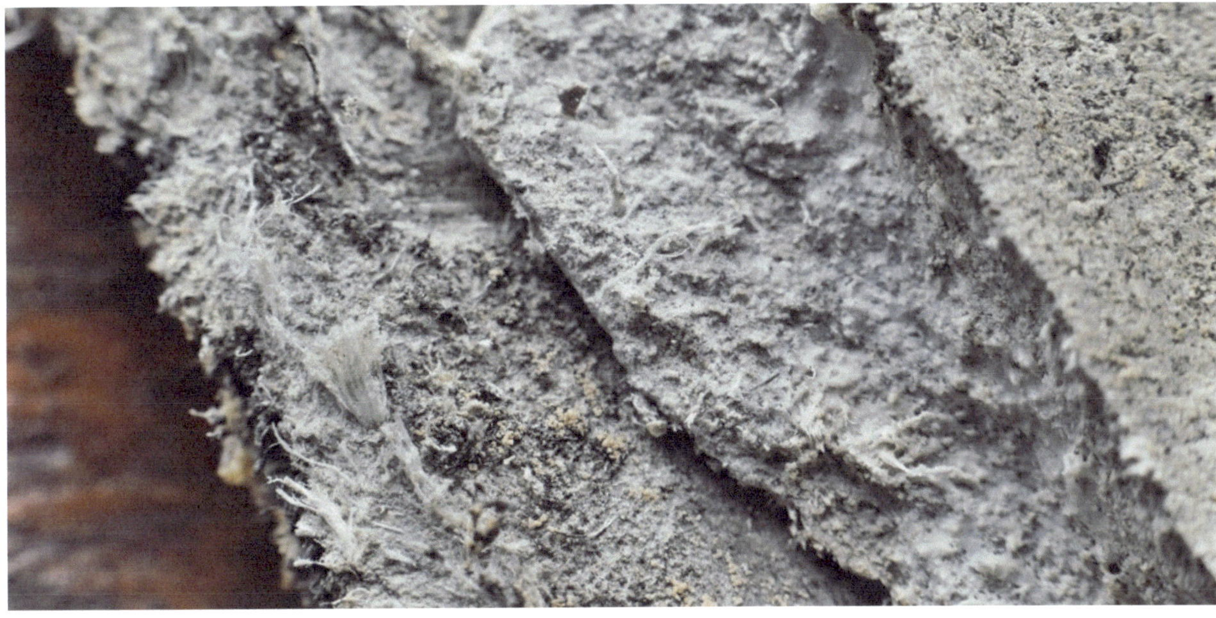

Admintag (2021). *What is Mesothelioma?* [online] Questions and Answers. [online] Available at: https://howtodoright.com/what-is-mesothelioma/

When people breathe the tiny fibers of asbestos, the lungs trap and accumulate them. Over time, inflammatory reactions set in, which lead to diseases like asbestosis (pulmonary fibrosis), chronic bronchitis, emphysema, plural effusions, lung cancer, plural plaques, mesothelioma, malignant mesothelioma, and death. While the most generic form of mesothelioma arises in pulmonary structures, it can form in tissues around the heart (pericardial mesothelioma), abdomen (peritoneal mesothelioma) and testicles (tunica vaginalis mesothelioma) as well (CDC, 2021).

High risk populations include persons in construction trades, boilermakers, shipyard workers, railroad workers, and U.S. Naval veterans (O'Reilly, et al., 2007).

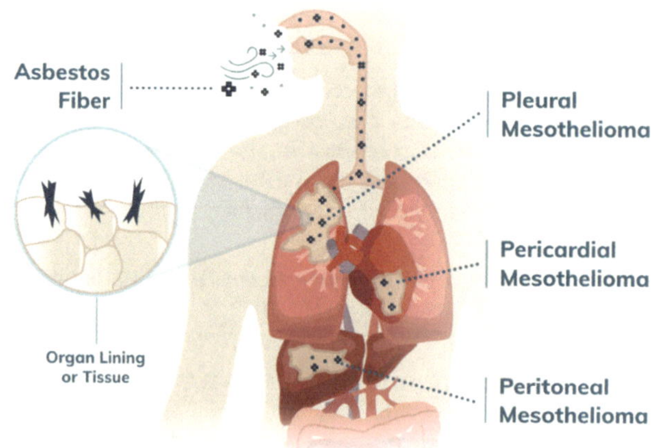

Inhaled asbestos fibers can lay dormant for many years causing inflammation and in some cases, mesothelioma, an often-lethal cancer affecting the pleura, pericardium, peritoneum, and testicles.

Molinari, L. and Stevenson, J. (2019). *Mesothelioma Cancer.* [online] Mesothelioma.com. Available at: https://www.mesothelioma.com/mesothelioma/

According to Bonafede, et al. (2018), due to the alarming consequences, latency time to disease manifestation, and the extraordinary number of exposed individuals "the risk of developing asbestos-related diseases among asbestos-exposed subjects is associated with high levels of psychological distress, despair, and mental health difficulties."

The U.S. Department of Health and Human Services classifies asbestos as a human carcinogen (National Cancer Institute, 2017).

Shipyards and Asbestos

The industrial applications of asbestos skyrocketed during World War II. According to Munz and Pacheco (2023) the U.S. Navy mandated the use of asbestos in shipbuilding and estimate that during World War II 4.5 million men and women endured high asbestos exposure risk.

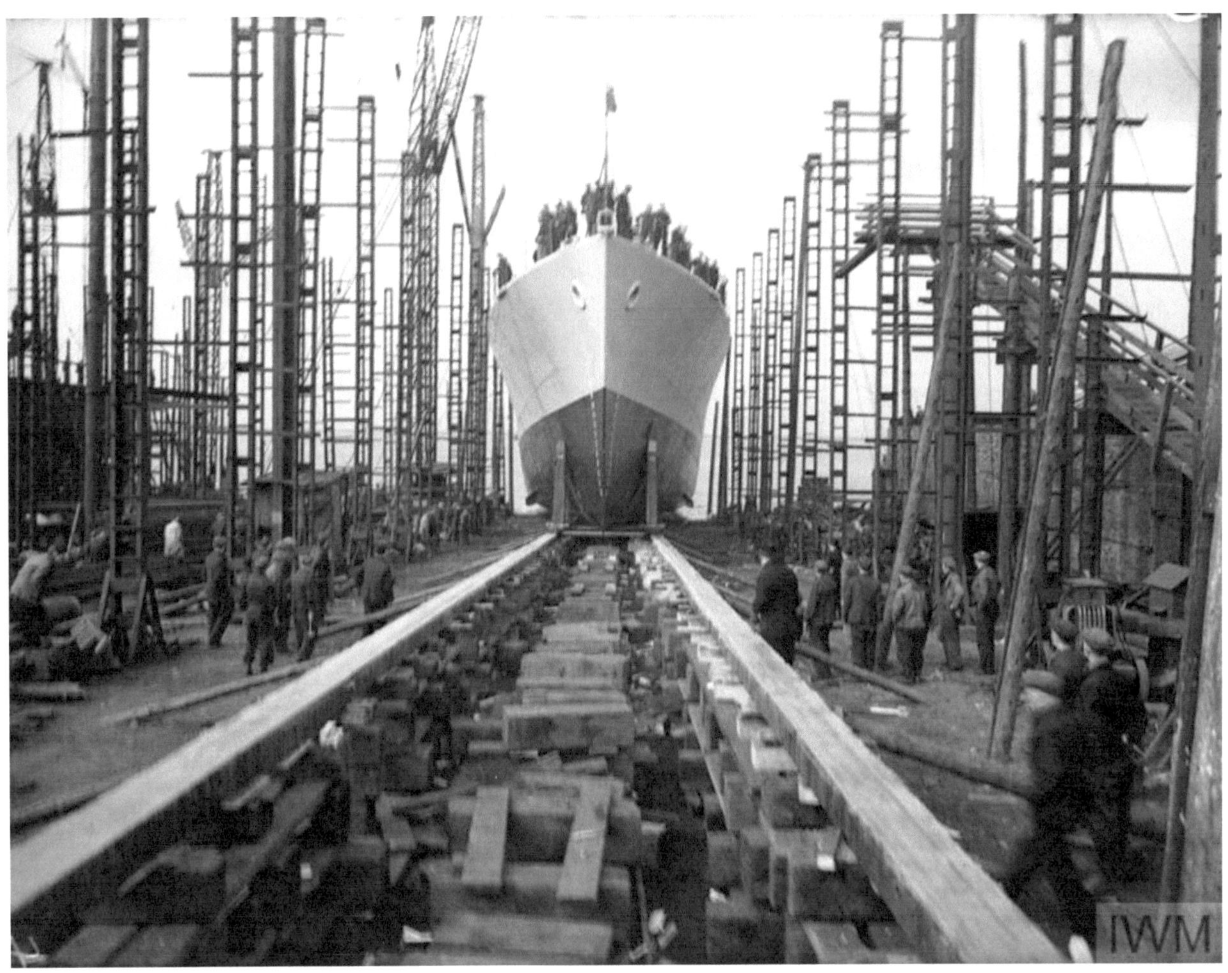

Imperial War Museums. (2023). *DESTROYER LAUNCHED BY MRS A V ALEXANDER. 23 MARCH 1943, LEITH. THE LAUNCH OF THE NEW DESTROYER, HMS LOCH ACHANALT BY THE WIFE OF THE FIRST LORD OF THE ADMIRALTY.* [online] Available at: https://www.iwm.org.uk/collections/item/object/205154687

Asbestos was considered a critical element in the shipbuilding industry, especially in the military, because of its ability to resist heat and prevent fires that were disastrous for vessels at sea (Munz, Pacheco and Waterman, 2023). Asbestos resists corrosion and hot temperatures, which made it an ideal material for use in the shipbuilding industry. It was used to prevent fires by insulating boilers, incinerators, hot water pipes and steam pipes. In 1943, one in 500 shipyard workers was an asbestos insulator. The job required them to handle asbestos directly by cutting, sanding, and fitting insulation to various components of ships (Munz and Pacheco, 2023).

During World War II and beyond shipyard workers shouldered the responsibility of constructing and maintaining wartime vessels and, in doing so, encountered repeated exposure to asbestos over months and years with no or inadequate PPE and insufficient ventilation. The tasks forced personnel into close contact with asbestos laden material for extended periods. However, workers displayed few symptoms from their prolonged exposure, as latency from exposure to disease manifestations can take forty years leaving workers grappling with the consequences long after their service ended. This exposure resulted in a tragic legacy of occupational diseases while simultaneously driving the push for safer working conditions and stricter safety regulations (National Cancer Institute, 2017).

International research indicates that asbestos-related disease is by no means confined to the United States and suggests that diseases may extend beyond those associated with the mesothelium. Investigators in Italy report increased incidence of laryngeal cancers in addition to mesothelioma, lung cancer and asbestosis among Genoa, Italy shipyard workers. In 2008, The Ulster Medical Society reported increased asbestosis in shipbuilders working in Northern Ireland. Velasco-Garcia, et al published data regarding asbestosis in Spanish populations in 2017. The European Union (EU) reported that 78% of cancers recognized as occupational relate back to asbestos and in 2019 alone more than 70,000 EU workers died from asbestos-related exposure (Munz, Pacheco and Waterman, 2023).

Although the Environmental Protection Agency (EPA) has banned asbestos in most commercial applications, it can still be found in lesser amounts in car parts, fire safety products, laboratory equipment, construction materials and fertilizers (Weyant, 2018). Homes, industrial structures, and commercial buildings including schools built between 1870 and 1990 contain varying amounts of asbestos products that require asbestos abatement also known as asbestos remediation (360training, 2021). The Occupational Safety and Health Administration (OHSA) regulates asbestos abatement requiring strict compliance procedures to fully contain disturbed asbestos materials to protect workers, persons at risk for contact with abated debris and the environment (OSHA, n.d.).

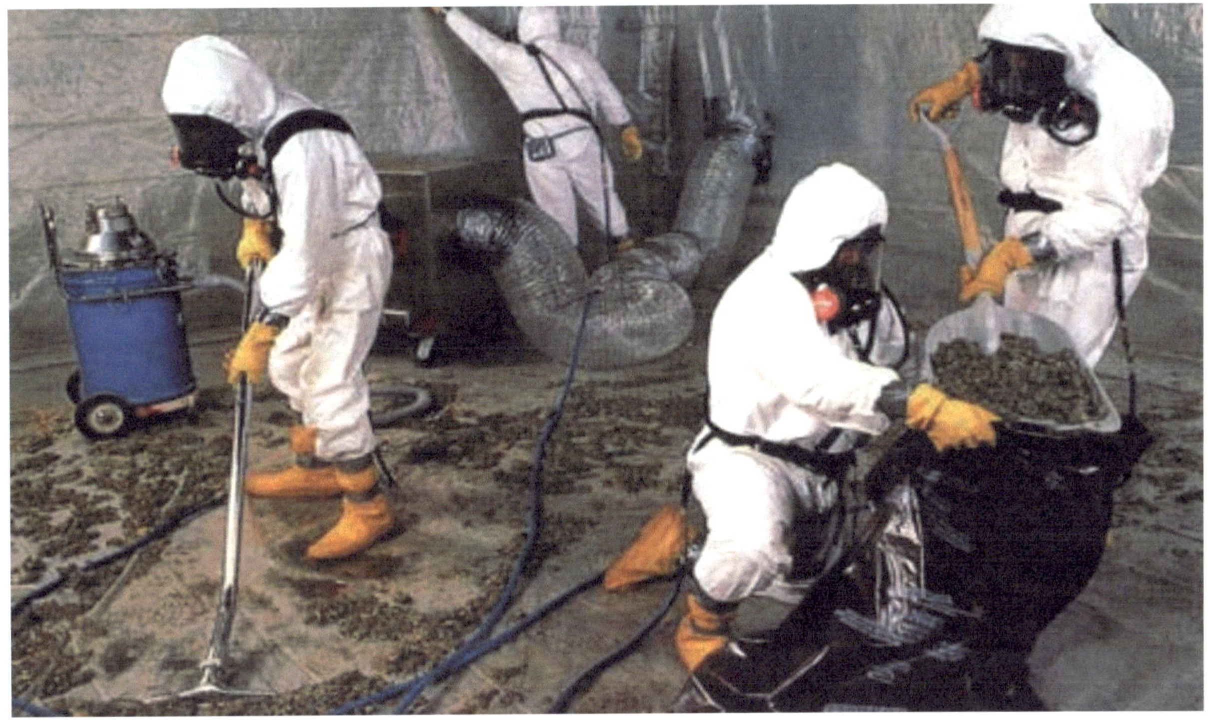

Asbestos Removal 12 (2013). *Asbestos Removal12: Asbestos Abatement Services*. [online] Available at: http://asbestosremoval12.blogspot.com/2013/02/asbestos-abatement-services.html

Work Environment as a Social Determinant of Health

Policies, politics, and governance

The United States took its first steps towards regulating asbestos use with the Clean Air Act of 1970 which classified asbestos as a hazardous air pollutant (US EPA, OCSPP, 2013a). In

1973, the EPA banned spray-applied surfacing asbestos-containing material for fireproofing and insulating purposes. In 1975, the EPA banned installation of asbestos pipe insulation and asbestos block insulation on facility components, such as boilers and hot water tanks (US EPA, OCSPP, 2013b).

Legal inveiglements have blocked EPA environmental protections in some instances. In 1989, the EPA attempted to ban most asbestos-containing products by issuing a final rule under Section 6 of Toxic Substances Control Act (TSCA). However, most of the original ban on the manufacture, importation, processing, or distribution in commerce for many of the asbestos-containing products originally covered in the 1989 final rule was *overturned in 1991 by the Fifth Circuit Court of Appeals.* As a result, the 1989 asbestos regulation only banned new uses of asbestos in products that would be initiated *for the first time* after 1989 and banned 5 other specific product types – flooring felt, rollboard, and corrugated, commercial, or specialty paper (US EPA, OCSPP, 2013b). In April 2019, the EPA issued a final rule to ensure that asbestos products that are no longer on the market cannot return to commerce without the EPA evaluating them and putting in place any necessary restrictions or prohibiting use (US EPA, OCSPP, 2013b).

The National Emission Standards for Hazardous Air Pollutants (NESHAP) established protocols for asbestos management during renovation and demolition projects to reduce airborne fiber release. Simultaneously, OSHA developed standards for occupational safety, imposing exposure limits, protective measures, and employee training (US EPA, OCSPP, 2013a).

Work Environment as a Social Determinant of Health

Conclusions

The COVID-19 pandemic and the asbestos debacle illuminate the resilience and dedication of workers in the face of adversity. Healthcare workers demonstrated unwavering commitment to patient care often at great personal sacrifice while industrial workers unknowingly confronted the dangers of asbestos exposure with diligence and fortitude, often as a patriotic duty to the WWII war effort. These crises underscore the importance of prioritizing worker safety, physical well-being, worker mental health and access to the full spectrum of healthcare. Their history prompts calls for improved occupational health and safety measures and heightened awareness of the long-term consequences of workplace hazards. By learning from these experiences and implementing proactive measures, advocacy for worker justice poses the potential to construct a future where every individual contributes to their fullest workplace potential without compromising health and well-being and devoid of economic sacrifice.

Questions for Further Consideration:

1. Describe ways healthcare workers and other workers support one another to prevent burnout? Use valid internet resources to support the evidence.
2. Have you witnessed policy changes in response to poor work conditions? If so, what changed? Did changes successfully mitigate unacceptable working conditions?
3. Are lawmakers advocating for healthy work environments in your locality? Are they legislating for everyone receiving a living wage?
4. Imagine you are a worker in an unsafe condition or not making a living wage. What are ways in which you as the employee could advocate for you and your fellow employees?

Sentinel Readings for a Deeper Dive:

Hargreaves, Sally (2019). *Occupational health outcomes among international migrant workers: a systematic review and meta-analysis* [Online]. Available at: https://www.ncbi.nlm.nih.gov/pmc/articles/PMC6565984/

Stressed out and burned out: the global primary care crisis. [Online]. Available at: https://www.commonwealthfund.org/publications/issue-briefs/2022/nov/stressed-out-burned-out-2022-international-survey-primary-care-physicians

Murthy, V.H. (2022). *Confronting health worker burnout and well-being.* [Online]. Available at: https://www.ncjm.org/doi/full/10.1056/NEJMp2207252

Granieri, A., Bonafede, M., Marinaccio, A., Iavarone, I., Marsili, D. and Franzoi, I.G. (2020). *SARS-CoV-2 and Asbestos Exposure: Can Our Experience with Mesothelioma Patients Help Us Understand the Psychological Consequences of COVID-19 and Develop Interventions?* [Online] Available at: https://www.frontiersin.org/articles/10.3389/fpsyg.2020.584320/full

References

360training (2021). *Asbestos Removal Process: What is Asbestos Abatement?* [online] Available at: https://www.360training.com/blog/asbestos-abatement [Accessed 24 Nov. 2023].

Admintag (2021). *What is Mesothelioma?* [online] Questions and Answers. Available at: https://howtodoright.com/what-is-mesothelioma/ [Accessed 23 Nov. 2023].

Armenti, K., Sweeney, M., Lingwall, C. and Yang, L. (2023). Work: A Social Determinant of Health Worth Capturing. *International Journal of Environmental Research and Public Health*, [online] Available at: https://doi.org/10.3390/ijerph20021199 [Accessed 2 November 2023].

Aronsson, G., Theorell, T., Grape, T., Hammarström, A., Hogstedt, C., Marteinsdottir, I., Skoog, I., Träskman-Bendz, L. and Hall, C. (2017). A systematic review including meta-analysis of work environment and burnout symptoms. *BMC Public Health*, [online] Available at: https://doi.org/10.1186/s12889-017-4153-7 [Accessed 28 October 2023].

Asbestos Removal 12 (2013). *Asbestos Removal12: Asbestos Abatement Services*. [online] Available at: http://asbestosremoval12.blogspot.com/2013/02/asbestos-abatement-services.html [Accessed 24 Nov. 2023].

Bartrip, P. (2004). History of asbestos related disease. *Postgraduate Medical Journal*, [online] Available at: https://doi.org/10.1136/pmj.2003.012526 Accessed 2 November 2023.

Bonafede, M., Ghelli, M., Corfiati, M., Rosa, V., Guglielmucci, F., Granieri, A., Branchi, C., Iavicoli, S. and Marinaccio, A. (2018). The psychological distress and care needs of mesothelioma patients and asbestos-exposed subjects: A systematic review of published studies. *American Journal of Industrial Medicine* [online] Available at: https://doi.org/10.1002/ajim.22831 [Accessed 2 November 2023].

CDC (2021). *Mesothelioma | CDC*. www.cdc.gov. [online] Available at: https://www.cdc.gov/cancer/mesothelioma/index.htm [Accessed 22 November 2023].

D'Couto, H. (2022). *Forcing my COVID patients to die alone is inhumane — and unnecessary*. [online] www.wbur.org. Available at: https://www.wbur.org/cognoscenti/2022/03/07/covid-patients-icu-dying-alone-helen-t-dcouto [Accessed 2 November 2023].

De Hert, S. (2020). Burnout in healthcare workers: Prevalence, impact and preventative strategies. *Local and Regional Anesthesia*, [online] 13(13), pp.171–183. doi: [Accessed 28 November 2023].

Edú-Valsania, S., Laguía, A. and Moriano, J.A. (2022). Burnout: A Review of Theory and Measurement. *International Journal of Environmental Research and Public Health*, [online] https://doi.org/10.3390/ijerph19031780 [Accessed 28 November 2023].

Hallett, N. (2022). Wage Theft and Worker Exploitation in Health Care. *AMA Journal of Ethics*, [online] https://doi.org/10.1001/amajethics.2022.890 [Accessed 28 November 2023].

Heiser, S. (2020). *New AAMC Report Confirms Growing Physician Shortage*. [online] AAMC. Available at: https://www.aamc.org/news/press-releases/new-aamc-report-confirms-growing-physician-shortage [Accessed 28 November 2023].

Hoban, R. (2022). *Within a decade, NC Could Be Short More than 21,000 Nurses*. North Carolina Health News. [online] Available at: https://www.northcarolinahealthnews.org/2022/03/02/within-a-decade-nc-could-see-nursing-shortage-of-more-than-21000/ [Accessed 28 November 2023].

Imperial War Museums. (2023). *DESTROYER LAUNCHED BY MRS A V ALEXANDER. 23 MARCH 1943, LEITH. THE LAUNCH OF THE NEW DESTROYER, HMS LOCH ACHANALT BY THE WIFE OF THE FIRST LORD OF THE ADMIRALTY.* [online] Available at: https://www.iwm.org.uk/collections/item/object/205154687 [Accessed 24 Nov. 2023].

Jewett, J.S., The Guardian, Christina (2021). *12 Months of Trauma: More Than 3,600 US Health Workers Died in Covid's First Year*. [online] KFF Health News. Available at: https://kffhealthnews.org/news/article/us-health-workers-deaths-covid-lost-on-the-frontline/[Accessed 2 November 2023].

Johns Hopkins Medicine (2019). *Occupational Lung Diseases*. [online] Available at: https://www.hopkinsmedicine.org/health/conditions-and-diseases/occupational-lung-diseases [Accessed 23 November 2023].

Könning, M. (2018). *Hazardous substances in welding fumes: How they affect the human body.* [online] SAFE WELDING. Available at: https://safe-welding.com/hazardous-substances-in-welding-fumes-how-they-affect-the-human-body/ [Accessed 23 November 2023].

Leo, C.G., Sabina, S., Tumolo, M.R., Bodini, A., Ponzini, G., Sabato, E. and Mincarone, P. (2021). Burnout among healthcare workers in the COVID 19 era: A review of the existing literature. *Frontiers in Public Health*, [online] Available at: doi: https://doi.org/10.3389/fpubh.2021.750529 [Accessed 2 November 2023].

Martin, B., Kaminski-Ozturk, N., O'Hara, C. and Smiley, R. (2023). Examining the Impact of the COVID-19 Pandemic on Burnout and Stress Among U.S. Nurses. *Journal of Nursing Regulation*, [online] Available doi: https://doi.org/10.1016/s2155-8256(23)00063-7 [Accessed 3 November 2023].

Mental Health America (2021). *The Mental Health of Healthcare Workers in COVID-19*. [online] Mental Health America. Available at: https://mhanational.org/mental-health-healthcare-workers-covid-19 [Accessed 2 November 2023].

Molinari, L. and Stevenson, J. (2019). *Mesothelioma Cancer*. [online] Mesothelioma.com. Available at: https://www.mesothelioma.com/mesothelioma/ [Accessed 2 November 2023].

Munz, A. and Pacheco, W. (2023). *Shipyards & Asbestos: Exposure Risks for Shipyard Workers*. [online] Mesothelioma Center - Vital Services for Cancer Patients & Families. Available at: https://www.asbestos.com/shipyards/ [Accessed 28 November 2023].

Munz, A., Pacheco, W. and Waterman, Y. (2023). *Shipyard Workers - Occupational Exposure, Studies & Lawsuits*. [online] Mesothelioma Center - Vital Services for Cancer Patients & Families. Available at: https://www.asbestos.com/occupations/shipyard-workers/ [Accessed 28 November 2023].

Mutikani, L. (2020). Millions of Americans join unemployment line as coronavirus savages economy. *Reuters*. [online] Available at: https://www.reuters.com/article/us-usa-economy-idUSKCN2250CS [Accessed 11 Nov. 2023].

National Cancer Institute (2017). *Asbestos Exposure and Cancer Risk Fact Sheet*. [online] National Cancer Institute. Available at: https://www.cancer.gov/about-cancer/causes-prevention/risk/substances/asbestos/asbestos-fact-sheet [Accessed 21 November 2023].

NIOSH (2020). *Falls in the Workplace | NIOSH | CDC* www.cdc.gov. [online] Available at: https://www.cdc.gov/niosh/topics/falls/default.html [Accessed 21 November 2023].

O'Reilly, K., Mclaughlin, A., Beckett, W. and Sime, P. (2007). Asbestos-Related Lung Disease. *American Family Physician*, [online] Available at: https://www.aafp.org/pubs/afp/issues/2007/0301/p683.html [Accessed 2 November 2023].

OSHA (n.d.). *Chemical Hazards and Toxic Substances - Overview | Occupational Safety and Health Administration*. [online] Available at: https://www.osha.gov/chemical-hazards [Accessed 23 November 2023].

OSHA (n.d.). *1926.1101 - Asbestos | Occupational Safety and Health Administration*. [online] Available at: https://www.osha.gov/laws-regs/regulations/standardnumber/1926/1926.1101 [Accessed 23 November 2023].

OSHA (n.d.). *Transitioning to Safer Chemicals: A Toolkit for Employers and Workers | Occupational Safety and Health Administration.* [online] Available at: https://www.osha.gov/safer-chemicals [Accessed 23 November 2023].

Shanafelt, T., Ripp, J. and Trockel, M. (2020). Understanding and Addressing Sources of Anxiety Among Health Care Professionals During the COVID-19 Pandemic. *JAMA*, [online] Available at: https://doi.org/10.1001/jama.2020.5893 [Accessed 25 October 2023].

Shanafelt, T., West, C., Sinsky, C., Trockel, M., Tutty, M., Satele, D., Carlasare, L. and Dyrbye, L. (2019). Changes in Burnout and Satisfaction with Work-Life Integration in Physicians and the General US Working Population between 2011 and 2017. *Mayo Clinic Proceedings*, [online] Available at: https://doi.org/10.1016/j.mayocp.2018.10.023 [Accessed 24 October 2023].

Steege, A., Silver, S., Mobley, A. and Sweeney, M. (2023). *Work as a Key Social Determinant of Health: The Case for Including Work in All Health Data Collections | Blogs | CDC.* [online] Centers for Disease Control and Prevention. Available at: https://blogs.cdc.gov/niosh-science-blog/2023/02/16/sdoh/ [Accessed 24 October 2023].

The Economist. (2020). *Health workers become unexpected targets during covid-19.* [online] Available at: https://www.economist.com/international/2020/05/11/health-workers-become-unexpected-targets-during-covid-19 Accessed 25 October 2023].

US EPA, OCSPP (2013a). *Asbestos Laws and Regulations | US EPA.* [online] US EPA. Available at: https://www.epa.gov/asbestos/asbestos-laws-and-regulations [Accessed 23 November 2023].

US EPA,OCSPP (2013b). *EPA Actions to Protect the Public from Exposure to Asbestos | US EPA.* [online] US EPA. Available at: https://www.epa.gov/asbestos/epa-actions-protect-public-exposure-asbestos [Accessed 23 November 2023].

Weyant, C. (2018). *6 Products That Still Contain Asbestos.* [online] ConsumerSafety.org. [online] Available at: https://www.consumersafety.org/news/6-products-that-still-contain-asbestos/ [Accessed 23 November 2023].

World Health Organization (2023). *Occupational Hazards in the Health Sector.* [online] Available at: https://www.who.int/tools/occupational-hazards-in-health-sector [Accessed 21 November 2023].

Lexicon of Listed Terms and Agencies:

- **EPA** the United States Environmental Protection Agency serves to protect human health and the environment

- **Frontline Workers** are employees who were required to go to their place of employment during the Covid-19 Pandemic.

- **Mental Health America** is nonprofit who was created to promote mental health, well-being, and illness prevention in the US.

- **Migrant Workers** are international migrants who are currently employed or are looking for employed in the country they currently reside in and is not their home country.

- **National Domestic Workers Alliance (NDWA)** is an organization that works to gain labor rights and protections for nannies, housecleaners, and homecare workers.

- **Occupational Safety and Health Act (OSHA) of 1970** was passed by Congress to ensure all workers have safe working conditions. It provides guidance to employers and employees.

- **Personal Protective Equipment (PPE)** describes equipment worn to minimize exposure to hazards. For healthcare workers, this commonly meant respirators, isolation gowns, gloves, and foot and eye protection.

- **US Consumer Product Safety Commissions (CPSC)** is a federal agency formed to protect the public against risks of injury or death from consumer products.

- **World Health Organization (WHO)** is a United Nations agency that connects people and organizations all over the world to promote health for all and help serve the vulnerable.

AUTHOR'S BIO SKETCH

Andrea Lynde, DO

Dr. Lynde was raised in Puyallup, WA and attended a local college where she met her future husband. Andrea attended medical school at the Pacific Northwest University of Health Sciences in Yakima, Washington. Following graduation, Dr. Lynde continued her medical education at the Community Health Care Family Medicine residency program in Tacoma. Dr. Lynde's dream from an early age was to give back to a community that had helped her family during demanding situations. In her free time, Andrea enjoys bowling, planning Disney trips and designing and making shirts for herself and her friends.

Chapter 10

Water and Sanitation as Social Determinants of Health

Ariahnna Croskey, DO, Author
James Lenhart, MD, MPH, Editor

"Water is life, and clean water means health."
- Audrey Hepburn, UNICEF Goodwill Ambassador 1988-1993

Water and Sanitation as Social Determinants of Health

The World Medical Association's Statement on Water and Health (Wma.net., 2014) confirmed the vital role water plays in human health, "An adequate supply of fresh (i.e., clean potable and uncontaminated) water is essential for individual and public health, as well as being a social determinant of health." The United Nations General Assembly (2015) affirmed the right to clean water and that "clean drinking water and sanitation are essential to the realization of human rights." Disparities in the actualization of this fundamental right and the resulting health outcomes underscore and refine its importance as a social determinant of health. Social determinants of health are often interrelated, and in the United States the quality of water accessible to people depends on socioeconomic status, geographic location, and race.

Water and Sanitation as Social Determinants of Health

In the context of Health

Contaminated water serves as a vector for diarrheal illnesses such as cholera, typhoid fever, hepatitis A, and dysentery, as well as other diseases like polio, legionella, and parasitic infections (WHO, 2022). Links between contaminated water supplies and illness were first recognized in the late nineteenth century, which led to improved water sanitation and significant declines in waterborne illnesses in areas where implemented (Tulchinsky, 2018). For example, the incidence of typhoid fever dropped from 30/100,000 people in the U.S. at the turn of the 20th century to negligible rates by 1950 following chlorination of water **Figure 1** (CDC, 1998). The U.S. Congress passed The Safe Drinking Water Act (SDWA) in 1974 permitting the Environmental Protection Agency to establish and enforce safe drinking water standards (EPA, 2022a). Since passing, the incidence of water borne disease outbreaks in the U.S. has declined, however, the law delegates much of its monitoring requirements to states, creating, at times, a confusing and complicated system of standards that must be adhered to and enforced. Although it has proven valuable in the safety standards it specifies, the law's administration and enforcement pose tremendous challenges (Weinmeyer et al., 2014).

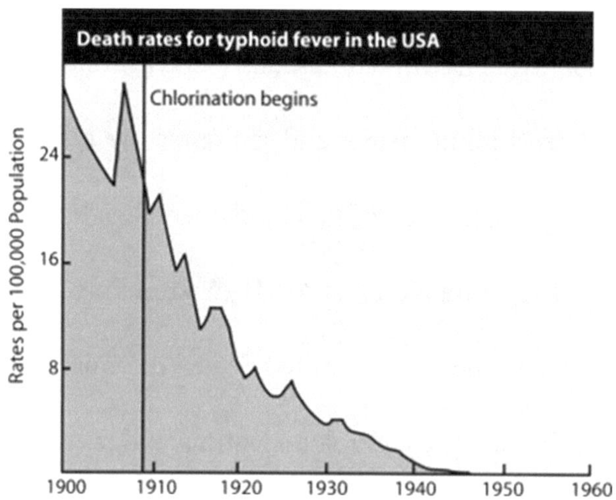

Figure 1. Death rates from typhoid fever following introduction of water chlorination. Summary of Notifiable Diseases, United States, 1997. (CDC, 1998).

Tulchinsky, T.H. (2018). *John Snow, Cholera, the Broad Street Pump; Waterborne Diseases Then and Now. Case Studies in Public Health*, [online] Available at: https://www.ncbi.nlm.nih.gov/pmc/articles/PMC7150208/ [Accessed Feb – Mar 2023].

While the morbidity and mortality rates are much lower in developed countries than in developing regions (Reiner et al., 2020), there are still an estimated 16.4 million cases of acute gastroenteritis per year attributable to community water supplies in the U.S. (Allaire, Wu and Lall, 2018). Ineffective water management triggers approximately 20 legionella outbreaks annually in the U.S. with an overall mortality rate of around 10% (CDC, 2021b).

According to the EPA, agricultural runoff is the leading cause of surface water pollution affecting the quality of source water available to rural and urban areas (EPA, 2022b). An Environmental Working Group (2010) study revealed rising nitrate contamination levels in states with significant levels of agricultural land use with the small, rural communities most likely to be affected, except in California where densely populated areas are surrounded by crop acreage (Schechinger, 2020).

The United States boasts more than 330 million acres of agricultural land producing abundant, high quality food products. When improperly managed activities from working farms and ranches can affect water quality and endanger human health. According to the Environmental Protection Agency (EPA, 2022c) five agricultural processes impact water quality:

Animal Feeding Operations: By confining animals in small areas or lots, farmers and ranchers can efficiently feed and support livestock. But these confined areas become major sources of animal waste. An estimated 238,000 working farms and ranches in the United States are considered animal feeding operations, generating about 500 million tons of manure each year. Runoff from poorly managed facilities can carry pathogens such as bacteria and viruses, nutrients, and oxygen-demanding organics and solids that contaminate shell fishing areas and cause other water quality problems.
Livestock Grazing: Overgrazing exposes soils, increases erosion, encourages invasion by undesirable plants, destroys fish habitat, and may destroy streambanks and floodplain vegetation necessary for habitat and water quality filtration.
Irrigation: Excessive irrigation can affect water quality by causing erosion, transporting nutrients, pesticides, and heavy metals, or decreasing the amount of water that flows naturally in streams and rivers. It can also cause a buildup of selenium, a toxic metal that can harm waterfowl reproduction.
Pesticides: Insecticides, herbicides, and fungicides are used to kill agricultural pests. These chemicals enter and contaminate water through direct application, runoff, and atmospheric deposition. They poison fish and wildlife, contaminate food sources, and destroy the habitat that animals use for protective cover.
Nutrients: Farmers apply nutrients such as phosphorus, nitrogen, and potassium in the form of chemical fertilizers, manure, and sludge. They may also grow legumes and leave crop residues to enhance production. When these sources exceed plant needs, or are applied just before it rains, nutrients wash into aquatic ecosystems (EPA, 2022c).
EPA (2022c). Protecting Water Quality from Agricultural Runoff [online] Available a: https://www.epa.gov/sites/default/files/2015-09/documents/ag_runoff_fact_sheet.pdf

Given the extraordinary prospect for water contamination through agriculture and industry, and the need for clean water, measures developed by the EPA to reduce pollution and treat contaminated water establishes the need for enforceable actions that ensure sustainable, safe water.

Water treatment requires careful analysis for contamination and subsequent mitigation of potentially harmful substances responsible for disease. For example:

- *Arsenic:* groundwater may naturally contain arsenic. Arsenic causes skin, lung, and bladder cancer as well as neurologic and cardiovascular disorders (ATSDR, (2021).
- *Nitrates:* fertilizer and manure entering water sources from agricultural run-off pollute water exposing residents to risks of colorectal cancer, thyroid disease, and neural tube birth defects in neonates (Schechinger, 2020). Infants fed formula prepared with nitrate contaminated water risk development of methemoglobinemia also known as "blue baby syndrome" a potentially fatal condition (Knobeloch, et al., 2000).
- *Lead:* according to the CDC, the most common sources of lead in drinking water are lead pipes, faucets, and plumbing fixtures (CDC, 2023). In 1986 Congress amended the Safe Drinking Water Act, prohibiting the use of pipes, solder or flux that were not "lead free" in public water systems or plumbing in facilities supplying water for human consumption (EPA, 2023). The toxic health effects of lead extend to every organ system. Due to increased intestinal absorption compared to adults, children are particularly vulnerable to lead toxicity. Neurologic effects in children include lifelong learning disabilities. Exposure to lead increases risk of all forms of cancers (ATSDR, 2021).
- *Per - and polyfluoroalkyl substances (PFAS):* PFAS include a group of chemicals used to make fluoropolymer coatings and products that resist heat, oil, stains, grease, and water including clothing, furniture, adhesives, food packaging, heat-resistant non-stick cooking surfaces, and

the insulation of electrical wire (CDC, 2022). According to the CDC, the human health effects from exposure to low environmental levels of PFAS are uncertain. Studies of laboratory animals given substantial amounts of PFAS indicate that some PFAS may affect growth and development. In addition, these animal studies signal that PFAS may affect reproduction, thyroid, immune system, and hepatic function (CDC, 2022). Due to significant concerns, yet unknown harms, the Environmental Protection Agency proposes a rule that sets maximum contaminant levels of PFAS and requires public water works to screen for and reduce these levels (EPA, 2023b).

Water treated *incorrectly* poses negative health effects. Over chlorination results in disinfection byproducts or DBPs. When excessive chlorine reacts with organic materials, carcinogenic chemicals, primarily in the form of substances called trihalomethanes are created. Chronic exposure to trihalomethanes can cause cancer, hepatic injury, and nervous system dysfunction (CDC, 2021a).

The clean water challenges outlined underscore the need for local and regional implementation of EPA (SDWA) standards, public health policy compliance, and uniform governance that ensure equitable distribution of resources including non-discriminatory standards and policies. Regrettably, evidence shows that within the United States rural, low income, and minority communities are frequent victims of unhealthy water.

Water and Sanitation as Social Determinants of Health

In the context of Geographic and Socioeconomic Inequalities

Eighty-seven percent of the U.S. population relies on public water supplies, while the remaining 13% use domestic wells. Most communities get water from large municipal water systems, with 9% of community water suppliers servicing 79% of the population (Center for

Sustainable Systems, 2021). A study published in The Proceedings of the National Academy of Sciences cross referenced violations of the SDWA from 1982-2015 using US Census data (2021). The findings concluded that low-income, rural communities faced increased vulnerability to SDWA violations. The study cited technical capacity, inadequate revenue streams, private versus public ownership (private less likely to violate) and resource justice as factors predisposing to Safe Water Act Violations (Allaire, Wu and Lall, 2018). Compliance gaps are represented in **Figure 2**.

Figure 2. EPA SDWA compliance gaps

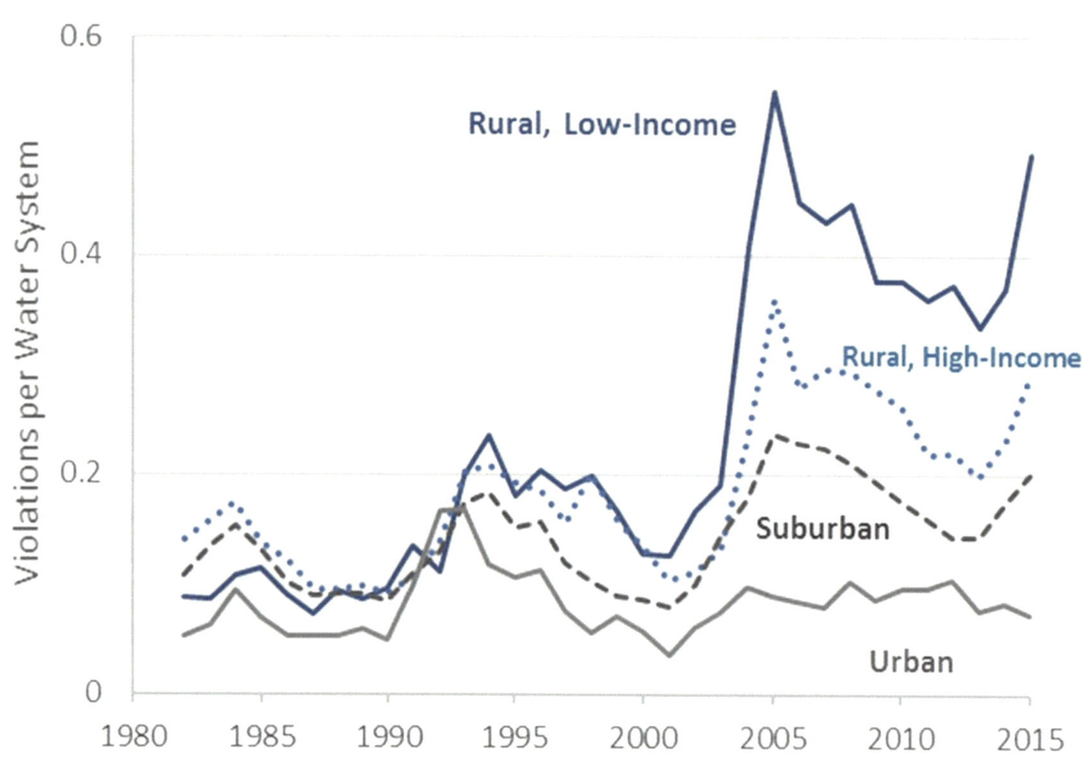

Figure 2. Total violations per water system, by housing density category and income group.

Allaire, M., Wu, H. and Lall, U. (2018) National trends in drinking water quality violations. *Proceedings of the National Academy of Sciences*, [online] Available at: https://www.pnas.org/content/115/9/2078.short?rss=1

While those living in small rural communities are more likely to consume water from SDWA violated sources, more vulnerable still are people that do not have access to a community water supply. Private wells and other small drinking water systems do not fall under the SDWA and are often contaminated with bacteria and chemicals. Estimates reveal that 15% of the US population is not served by approved public water systems (CDC, 2009). While it can be difficult to collect data about these unregulated wells, a 2009 study by the U.S. Geological Survey evaluated water from over 2,000 private wells across the country and found that 23% of them contained at least one contaminant at a potentially harmful level (USGS, 2018). Those living in low-income rural communities are more likely to experience inequities in access to clean water due to economic and environmental factors placing them at risk for water-borne illness, disease, and death.

Water and Sanitation as a Social Determinant of Health

In the context of racial and socioeconomic inequalities

Systemic racism and water intersect irrefutably to result in unfit, unsafe water in several regions of the United States. Rural and urban areas with high minority populations are disproportionately affected underscoring systemic racial inequalities in the availability of clean, safe water.

Rural Areas

According to Schaider and Swetschinski (2019), low-income and minority communities often face excessive polluted water exposures. In a nationwide analysis, 5.6 million Americans relied on a public water supply with an average nitrate concentration ≥ 5 mg/L. Epidemiological studies suggest that long-term exposure to water with nitrate concentrations above 5 mg/L may be associated with some types of cancer, birth defects, and preterm birth. Schaider's and Swetschinski's research showed that people of Hispanic origin and poverty were significantly vulnerable to exposure to water having elevated nitrate levels. Community Water Systems (CWSs) "in the top quartile of Hispanic residents exceeded 5 mg/L nearly three times as often as CWSs serving the lowest quartile" (Schaider and Swetschinski, 2019).

Balazs, et al., (2011) studied nitrate levels in persons living in California's San Joaquin Valley an area known as an urban-agricultural interface; Hispanics were disproportionately affected by high nitrates levels, whereas as home ownership (considered an indicator of wealth and political empowerment) was inversely associated with elevated nitrate levels (Balazs, et al., 2011).

Urban Areas

A 2017 study examined the water quality of Black peri-urban neighborhoods in North Carolina excluded from municipal water services, most getting water from private wells. The research compared Black peri-urban neighborhoods water quality against that of adjacent neighborhoods receiving municipal services. 29.2% of the samples from excluded neighborhoods tested positive for coliform bacteria, while only 0.56% of the samples from the municipal supply were affected (Stillo and Gibson, 2017).

Many low-income communities with community water services (CWSs) suffer from poorly maintained water system infrastructure as well as administrative failure to invest in scheduled maintenance or repair of failing systems. The Drinking Water State Revolving Fund (DWSRF) is the largest source of government aid for repair and maintenance of drinking water systems. The DWSRF financial assistance program aims to aid CWSs achieve the health protection aims of the EPA's SDWA. As an arm of the Environmental Protection Agency, it provides loans to municipalities in need of capital to invest in water infrastructure. The CWS must pay back these loans, with the accumulated interest revolving back to DWSRF to fund other CWS projects (EPA, 2015).

The Environmental Policy Innovation Center in conjunction with the University of Michigan (Hansen, 2021) analyzed the distribution of DWSRF funding. Their research concluded that small communities and those with higher minority populations were less likely to receive aid, due to a variety of factors including limited ability to pay back DWSRF loans. This data establishes a pattern of financial discrimination perpetuating underinvestment in water systems that supply safe drinking water for needy low income, minority communities.

While underinvestment in water infrastructure is more common in smaller communities, when it does occur in large urban areas, the consequences can be severe and affect thousands of people. The water crises in Flint, Michigan and Jackson Mississippi pose striking examples.

Jackson, Mississippi is a majority (83%) Black city in the U.S. struggling to provide residents with safe water for decades. Residents must deal with frequent water shutoffs, boil water advisories, and visibly dirty water coming from their pipes, with water advisories twice as frequent in the city's poorest zip codes (Samuels, et al 2022). SWDA violations were noted by the EPA as far back as 2015, and in October of 2020 the EPA launched a formal investigation into these repeated issues (Environmental Protection Agency, 2020 and Nilsen and Babineau, 2022).

> Though the water problems have grown more acute in recent years, they are not new. Residents have dealt with frequent boil water notices for decades. Officials have warned of risks to the water system since the 1970s, and pipes throughout the capital city have not been properly maintained since the 1950s.
>
> Local leadership has struggled to deal with the City's water problems, owing in part to Jackson's dwindling tax base. After desegregation, white middle- and upper-class families began fleeing Jackson for the outlying suburbs, taking much of the City's tax base with them.
>
> Pittman, A. (2022) EPA Investigating Mississippi for Civil Rights Violations Over Jackson Water Crisis. [online] Available at: https://www.mississippifreepress.org/28565/epa-investigating-mississippi-for-civil-rights-violations-over-jackson-water-crisis
>
> - Mississippi Free Press, October 20, 2022

Flooding pushed the Jackson, Mississippi's fragile water system infrastructure over the edge in August of 2022 when damage to one of the plants made water unsafe for drinking for 45 days (Moore, 2022). Jackson's tenuous water system meant regular boil water advisories throughout the city, with the Mississippi State Department of Health website citing five advisories active in March of 2023 and a water conservation advisory in place for the entire city as well (MSDH, 2023). This crisis gained national attention, and the city received federal grant money to help replace its aged infrastructure. The 2022 summer outage and the state of governmental affairs leading up to it, forced an ongoing EPA investigation to determine if state and local officials used prior aid money in a way that discriminated against Jackson's non-white residents (Adams, 2023). Health consequences due to Jackson's water crisis include lead poisoning resulting in neurologic injury and learning disabilities in children and E. coli sepsis leading to death (Rayasam, 2022).

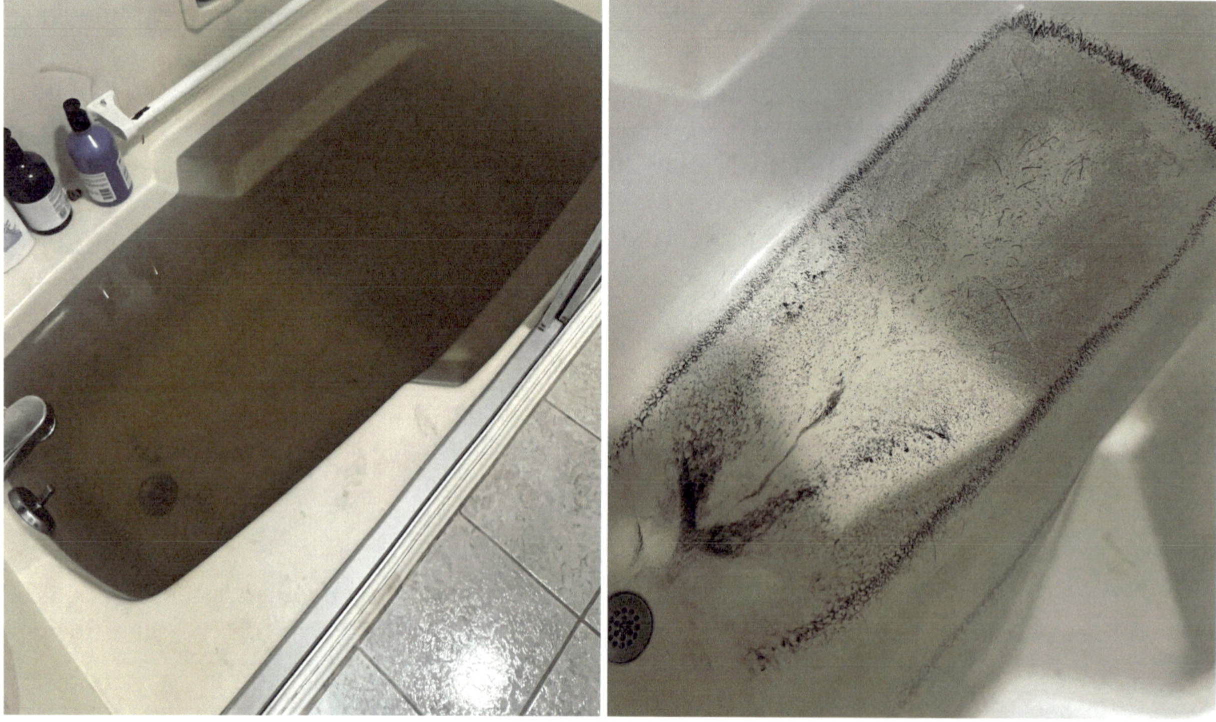

What to expect when you draw a bath in Jackson, Mississippi, 2022.

Samuels, R., Martinez, E. and Lott, J. (2022) *The problem in the pipes.* The Washington Post. [online] Available at: https://www.washingtonpost.com/nation/interactive/2023/jackson-mississippi-water-crisis/ [Accessed Mar - June 2023].

In 2014 Flint, Michigan embraced a cost saving measure that switched pre-treated Detroit city water to water sourced from the Flint River. Inadequate testing and treatment of the water resulted in a series of major water quality and health issues for Flint residents – issues that were chronically ignored, overlooked, and discounted by government officials even as complaints mounted that the foul-smelling, discolored, and off-tasting water piped into Flint homes for 18 months caused rashes, hair loss and itches (Denchak, 2018).

Concerned citizens protested, brought jugs of yellow to brown tap water to events and complained of rashes and hair loss, but went unheeded and were reassured that the water was safe (Denchak, 2018). Then, Hanna-Attisha, et al. (2016) local Flint pediatricians brought the legitimacy of the allegations to light. Conducting a study, they found increased incidence of elevated blood lead levels in Flint children, with the poorest neighborhoods in the city being the most affected. When they went public with the findings, a representative from the State of Michigan accused them of "splicing and dicing data" and "causing near hysteria" (Gross, 2018).

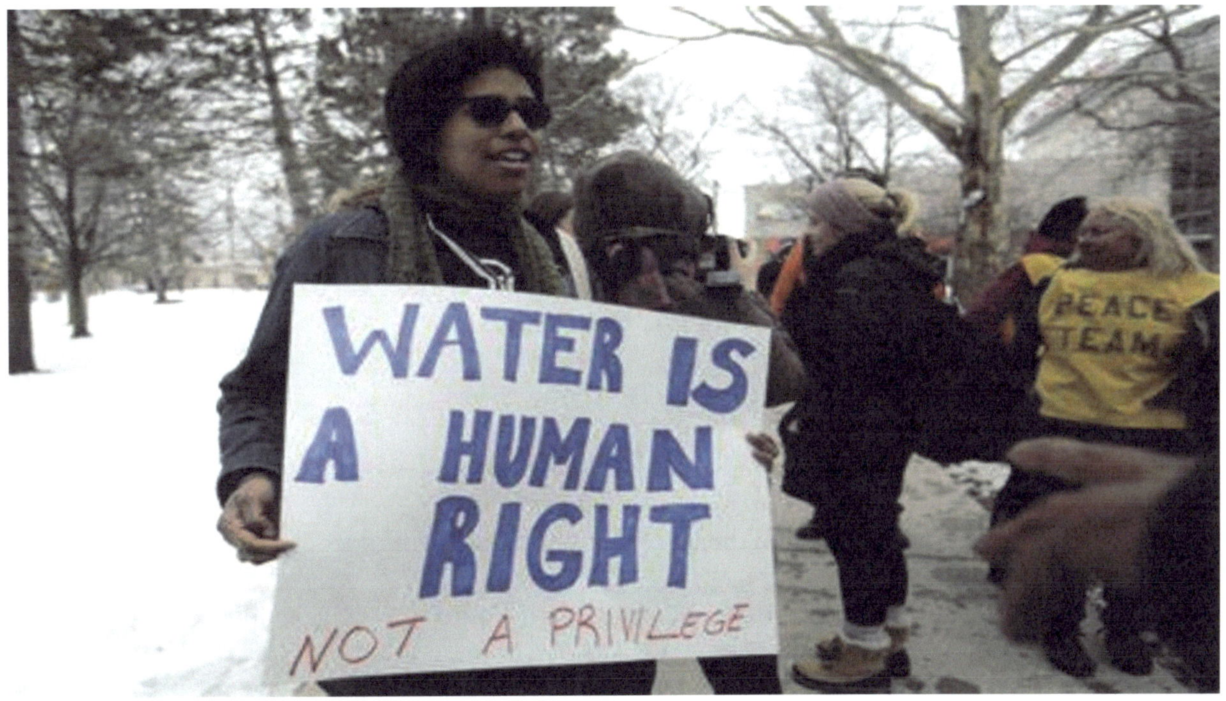

Newsweek, 2016. Flint Families Sue Michigan Governor Over Water Crisis [online] Available at: [https://www.newsweek.com/flint-families-sue-michigan-governor-over-water-crisis-434714

Unfortunately, lead contamination was not the end of the Flint water saga. In addition to not treating the water with anti-corrosives, the Flint CWS did not adequately chlorinate it, leading to the third largest outbreak of legionnaire's disease in U.S. history, which resulted in multiple deaths (Smith, 2019).

Financial aid was provided only after state and city officials were sued and mandated by a federal judge to supply bottled water to residents in late 2016 (Denchak, 2018). A settlement reached in March of 2017 guaranteed that the lead pipes would be replaced within three years [Suh, 2017]. As of November 2022, 95 percent of the city's pipes have been replaced, with an added motion filed by activist groups that month to compel the city to complete the work (Thompson and Ruble, 2022).

The Michigan Civil Rights Commission (2017) cites the city and the state government responses to the crisis as examples of systemic racism. The tragedy that took place in Flint and the government's attempt to conceal its ineptitude gained national attention and now serves as a sobering example of the inequities faced by impoverished minority communities. Were it any solace, the Flint crisis serves as an impetus to examine the quality of water provided in similar communities across the country and inspired many of the large national studies cited above.

Water and Sanitation as Social Determinants of Health

Politics, policies, and governance

Access to clean water in the U.S. is intimately connected to governmental regulations through the EPA, state enforcement of those regulations, and state and federal investments in water treatment plants and other infrastructure. Considering the growing evidence that smaller community water systems struggle more to support regulatory compliance, in 2020 the EPA launched the Compliance Advisors for Sustainable Water Systems. So far, this program has provided technical aid, operator training, resource evaluations, and other assistance to approximately two hundred small community water systems, with promising results. One example of this success is the program's involvement with a Tribal system in New Mexico that operates ten small community water systems and had been out of compliance for over ten years. With the program's help 96% percent of the system's drinking water deficiencies have been resolved (US EPA, O 2015). Equitable access to clean water is possible with proper government help and allocation of resources where they are needed the most.

Access to safe, clean water is a fundamental human right and an important social determinant of health. Research shows that inequities in access to clean water plague water system management in the United States, putting low income, rural and agricultural, and minority communities at risk for a multitude of negative health effects. More government investment in water infrastructure in these areas is needed and has the potential to be effective in addressing injustices when resources are distributed equitably.

Questions for Further Consideration:

1. In what ways can healthcare professionals support efforts to improve their local drinking water supplies?
2. Is inferior quality drinking water affecting the health of your patient population? And if so, are there ways you can help mitigate it?
3. What advocacy opportunities are available near you, and what are their aims to improve local water quality?
4. Do your local politicians or community leaders support outdated water infrastructure improvements in your area? Does this issue come up in elections as often as you think it should?

Sentinel Readings for a Deeper Dive

National trends in drinking water quality violations Available at:
https://www.pnas.org/doi/10.1073/pnas.1719805115#body-ref-r2

The Problems in the Pipes (As government at every level tries to untangle generations of systemic failure, residents in Jackson, Miss., still have no reliable water) [online] Available at: https://www.washingtonpost.com/nation/interactive/2023/jackson-mississippi-water-crisis/

Rural Water Supplies and Water-Quality Issues. CDC [online] Available at: https://www.cdc.gov/nceh/publications/books/housing/cha08.htm

Hanna-Attisha, M. (2016). *Elevated Blood Lead Levels in Children Associated with the Flint Drinking Water Crisis: A Spatial Analysis of Risk and Public Health Response.* [online] Available at: https://pubmed.ncbi.nlm.nih.gov/26691115/

EPA (2022). *National Enforcement and Compliance Initiative: Reducing Noncompliance with Drinking Water Standards at Community Water Systems* [online] Available at: https://www.epa.gov/enforcement/national-enforcement-and-compliance-initiative-reducing-noncompliance-drinking-water

References

Adams, C. (2023) *Jackson's water crisis persists as national attention and help fade away.* NBC News. [online] Available at: https://www.nbcnews.com/news/nbcblk/jackson-mississippi-still-dealing-water-crisis-rcna65563 [Accessed Mar - June 2023].

Allaire, M., Wu, H. and Lall, U. (2018) National trends in drinking water quality violations. *Proceedings of the National Academy of Sciences*, [online] Available at: https://www.pnas.org/content/115/9/2078.short?rss=1 [Accessed Mar - June 2023].

ATSDR, (2021) *Arsenic Toxicity: What are the Physiologic Effects of Arsenic Exposure? | Environmental Medicine* [online] www.atsdr.cdc.gov. Available at: https://www.atsdr.cdc.gov/csem/arsenic/physiologic_effects.html. [Accessed Mar - June 2023].

Balazs, C., Morello-Frosch, R., Hubbard, A. and Ray, I. (2011) Social Disparities in Nitrate-Contaminated Drinking Water in California's San Joaquin Valley. *Environmental Health Perspectives*, 119(9), pp.1272–1278. [online] Available at: https://pubmed.ncbi.nlm.nih.gov/21642046/ [Accessed Mar - June 2023].

CDC (1998) *Summary of Notable Diseases.* [online] Available at: https://www.cdc.gov/mmwr/preview/mmwrhtml/00056071.htm [Accessed Mar - June 2023].

CDC (2009) *Rural Water supplies and Water Quality Issues* [online] Available at: https://www.cdc.gov/nceh/publications/books/housing/cha08.htm [Accessed Mar - June 2023].

CDC (2021a) *Disinfection By-products (DBPs) Factsheet | National Biomonitoring Program* [online] www.cdc.gov. Available at: https://www.cdc.gov/biomonitoring/THM-DBP_FactSheet.html [Accessed Mar - June 2023].

CDC (2021b) *Preventing Legionnaires' Disease*. [online] Centers for Disease Control and Prevention. Available at: https://www.cdc.gov/vitalsigns/legionnaires/index.html#:~:text=About%205%2C000%20people%20are%20diagnosed [Accessed Mar - June 2023].

CDC (2022) *Per- and Polyfluorinated Substances (PFAS) Factsheet | National Biomonitoring Program | CDC*. [online] Available at: https://www.cdc.gov/biomonitoring/PFAS_FactSheet.html#:~:text=Print [Accessed Mar - June 2023].

CDC (2023) *Lead in Drinking Water* [online] Available at: https://www.cdc.gov/nceh/lead/prevention/sources/water.htm [Accessed Mar - June 2023].

Center For Sustainable Systems, University of Michigan (2021) *U.S. Water Supply and Distribution Factsheet*. [online] Available at: https://css.umich.edu/publications/factsheets/water/us-water-supply-and-distribution-factsheet [Accessed Mar - June 2023].

Denchak, M. (2018) *Flint water crisis: Everything you need to know*. [online] NRDC. Available at: https://www.nrdc.org/stories/flint-water-crisis-everything-you-need-know [Accessed Mar - June 2023].

Environmental Protection Agency (2020) *NEIC Civil Investigation Report, City of Jackson Water System*. [online] Available at: https://www.epa.gov/system/files/documents/2021-07/neic-civil-investigation-report_city-of-jackson-public-water-system.pdf [Accessed Mar - June 2023].

Environmental Working Group (2010) *State of American Drinking Water: EWG's Tap Water Database*. [online] Available at: https://www.ewg.org/tapwater/state-of-american-drinking-water.php [Accessed Mar - June 2023].

EPA (2015) *How the Drinking Water State Revolving Fund Works*. [online] Available at: https://www.epa.gov/dwsrf/how-drinking-water-state-revolving-fund-works#tab-1 [Accessed Mar - June 2023].

EPA (2022a) *Safe Water Drinking Act* [online] Available at: https://www.epa.gov/sdwa [Accessed Mar - June 2023].

EPA (2022b) *Nonpoint Source: Agriculture* [online] Available at: https://www.epa.gov/nps/nonpoint-source-agriculture [Accessed Mar - June 2023].

EPA (2022c) *Protecting Water Quality from Agricultural Runoff* [online] Available a: https://www.epa.gov/sites/default/files/2015-09/documents/ag_runoff_fact_sheet.pdf [Accessed Mar - June 2023].

EPA (2023a) *Use of Lead Free Pipes, Fittings, Fixtures, Solder, and Flux for Drinking Water* [online] Available at: https://www.epa.gov/sdwa/use-lead-free-pipes-fittings-fixtures-solder-and-flux-drinking-water [Accessed Mar - June 2023].

EPA (2023b) *Key EPA Actions to Address PFAS* [online] Available at; https://www.epa.gov/pfas/key-epa-actions-address-pfas [Accessed Mar - June 2023].

Gross, T. (2018) NPR Choice page. *NPR.org*. [online] Available at: https://www.npr.org/sections/health-shots/2018/06/25/623126968/pediatrician-who-exposed-flint-water-crisis-shares-her-story-of-resistance [Accessed Mar - June 2023].

Hansen, K. (2021) *Drinking Water Equity: Analysis and Recommendations for the Allocation of the State Revolving Funds*. [online] Environmental Policy Innovation Center. Available at: https://www.policyinnovation.org/publications/drinking-water-equity?rq=drinking%20water%20state%20revolving%20funds [Accessed Mar - June 2023].

Hanna-Attisha, M., LaChance, J., Sadler, R.C. and Champney Schnepp, A. (2016) Elevated Blood Lead Levels in Children Associated with the Flint Drinking Water Crisis: A Spatial Analysis of Risk and Public Health Response. *American Journal of Public Health* [online] Available at: https://pubmed.ncbi.nlm.nih.gov/26691115/ [Accessed Mar - June 2023].

Knobeloch, L., Salna, B., Hogan, A., Postle, J. and Anderson, H. (2000). Blue babies and *nitrate*-contaminated well water. *Environmental Health Perspectives*, [online] 108(7), pp.675–678. Available at: https://www.ncbi.nlm.nih.gov/pmc/articles/PMC1638204/. [Accessed Mar - June 2023].

Lott, J. (2023) *The problems in the pipes*. [online] Washington Post. Available at: https://www.washingtonpost.com/nation/interactive/2023/jackson-mississippi-water-crisis/ [Accessed Mar - June 2023].

Michigan Civil Rights Commission (2017) *Systemic Racism Through the Lens of Flint, Michigan Civil Rights Commission*. [online] Available at: https://www.michigan.gov/-/media/Project/Websites/mdcr/mcrc/reports/2017/flint-crisis-report-edited.pdf?rev=4601519b3af345cfb9d468ae6ece9141. [Accessed Mar - June 2023].

MSDH Mississippi State Department of Health (2023). *Boil Water Notices*. [online] Available at: https://www.msdh.state.ms.us/msdhsite/_static/23,0,148.html#page_end [Accessed 15 Mar. 2023].

Moore, Y. (2022) *Jackson, Mississippi Water Crisis - Center for Disaster Philanthropy*. [online] Center for Disaster Philanthropy. Available at: https://disasterphilanthropy.org/disasters/jackson-mississippi-water-crisis/ [Accessed Mar - June 2023].

Nilsen, E. and Babineau, A. (2022). *EPA launches federal civil rights investigation over Jackson water crisis*. [online] CNN. Available at: https://www.cnn.com/2022/10/20/us/jackson-mississippi-water-crisis-epa-civil-rights-investigation-reaj/index.html [Accessed 24 June 2023].

Pittman, A. (2022) *EPA Investigating Mississippi for Civil Rights Violations Over Jackson Water Crisis*. [online] Available at: https://www.mississippifreepress.org/28565/epa-investigating-mississippi-for-civil-rights-violations-over-jackson-water-crisis [Accessed 24 June 2023]

Rayasam, R. (2022). *In Jackson, the Water Is Back, but the Crisis Remains*. [online] KFF Health News. Available at: https://kffhealthnews.org/news/article/jackson-mississippi-bottled-water-crisis/ [Accessed 18 January 2024].

Reiner, R. et al. (2020) *Mapping geographical inequalities in childhood diarrhoeal morbidity and mortality in low-income and middle-income countries, 2000–17: analysis for the Global Burden of Disease Study 2017*. [online] Available at: https://www.thelancet.com/journals/lancet/article/PIIS0140-6736(20)30114-8/fulltext [Accessed Mar - June 2023].

Samuels, R., Martinez, E. and Lott, J. (2022) *The problem in the pipes*. The Washington Post. [online] Available at: https://www.washingtonpost.com/nation/interactive/2023/jackson-mississippi-water-crisis/ [Accessed Mar - June 2023].

Schaider, L.A., Swetschinski, L., Campbell, C. and Rudel, R. (20). *Environmental justice and drinking water quality: are there socioeconomic disparities in nitrate levels in U.S. drinking water?* [online] Available at: https://ehjournal.biomedcentral.com/articles/10.1186/s12940-018-0442-6 [Accessed Mar - June 2023].

Schechinger, A. (2020) *EWG Investigation: Across Farm Country, Nitrate Pollution of Drinking Water for More Than 20 million Americans is Getting Worse*. [online] Available at: https://www.ewg.org/interactive-maps/2020-nitrate-pollution-of-drinking-water-for-more-than-20-million-americans-is-getting-worse/#:~:text=Nitrate%20is%20a%20primary%20chemical [Accessed Mar - June 2023].

Smith, A., Huss, A., Dorevitch, S., Heijnen, L., Arntzen, V., Davies, M., Mirna, Ry Van Beest Holle, R.-D., Fujita, Y., Verschoor, A., Raterman, B., Oesterholt, F., Heederik, D. and Medema, G. (2019). Multiple Sources of the Outbreak of Legionnaires' Disease in Genesee County, Michigan, in 2014 and 2015. *Environmental Health Perspectives*. [online] Available at:

https://www.ncbi.nlm.nih.gov/pmc/articles/PMC6957290/pdf/ehp-127-127001.pdf [Accessed Mar - June 2023].

Stillo, F. and MacDonald Gibson, J. (2017) Exposure to Contaminated Drinking Water and Health Disparities in North Carolina. *American Journal of Public Health*. [online] Available at: https://pubmed.ncbi.nlm.nih.gov/27854523/ [Accessed Mar - June 2023].

Suh, R. (2017) *A Major Step Forward in the Flint Water Crisis*. [online] Available at: https://www.nrdc.org/experts/rhea-suh/major-step-forward-flint-water-crisis [Accessed Mar - June 2023].

Thompson, C. and Ruble, K. (2022) *Coalition sues to force Flint to finish replacing lead water lines*. [online] Available at: https://www.detroitnews.com/story/news/michigan/flint-water-crisis/2022/11/02/coalition-sues-to-force-flint-to-finish-replacing-lead-water-lines/69614478007/#:~:text=%E2%80%9CMore%20than%2095%25%20of%20lead [Accessed Mar - June 2023].

Tulchinsky, T. (2018) *John Snow, Cholera, the Broad Street Pump; Waterborne Diseases Then and Now. Case Studies in Public Health*, [online] Available at: https://www.ncbi.nlm.nih.gov/pmc/articles/PMC7150208/ [Accessed Mar - June 2023].

United Nations General Assembly, (2015) *Human right to water and sanitation | International Decade for Action 'Water for Life' 2005-2015*. [online] Available at: https://www.un.org/waterforlifedecade/human_right_to_water.shtml. [Accessed Mar - June 2023].

US Census Bureau, (2021) *Quick Facts, Flint City MI*. [online] Available at: https://www.census.gov/quickfacts/flintcitymichigan? [Accessed Mar - June 2023].

US EPA, O. (2015). *Region 6 Tribal Program*. [online] www.epa.gov. Available at: https://www.epa.gov/tribal/region-6-tribal-program [Accessed 19 Jan. 2024].

USGS Water Science School, (2018) Contamination in U.S. Private Wells | U.S. Geological Survey. *USGS* [online] Available at: https://www.usgs.gov/special-topics/water-science-school/science/contamination-us-private-wells [Accessed Mar - June 2023].

Weinmeyer, R., Norling, A., Kawarski, M. and Higgins, E. (2014). The Safe Drinking Water Act of 1974 and Its Role in Providing Access to Safe Drinking Water in the United States. *AMA Journal of Ethics*, [online] Available at: https://journalofethics.ama-assn.org/article/safe-drinking-water-act-1974-and-its-role-providing-access-safe-drinking-water-united-states/2017-10. [Accessed Mar - June 2023].

WHO (2022). *Diarrhoeal disease.* [online] Available at: https://www.who.int/news-room/fact-sheets/detail/diarrhoeal-disease#:~:text=Diarrhoeal%20disease%201%20Scope%20of%20diarrhoeal%20disease%20Diarrhoeal [Accessed Mar - June 2023].

WMA.net. (2014). *WMA - The World Medical Association-WMA Statement on Water and Health.* [online] Available at: https://www.wma.net/policies-post/wma-statement-on-water-and-health/ [Accessed Mar - June 2023].

Lexicon of Listed Terms and Agencies

- **Community Water Source (CWS)** refers to a system that supplies the same population with water year-round and serves at least 25 people or 15 residences.
- **Environmental Policy Innovation Center** an organization that helps craft government policies to improve the speed and scale of conservation.
- **Environmental Protection Agency (EPA)** is an American government agency that develops standards and regulations to protect people and the environment from significant health risks. This organization also conducts environmental research and enforces regulations.
- **Environmental Working Group** is an American non-profit group specializing in research and advocacy in the areas of toxic chemicals, drinking water contaminants, and other environmental concerns.
- **Ground Water** is the other main water source for community water supplies, and is water drawn from subterranean deposits.
- **Surface Water** is water from rivers, lakes, ice, and snow and is one of the two main source types for community water supplies.
- **The Agency for Toxic Substances and Disease Registry (ATSDR)** is an advisory agency that is part of the US Department of Health and Human Services that creates profiles of toxic substances and conducts research regarding hazardous exposures.
- **The Safe Drinking Water Act (SDWA)** was passed by the US Congress in 1974 that gives the EPA the authority to set national health-based standards for drinking water.
- **The US Geological Survey** is a government agency that studies US landscapes, natural resources, and the hazards that threaten them.
- **WaterAid** is an international organization that focuses on water, sanitation, and hygiene education founded in 1981.

AUTHOR'S BIO SKETCH

Ariahnna Croskey, DO

Dr. Croskey is originally from Oakland Township, MI, and received her undergraduate degree in biology locally at Oakland University. She completed medical school at Michigan State University and completed her residency in Family Medicine at University of Washington affiliated Community Health Care in Tacoma. She is passionate about collaborating with underserved communities and will be working in a low-income Health Professions Shortage Area after graduation. In her free time, she enjoys ballroom dancing with her husband, running, hiking, knitting, and game nights with friends.

Chapter 11

Employment as a Social Determinant of Health

Naomi Epstein, MD, Author
Amanda Wolf, MD, Editor

"Everyone has the right to work, to free choice of employment, to just and favourable conditions of work and to protection against unemployment"
- The Universal Declaration of Human Rights United Nations General Assembly, 1948

Employment as a Social Determinant of Health

The social determinants of health are "the non-medical factors that influence health outcomes" (World Health Organization, 2023). These include "conditions in which people are born, grow, work, live, and age, and the wider set of forces and systems shaping the conditions of daily life" (World Health Organization, 2023). Employment falls into many of these categories including how individuals work and live, and how they can provide for themselves and their families. Employment is therefore a critical social determinant of health. Investigating that further, this chapter explores employment's effects on physical and emotional health, access to care, poverty, and standard of living.

Employment as a Social Determinant of Health

In the context of Health

Employment exerts its impact on health in many ways. Unemployment has negative health effects, both physical and emotional (Marmot and Wilkinson, 2003). One study analyzing employment status and its effect on health found that, "Adverse health outcomes increased with unemployment duration and were highest for those unable to work," (Silver, Li, and Quay, 2021). In analyzing unemployment's impact, Driscoll and Bernstein (2012) showed that affordability of healthcare costs modifies health outcomes. Logic follows that unemployment reduces funds available to meet these expenses. Hospital stays, doctor's visits, imaging, labs, and ancillary services like physical and occupational therapy or wound care are tied to forms of reimbursement. During unemployment, money limits expenditures to priority necessities like food and housing with often little left over to meet healthcare needs.

Linn, Sandifer, and Stein (1985) tied unemployment to negative mental health effects, "After unemployment, symptoms of somatization, depression, and anxiety were significantly greater in the unemployed than employed." The authors further hypothesized that unemployed persons lack the cognitive satisfaction derived from productivity, which contributes to states of somatization, anxiety, depression, and low self-esteem.

Work circumstances and working conditions affect the health of the employed as well. According to Marmot and Wilkinson *The Solid Facts* (2003), people with high demand-low control jobs experience negative health consequences. Specifically, having little control over one's job increases cardiovascular risk. A considerable proportion of jobs fall into this category. Many undocumented workers are unable to control their work environment due to fear of repercussions. For example, migrant workers are in physically demanding jobs over which they have limited control, and for those with the added stress of being undocumented, cardiovascular risks are intensified. Even those in well-respected jobs such as medical residency may feel little control over their work and schedule, increasing the risk for cardiovascular disease (Marmot and Wilkinson, 2003).

In addition to direct threats of employment/unemployment on physical and mental well being, there are indirect risks. These include the ability to find time to exercise and afford healthy food. "Unhealthy diet and lack of physical activity are leading global risks to health," according to the World Health Organization (2020). People who work long hours or at two jobs may not have time for exercise. When it comes to healthy diets, the World Bank (2023) found that "42% - or

3.14 billion - of the global population could not afford a healthy diet in 2021" In the U.S. specifically, "4 million people could not afford a healthy diet in 2021" (World Bank, 2023). A healthy diet "meets nutritional standards set by dietary guidelines" (FAO, 2023). The FAO emphasizes, however, that a healthy diet need not be extravagant, it simply must meet established dietary guideline standards.

Dietary Guidelines for Americans, 2020 - 2025

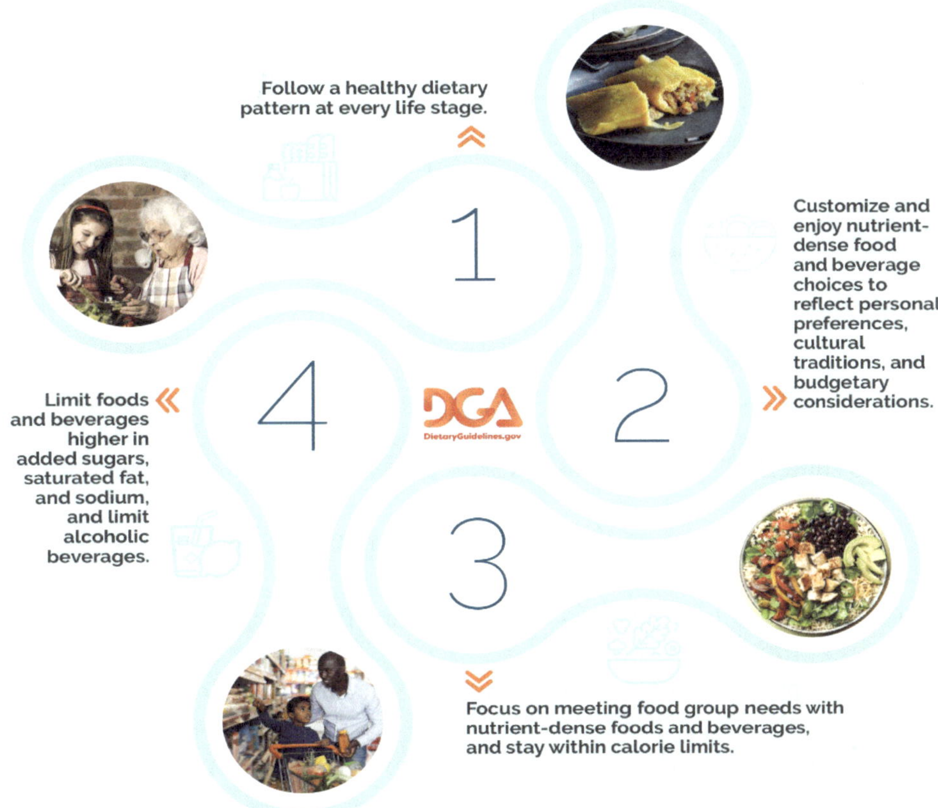

The Guidelines
Make every bite count
with the Dietary Guidelines for Americans. Here's how:
Follow a healthy dietary pattern at every life stage.
1
Customize and enjoy nutrient-dense food and beverage choices to reflect personal preferences, cultural traditions, and budgetary considerations.
2
DGA
DietaryGuidelines.gov
3
Focus on meeting food group needs with nutrient-dense foods and beverages, and stay within calorie limits.
4
Limit foods and beverages higher in added sugars, saturated fat, and sodium, and limit alcoholic beverages.

Dietary Guidelines for Americans (n.d.). *Downloadable Graphics | Dietary Guidelines for Americans*. [online] Available at: https://www.dietaryguidelines.gov/resources/downloadable-graphics#infographics

Underemployed or unemployed individuals struggle to afford healthy food to meet dietary guidelines. Working multiple jobs to purchase nutritious foods and make ends meet, reduces time to exercise, sleep, capture family time and recreational experiences further impacting individual health. Employment status affects health status in many ways in terms physical and mental health, through healthy diet, regular exercise, and sufficient rest as well as access to care.

Employment as a Social Determinant of Health

In the context of Access to Care

The World Health Organization (1948) declared, "The enjoyment of the highest attainable standard of health is one of the fundamental rights of every human being without distinction of race, religion, political belief, economic or social condition." The World Health Organization (2022) further elaborated, "Acknowledging health as a human right recognizes a legal obligation on states to ensure access to timely, acceptable, and affordable health care." In alignment with WHO proclamations, many countries embrace concepts of national or universal healthcare (The Commonwealth Fund, 2020b).

In the United States, gainful employment awards the right to affordable healthcare – thus, healthcare access is conferred by employment status, rather than granted as a human right (Institute of Medicine (US) Committee on Employment-Based Health Benefits, Field, and Shapiro, 2018). This stance dates to conclusion of World War II, when the U.S. diverged from many countries that established healthcare policy in alignment with WHO depositions (Institute of Medicine (US) Committee on Employment-Based Health Benefits, Field, and Shapiro (2018). According to Keisler-Starkey and Bunch (2021), "In 2020, 87.0 percent of full-time, year-round workers had private insurance coverage, up from 85.1 percent in 2018. In contrast, those who worked less than full-time, year-round were *less* likely to be covered by private insurance in 2020 than in 2018 (68.5

percent in 2018 and 66.7 percent in 2020)," which marginalized the imperative for affordable access to care for many individuals, *even those employed.* Furthermore, in 2020 8.6 percent of people, or 28 million people in the US. did not have health insurance at any point during the year Keisler-Starkey and Bunch (2021). The extraordinary costs of healthcare in the U.S. further exacerbates the dilemma of access to care for those without health insurance coverage (Kissell, 2022). In the circumstance of those *with* health insurance, exclusions and limitations to coverage and deductibles make healthcare unaffordable despite some forms of indemnification (Organisation for Economic Co-operation and Development, 2022).

Internationally, there are many different systems for providing access to healthcare, and not all are tied to employment (The Commonwealth Fund, 2020a). In fact, the U.S. is the only high-income country that does not guarantee health coverage (Gunja, Gumas, and Williams, 2023).

The U.S. is the only high-income country that does not guarantee health coverage.

Percent of total population with health insurance coverage

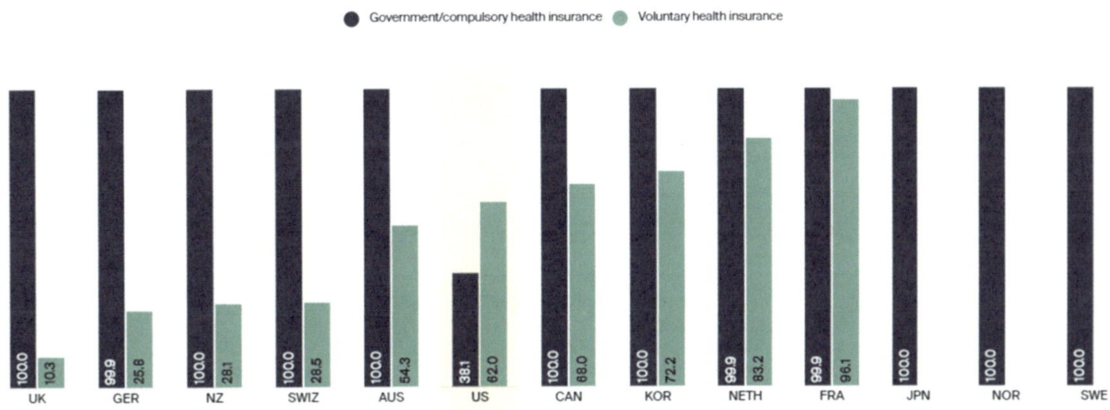

Notes: Government/compulsory health insurance data: 2021 data for AUS, CAN, FRA, NZ, and NOR; 2020 data for GER, KOR, NETH, SWE, SWIZ, UK, and US; 2019 data for JPN. Voluntary health insurance coverage data: 2021 data for AUS, CAN, and NZ; 2020 data for GER, KOR, NETH, and US; 2019 data for UK; 2017 data for FRA and SWIZ. Government health insurance refers to public benefit basket covering a minimum set of health services. Voluntary health insurance refers to payments for private insurance premiums, which grant coverage for services from private providers. See more information on definitions here: https://www.oecd.org/health/Spending-on-private-health-insurance-Brief-March-2022.pdf.

Data: OECD Health Statistics 2022.

Gunja, M., Gumas, E. and Williams II, R. (2023). *U.S. Health Care from a Global Perspective, 2022: Accelerating Spending, Worsening Outcomes*. [online] The Commonwealth Fund. Available at: https://www.commonwealthfund.org/publications/issue-briefs/2023/jan/us-health-care-global-perspective-2022

The imposition of full-time employment on access to affordable care plays significantly on health outcomes in the United States compared to other high income countries. For example, the U.S. has the *highest rate of infant and maternal deaths* (Gunja, Gumas, and Williams, 2023).

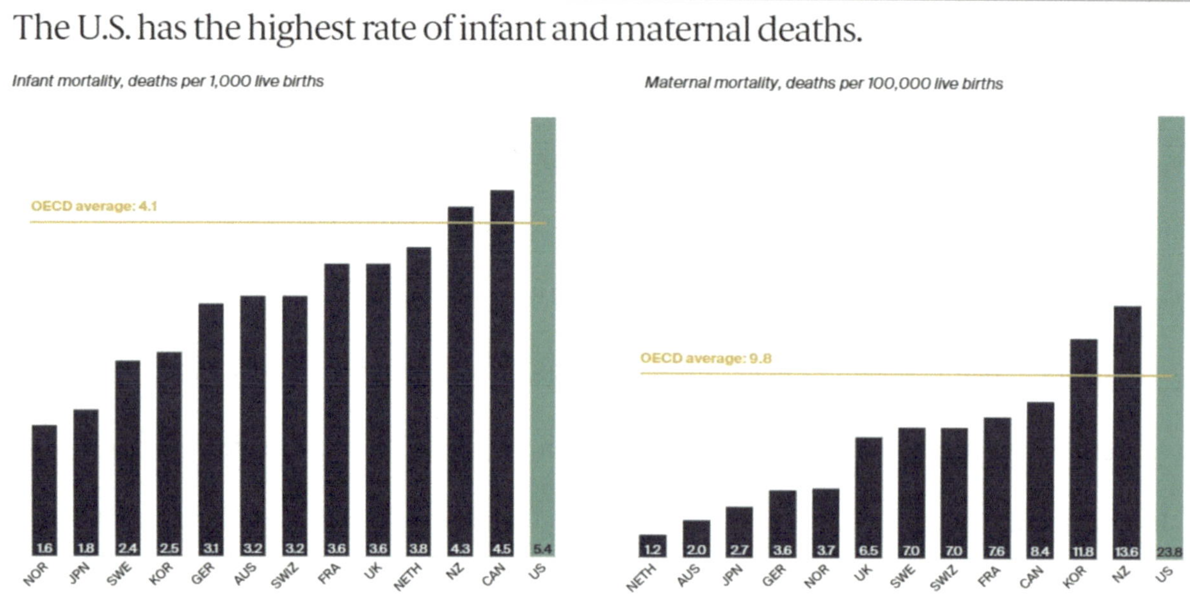

Notes: Infant mortality rates reflect no minimum threshold or gestation period or birthweight. Infant mortality 2021 data for FRA and SWIZ; 2020 data for AUS, CAN, GER, JPN, KOR, NETH, NOR, SWE, UK, and US; 2018 data for NZ. Maternal mortality 2020 data for AUS, CAN, GER, JPN, KOR, NETH, NOR, SWE, and US; 2019 data for SWIZ; 2018 data for NZ, 2017 data for UK; 2015 data for FRA. OECD average reflects the average of 38 OECD member countries.

Data: OECD Health Statistics 2022.

Source: Munira Z. Gunja, Evan D. Gumas, and Reginald D. Williams II, *U.S. Health Care from a Global Perspective, 2022: Accelerating Spending, Worsening Outcomes* (Commonwealth Fund, Jan. 2023). https://doi.org/10.26099/8ejy-yc74

Gunja, M.Z., Gumas, E.D. and Williams II, R.D. (2023). *U.S. Health Care from a Global Perspective, 2022: Accelerating Spending, Worsening Outcomes*. [online] The Commonwealth Fund. Available at: https://www.commonwealthfund.org/publications/issue-briefs/2023/jan/us-health-care-global-perspective-2022

According to Gunja, Gumas, and Williams (2023), compared to other OECD countries, the U.S. has the *highest avoidable deaths per 100,000 population* (deaths from conditions that are preventable and treatable), *deaths from assaults* (deaths from physical assault, including gun violence), *rates of obesity* (BMI greater than 30 kg/m^2), *adults with multiple chronic conditions* (two or more such as asthma, cancer, heart disease, hypertension), *deaths due to COVID-19* and *high suicide rates*. Reliance on employer provided health insurance and access to affordable care in the U.S. reflects as well on the low rates of physician visits and number of practicing physicians compared to other high-income countries.

Taken in aggregate the bottom-line reverts to healthy life-expectancy and life expectancy. U.S. life expectancy at birth is three years lower than the OECD average according to Gunja, Gumas, and Williams (2023). In the United States, life expectancy is inextricably tied to long term, full-time employment that provides health insurance as an employer benefit, not the principle that healthcare is a human right nor the responsibility of government.

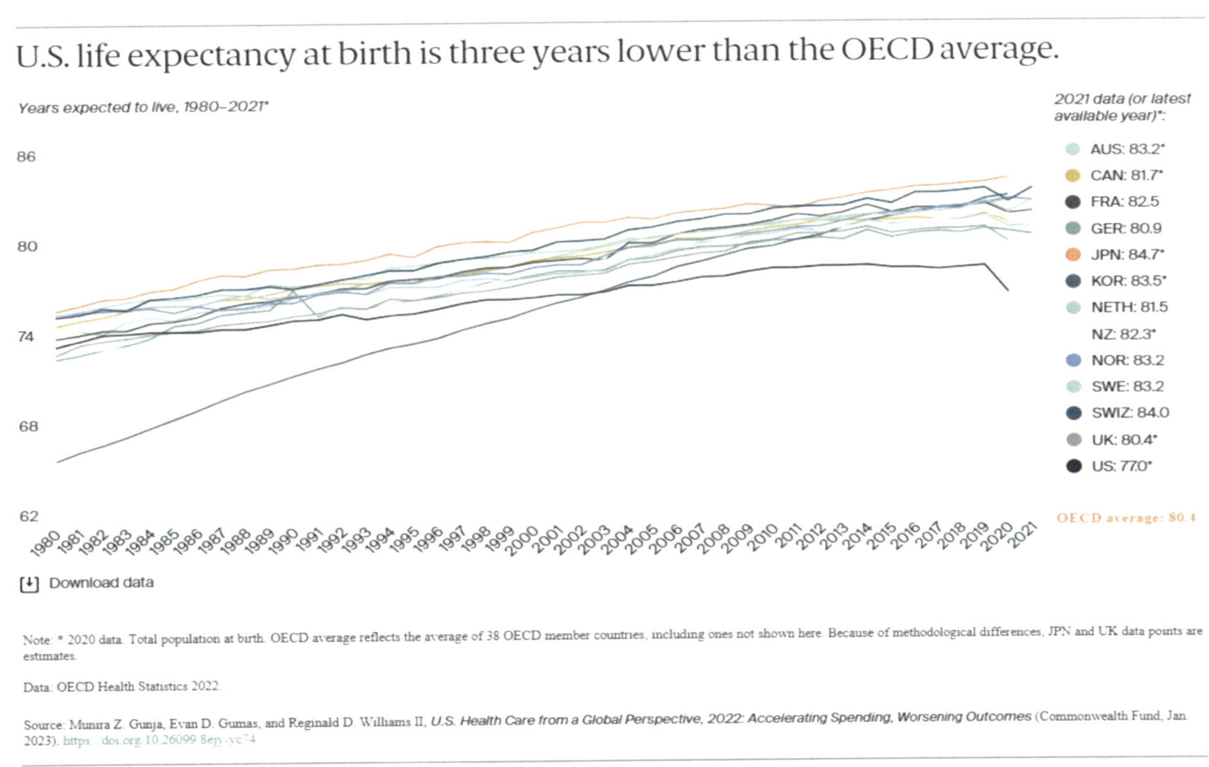

Gunja, M.Z., Gumas, E.D. and Williams II, R.D. (2023). *U.S. Health Care from a Global Perspective, 2022: Accelerating Spending, Worsening Outcomes*. [online] The Commonwealth Fund. Available at: https://www.commonwealthfund.org/publications/issue-briefs/2023/jan/us-health-care-global-perspective-2022

In 2010, the United States Congress passed the Affordable Care Act (ACA), enshrining employer shared responsibility provisions with specific language connecting employment and access to healthcare (IRS, 2016). The wording obliges "certain employers" (called applicable large employers or ALEs) to offer health coverage that is "affordable" and that provides "minimum value" to full-time employees and offers "coverage to the full-time employees' dependents" (IRS, 2016). According to Dillender, Heinrich, and Houseman (2023), the ACA intended to increase employer-sponsored health insurance and thereby improve workers' compensation and the quality of jobs, particular for low-wage workers.

The ACA mandates that companies with more than 50 full-time employees (defined as working greater than 30 hours per week) must provide some form of health insurance to their employees or pay fines if they fail to comply. The mandated requirements created chilling effects for corporations by increasing the cost of doing business, impacting competitive price advantages, and eroding profits.

Some companies fired back with strategies to circumvent the imposed mandates.

Firing back at the ACA

- Passing along the premium costs to workers in the form of lower real wages or other reduced benefits.
- Increasing the use of workers in staffing arrangements not covered by the employer mandate.
- Reducing weekly hours below 30 or shifting the mix of staffing toward greater use of on-call, direct-hire and agency temporaries.
- Outsourcing certain tasks to firms with fewer than 50 full-time employees.
- Increasing the share of low-hours, part-time (defined as averaging less than 30 hours per week); temporary; and contract employment.

Dillender, M., Heinrich, C. and Houseman, S. (2023). Effects of the Affordable Care Act on Part-Time Employment: Early Evidence. [online] Cato.org. Available at: https://www.cato.org/research-briefs-economic-policy/effects-affordable-care-act-part-time-employment-early-evidence [Accessed 4 Dec. 2023].

These draconian retaliations imposed significant hardships for many employees and produced unintended consequences of the ACA for those most in need of health insurance. According to Even and Macpherson (2018), the "use involuntary part-time employment (IPT) in 2015 exceeded predictions based on economic conditions and the structure of the labor market. Of greater importance, using difference-in-difference methods, they found that the increase in the probability of IPT employment since passage of the ACA was greater in occupations with a larger share of workers affected by the mandate." The authors' estimates suggest that 700,000 additional workers without a college degree are in IPT employment because of the ACA employer mandate.

Employed vulnerable populations – those with unstable jobs, low-wage jobs, migrant workers, and undocumented workers – face daunting challenges accessing healthcare in the United States. "To care for the lower income residents, including undocumented immigrants, the U.S. relies on a patchwork system of safety-net providers, including public and not-for-profit hospitals, federally qualified community health centers (FQHCs), and migrant health centers," (Alarcon, 2022). All-important continuous primary and preventive care evades susceptible populations (American Family Physicians, 2019). According to Berk and Schur (2001) undocumented immigrants face exceptional circumstances. Their research discovered that 39% of undocumented adult immigrants expressed fear of accessing medical services due to undocumented status and the dread of recriminations including deportation.

Health care costs reflected in dollars and cents for Federal minimum wage jobs at $7.25/hour translates into $15,080 per year on full time forty hours per week. According to the World Bank Open Data (2023) per capita national health expenditures in the U.S. (the cost of care per individual) was $11,702).

Employment as a Social Determinant of Health

In the context of Poverty and Standard of Living

At its most basic, employment should permit individuals to earn a living wage that propels them beyond the brink of poverty and pay check to pay check subsistence. In the most favorable circumstance, employment provides expansive benefits like health insurance, paid time off, retirement packages, as well as job and wage security.

Based on employment history throughout the prior 100 years, in 1948 The United Nations General Assembly Universal Declaration of Human Rights etched into history the privilege for individuals to join unions, "Everyone has the right to form and to join trade unions for the protection of his interests," United Nations (1948). The American Federation of Labor (AFL-CIO, 2019) asserts that unions give workers a collective voice in negotiations with employers, leading to better employment and protections through empowerment and advocacy for economic justice within a democratic process.

Supporting the perspective of the Universal Declaration and the American Federation of Labor, a recent in-depth analysis from the U.S. Department of Treasury demonstrates the power of unions to address and influence negative employment trends by raising middle-class wages, improving work environment, and promoting demographic equality. "The Treasury Department released a first-of-its-kind report on labor unions, highlighting the evidence that unions serve to strengthen the middle class and grow the economy at large. Over the last half century, middle-class households have experienced stagnating wages, rising income volatility, and reduced intergenerational mobility, even as the economy as a whole has prospered," (Feiveson, 2023).

The Treasury analysis evaluated organized labor impact on income inequality, wages of non-union versus union workers, working environments, non-wage compensation (benefits like health insurance, paid time off), workplace equality, and the phenomenon of spillover – the effect of union employment benefits on nonunionized companies in competition with unionized workplaces, coercing non-union shops to raise wages, change hiring practices, and improve workplace environments to attract workers in concert and competitive with union shops.

The following table summarizes the highlights of the U.S. Department of Treasury report.

Labor Unions and the U.S. Economy

Income Inequality

Union membership in the U.S. peaked in the 1950s at 1/3 of the workforce. As union membership over subsequent decades steadily declined, income inequality steadily rose following the 1970s.

During the same period median family income stagnated, income became more volatile, time spent on vacation fell and middle-class Americans became less prepared for retirement. In 2022, union membership plateaued at 10 percent of workers while the top one percent of income earners earned almost 20 percent of total income. The Treasury report asserts that unions have the potential to address these negative trends by raising middle-class wages, improving work environments, and promoting demographic equality.

Wages

Union workers enjoy the "union wage premium" – the amount that union members make beyond non-union members. Analyzed from various methodologies the union wage premium amounts to 15 percent, with a larger effect for those long-tenured.

Work Environments

Studies find that 80 percent of people who like their jobs cite non-wage reasons as the primary cause of their satisfaction and the same percentage of people who *dislike* their jobs cite non-wage reasons to explain their dissatisfaction. Non-wage benefits affect worker well-being. Benefits, such as healthcare insurance and retirement benefits, represent components of compensation packages and confer substantial monetary value. Features of work environments, like flexible scheduling or workplace safety regulations, may not have direct monetary value but are highly valued by workers. In collective bargaining deliberations, unions enjoy a place at the table to negotiate wage and non-wage compensation unlike non-union employees.

Workplace Equality

Unions promote within-firm equality by adopting explicit anti-discrimination measures, supporting anti-discrimination legislation and enforcement, and promoting wage-setting practices that are less susceptible to implicit bias. Union membership is equal across men and women. In 2021, Black men had a particularly high union representation rate at 13 percent, compared to the population average of 10 percent.

Spillover Effects

In addition to the spillover effects noted above this table, unions drive workplace norms by lobbying for workplace safety and advocating for changes in minimum wage laws. Unions produce benefits for communities that extend beyond individual workers and employers by enhancing social capital and civic engagement. Union members vote 12 percentage points more often than nonunion members. Union members are more likely to donate to charity, attend community meetings, participate in neighborhood projects, and volunteer for an organization.

Feiveson, L. (2023). *Labor Unions and the U.S. Economy*. [online] U.S. Department of the Treasury. Available at: https://home.treasury.gov/news/featured-stories/labor-unions-and-the-us-economy

The following Bureau of Statistic figure further illustrates the dynamic power of union membership. In this instance influence on fringe benefits and amenities (Feiveson, 2023).

Fringe Benefits & Amenities Union vs. Non-union Employment Compared

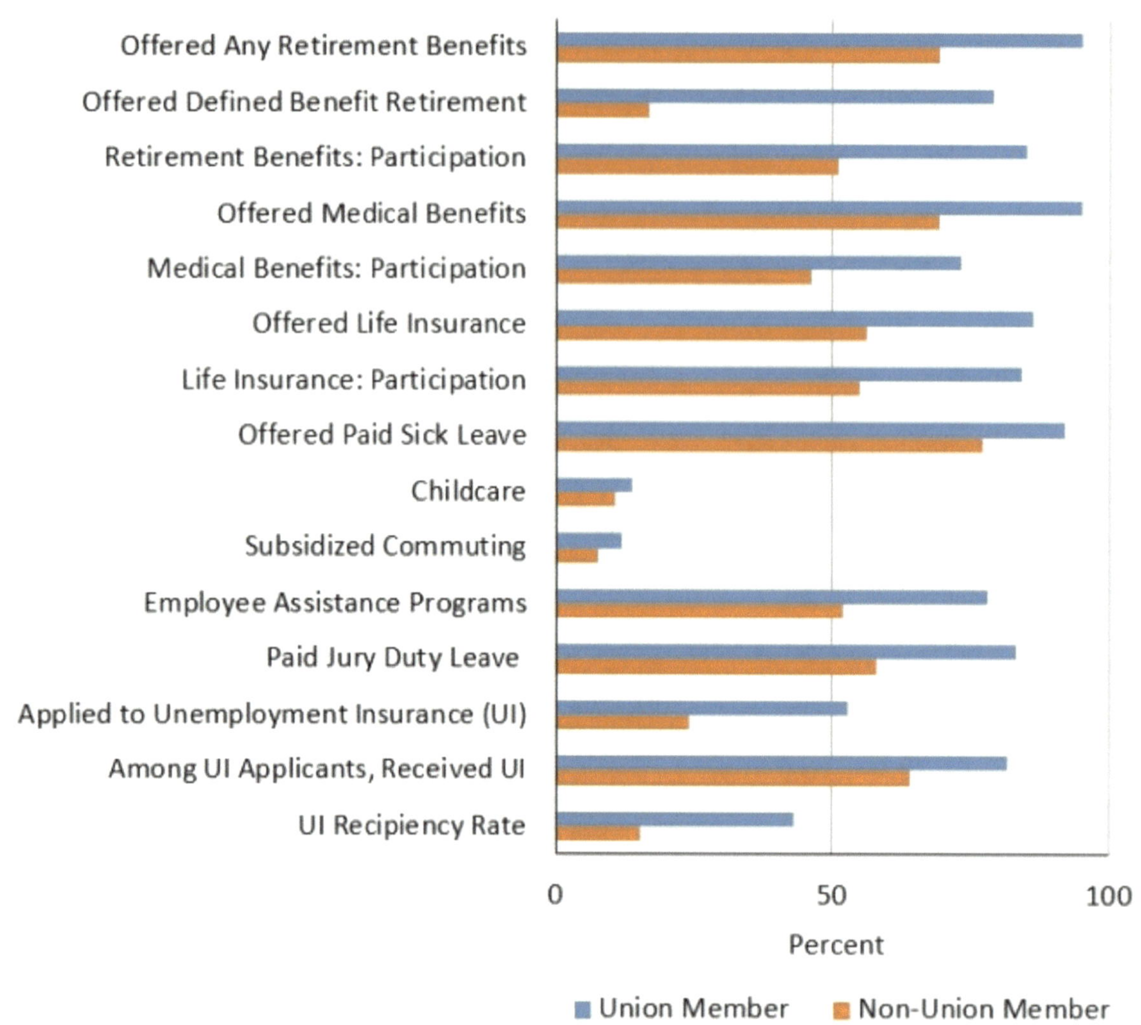

Feiveson, L. (2023). *Labor Unions and the U.S. Economy*. [online] U.S. Department of the Treasury. Available at: https://home.treasury.gov/news/featured-stories/labor-unions-and-the-us-economy

The 2023 United Auto Workers Strike

The six-week United Auto Workers (UAW) strike in the summer months of 2023, illustrates the extraordinary power of unions when applied with convincing data and a determined voice. "Capitalizing on the industry's high profits, a tight labor market, and support from President

Biden, the union forced the Big Three automakers to make big concessions not just on wage rates but in other areas too" (Cassidy, 2023).

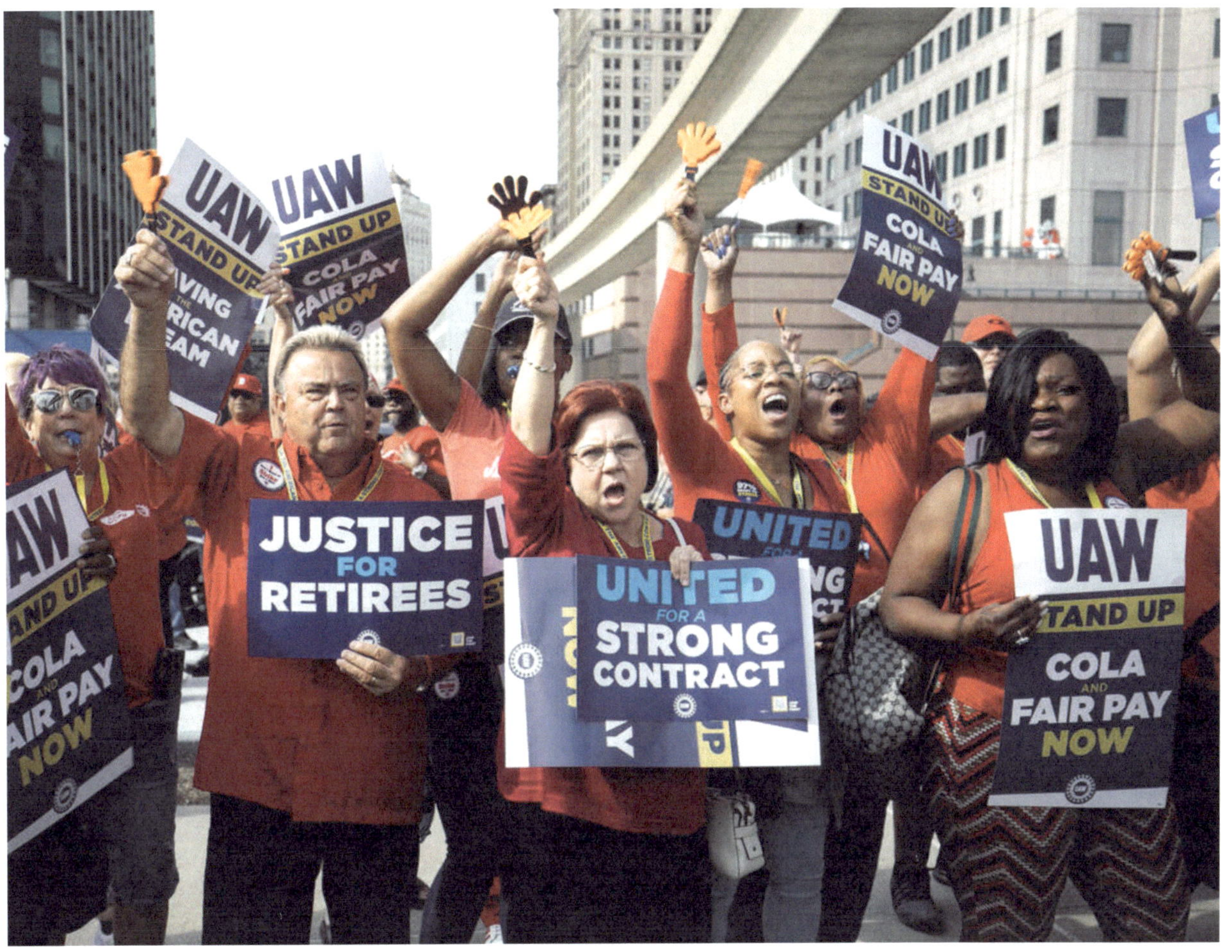

Domonoske, C. (2023). *The UAW Won Big in the Auto Strike — but What Does It Mean for the Rest of us?* [online] NPR. Available at: https://www.npr.org/2023/11/12/1211602392/uaw-auto-strike-deals-ratified-big-three-shawn-fain
Bill Pugliano/Getty Images, 2013.

According to Cassidy (2023), Shawn Fain, the leader of the U.A.W., has hailed the outcome of the strike as a major win for the entire labor movement. Like the recent deals between the Teamsters and UPS, health-care workers and Kaiser Permanente, and the Writers Guild and the Hollywood studios, the tentative agreement between the U.A.W. and the Big Three demonstrates that, "even in the fissured and outsourced economy of the twenty-first century, organized labor can still wield considerable power, especially in favorable economic conditions. That is not a surprise to anybody familiar with labor history, but it is a lesson that in recent decades has often been lost, or deliberately obscured" (Cassidy, 2023). Predictably the UAW, Teamsters, Kaiser, and Writers Guild contracts will propel a "spillover" effect of similar concessions and benefits for other employees fortunate to be represented by organized labor.

What The U.A.W. Won

Going into the strike, the media attention focused on four of the U.A.W.'s basic demands: sharply higher wages, including the restoration of automatic cost-of-living adjustments; the elimination of a two-tier pay system that was introduced more than fifteen years ago; a pathway to unionize new electric-vehicle plants; and the restoration of defined pensions and health insurance for union retirees. In the first three areas, the union appears to have achieved what it wanted. Only around retiree benefits did the auto companies manage to hold the line.

Under the new labor contract with Ford, which served as the model for the agreements with Stellantis and G.M., fully vested production-line workers will receive cumulative hourly pay increases of about twenty-seven per cent, and some members of skilled trades will receive raises of more than thirty per cent. All union members will also receive annual cost-of-living adjustments based on the rate of consumer-price inflation. Taken together, these provisions will raise the top hourly wages of Ford production workers from $32.05 to $42.60 during the contract, which will run until 2028, and the hourly wages of skilled workers from $36.96 to $50.97, the union said.

The agreement will also shorten the time it takes for new hires to be paid full wages. Under a two-tier pay system that was introduced in 2007, newer Ford workers received half as much pay as older workers, and it took them eight years to make up the difference. Going forward, new hires will be paid eighty-five per cent of the top rate after two years, and a hundred per cent after three years. Between now and October, 2025, according to the union, some Ford workers will see their hourly wages double under this provision.

Cassidy, J. (2023). *What the U.A.W. Won.* [online] The New Yorker. Available at: https://www.newyorker.com/news/our-columnists/what-the-uaw-won

Employment as a Social Determinant of Health

In the context of Minimum, Subminimum, and Living Wages

The U.S. defines wages in three categories – minimum, subminimum, and living.

Minimum Wage:

The Federal minimum wage provisions for covered nonexempt employees are contained in the Fair Labor Standards Act (FLSA). The Fair Minimum Wage Act of 2007 included phased increases to the Federal minimum wage.

- For work performed on or after July 24, 2009, the Federal minimum wage is $7.25 per hour.
- Many states have minimum wage laws. Where an employee is subject to both the state and Federal minimum wage laws, *the employee is entitled to the higher of the two minimum wages.*
- Various minimum wage exceptions apply under specific circumstances to workers with disabilities, full time students, youth under age 20 in their first 90 consecutive calendar days of employment, tipped employees and student-learners.
- A tipped employee means any employee engaged in an occupation in which he or she customarily and regularly receives more than $30 a month in tips.

United States Department of Labor (2009). elaws - Fair Labor Standards Act Advisor. [online] Dol.gov. Available at: https://webapps.dol.gov/elaws/faq/esa/flsa/001.htm

Federal Fair Minimum Wage Act 2007

The stipulations of the Federal Fair Minimum Wage Act of 2007 have not changed. Nor has the Federal minimum wage of $7.25 per hour increased since 2009. Compensation for a full-time worker at the 2009 minimum wage computes to $15,080 annually ($7.25 x 2080). According to the Office of Assistant Secretary for Planning and Evaluation (2023), the HHS Poverty Guideline for a family of three across the U.S. is $24,860 ($14,580 for a family of 1). According to the CPI Inflation Calculator, $7.25 in 2009 is worth $10.40 in 2023.

Office of the Assistant Secretary for Planning and Evaluation (2023). *Poverty guidelines*. [online] ASPE. Available at: https://aspe.hhs.gov/topics/poverty-economic-mobility/poverty-guidelines

CPI Inflation Calculator (2023). *$7.25 in 2009 → 2021 | Inflation Calculator*. [online] www.in2013dollars.com. Available at: https://www.in2013dollars.com/us/inflation/2009?amount=7.25

Subminimum Wage:

The Fair Labor Standards Act (FLSA) provides for the employment of certain individuals at wage rates *below the statutory minimum*. Such individuals include student-learners (vocational education students), as well as full-time students employed in retail or service establishments, agriculture, or institutions of higher education. Also included are individuals whose earning or productive capacities are impaired by a physical or mental disability, including those related to age or injury, for the work to be performed. Employment at less than the minimum wage is authorized to prevent curtailment of opportunities for employment. Such employment is permitted only under certificates issued by the Wage and Hour Division.

U.S. Department of Labor (n.d.). *Subminimum Wage | U.S. Department of Labor*. [online] www.dol.gov. Available at: https://www.dol.gov/agencies/whd/special-employment

Many U.S. states progressively structure and annually review wage rates well beyond Federal minimum levels – Washington $15.74, Oregon $13.50, New Jersey $14.13, Colorado $13.65, Arizona $13.85, among others. On the contrary, many more states subscribe to Federal minimums – Mississippi, North Carolina, Kansas, Alabama, Georgia, Kentucky, South Carolina, Wyoming, and many others to name a few (Konish, 2023).

Living Wage:

Led by Amy Glasmeier, PhD and professor of Economic Geography and Regional Planning at Massachusetts Institute of Technology, researchers and policy activists have promoted the concept of the living wage since 2004 (Living Wage Calculator, 2019).

The Living Wage

Analysts and policy makers often compare income to the federal poverty threshold in order to determine an individual's ability to live within a certain standard of living. However, *poverty thresholds do not account for living costs beyond a basic food budget.* The federal poverty measure does not take into consideration costs like childcare and health care that not only draw from one's income, but also are determining factors in one's ability to work and to endure the potential hardships associated with balancing employment and other aspects of everyday life. Further, *poverty thresholds do not account for geographic variation in the cost of essential household expenses.*

The living wage model is an alternative measure of basic needs. It is a *market-based approach that draws upon geographically specific expenditure data related to a family's minimum food, childcare, health insurance, housing, transportation, and other basic necessities (e.g., clothing, personal care items, etc.) costs.* The living wage draws on these cost elements and the rough effects of income and payroll taxes to determine the minimum employment earnings necessary to meet a family's basic needs while also maintaining self-sufficiency.

The living wage model generates a cost-of-living estimate that exceeds the federal poverty thresholds. As calculated, the living wage estimate accounts for the basic needs of a family. The living wage model does not include funds that cover what many may consider as necessities enjoyed by many Americans.

Living Wage Calculator (2019). *Living Wage Calculator.* [online] Available at: https://livingwage.mit.edu/pages/about [Accessed 11 December 2023].

Declaring that a living wage is an "essential aspect of decent work to ensure that all workers, families and communities can live in dignity" and that "minimum wages do not always allow for a decent living" the United Nations fully supports living wage concepts. The U.N. further asserts that living wages directly advance the Global Compact Sustainable Development Goals – Goal 1: No Poverty, Goal 5: Gender Equality, Goal 8: Decent Work and Economic Growth and Goal 10: Reduced Inequalities" (United Nations, n.d.).

Employment as a Social Determinant of Health

Policy, Politics and Governance

Although both Republicans and Democrats in the U.S. Senate allegedly support minimum wage increases, on March 4th 2021 the Senate voted down an amendment to increase the Federal minimum wage to $15 an hour by 2025. The wage increase came as a provision of President Biden's $1.9 trillion COVID-19 stimulus package. The vote to increase failed by a margin of 58 - 42 with eight democrats joining with republicans to defeat it – Senators Joe Manchin III of West Virginia, Kyrsten Sinema of Arizona, Jeanne Shaheen and Maggie Hassan of New Hampshire, Tom Carper and Chris Coons of Delaware, and Jon Tester of Montana (Cochran and Edmondson, 2021).

The U.S. minimum wage of $7.25/hour stands pat since the last increase that went into effect in 2009. It translates to $15,080 annually. The federal poverty level for a single individual is $14,580 and $24,860 for a family of three.

On the contrary, the U.S. Office of Personnel Management (OPM) announced January 20, 2022 that Federal civilian employees in the United States will be paid at least $15.00/hour. "The Departments of Agriculture, Commerce, Defense, Interior, Treasury, and Veterans Affairs collectively employ the vast majority of the people who are currently paid below $15 per hour, but the $15 minimum hourly rate policy applies to all agencies excluding the U.S. Postal Service and Postal Regulatory Commission" (U.S. Office of Personnel Management, 2022). Fifteen dollars per hour equates to $31,200 annually for full time employees. According to FEHB (n.d.), the Federal Employee's Health Benefit program offers federal employees a choice of multiple health insurance plans at a reduced rate and paid with pre-tax dollars. The U.S. Government pays 72-75% of the premiums for each plan and employees are responsible for the remainder of the premium.

In December 2023, the U.S. Congress passed the National Defense Authorization Act, which authorized, in addition to billions in defense related spending, a 5.2% pay raise for service members and civilian defense employees (Kheel, 2023). In 2024, an enlisted service member with a paygrade of E-1 will receive an estimated $2,017.32 per month in basic pay ($24,207.84 annually). Meanwhile, a more senior enlisted person with a paygrade of E-6, who has more than a decade of service, will earn an estimated $4,387.92 monthly or $52,655.04 annually (Military.com Network, 2023a).

Basic Military Pay or "base pay" is the standard amount of compensation for military personnel based on each individual pay grade. It amounts to *compensation before additional allowances* such as Basic Allowance for Housing, Basic Needs Allowance, Cost of Living Allowance, clothing, bonuses for reenlistment and special pay for certain assignments. Most *allowances are non-taxable*, adding significantly to net income (Military.com Network, 2023b).

Uniformed Service members and family members also benefit from fully paid health and dental insurance including prescriptions through Tricare (Tricare, 2019).

According to Institute of Medicine (US) Committee on Employment-Based Health Benefits, Field, M. and Shapiro, H. (2018), "The current U.S. system of voluntary employment-based health benefits is not the consequence of an overarching and deliberate plan or policy.

Rather, it reflects a gradual accumulation of factors: innovations in health care finance and organization, conflicting political and social principles, coincidences of timing, market dynamics, programs stimulated by the findings of health services research, and spillover effects of tax and other policies aimed at different targets." This hodge-podge leaves millions of Americans devoid of the 1948 World Health Organization declaration that health is a human right – "The enjoyment of the highest attainable standard of health is one of the fundamental rights of every human being without distinction of race, religion, political belief, economic or social condition" and sets the table for health outcomes that are anything but the envy of the world.

Questions for Further Consideration:

1. Compare and contrast international employee benefits of several high-income countries.
2. Explore The Common Wealth Fund at: https://www.commonwealthfund.org/international-health-policy-center/system-features/how-does-universal-health-coverage-work Create a table that compares various health systems with a focus on healthcare finance - government versus employer funded.
3. Health care for "undocumented" employees challenges employers, employees, and the U.S. government. How do various European countries manage health care finance for ex-patriots?
4. Should employers (enterprise, industry, business) or the government be responsible for funding health care?

Sentinel Readings for a Deeper Dive

CDC (2022). *NIOSH Study Examines Relationship between Employment Status, Healthcare Access, and Health Outcomes*. [online] Available at: https://www.cdc.gov/niosh/updates/upd-11-18-21.html [Accessed 9 Nov. 2023].

Marmot, M. and Wilkinson, R. (2003). *The solid facts: Social determinants of health*. 2nd ed. Copenhagen: Centre for Urban Health, World Health Organization. [online} Available at: https://iris.who.int/bitstream/handle/10665/108082/9289012870-eng.pdf?sequence=1&isAllowed=y [Accessed 8 November 2023].

The Commonwealth Fund (2020). *How does universal health coverage work?* [online] www.commonwealthfund.org. Available at: https://www.commonwealthfund.org/international-health-policy-center/system-features/how-does-universal-health-coverage-work [Accessed 3 December 2023].

The Commonwealth Fund (2020b). *International Health Care System Profiles*. [online] www.commonwealthfund.org. Available at: https://www.commonwealthfund.org/international-health-policy-center/system-profiles [Accessed 3 December 2023].

Cassidy, J. (2023). *What the U.A.W. Won*. [online] The New Yorker. Available at: https://www.newyorker.com/news/our-columnists/what-the-uaw-won {Accessed 5 December 2023].

References

AFL-CIO (2019). *What Unions Do | AFL-CIO*. [online] Aflcio.org. Available at: https://aflcio.org/what-unions-do [Accessed 13 December 2023].

Alarcon, F.J. (2022). The Migrant Crisis and Access to Health Care. *Delaware journal of public health*, [online] doi: https://www.ncbi.nlm.nih.gov/pmc/articles/PMC9621574/ [Accessed 8 November 2023].

American Academy of Family Physicians (2019). *Health Care for All: A Framework for Moving to a Primary Care-Based Health Care System in the United States*. [online] Aafp.org. Available at: https://www.aafp.org/about/policies/all/health-care-for-all.html [Accessed 8 December 2023].

Berk, M.L. and Schur, C.L. (2001). The Effect of Fear on Access to Care Among Undocumented Latino Immigrants. *Journal of Immigrant Health*, [online] Available at: http://www.jstor.org/stable/45436762 [Accessed 8 November 2023].

Cassidy, J. (2023). *What the U.A.W. Won*. [online] The New Yorker. Available at: https://www.newyorker.com/news/our-columnists/what-the-uaw-won [Accessed 13 December 2023].

Cochrane, E. and Edmondson, C. (2021). Minimum Wage Increase Fails as 7 Democrats Vote against the measure. *The New York Times*. [online] Available at: https://www.nytimes.com/2021/03/05/us/minimum-wage-senate.html [Accessed 13 December 2023].

CPI Inflation Calculator (2023). *$7.25 in 2009 → 2021 | Inflation Calculator*. [online]. Available at: https://www.in2013dollars.com/us/inflation/2009?amount=7.25 [Accessed 13 December 2023].

Dietary Guidelines for Americans (n.d.). *Downloadable Graphics | Dietary Guidelines for Americans*. [online] Available at: https://www.dietaryguidelines.gov/resources/downloadable-graphics#infographics [Accessed 3 Dec. 2023].

Dillender, M., Heinrich, C. and Houseman, S. (2023). *Effects of the Affordable Care Act on Part-Time Employment: Early Evidence*. [online] Available at: https://www.cato.org/research-briefs-economic-policy/effects-affordable-care-act-part-time-employment-early-evidence [Accessed 4 Dec. 2023].

Domonoske, C. (2023). *The UAW Won Big in the Auto Strike — but What Does It Mean for the Rest of us?* [online] NPR. Available at: https://www.npr.org/2023/11/12/1211602392/uaw-auto-strike-deals-ratified-big-three-shawn-fain [Accessed 13 December 2023].

Driscoll, A. and Bernstein, A. (2012). Health and Access to Care among Employed and Unemployed Adults: United States, 2009-2010. *NCHS data brief*, [online] Available at: https://pubmed.ncbi.nlm.nih.gov/22617552/ [Accessed 7 November 2023].

Even, W.E. and Macpherson, D.A. (2018). The Affordable Care Act and the Growth of Involuntary Part-Time Employment. *ILR Review* [online] Available at: https://doi.org/10.1177/0019793918796812 [Accessed 7 November 2023].

FAO (2023). The State of Food Security and Nutrition in the World 2023. [online] Available at: https://doi.org/10.4060/cc3017en [Accessed 8 November 2023].

Feiveson, L. (2023). *Labor Unions and the U.S. Economy*. [online] U.S. Department of the Treasury. Available at: https://home.treasury.gov/news/featured-stories/labor-unions-and-the-us-economy [Accessed 12 November 2023].

Gunja, M.Z., Gumas, E.D. and Williams II, R.D. (2023). *U.S. Health Care from a Global Perspective, 2022: Accelerating Spending, Worsening Outcomes*. [online] The Commonwealth Fund. Available at: https://www.commonwealthfund.org/publications/issue-briefs/2023/jan/us-health-care-global-perspective-2022 [Accessed 9 November 2023].

Institute of Medicine (US) Committee on Employment-Based Health Benefits, Field, M.J. and Shapiro, H.T. (2018). *Origins and Evolution of Employment-Based Health Benefits*. [online] Available at: https://www.ncbi.nlm.nih.gov/books/NBK235989/ [Accessed 9 November 2023].

IRS (2016). *Questions and Answers on Employer Shared Responsibility Provisions Under the Affordable Care Act | Internal Revenue Service*. [online] Available at: https://www.irs.gov/affordable-care-act/employers/questions-and-answers-on-employer-shared-responsibility-provisions-under-the-affordable-care-act [Accessed 12 November 2023].

Keisler-Starkey, K. and Bunch, L. (2021). *Health Insurance Coverage in the United States: 2020*. [online] The United States Census Bureau. [online] Available at: https://www.census.gov/library/publications/2021/demo/p60-274.html [Accessed 12 November 2023].

Kheel, R. (2023). *Biggest Military Pay Raise in 2 Decades Finalized in Newly Released Defense Bill*. [online] Military.com. Available at: https://www.military.com/daily-news/2023/12/07/military-pay-raise-2024-will-be-52-under-newly-unveiled-defense-bill.html [Accessed 16 December 2023].

Kissell, C. (2022). *What Happens If You Don't Have Health Insurance? – Forbes Advisor*. [online] www.forbes.com. Available at: https://www.forbes.com/advisor/health-insurance/what-happens-if-you-dont-have-health-insurance/ [Accessed 12 November 2023].

Konish, L. (2023). *These states are raising their minimum wages in 2023. Chart shows where workers can expect higher pay*. [online] CNBC. Available at: https://www.cnbc.com/2023/01/01/these-states-will-raise-their-minimum-wages-in-2023.html [Accessed 16 December 2023].

Linn, M., Sandifer, R. and Stein, S. (1985). Effects of Unemployment on Mental and Physical Health. *American journal of public health*, [online] Available at: https://doi.org/10.2105/ajph.75.5.502 [Accessed 12 November 2023].

Living Wage Calculator (2019). *Living Wage Calculator*. [online] Mit.edu. Available at: https://livingwage.mit.edu/pages/about [Accessed 16 December 2023].

Marmot, M. and Wilkinson, R. (2003). *The solid facts: Social determinants of health*. 2nd ed. Copenhagen: Centre for Urban Health, World Health Organization. [online} Available at: https://iris.who.int/bitstream/handle/10665/108082/9289012870-eng.pdf?sequence=1&isAllowed=y [Accessed 8 November 2023].

Military.com Network (2023a). *2021 Military Pay Charts*. [online] Available at: https://www.military.com/benefits/military-pay/charts [Accessed 16 December 2023].

Military.com Network (2023b). *Basic Pay*. [online] Military.com. Available at: https://www.military.com/benefits/military-pay/basic-pay [Accessed 16 December 2023].

Office of the Assistant Secretary for Planning and Evaluation (2023). *Poverty guidelines*. [online] ASPE. Available at: https://aspe.hhs.gov/topics/poverty-economic-mobility/poverty-guidelines [Accessed 9 November 2023].

Organisation for Economic Co-operation and Development (2022). *Health resources - health spending - OECD data.* [online] Organisation for Economic Co-operation and Development. Available at: https://data.oecd.org/healthres/health-spending.htm [Accessed 9 November 2023].

Silver, S., Li, J. and Quay, B. (2021). Employment status, unemployment duration, and health-related metrics among US adults of prime working age: Behavioral Risk Factor Surveillance System, 2018–2019. *American Journal of Industrial Medicine* [online] Available at: https://doi.org/10.1002/ajim.23308 [Accessed 9 November 2023].

The Commonwealth Fund (2020a). *How does universal health coverage work?* [online] www.commonwealthfund.org. Available at: https://www.commonwealthfund.org/international-health-policy-center/system-features/how-does-universal-health-coverage-work [Accessed 10 November 2023].

The Commonwealth Fund (2020b). *International Health Care System Profiles*. [online] www.commonwealthfund.org. Available at: https://www.commonwealthfund.org/international-health-policy-center/system-profiles [Accessed 3 December 2023].

Tricare (2019). *Home | TRICARE*. [online] Available at: https://www.tricare.mil/ [Accessed 17 Dec. 2023].

U.S. Department of Labor (n.d.). *Subminimum Wage | U.S. Department of Labor*. [online] www.dol.gov. Available at: https://www.dol.gov/agencies/whd/special-employment [Accessed 13 December 2023].

U.S. Office of Personnel Management. (2022). *RELEASE: OPM Announces $15 Minimum Wage for U.S. Federal Civilian Employees*. [online] Available at: https://www.opm.gov/news/releases/2022/01/release-opm-announces-dollar15-minimum-wage-for-us-federal-civilian-employees/ [Accessed 13 December 2023].

United Nations (n.d.). *Living Wage | UN Global Compact*. [online] Available at: https://unglobalcompact.org/what-is-gc/our-work/livingwages [Accessed 13 December 2023].

United Nations (1948). *Universal Declaration of Human Rights*. [online] United Nations. Available at: https://www.un.org/en/about-us/universal-declaration-of-human-rights [Accessed 6 November 2023].

United States Department of Labor (2009). *elaws - Fair Labor Standards Act Advisor*. [online] Available at: https://webapps.dol.gov/elaws/faq/esa/flsa/001.htm [Accessed 13 December 2023].

World Bank. (2023). *Food Prices for Nutrition DataHub: Global Statistics on the Cost and Affordability of Healthy Diets*. [online] Available at: https://www.worldbank.org/en/programs/icp/brief/foodpricesfornutrition [Accessed 8 November 2023].

World Health Organization (1948). *Constitution of the World Health Organization*. [online] World Health Organisation. Available at: https://www.who.int/about/accountability/governance/constitution [Accessed 6 November 2023].

World Health Organization (2020). *Healthy Diet*. [online] World Health Organisation. Available at: https://www.who.int/news-room/fact-sheets/detail/healthy-diet [Accessed 6 November 2023].

World Health Organisation (2022). *Human Rights and Health*. [online] World Health Organisation. Available at: https://www.who.int/news-room/fact-sheets/detail/human-rights-and-health [Accessed 6 November 2023].

World Health Organization (2023). *Social Determinants of Health*. [online] Available at: https://www.who.int/health-topics/social-determinants-of-health#tab=tab_1 [Accessed 7 November 2023].

Lexicon of Listed Terms and Agencies

- **CDC – Centers for Disease Control** CDC is the nation's leading science-based, data-driven, service organization that protects the public's health. For more than 70 years, we have put science into action to help children stay healthy so they can grow and learn; to help families, businesses, and communities fight disease and stay strong; and to protect the public's health.

- **IRS – Internal Revenue Service** the IRS is a bureau of the Department of the Treasury and one of the world's most efficient tax administrators.

- **UAW** – The International Union, United Automobile, Aerospace and Agricultural Implement Workers of America (UAW) is one of the largest and most diverse unions in North America, with members in every sector of the economy.

  UAW-represented workplaces range from multinational corporations, small manufacturers and state and local governments to colleges and universities, hospitals, and private non-profit organizations.

  The UAW has more than 400,000 active members and more than 580,000 retired members in the United States, Canada, and Puerto Rico.

- **UN – United Nations** one place where the world's nations can gather, discuss common problems, and find shared solutions.

- **United States Department of Labor** to foster, promote, and develop the welfare of the wage earners, job seekers, and retirees of the United States; improve working conditions; advance opportunities for profitable employment; and assure work-related benefits and rights.

- **WHO – World Health Organization** an organization of professionals committed to integrity and excellence in health. With a spirit of collaboration and a steadfast commitment to science, we are trusted to care for the world's health.

AUTHOR'S BIO SKETCH

Naomi Epstein, MD

Dr. Epstein grew up in the San Francisco Bay area. She attended Harvey Mudd College as a joint biology-chemistry major, then did a post-baccalaureate program at San Francisco State University. She enrolled in medical school at the University of South Florida, where she matriculated in the SELECT pathway, completing preclinical courses in Tampa and clinical rotations in Allentown, Pennsylvania. Through the SELECT curriculum she acquired training in leadership, values-based patient-centered care, and health systems in addition to her clinical experiences. Dr. Epstein is passionate about helping underserved individuals and patient advocacy. She intends to pursue her interests with a special focus on women's health in her professional future. In her free time, she enjoys cooking and baking, aerial silks, and languages which help her gain an understanding of diverse cultures and traditions.

Chapter 12

Healthcare Access as a Social Determinant of Health

Sylvia Otto, DO, Author
Dylan Peterson, MD, Editor

"Of all forms of discrimination and inequalities, injustice in health is the most shocking and inhumane."

-Martin Luther King Jr.

Healthcare Access as a Social Determinant of Health

In the context of Access to Care

The University of Missouri School of Medicine defines healthcare access as the "ability to obtain healthcare services such as prevention, diagnosis, treatment and management of diseases, illness, disorders, and other health-impacting conditions" (University of Missouri, 2020). They further declare that for healthcare to be accessible it must be affordable and convenient. Socioeconomic status, regional resources, health insurance availability, policy and politics contribute to the accessibility of health care. This essay explores how the broad array of healthcare access drivers, including policies and politics, influence health outcomes and provides for comparison, international population health status.

Absence of health insurance ranks as an uppermost barrier to health care and contributes significantly to health disparities. Most high-income countries have universal healthcare where the country's government bears the financial burden of the health insurance rather than the individual. The United States stands alone. It is the only high-income country that does not guarantee health care coverage to its residents (Gunja, Gumas, and Williams, 2023) (**Figure 1**).

According to a 2022 Gallup poll (Brenan, 2023), 57% of the United States population viewed healthcare as the responsibility of the federal government (**Figure 2**). However, in the same poll, 53% of the U.S. population preferred a system based on private insurance (**Figure 3**).

Figure 1.

The U.S. is the only high-income country that does not guarantee health coverage.

Percent of total population with health insurance coverage

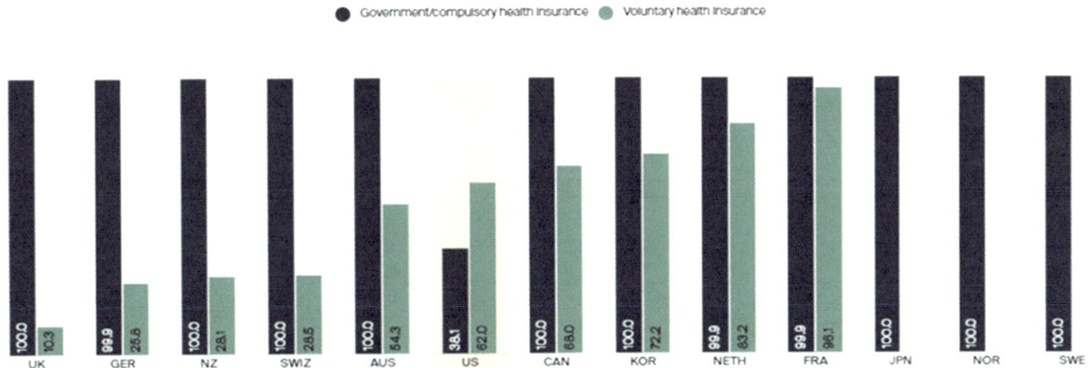

Notes: Government compulsory health insurance data: 2021 data for AUS, CAN, FRA, NZ, and NOR; 2020 data for GER, KOR, NETH, SWE, SWIZ, UK, and US; 2019 data for JPN. Voluntary health insurance coverage data: 2021 data for AUS, CAN, and NZ; 2020 data for GER, KOR, NETH, and US; 2019 data for UK; 2017 data for FRA and SWIZ. Government health insurance refers to public benefit basket covering a minimum set of health services. Voluntary health insurance refers to payments for private insurance premiums, which grant coverage for services from private providers. See more information on definitions here: https://www.oecd.org/health/Spending-on-private-health-insurance-Brief-March-2022.pdf.

Data: OECD Health Statistics 2022.

Source: Munira Z. Gunja, Evan D. Gumas, and Reginald D. Williams II, *U.S. Health Care from a Global Perspective, 2022: Accelerating Spending, Worsening Outcomes* (Commonwealth Fund, Jan. 2023). https://doi.org/10.26099/8ejy-yc74

Gunja, M., Gumas, E. and Williams, R. (2023). *U.S. Health Care from a Global Perspective, 2022: Accelerating Spending, Worsening Outcomes*. [online] www.commonwealthfund.org. Available at: https://www.commonwealthfund.org/publications/issue-briefs/2023/jan/us-health-care-global-perspective-2022#1

Figure 2.

Majority in U.S. Say Healthcare Is Federal Government's Responsibility

Do you think it is the responsibility of the federal government to make sure all Americans have healthcare coverage, or is that not the responsibility of the federal government?

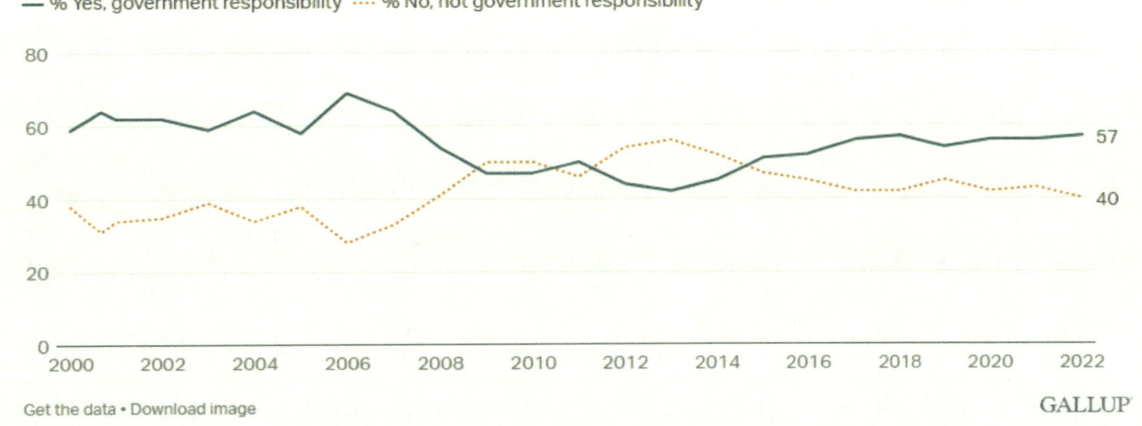

Brenan, M. (2023). *Majority in U.S. Still Say Gov't Should Ensure Healthcare*. [online] Gallup.com. Available at: https://news.gallup.com/poll/468401/majority-say-gov-ensure-healthcare.aspx.

Figure 3.

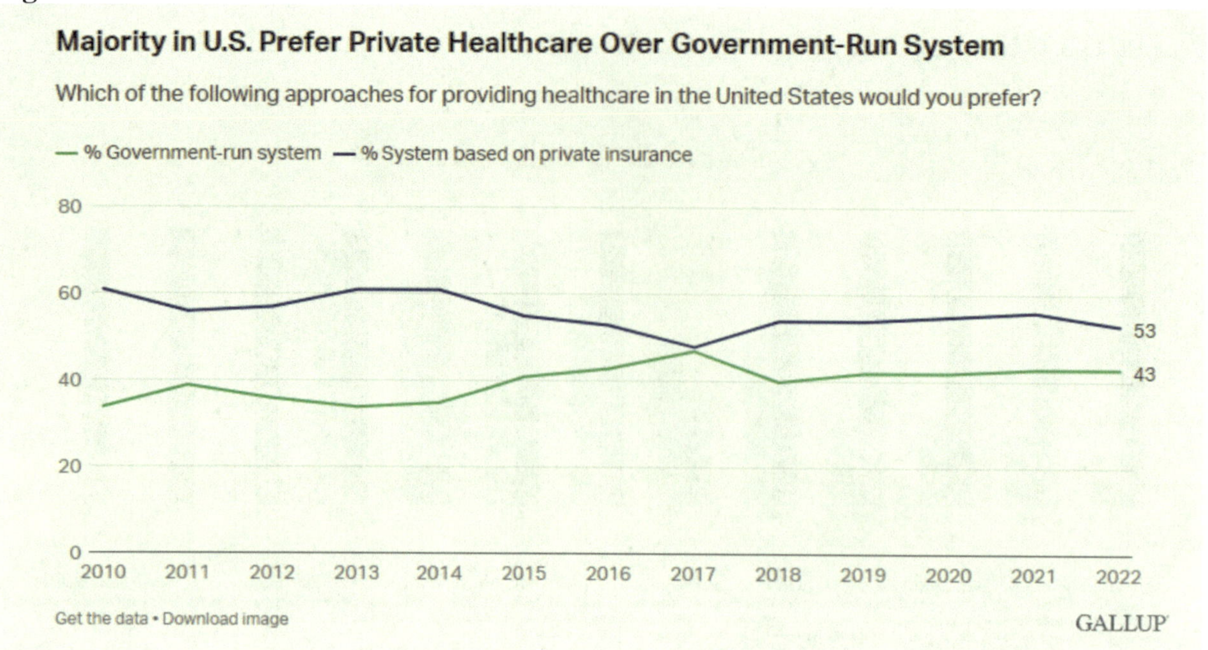

Brenan, M. (2023). *Majority in U.S. Still Say Gov't Should Ensure Healthcare.* [online] Gallup.com. Available at: https://news.gallup.com/poll/468401/majority-say-gov-ensure-healthcare.aspx.

Even though the U.S. does not make available health insurance coverage for all, some government funded healthcare insurance plans provide coverage for specific populations. Programs include Children's Health Insurance Program (CHIP), Medicare, Medicaid and military beneficiaries. These government funded health care programs increase access to care for vulnerable populations that qualify (children, pregnant mothers, elderly, disabled). According to Healthy People 2030 (n.d.), uninsured people from 60 to 64 years of age who became eligible for Medicare at age 65 increased their use of clinical services. Similar studies found that providing Medicaid to previously uninsured adults increased the rate of detecting diabetes and receiving diabetic treatment (Healthy People 2030, n.d.). Despite clear evidence for the effectiveness of government programs, barriers like means testing derail availabilty to those who may need it most.

In the United States, recipients of government assistance must prove eligibility through means testing. Means testing is a procedure used to determine financial and personal need for assistance with an alleged goal of reducing poverty and providing availability of essential goods and services.

Although means testing endures scrutiny and criticism on political and policy levels, means-tested entitlement programs delineate the core of the nation's social safety net, according to the House Committee on the Budget (2017). They deliver vital assistance that protects millions of Americans from entering poverty, while providing ongoing safety and stability for individuals and families facing poverty. Means-tested entitlement programs fall into two major categories – health programs (i.e., Medicaid, Children's Health Insurance Program, and Affordable Care Act subsidies) and income security programs (i.e., nutrition assistance, Supplemental Security Income (SSI), the Earned Income Tax Credit (EITC), and the Child Tax Credit (CTC). Also included are pensions for low-income veterans. Eligibility for means-tested entitlement programs varies by plan. However, across the board they primarily benefit individuals and families living at or near the federal poverty level (FLP) (House Committee on the Budget, 2017).

Detractors assert means testing at or near the FLP excludes health insurance coverage for millions of Americans. To support this contention, the Centers for Disease Control and Prevention reported in the National Health Interview Survey (2022) that despite government coverage safety nets, 10.1% or 23.4 million indiviudals under the age of 65 in the United States were uninsured at the time of the interview (National Health Interview Survey, 2022). Furthermore, 4.2% of children (2.7 million) under the age of 18 were uninsured at the time of the interview (National Health Interview Survey, 2022). Detractors further contend that means testing to prove eligibility for healthcare access deeply offends the precept of healthcare as a human right (United Nations, 1948).

To track health care data, The National Center for Health Statistics (NCHS) conducts the National Health Interview Survey (NHIS) to monitor U.S. health status. The NHIS collects comprehensive data annually on a broad range of health topics through personal household interviews. Survey results are instrumental in supplying data to track health status, health care access, and progress toward achieving national health goals (CDC, 2023).

The Affordable Care Act (ACA) led to significant improvement in health care coverage through Medicaid expansion to include adults with incomes at or below 138% of the federal poverty level (Garfield, Orgera, and Damico, 2019). It provides tax credits for those individuals with incomes between 100-400% of the federal poverty level to make private insurance in the individual market more attainable (Garfield, Orgera, and Damico, 2019). Affordable healthcare coverage continues to be out of reach for many Americans, however, as not all 50 states have adopted Medicaid expansion, some individuals remain ineligeble for financial assistance and many are not able to afford healthcare coverage despite the financial assistance (Garfield, Orgera, and Damico, 2019). The Kaiser Family Foundation (2022) publication *Status of State Medicaid Expansion Decisions:Interpretive Map* revealed that twelve states had not yet adopted the Medicaid expansion (**Figure 4**).

Figure 4.

Status of State Medicaid Expansion Decisions

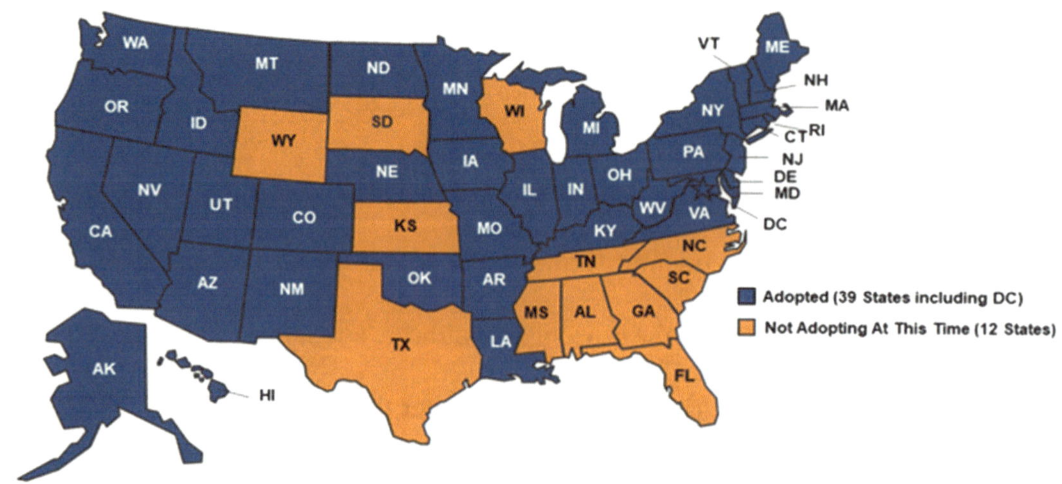

NOTES: Current status for each state is based on KFF tracking and analysis of state activity. See link below for additional state-specific notes.
SOURCE: "Status of State Action on the Medicaid Expansion Decision," KFF State Health Facts, updated July 21, 2022 https://www.kff.org/health-reform/state-indicator/state-activity-around-expanding-medicaid-under-the-affordable-care-act/

KFF

The Agency for Healthcare Research and Quality (AHRQ) states that "access to health care means having the timely use of personal health services to achieve the best health outcome" (AHRQ, 2018). Access includes four elements: *services* (having a usual source of care); *timeliness* health care when needed); *workforce* (qualified and culturally competent providers) and *coverage* (insurance that facilitates entry into the healthcare system) (AHRQ, 2018).

Healthcare Coverage

Cited by the AHRQ (2018), health insurance inequities include race/ethnicity as well as socioeconomic status. **Figure 5** details the disproportionate impact of race and ethnicity on insurance coverage. The graph illustrates the favorable impact of Obama Care as well beginning with passage in 2013.

Figure 5.

People under age 65 who were uninsured at the time of interview, by race/ethnicity, 2010-2015 Q3

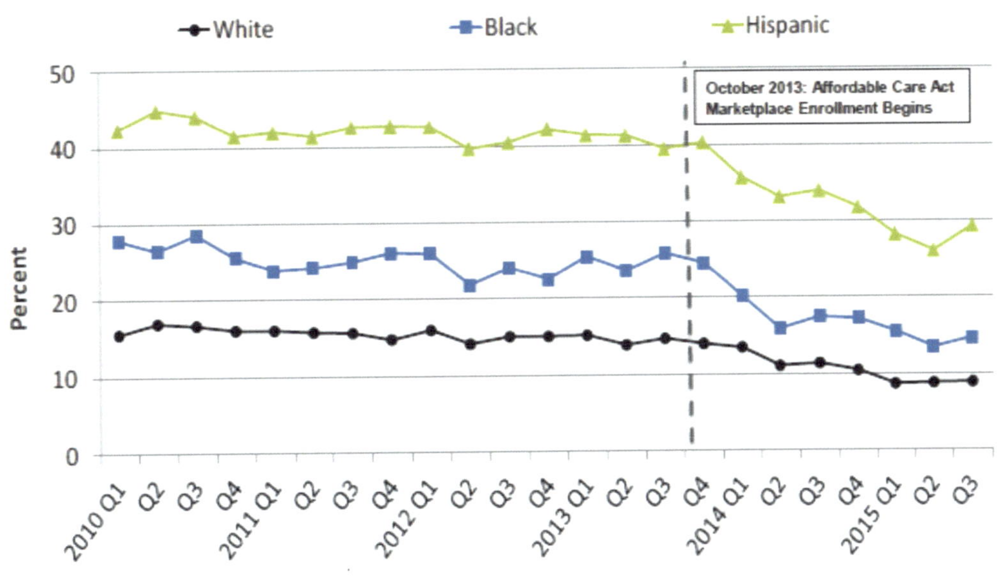

Agency for Healthcare Research and Quality(AHRQ) (2018). *Elements of Access to Health Care | Agency for Health Research and Quality*. [online] www.ahrq.gov. Available at: https://www.ahrq.gov/research/findings/nhqrdr/chartbooks/access/elements.html

Poverty weighs heavily on access to coverage. **Figure 6** illustrates poverty's impact on health insurance coverage as well as the mitigative effects of Obama Care in 2013 (AHRQ, 2018).

Figure 6.

People under age 65 who were uninsured at the time of interview, by poverty status, 2010-2015 Q3

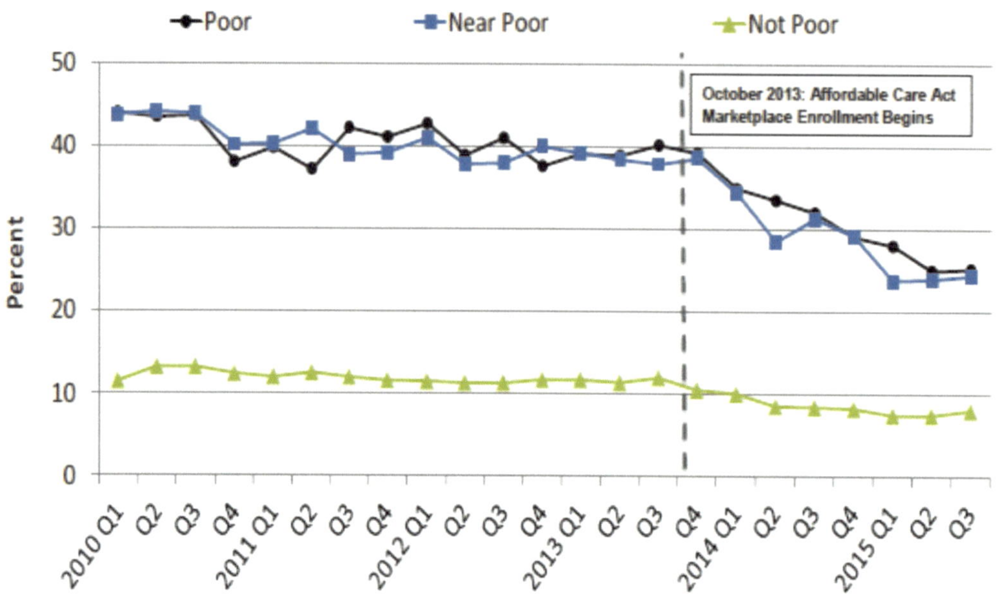

Agency for Healthcare Research and Quality (AHRQ) (2018). *Elements of Access to Health Care | Agency for Health Research and Quality*. [online] www.ahrq.gov. Available at: https://www.ahrq.gov/research/findings/nhqrdr/chartbooks/access/elements.html

According to Gunja, Gumas, and Williams (2023), the United States lags other high-income countries in life expectancy, avoidable deaths, obesity, and maternal and infant mortality. Uninsured healthcare status contributes to these statistics. Uninsured adults and children are less likely to receive preventative services such as immunizations, dental care, and health assessment screenings (Healthy People 2030, n.d.). Additionally, individuals often choose to postpone care or treatment because out-of-pocket costs are prohibitive for both insured and uninsured individuals as diagrammed in **Figure 7** (Garfield, Orgera, and Damico, 2019).

Figure 7.

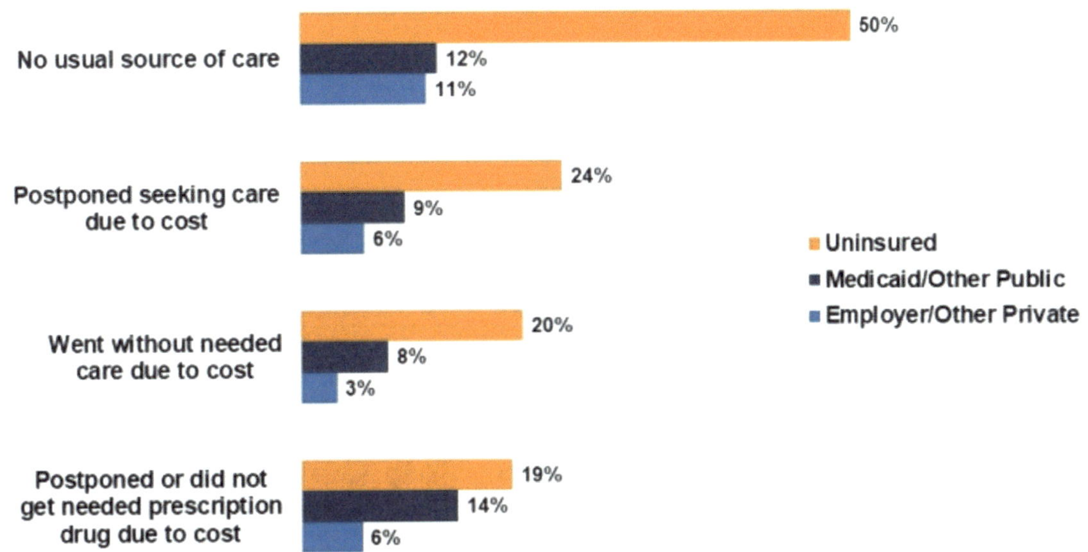

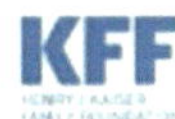

Garfield, R., Orgera, K. and Damico, A. (2019). *The Uninsured and the ACA: A Primer – Key Facts about Health Insurance and the Uninsured amidst Changes to the Affordable Care Act - How does lack of insurance affect access to care?* The Henry J. Kaiser Family Foundation. [online] Available at: https://www.kff.org/report-section/the-uninsured-and-the-aca-a-primer-key-facts-about-health-insurance-and-the-uninsured-amidst-changes-to-the-affordable-care-act-how-does-lack-of-insurance-affect-access-to-care/

Healthcare Services

When it comes to availability of healthcare services, the United States falls behind other high-income countries with below average number of practicing physicians per capita compared to other Organization for Economic Co-operation and Development (OECD) countries as illustrated in **Figure 8** (Gunja, Gumas and Williams, 2023). Clinician availability causes Americans to visit physicians less frequently than other high-income countries with only four visits per person per year on average compared to OECD average of 5.7 (Gunja, Gumas and Williams, 2023).

Figure 8.

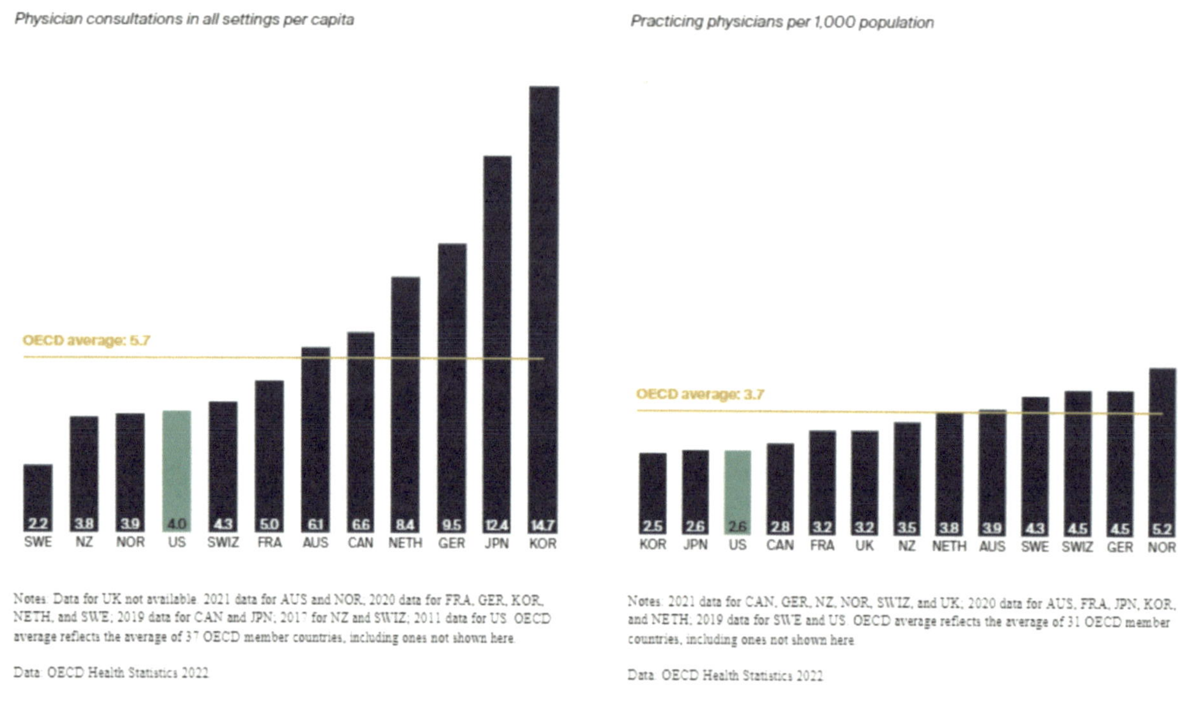

Gunja, M., Gumas, E. and Williams, R. (2023). *U.S. Health Care from a Global Perspective, 2022: Accelerating Spending, Worsening Outcomes*. [online] www.commonwealthfund.org. Available at: https://www.commonwealthfund.org/publications/issue-briefs/2023/jan/us-health-care-global-perspective-2022#1

Provider shortages disproportionately affect patients with government insurance plans such as Medicaid that provide marginal reimbursement, which leads to reduced plan acceptance by physicians, creates longer wait times and promotes delayed care (Healthy People 2030, 2023).

Fianlly, the United States has just 2.8 hospital beds per 1,000 population, which is lower than the OECD average of 4.3 hospital beds per 1,000 population (Gunja, Gumas and Williams, 2023) further impacting availabilty of healthcare services.

Healthcare Access as a Social Determinant of Health

In the context of Well-being

International comparisons of access to health care services aside, how do developed countries compare with respect to overall population well-being? Do variations in access to health care services and other dimensions of health care systems translate into disparities in health outcomes?

The United States' health care spending both per person and as a percent of gross domestic product (GDP) is higher than other high-income countries despite being the only developed country that does not have universal health coverage (Gunja, Gumas and Williams, 2023).

Figure 9.

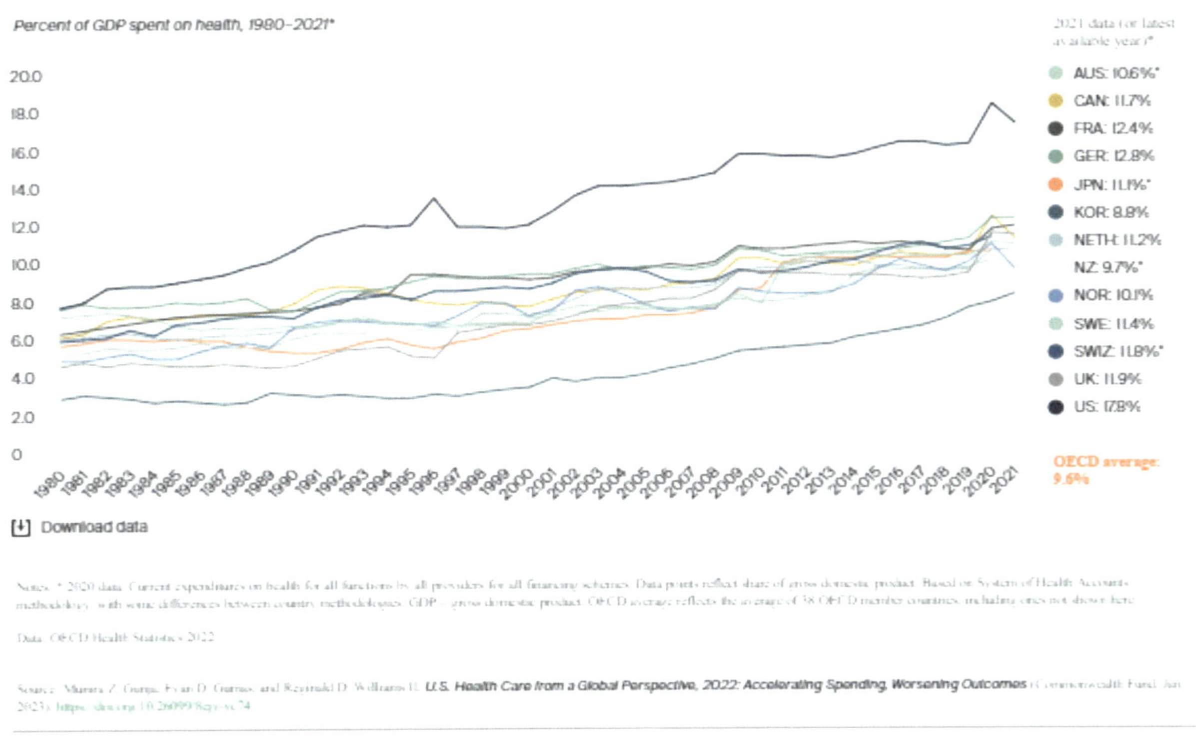

Gunja, M., Gumas, E. and Williams, R. (2023). *U.S. Health Care from a Global Perspective, 2022: Accelerating Spending, Worsening Outcomes*. [online] www.commonwealthfund.org. Available at: https://www.commonwealthfund.org/publications/issue-briefs/2023/jan/us-health-care-global-perspective-2022#1

According to the data graphed in **Figure 9**, the U.S. spends 17.8% of its GDP on healthcare compared to other representative high-income countries like Korea 8.8%, Norway 10.1%, Japan 11.1%, Canada 11.7%, and Germany 12.8% (Gunja, Gumas and Williams, 2023).

Paradoxically, high national spending on healthcare does not translate to better health outcomes comparing the Unites States to other high-income states including Australia, Canada, France, Germany, Japan, the Netherlands, New Zealand, Norway, South Korea, Sweden, Switzerland, and the United Kingdom (Gunja, Gumas and Williams, 2023).

Return on Investment?

The Commonwealth Fund (2023) reported in *U.S. Health Care from a Global Perspective* that "individuals in the United States experience the worst health outcomes overall of any high-income nation."

Despite high U.S. spending, Americans experience worse health outcomes than their peers around world. For example, life expectancy at birth in the U.S. was 77 years in 2020 — three years lower than the OECD average. Provisional data shows life expectancy in the U.S. dropped even further in 2021.

Compared to other high-income countries, the U.S. has the highest death rates for avoidable or treatable conditions, the highest maternal and infant mortality, and among the highest suicide rates.

In the U.S., life expectancy masks racial and ethnic disparities. Average life expectancy in 2019 for non-Hispanic Black Americans (74.8 years) and non-Hispanic American Indians or Alaska Natives (71.8 years) is four and seven years lower, respectively, than it is for non-Hispanic whites (78.8 years).

Gunja, M., Gumas, E. and Williams, R. (2023). *U.S. Health Care from a Global Perspective, 2022: Accelerating Spending, Worsening Outcomes.* [online] www.commonwealthfund.org. Available at: https://www.commonwealthfund.org/publications/issue-briefs/2023/jan/us-health-care-global-perspective-2022#1

As a population health outcome, well-being looks beyond morbidity and mortality and investigates multiple dimensions of comprehensive health. The United States has the highest rate of people with multiple chronic conditions according to the Commonwealth Fund (Gunja, Gumas and Williams, 2023). Construe chronic medical cnditions as the construct of co-existent multiple chronic medical conditions like heart disease, diabetes, hypertension, and kidney failure. According to (Gunja, Gumas and Williams, 2023) adults in the U.S. are most likely to have multiple chronic medical conditions by international comparison (**Figure 10**).

Figure 10.

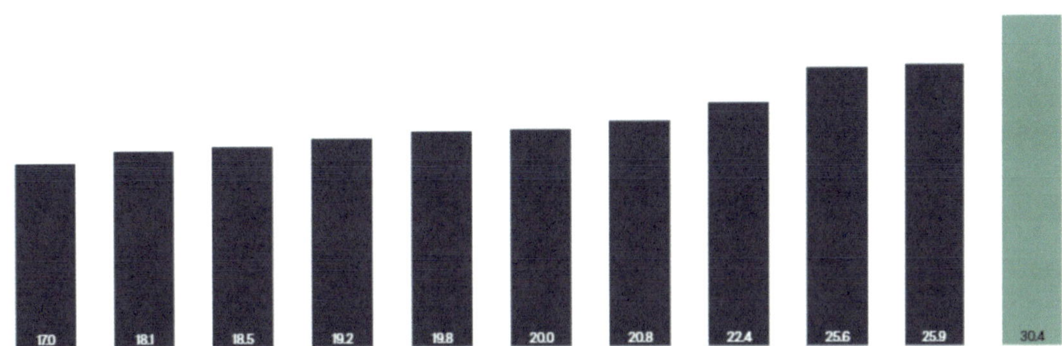

Gunja, M., Gumas, E. and Williams, R. (2023). *U.S. Health Care from a Global Perspective, 2022: Accelerating Spending, Worsening Outcomes*. [online] www.commonwealthfund.org. Available at: https://www.commonwealthfund.org/publications/issue-briefs/2023/jan/us-health-care-global-perspective-2022#1

Rates of obesity, suicide and assaults constitute measures of population well-being. According to the *U.S. Health Care from a Global Perspective, 2022: Accelerating Spending, Worsening Outcomes* by The Commonwealth Fund (Gunja, Gumas, and Williams, 2023).

The United States obesity rate is twice the OECD average (**Figure 11**). According to the CDC obesity is associated with high blood pressure, type 2 diabetes, heart attack, stroke, sleep apnea low quality life, depression and all cause mortality (CDC, 2022a).

Figure 11.

The U.S. obesity rate is nearly double the OECD average.

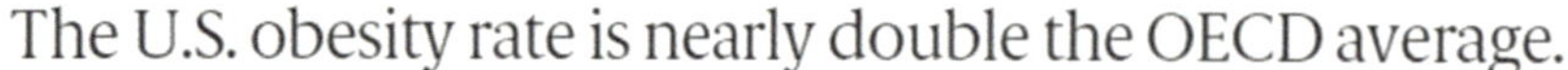

Percent of total population that is obese

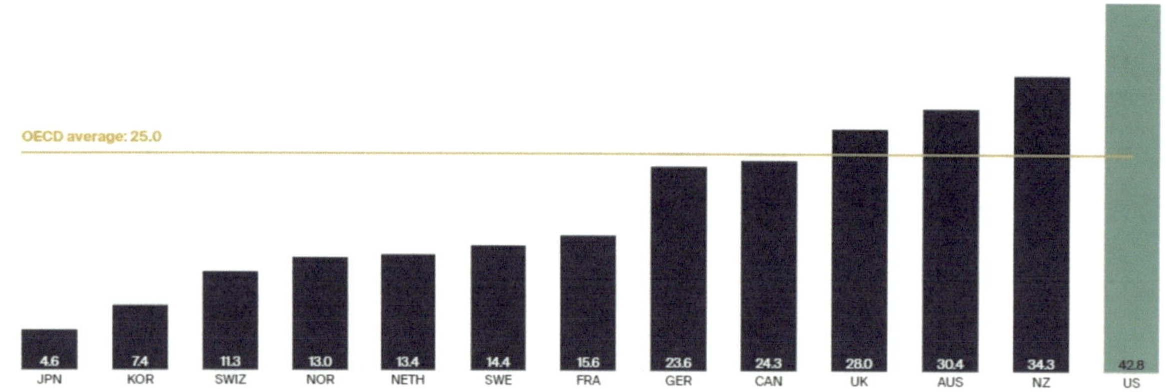

Notes: Obese defined as body-mass index of 30 kg/m² or more. Data reflect rates based on measurements of height and weight, except NETH, NOR, SWE, SWIZ, for which data are self-reported. (Self-reported rates tend to be lower than measured rates.) 2021 data for NZ; 2020 data for KOR, NETH, and SWE; 2019 data for CAN, JPN, NOR, UK, and US; 2017 data for AUS, FRA, and SWIZ; 2012 data for GER. OECD average reflects the average of 23 OECD member countries, including ones not shown here, which provide data on obesity rates.

Data: OECD Health Statistics 2022.

Source: Munira Z. Gunja, Evan D. Gumas, and Reginald D. Williams II, *U.S. Health Care from a Global Perspective, 2022: Accelerating Spending, Worsening Outcomes* (Commonwealth Fund, Jan. 2023). https://doi.org/10.26099/8ejy-yc74

Gunja, M., Gumas, E. and Williams, R. (2023). *U.S. Health Care from a Global Perspective, 2022: Accelerating Spending, Worsening Outcomes*. [online] www.commonwealthfund.org. Available at: https://www.commonwealthfund.org/publications/issue-briefs/2023/jan/us-health-care-global-perspective-2022#1

Suicide rates (**Figure 12**), which dramatically increased during the COVID-19 pandemic, show a high burden of mental illness. The U.S. has the third-highest suicide rate, while the U.K. has the lowest – half the U.S. rate (Gunja, Gumas and Williams, 2023).

According to the CDC (2022a), "suicide is rarely caused by a single circumstance or event. Instead, a range of factors – at the individual, relationship, community, and societal levels – increase risk."

The CDC proposes multiple risk factors leading to suicide (CDC, 2022b). These include previous suicide attempts, depression, chronic pain, legal problems, job loss, substance use, adverse childhood experiences, domestic violence, bullying, loss of relationships, lack of access to health care, community violence, and discrimination. *Taken in aggregate, these risks connect directly to the array of the social determinants of health.*

Figure 12.

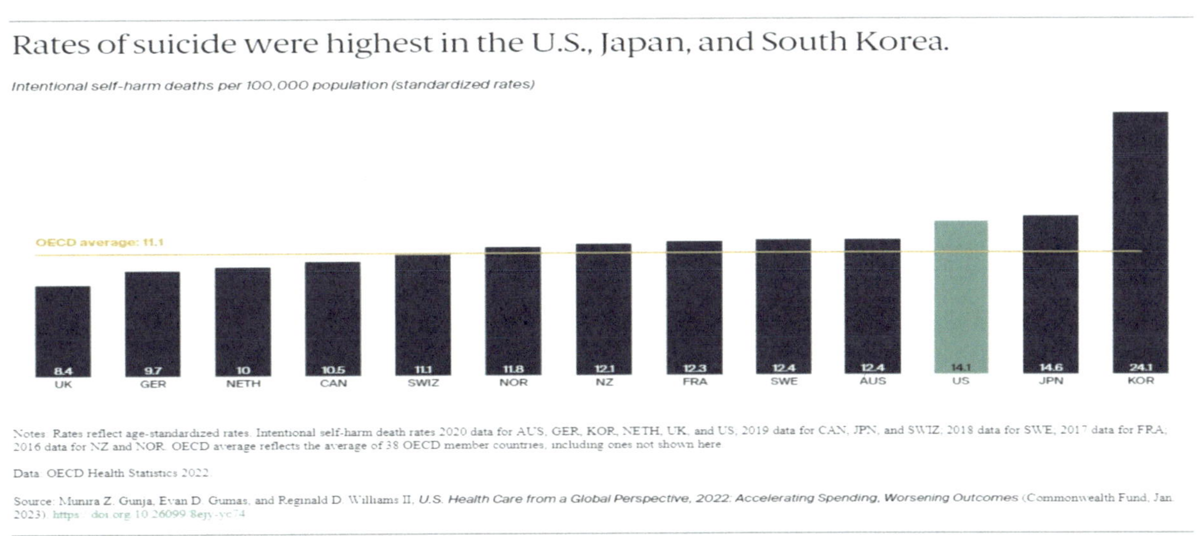

The U.S. is an outlier in deaths from physical assault, which includes gun violence. Its 7.4 deaths per 100,000 people (**Figure 13**) far exceeds the OECD average of 2.7.

Figure 13.

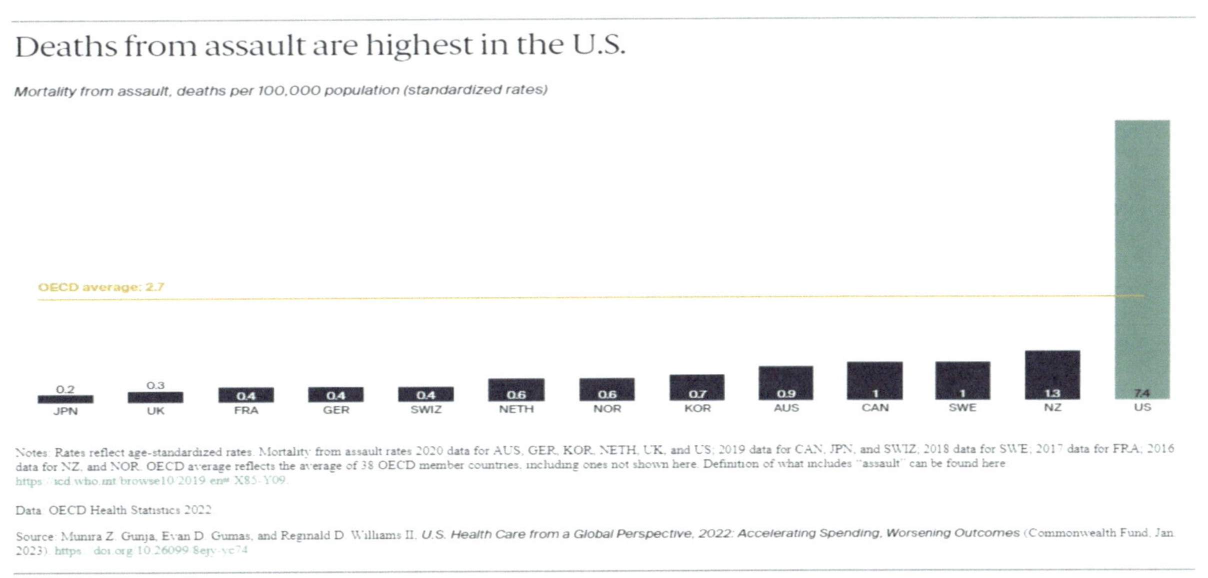

Figures 12 & 13 from Gunja, M., Gumas, E. and Williams, R. (2023). *U.S. Health Care from a Global Perspective, 2022: Accelerating Spending, Worsening Outcomes.* [online] www.commonwealthfund.org. Available at: https://www.commonwealthfund.org/publications/issue-briefs/2023/jan/us-health-care-global-perspective-2022#1

Healthcare Access as a Social Determinant of Health

In the context of Life-expectancy and Healthy life-expectancy

While the United States spends twice as much as the average OECD country, the life expectancy at birth is lower than the OECD average (**Figure 14**).

Figure 14.

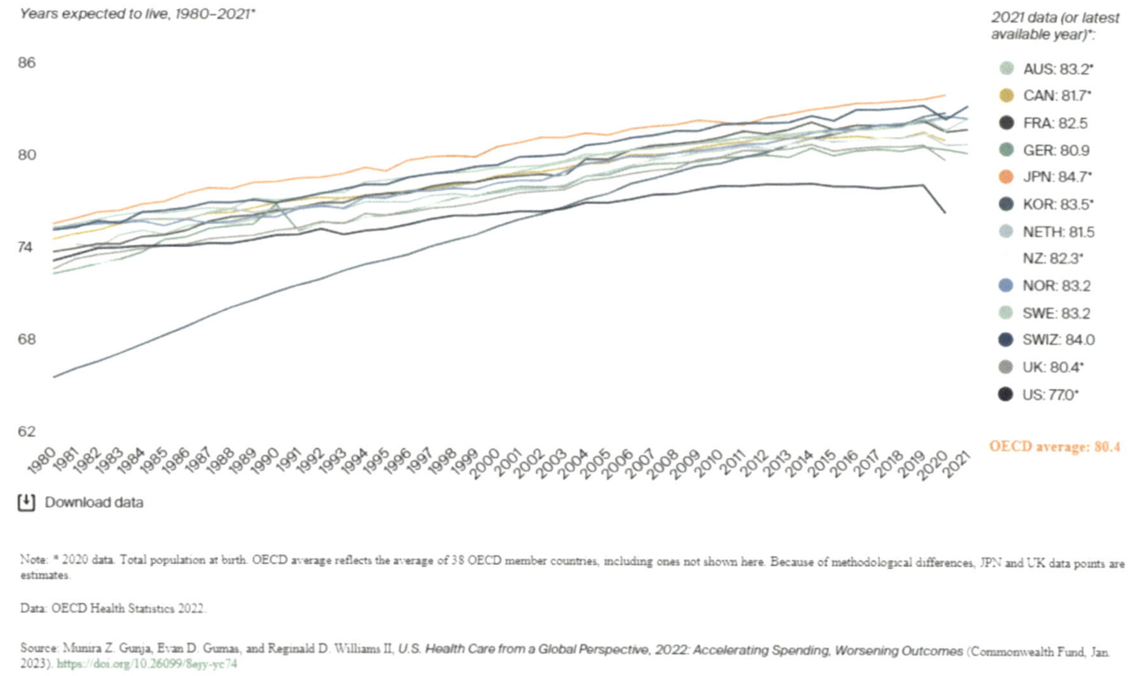

Gunja, M., Gumas, E. and Williams, R. (2023). *U.S. Health Care from a Global Perspective, 2022: Accelerating Spending, Worsening Outcomes*. [online] www.commonwealthfund.org. Available at: https://www.commonwealthfund.org/publications/issue-briefs/2023/jan/us-health-care-global-perspective-2022#1

According to Shmerling (2022), life expectancy rose in the U.S. for over 100 years. Citing National Center for Health Statistics, life expectancy was 47 years in 1900, 68 years in 1950, and 79 years in 2019, but it fell to 77 in 2020 and dropped further, to just over 76, in 2021.

Citing the same data, Shmerling further notes some groups fare better than others:

- Life expectancy for American Indian and Alaska Native populations fell more than other ethnic groups to 65.2 years.

- Life expectancy for white Americans (76.4 years) is longer than that of Black Americans (70.8 years).
- For Asian Americans, life expectancy is 83.5 years, the longest among ethnic groups. Hispanic Americans had the next longest life expectancy at 77.7 years.
- Life expectancy for women (79.1 years) and for men (73.2 years) reveals a significant gender gap (Shmerling, 2022).

Ethnic groups experienced much larger drops in life expectancy over the last two years: 6.6 years for American Indian/Alaskan Native populations; 4.2 years for Hispanic Americans; 4.0 years for Black Americans; 2.4 years for white Americans; 2.1 years for Asian Americans.

Why is life expectancy falling in the US?

COVID- 19, drug overdoses, and accidental injury accounted for 2/3 of the decline in life expectancy, according to the National Center for Health Statistics 2021 report. Increased rates of deaths due to heart disease, liver disease and suicides further explain the decline.

The alarming disparities in life expectancy experienced by ethnic groups can be explained by the ***social determinants of health***. Those with the shortest life expectancy in the U.S. have the most poverty, face the most food insecurity, and have less or no access to health care, all factors that contribute to lower life expectancy. Groups with lower life expectancy have higher risk jobs that cannot be performed virtually, live in more crowded settings, and have less access to vaccination, which increases the risk of becoming sick with or dying of COVID-19.

Notably, life expectancy varies widely by state. Lower life expectancy in southern states raises the possibility that politics, vaccination policies, pollution, climate, or other variable factors contribute to discrepancies in life expectancies.

Shmerling, R. (2022). *Why life expectancy in the US is falling.* Harvard Health Publishing Harvard Medical School [online] Available at: https://www.health.harvard.edu/blog/why-life-expectancy-in-the-us-is-falling-202210202835

Robert Shmerling, MD acts as the Senior Faculty Editor of Harvard Health Publishing, Harvard Medical School.

Gunja, Gumas, and Williams (2023) define avoidable mortality as deaths that are preventable and treatable. Preventable deaths are avoided through effective public health measures and through primary prevention, such as nutritional diet and exercise. Treatable mortality is avoided through prompt and effective health care interventions, including regular exams, screenings, and treatment. Since 2015, avoidable deaths have been on the rise in the U.S., which had the highest rate in 2020 of all the countries in their analysis (Gunja, Gumas, and Williams, 2023).

Figure 15.

Avoidable deaths per 100,000 population in the U.S. are higher than the OECD average.

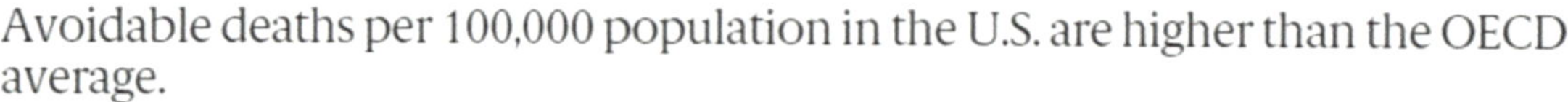

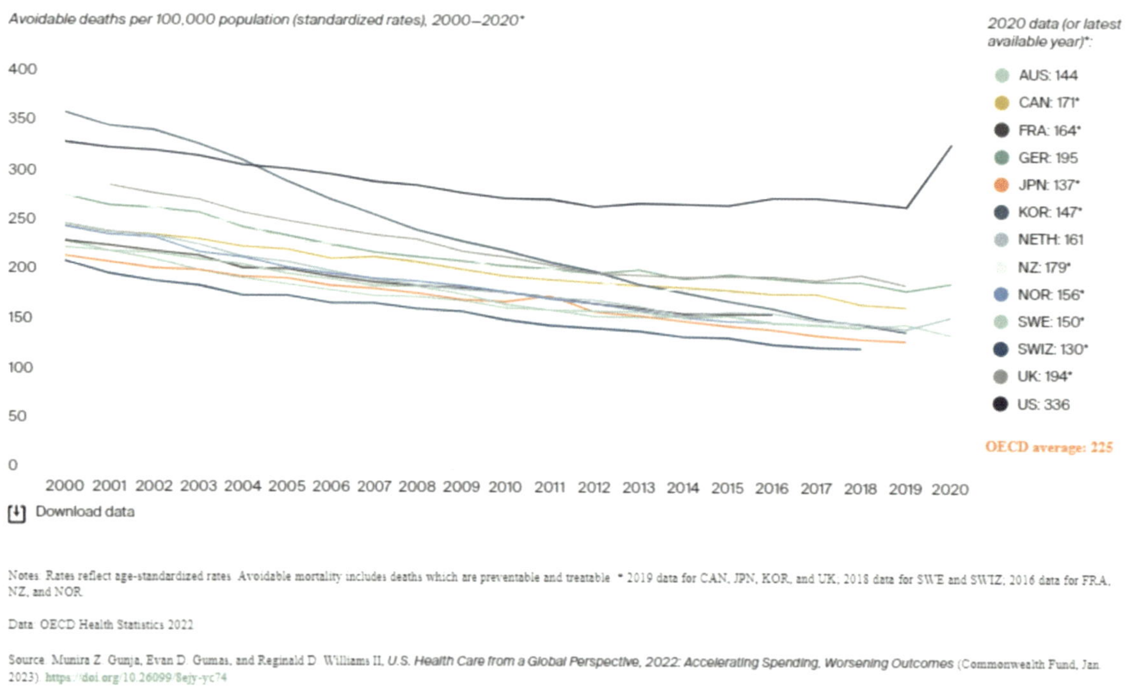

Gunja, M., Gumas, E. and Williams, R. (2023). *U.S. Health Care from a Global Perspective, 2022: Accelerating Spending, Worsening Outcomes*. [online] www.commonwealthfund.org. Available at: https://www.commonwealthfund.org/publications/issue-briefs/2023/jan/us-health-care-global-perspective-2022#1

The US owns the highest rate of avoidable deaths per 100,000 population at 336 compared to the OECD average of 225 per 100,000.

Using Commonwealth Fund and OECD definitions, deaths from COVID-19 are both avoidable and preventable. According to the Commonwealth Fund (2023), since the beginning of the pandemic, the United States experienced more deaths related to COVID-19 than any other high-income nation. For every 1 million cases of COVID-19 in the United States between January 22, 2020 and January 18, 2023, there were more than 3,000 deaths (**Figure 16**). Data shows this is no wonder, the United States lags many of high-income nations in its number of residents that are fully vaccinated against COVID-19 (Gunja, Gumas, and Williams, 2023).

Figure 16.

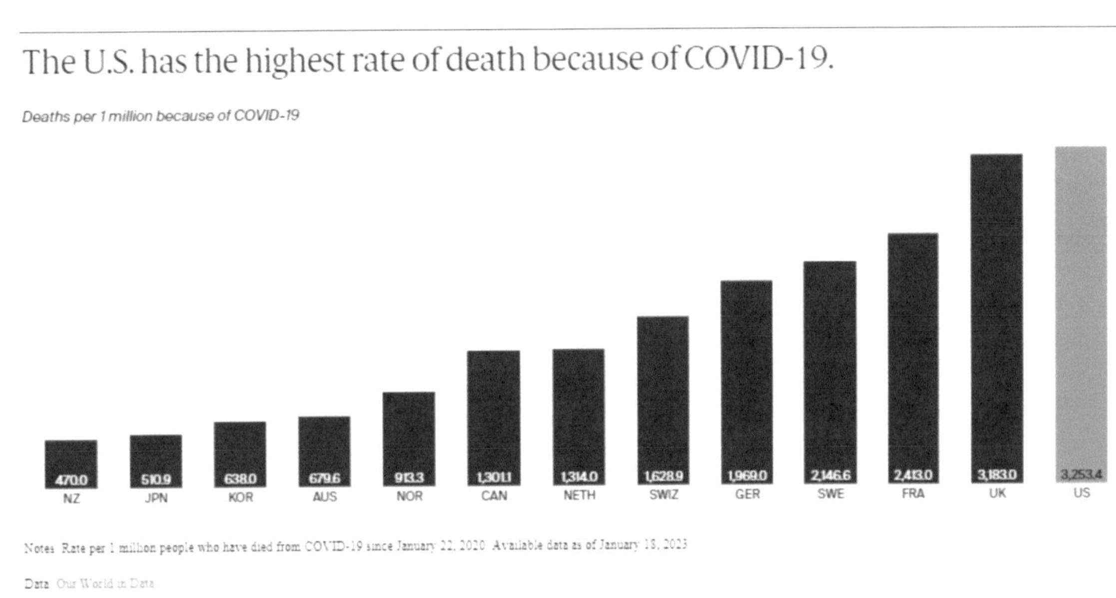

Gunja, M., Gumas, E. and Williams, R. (2023). *U.S. Health Care from a Global Perspective, 2022: Accelerating Spending, Worsening Outcomes*. [online] www.commonwealthfund.org. Available at: https://www.commonwealthfund.org/publications/issue-briefs/2023/jan/us-health-care-global-perspective-2022#1

Healthcare Access as a Social Determinant of Health

Politics, policies, and governance

Gallup began polling U.S. partisans in 2001 discovering considerable variance. 79% of Democrats on average have asserted it is the government's obligation to ensure healthcare for all, while an average of 71% of Republicans said the opposite over the same period. 56% of independents have said it is a governmental obligation (Brenan, 2023). Nonetheless, according to Brenan, the majority in the U.S. say the government should ensure healthcare.

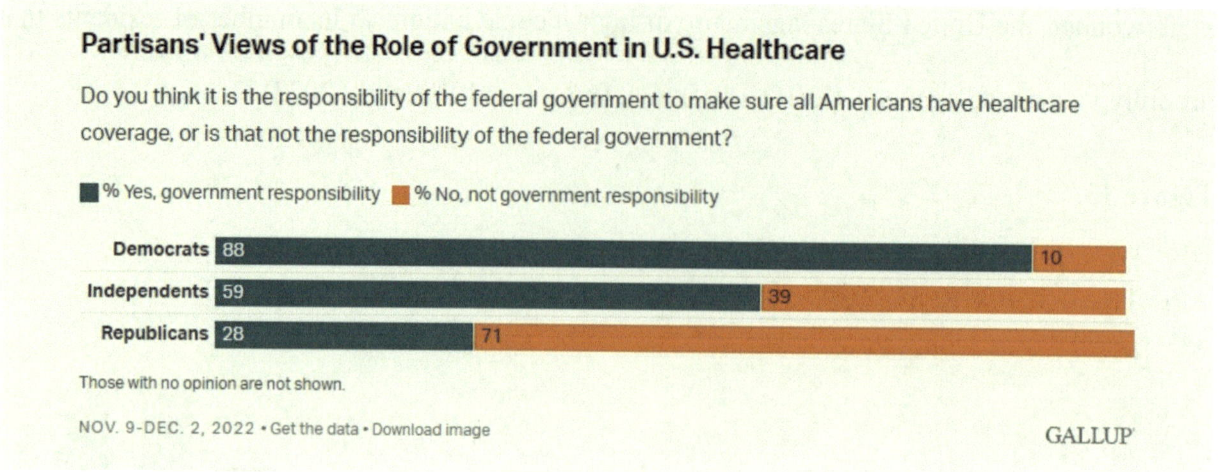

Brenan, M. (2023). *Majority in U.S. Still Say Gov't Should Ensure Healthcare.* [online] Gallup.com. Available at: https://news.gallup.com/poll/468401/majority-say-gov-ensure-healthcare.aspx

Partisan's preference for type healthcare (government vs. private) paints a slightly different, yet similar picture – Democrats opting for a government run system (72%), Republicans preferring private (83%) and Independents 50% for private insurance according to Gallup polling (Brenan, 2023).

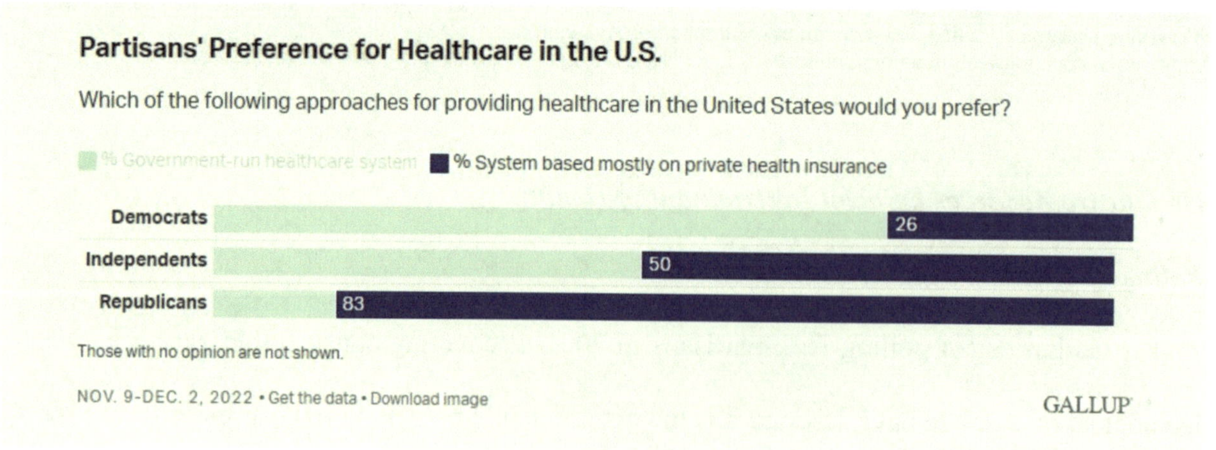

Brenan, M. (2023). *Majority in U.S. Still Say Gov't Should Ensure Healthcare.* [online] Gallup.com. Available at: https://news.gallup.com/poll/468401/majority-say-gov-ensure-healthcare.aspx

The Right to Abortion

Over the past fifty years, the Supreme Court of the United States (SCOTUS) has ruled on two cases affecting women's rights to make health care decisions – *Roe v. Wade* (1973) granted women the right to abortion. *Dobbs, State Health Officer of the Mississippi Department of Health et al v. Jackson Women's Health Organization et al* (The Supreme Court of the United States, 2022) revoked the right to that decision.

In 1973, the United States Supreme Court ruled in *Roe v. Wade* that women had the right to reproductive decision making (Center for Reproductive Rights, 2023). This ruling found that the "liberty" guaranteed for all Americans under the Fourteenth Amendment of the United States Constitution extended to women's right to decide whether to continue or terminate a pregnancy. *Roe v. Wade* acknowledged that the decision whether to continue or end a pregnancy belonged to the individual, not the government (Center for Reproductive Rights, 2023).

In December 2021, Mississippi's Gestational Age Act was argued in *Dobbs, State Health Officer of the Mississippi Department of Health et al v. Jackson Women's Health Organization et al* (SCOTUS, 2022). Mississippi's Gestational Act provides that "[e]xept in a medical emergency or in the case of severe fetal abnormality, a person shall not intentionally or knowingly perform…or induce an abortion of an unborn human being if the probable gestational age of the unborn human being has been determined to be greater than fifteen (15) weeks." (SCOTUS, 2022).

In June 2022 America's healthcare landscape changed drastically when the Supreme Court's ruling in *Dobbs v. Jackson Women's Health Organization* overturned the 1973 *Roe v Wade* ruling (Center for Reproductive Rights, 2023). With this ruling the United States Supreme Court revoked women's constitutional right to abortion reasoning that the Constitution does not protect the right to abortion (The National Constitution Center, 2022). Further, the Dobbs decision conceded the regulation of abortion to the individual States (SCOTUS, 2022).

Although little discussed as the decision rolled out in popular media, the SCOTUS ruling holds language conferring *criminality* to anyone seeking or performing an abortion, granting significant power to States outlawing the procedure (see ruling excerpts in italicized text below).

Dobbs v. Jackson Women's Health Organization - SCOTUS (2022)

Arguing:

First, the Court reviews the standard that the Court's cases have used to determine whether the Fourteenth Amendment's reference to "liberty" protects a particular right.

Next, the Court examines whether the right to obtain an abortion is rooted in the Nation's history and tradition and whether it is an essential component of "ordered liberty."

History and tradition that map the essential components of the Nation's concept of ordered liberty, the Court finds the Fourteenth Amendment clearly does not protect the right to an abortion. Until the latter part of the 20th century, there was no support in American law for a constitutional right to obtain an abortion. No state constitutional provision had recognized such a right. Until a few years before Roe, no federal or state court had recognized such a right. Nor had any scholarly treatise. Indeed, abortion had long been a crime in every single State. At common law, abortion was criminal in at least some stages of pregnancy and was regarded as unlawful and could have very serious consequences at all stages. American law followed the common law until a wave of statutory restrictions in the 1800s expanded criminal liability for abortions. By the time, the Fourteenth Amendment was adopted, three-quarters of the States had made abortion a crime at any stage of pregnancy. This consensus endured until the day Roe was decided. Roe either ignored or misstated this history, and Casey declined to reconsider Roe's faulty historical analysis.

Finally, the Court considers whether a right to obtain an abortion is part of a broader entrenched right that is supported by other precedents

Held: The Constitution does not confer a right to abortion; *Roe* and *Casey* are overruled; and the authority to regulate abortion is returned to the people and their elected representatives.

SCOTUS (2022). *Dobbs v. Jackson Women's Health Organization.* [online] Available at: https://www.supremecourt.gov/opinions/21pdf/19-1392_6j37.pdf [Accessed 1 October 2023].

Those states looking to restrict abortions used this ruling to embed new and existing legislation (KFF, 2023a). As of August 23, 2023, fifteen states had completely banned abortions, four states had put in place regulations to limit abortions to between six- and twelve- weeks' gestation, six states limited abortions to between 16- and 22- weeks' gestation, and 26 states as well as D.C. allowed abortion beyond 22 weeks gestation **Figure 17** (KFF, 2023a)

Figure 17.

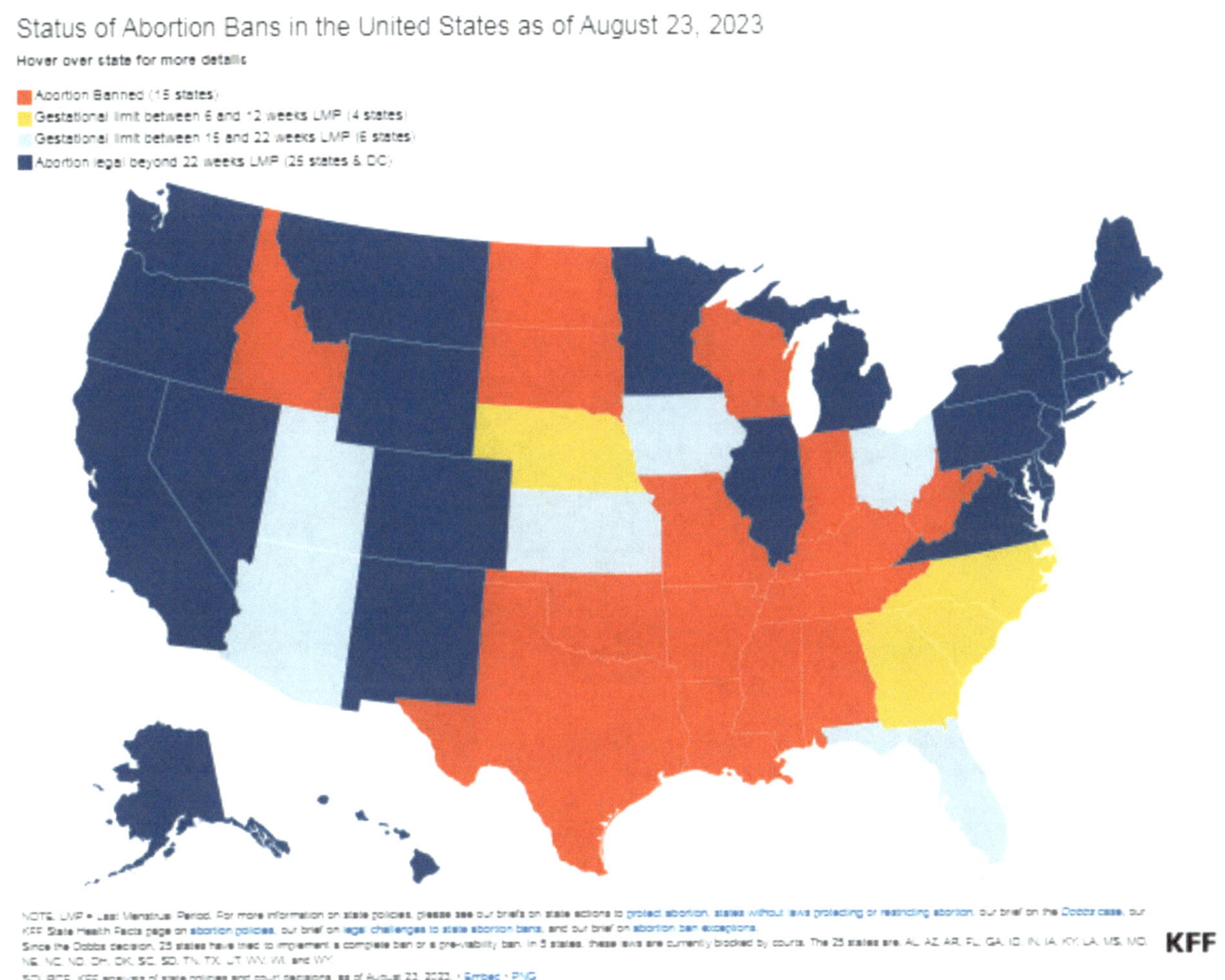

KFF (2023a). Abortion in the United States Dashboard [online] Available at: https://www.kff.org/womens-health-policy/dashboard/abortion-in-the-u-s-dashboard/

Since *Dobbs* Twenty States without active abortion bans have implemented at least one restriction applied to abortion regulations (KFF, 2023b) (**Figure 18**). Restrictions include ultrasound requirements, limiting medication abortions to only those prescribed by a physician, banning telemedicine appointments for medication abortions, requiring multiple clinic trips or specific regulations on the time between counseling appointment and termination of pregnancy (KFF, 2023b).

Figure 18.

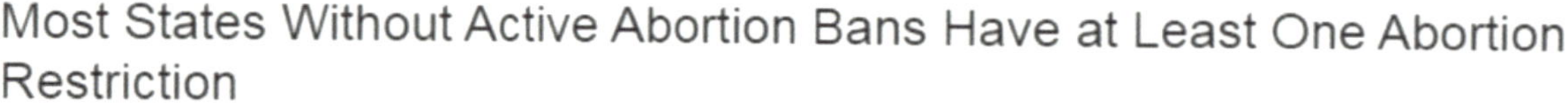

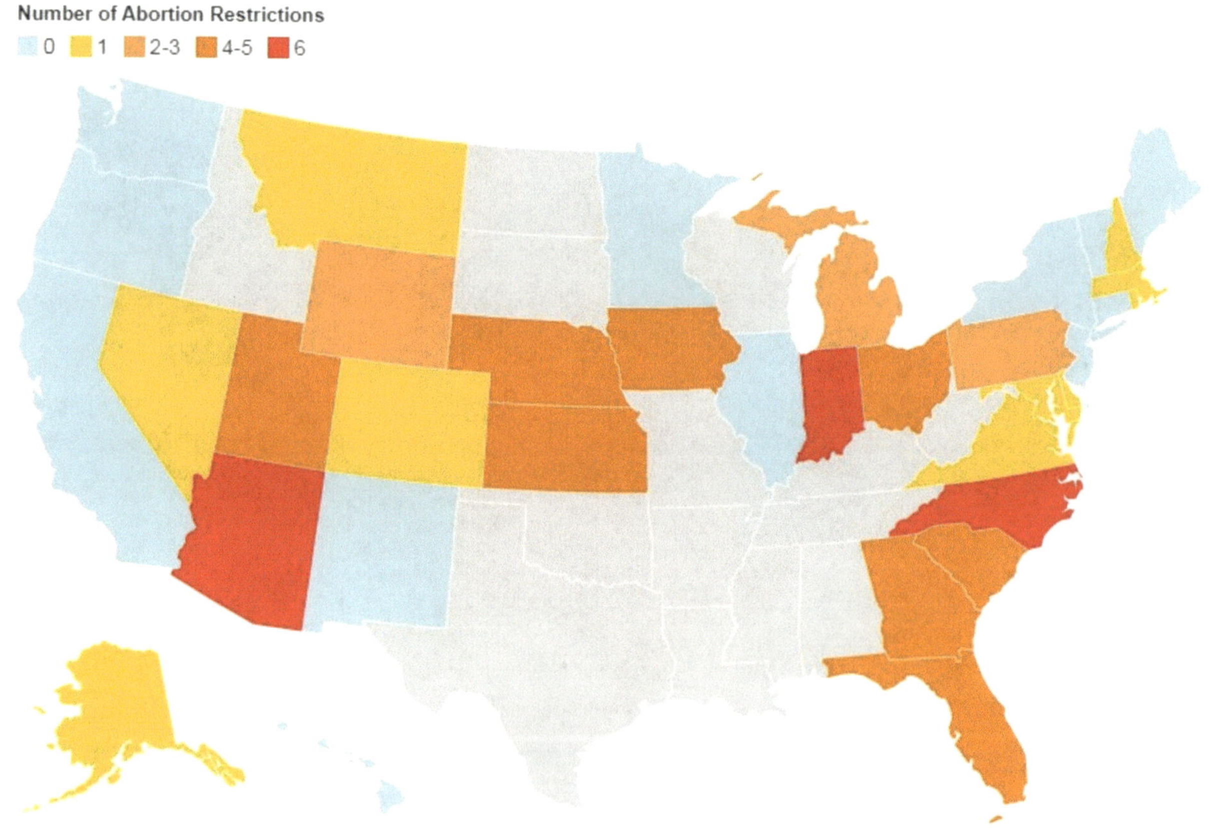

NOTE: Abortion restriction indicators include 6 main categories: pre-viability gestational limits, waiting periods, ultrasound requirements, requirements that physicians provide abortion care, limits on telemedicine care, and parental notification or consent requirements.
In Colorado, Delaware, Maryland, Massachusetts, Montana, New Hampshire, Rhode Island, and Virginia the only restrictions are parental notification/consent requirements.

SOURCE: KFF Analysis of State Laws; Planned Parenthood, Parental Consent and Notification Laws; Center for Reproductive Rights, Abortion Laws by State • PNG

KFF

KFF (2023b). *A Year After Dobbs: Policies Restricting Access to Abortion in States Even Where It's Not Banned.* [online] Available at: https://www.kff.org/policy-watch/year-after-dobbs-policies-restricting-access-to-abortion/ [Accessed 30 August 2023].

Individual state regulations on abortions place significant barriers to healthcare access for women living in abortion restricted areas. They increase the existing disparities and inequities in those states by further curtailing access to maternal health and reproductive services as well as access to abortion (Seervai, et al., 2023). These restrictions disproportionately affect women facing other social determinants of health barriers including race, unemployment, transportation, poverty and the likelihood of being uninsured (Seervai, et al., 2023).

Compared to other high-income countries, women in the United States are more likely to experience financial burden when seeking reproductive health care, especially abortions, which in the United States can range in cost from $0 to $3,700 based on insurance status, geographic region, and procedure type (Seervai, et al., 2023). Women seeking abortion services out of state may need to travel significant distances due to state bans and restrictions, which imposes the added costs for transportation (Seervai, et al., 2023).

Even in states where abortion is legal, cost is a significant factor for women. According to Planned Parenthood (2022), a medication abortion costs about eight-hundred dollars, while an in-clinic abortion in the first trimester runs $600.00. Second semester terminations cost more. Out of pocket expense may be much less depending on availability and type of insurance.

Criminal Penalties

In many states where abortions are banned, regulations put providers at risk of criminal penalties. For example, some states allow for the removal of a dead fetus, however some individuals may be denied care if there continues to be detectable fetal cardiac activity or until the miscarriage puts the pregnant individual at risk of death (KFF, 2023b). In Idaho, there exists no explicit medical exemption in its abortion ban, instead it allows physicians to assert a defense for criminal prosecution if by their medical judgment they found performing the abortion was "necessary to prevent the death of the pregnant woman" (KFF, 2023b). Abortion restrictions are not clear or may be contradictory in some states causing providers to delay miscarriage management care in fear of criminal prosecution (KFF, 2023b).

According to Zablocki and Sutrina (2022), "states also vary widely when it comes to the criminal penalties imposed for an illegal abortion (**Figure 19**). Depending on the state, a person may be fined anywhere from $1,000 to $100,000. In addition to monetary penalties, a provider's license is also at risk. And, depending on the state, a person convicted of an illegal abortion may face the possibility of incarceration anywhere from a few months to life in prison," as follows:

Figure 19.

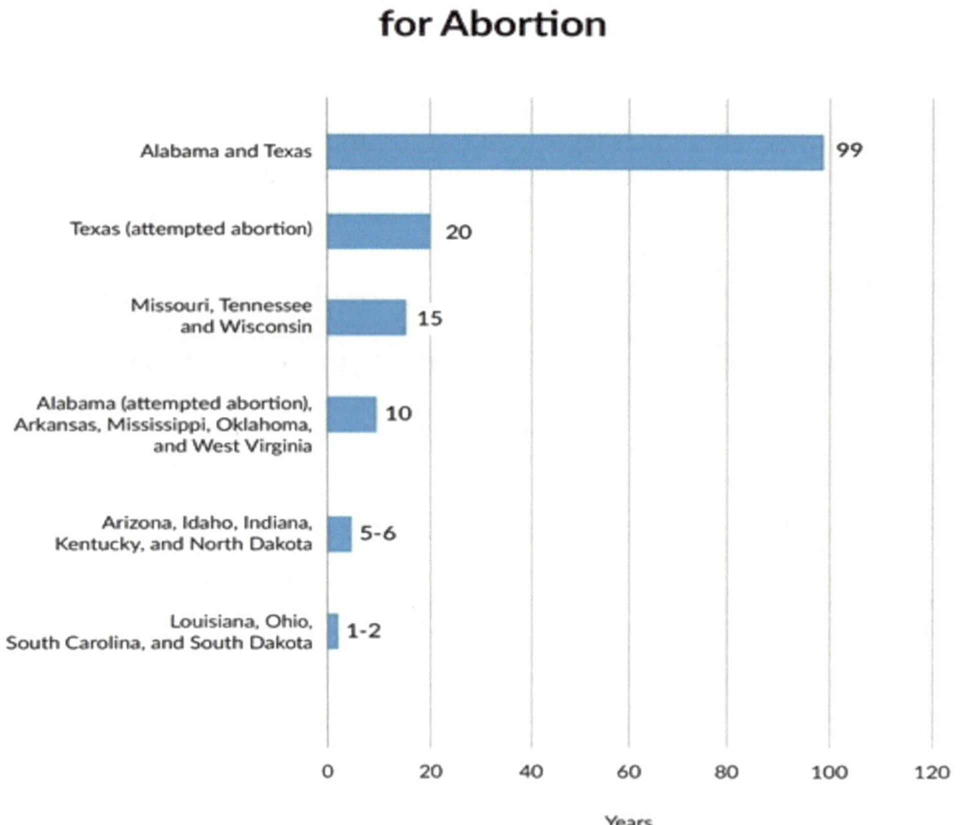

Zablocki, A. and Sutrina, M. (2022). *The Impact of State Law Criminalizing Abortion* LexisNexis [online] Available at: https://www.lexisnexis.com/community/insights/legal/practical-guidance-journal/b/pa/posts/the-impact-of-state-laws-criminalizing-abortion

Citing the Commonwealth Fund *Limiting Abortion Access for American Women Impacts Health, Economic Security: An International Comparison,* "Research shows restricted access to abortion is associated with negative social and health-related consequences for pregnant women and can result in adverse birth outcomes" (Seervai, et al., 2023).

The United States has the highest rate of infant and maternal mortality, with 23.8 maternal deaths per 100,000 live births compared to the OECD average of 9.8 maternal deaths per 100,000 live births ((Gunja, Gumas, and Williams, 2023) (**Figure 20**). Research at the Commonwealth Fund predicts this rate will rise in coming years as state mandates limit access to reproductive healthcare and reproductive rights. Further, they foresee disproportionate effect on women experiencing other socioeconomic barriers to healthcare access (Gunja, Gumas, and Williams, 2023).

Figure 20.

The U.S. has the highest rate of infant and maternal deaths.

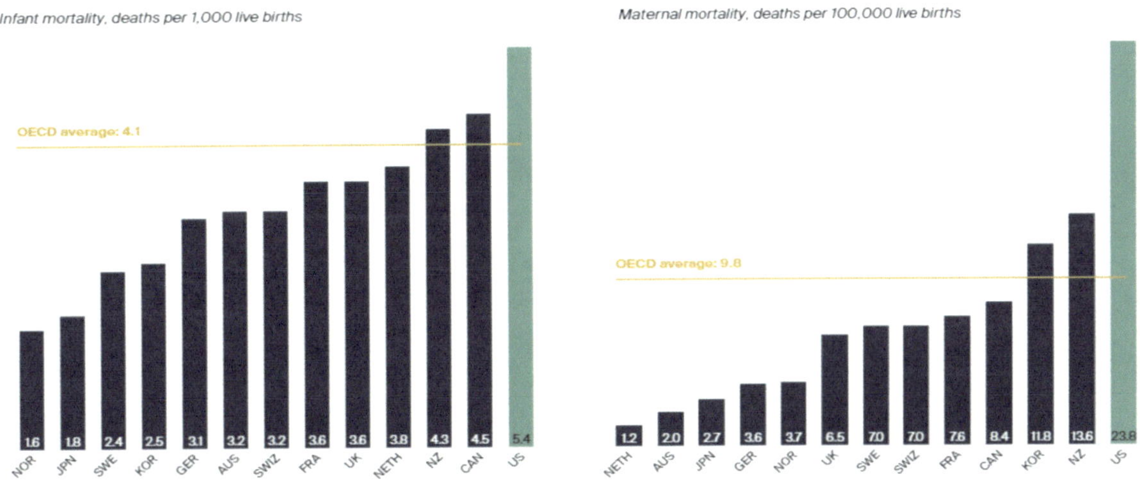

Notes: Infant mortality rates reflect no minimum threshold or gestation period or birthweight. Infant mortality 2021 data for FRA and SWIZ; 2020 data for AUS, CAN, GER, JPN, KOR, NETH, NOR, SWE, UK, and US; 2018 data for NZ. Maternal mortality 2020 data for AUS, CAN, GER, JPN, KOR, NETH, NOR, SWE, and US; 2019 data for SWIZ; 2018 data for NZ, 2017 data for UK; 2015 data for FRA. OECD average reflects the average of 38 OECD member countries.

Data: OECD Health Statistics 2022.

Source: Munira Z. Gunja, Evan D. Gumas, and Reginald D. Williams II, *U.S. Health Care from a Global Perspective, 2022: Accelerating Spending, Worsening Outcomes* (Commonwealth Fund, Jan. 2023). https://doi.org/10.26099/8ejy-yc74

Gunja, M., Gumas, E. and Williams, R. (2023). *U.S. Health Care from a Global Perspective, 2022: Accelerating Spending, Worsening Outcomes*. [online] www.commonwealthfund.org. Available at: https://www.commonwealthfund.org/publications/issue-briefs/2023/jan/us-health-care-global-perspective-2022#1

Social Spending Predicts Health Outcomes

According to Countryeconomy.com (2016) and Our World in Data (2016), the United States boasted a nineteen trillion-dollar economy, significantly besting the next highest high-income economies like Japan (5 trillion), Germany (3.5 trillion), the United Kingdom (2.7 trillion) and South Korea (1.5 trillion). During that same period, the United States devoted 19.2% of its GDP to public social spending compared to France (31.55%), Italy (28.9%), Denmark (28.7%), Germany (25.3%) and Norway (25.7). The OECD defines "social spending as the provision of public or private agencies of benefits to, and financial contributions targeted at, households and individuals in order to provide support during circumstances which adversely affect their welfare."

Figure 21.

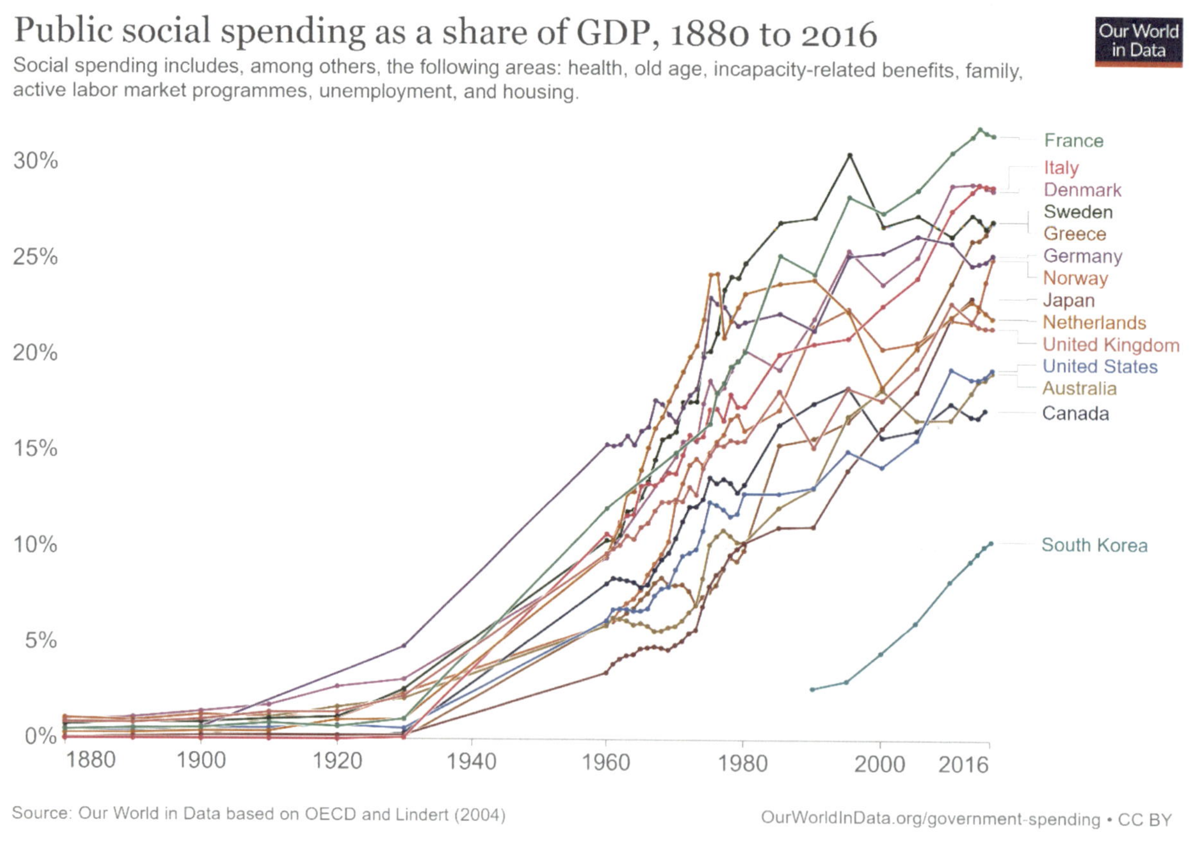

Our World in Data (n.d.). Public social spending as a share of GDO, 1880 to 2016. [online] Available at: https://ourworldindata.org/grapher/social-spending-oecd-longrun

Health outcomes data from the Organization for Economic Co-operation and Development (OECD) (2023), indicates that public social spending improves health outcomes. For example, countries dedicating significant percentages of GDP to public social spending in 2016 (France, Italy, Denmark, and Sweden) predicted favorable indices of infant and maternal mortality and life expectancy compared to the United States five years later in 2021 (**Table 1**).

Table 1.

Country	Social Spending % GDP 2016	GDP 2016	Infant Mortality 1000 Live Births 2021	Maternal Mortality 1000 Live Births 2021	Life Expectancy Years	% GDP on Education	% Population Tertiary Education
France	31.55	$2,472,282M	3.7	ND	82.4	5.5	50.3
Italy	28.87	$1,876,554M	2.3	2.7 (2020)	82.7	4.3	28.3
Denmark	28.68	$313,116M	2.4	0	81.5	6.4	49
Sweden	27.1	$515,655M	1.8	2.6	83.1	7.2	49.2
Greece	27.3	$193,097M	3.5	3.5 (2020)	80.2	4.4	44.2
Germany	25.3	$3,468,896M	3.0	3.5	80.8	4.7	35
Norway	25.7	$370,957M	1.7	3.7	83.2	5.9	55
Japan	23	$5,003,678M	1.7	3.4	82.7	3.4	64.8
Netherlands	22	$783,844M	3.3	2.8	81.4	5.3	55.6
UK	21.5	$2,709,678M	4.0	ND	81 (2020)	5.5	57.5
USA	19.2	$18,804,900 M	5.4 (2020)	23.8 (2020)	76.4	6.1	51.7
Australia	19.2	$1,263,521M	3.3	3.5	83.3	6.1	54.31
Canada	17.2	$1,527,996M	4.5 (2020)	8.4 (2020)	81.8	5.2	66.7
South Korea	10.36	$1,500,030M	2.4	8.8	83.6	4.7	69.29

Countryeconomy.com. (2016). *GDP - Gross Domestic Product 2016 | countryeconomy.com*. [online] Available at: https://countryeconomy.com/gdp?year=2016 [Accessed 8 Oct. 2023].

CIA.gov. (n.d.). *Education expenditures - The World Factbook*. [online] Available at: https://www.cia.gov/the-world-factbook/field/education-expenditures/ [Accessed 8 October 2023].

OECD (2023). *Health Status*. [online] Oecd.org. [online] Available at: https://stats.oecd.org/Index.aspx?DataSetCode=HEALTH_STAT [Accessed 8 October 2023].

Our World in Data. (n.d.). Public social spending as a share of GDP. [online] Available at: https://ourworldindata.org/grapher/social-spending-oecd-longrun [Accessed 8 October 2023].

Wisevoter. (n.d.). Most Educated Countries 2023. [online] Available at: https://wisevoter.com/country-rankings/most-educated-countries/ [Accessed 8 October 2023].

As articulated throughout this text, many non-medical factors play together to deliver on the promise of quality health outcomes. Analysts bundle them as the social determinates of health

– poverty, education, food security, employment, transportation, healthcare access, housing and the like. Financial resource powers these determinants. Simply put, no money no mission. Public social spending provides the capital to ensure the social determinants of health are available to all irrespective of race, color, creed, culture, gender, income, education, and social positioning. The policies and politics of the United States fail to ensure those resources. Given the prowess of the United States economy, the outcome of U.S. infant and maternal mortality, life expectancy and many other indicators of health and healthy life expectancy seem utterly unacceptable.

Questions for Further Consideration:

1. In what way can healthcare providers increase healthcare access, especially to those individuals experiencing other social determinants of health?
2. The United States falls below other high-income countries in health outcomes, discuss possible reasons for this.
3. Healthcare costs are often given as rational for the United States not embracing universal healthcare. Discuss ways in which the United States can reduce healthcare costs. Specifically, what can healthcare providers do to reduces healthcare costs?
4. How can healthcare providers change state legislation on abortion bans and regulations?

Sentinel Readings for a Deeper Dive

A Year After Dobbs: Policies Restricting Access to Abortion in States Even Where It's Not Banned. Available at: https://www.kff.org/policy-watch/year-after-dobbs-policies-restricting-access-to-abortion/

Limiting Abortion Access for American Women Impacts Health, Economic Security: An International Comparison. [online] Available at: https://www.commonwealthfund.org/blog/2023/limiting-abortion-access-american-women-impacts-health-economic-security

Dobbs v. Jackson Women's Health Organization (2022). Available at: Dobbs v. Jackson Women's Health Organization | Constitution Center

U.S. Health Care from a Global Perspective, 2022: Accelerating Spending, Worsening Outcomes. Available at: https://www.commonwealthfund.org/publications/issue-briefs/2023/jan/us-health-care-global-perspective-2022#1

The Uninsured and the ACA: A Primer-Key Facts about Health Insurance and the Uninsured amidst Changes to the Affordable Care Act. Available at: The Uninsured and the ACA: A Primer – Key Facts about Health Insurance and the Uninsured amidst Changes to the Affordable Care Act – How does lack of insurance affect access to care? – 7451-14 | KFF

References

AHRQ (2018). *Elements of Access to Health Care | Agency for Health Research and Quality.* [online] www.ahrq.gov. Available at: https://www.ahrq.gov/research/findings/nhqrdr/chartbooks/access/elements.html [Accessed 28 August 2023].

Brenan, M. (2023). *Majority in U.S. Still Say Gov't Should Ensure Healthcare*. [online] Gallup.com. Available at: https://news.gallup.com/poll/468401/majority-say-gov-ensure-healthcare.aspx [Accessed 29 August 2023].

CDC (2022a). *Health Effects of Overweight and Obesity* [online] Available at: https://www.cdc.gov/healthyweight/effects/index.html [Accessed 29 September 2023].

CDC (2022b). *Suicide Prevention: Risk and Protective Factors* [online] Available at: https://www.cdc.gov/suicide/factors/index.html [Accessed 29 September 2023].

CDC (2023). *About the National Health Interview Survey* National Center for Health Statistics [online] Available at: https://www.cdc.gov/nchs/nhis/about_nhis.htm [Accessed 29 August 2023].

Center For Reproductive Rights (2022). *Roe v. Wade*. [online] Center for Reproductive Rights. Available at: https://reproductiverights.org/roe-v-wade/ [Accessed 30 August 2023].

CIA.gov. (n.d.). *Education expenditures - The World Factbook*. [online] Available at: https://www.cia.gov/the-world-factbook/field/education-expenditures/ [Accessed 8 October 2023].

Commonwealth Fund (2023). *U.S. Health Care from a Global Perspective, 2022: Accelerating Spending, Worsening Outcomes*. [online] Available at: https://www.commonwealthfund.org/publications/issue-briefs/2023/jan/us-health-care-global-perspective-2022#1 [Accessed 29 August 2023].

Countryeconomy.com. (2016). *GDP - Gross Domestic Product 2016* | countryeconomy.com. [online] Available at: https://countryeconomy.com/gdp?year=2016 [Accessed 8 Oct. 2023].

Garfield, R., Orgera, K. and Damico, A. (2019). *The Uninsured and the ACA: A Primer – Key Facts about Health Insurance and the Uninsured amidst Changes to the Affordable Care Act - How does lack of insurance affect access to care?* The Henry J. Kaiser Family Foundation. [online] Available at: https://www.kff.org/report-section/the-uninsured-and-the-aca-a-primer-key-facts-about-health-insurance-and-the-uninsured-amidst-changes-to-the-affordable-care-act-how-does-lack-of-insurance-affect-access-to-care/ [Accessed 29 August 2023].

Gunja, M., Gumas, E. and Williams, R. (2023). *U.S. Health Care from a Global Perspective, 2022: Accelerating Spending, Worsening Outcomes*. [online] www.commonwealthfund.org. Available at: https://www.commonwealthfund.org/publications/issue-briefs/2023/jan/us-health-care-global-perspective-2022#1 [Accessed 29 August 2023].

Healthy People 2030 (n.d.). *Access to Health Services - Healthy People 2030 | health.gov*. [online] Available at: https://health.gov/healthypeople/priority-areas/social-determinants-health/literature-summaries/access-health-services#cit2 [Accessed 29 August 2023].

House Committee on the Budget (2017). *What You Need to Know About Means-Tested Entitlements* [online] Available at: https://democrats-budget.house.gov/publications/report/what-you-need-know-about-means-tested-entitlements [Accessed 29 September 2023].

Kaiser Family Foundation (2022). *Status of State Medicaid Expansion Decisions: Interactive Map*. The Henry J. Kaiser Family Foundation. [online] Available at: https://www.kff.org/medicaid/issue-brief/status-of-state-medicaid-expansion-decisions-interactive-map/ [Accessed 29 August 2023].

KFF (2023a). Abortion in the United States Dashboard [online] Available at: https://www.kff.org/womens-health-policy/dashboard/abortion-in-the-u-s-dashboard/ [Accessed 30 August 2023].

KFF (2023b). *A Year After Dobbs: Policies Restricting Access to Abortion in States Even Where It's Not Banned.* [online] Available at: https://www.kff.org/policy-watch/year-after-dobbs-policies-restricting-access-to-abortion/ [Accessed 30 August 2023].

National Constitution Center – constitutioncenter.org. (2022). *Dobbs v. Jackson Women's Health Organization | Constitution Center*. [online] Available at: https://constitutioncenter.org/the-constitution/supreme-court-case-library/dobbs-v-jackson-womens-health-organization#:~:text=In%20Dobbs%2C%20the%20Supreme%20Court.

National Health Interview Survey (2022). *Health Insurance Coverage* CDC [online] Available at: https://www.cdc.gov/nchs/data/nhis/earlyrelease/Quarterly_Estimates_2023_Q11.pdf [Accessed 29 September 2023].

OECD (2023). *Health Status*. [online] Oecd.org. [online] Available at: https://stats.oecd.org/Index.aspx?DataSetCode=HEALTH_STAT [Accessed 8 October 2023].

Our World in Data. (n.d.). Public social spending as a share of GDP. [online] Available at: https://ourworldindata.org/grapher/social-spending-oecd-longrun [Accessed 8 October 2023].

Planned Parenthood (2022). How much does an Abortion Cost? [online] Available at: https://www.plannedparenthood.org/blog/how-much-does-an-abortion-cost [Accessed 1 October 2023].

SCOTUS (2022). *Dobbs, State Health Officer of the Mississippi Department of Health et al v. Jackson Women's Health Organization et al.* [online] Available at: https://www.supremecourt.gov/DocketPDF/19/19-1392/192717/20210917120823669_Dobbs%20Final%20Brief.pdf [Accessed 29 September 2023].

Seervai, S., Gunja, M., Zephyrin, L. and Williams, R. (2023). *Limiting Abortion Access for American Women Impacts Health, Economic Security: An International Comparison*. [online] Available at: https://www.commonwealthfund.org/blog/2023/limiting-abortion-access-american-women-impacts-health-economic-security [Accessed 30 August 2023].

Shmerling, R. (2022). *Why life expectancy in the US is falling.* Harvard Health Publishing Harvard Medical School [online] Available at: https://www.health.harvard.edu/blog/why-life-expectancy-in-the-us-is-falling-202210202835 [Accessed 30 September 2023].

The Supreme Court of the United States (2022). *Dobbs, State Health Officer of the Mississippi Department of Health et al v. Jackson Women's Health Organization et al.* [online] Available at: https://www.supremecourt.gov/DocketPDF/19/19-1392/192717/20210917120823669_Dobbs%20Final%20Brief.pdf [Accessed 29 September 2023].

United Nations (1948). *Universal Declaration of Human Rights*. [online] United Nations. Available at: https://www.un.org/en/about-us/universal-declaration-of-human-rights [Accessed 29 August 2023].

University of Missouri (2020). *Health Care Access - MU School of Medicine*. [online] medicine.missouri.edu. Available at: https://medicine.missouri.edu/centers-institutes-labs/health-ethics/faq/health-care-access [Accessed 29 August 2023].

Wisevoter. (n.d.). Most Educated Countries 2023. [online] Available at: https://wisevoter.com/country-rankings/most-educated-countries/ [Accessed 8 October 2023].

Zablocki, A. and Sutrina, M. (2022). *The Impact of State Law Criminalizing Abortion* LexisNexis [online] Available at: https://www.lexisnexis.com/community/insights/legal/practical-guidance-journal/b/pa/posts/the-impact-of-state-laws-criminalizing-abortion [Accessed 1 October 2023].

Lexicon of Listed Terms and Agencies

- **Centers for Disease Control and Prevention (CDC)** is a major operating component of the Department of Health and Human Services whose mission is to protect America from health, safety and security threats, both foreign and domestic. It is the nation's leading science-based, data-driven, service organization that protect's the public's health.

- **Center for Reproductive Rights** is a global human rights organization of lawyers and advocates who ensure reproductive rights are protected in law as fundamental human rights for the dignity, equality, health and well-being of every person.

- **Gallup** is a global analytic and advice firm that helps leaders and organizations solve thei most pressing problems.

- **Organization for Economic Co-operation and Development (OECD)** is an international organization that works with governments, policy makers and citizens to establish international standards that are focused on well-being for all.

- **The Agency for Healthcare Research and Quality (AHRQ)** is an agency under the Department of Health and Human Services whose mission is to produce evidence to make health care safer, higher quality, more accessible, equitable and afordable.

- **The Commonwealth Fund** is a private foundation thatthat aims to promote a high performing heath care system that achieves better access, improved quality and greater efficiency, particularly for society's most vulnerable.

- **The Kaiser Family Foundation (KFF)** is a non-profit organization focusing on national health issues, as well as the United State's role in global health policy. KFF serves as a non-partisan source of facts, analysis and journalism for policymakers, the media, the health policy community and the public.

- **The National Constitution Center** is a private, nonprofit organization that serves as America's leading platform for constitutional education and debate.

AUTHOR'S BIO SKETCH

Sylvia Otto, DO

Dr. Sylvia Otto is originally from Manitowoc, WI and attended the University of Wisconsin-Madison where she received her Bachelor of Science in Biochemistry. She completed medical school at Campbell University in rural Lillington, NC before pursuing her residency in Family Medicine at the University of Washington affiliated Community Health Care in Tacoma, WA. She is dedicated to caring for underserved patient populations and is proud to completing her training at a Federally Qualified Healthcare Center. When not at work, Dr. Otto enjoys traveling and exploring new restaurants with her husband, hiking, cross-stitching, and playing board games.

Chapter 13

Transportation as a Social Determinant of Health

James Pecsok, MD, Author
Laila Siddiqui, MD, Editor

"*Our transportation decisions determine much more than where roads or bridges or tunnels or rail lines will be built. They determine the connections and barriers that people will encounter in their daily lives...*"

- Elijah Cummings U.S. Congressman and Civil rights Activist

Transportation as a Social Determinant of Health

In the context of Well-being

An agricultural implement dealer in rural Kansas with high blood cholesterol quits drinking alcohol but does not take time to drive to the gym 25 minutes away to workout. A mother wishes to walk with her children to the science museum, but gangs hang out between her apartment and the metro bus stop making it a dangerous seven block trek from her home. An elderly man desires to exercise his golden retriever but is reluctant because his neighborhood doesn't have sidewalks and several pedestrians have been struck by cars during the past year. Every day, typical Americans make four trips and travel an average of 40 miles (BTS, 2017; Huxley-Reicher, 2022).

Transportation plays a key role in shaping health outcomes. Access to the social determinants of health – employment, education, healthcare, housing, and grocery markets to say nothing of important family, recreational, social, and spiritual engagements depend on efficiently moving from point A to point B. Many Americans make efforts to eat a balanced diet, exercise more, and cut back on unhealthy habits, and take for granted the dynamic impact transportation systems have on their health and well-being.

Before understanding how transportation impacts health outcomes, it is important to identify how people in the U.S. interact with its transportation infrastructure. This interaction depends on the built environment, which "touches all aspects of our lives, encompassing the buildings we live in, the distribution systems that provide us with water and electricity, and the roads, bridges, and transportation systems we use to get from place to place" (US EPA, 2023). According to Hinton and Artiga (2018), socioeconomic status, and the presence of physical, emotional, or mental incapacities form an essential element of the human - transportation interaction. For instance, a software developer working in the suburbs of Denver can safely bike to the commuter bus-stop or engage Uber or Lyft without disrupting her work day. However, a part-time grocery store clerk living in a poor neighborhood on the edge of poverty may have a completely unique experience. She feels unsafe taking the bus or struggles to find an accessible, efficient bus route. Her below the poverty line income makes owning an automobile prohibitive. These obstacles contribute to lost work hours, increased life stress, and decreased income.

This chapter discusses the strategies utilized historically to develop the U.S. transportation infrastructure, followed by dialogue on transportation's place as a social determinant of health and vital role in individual and community well-being, then closes with optimistic perspectives for the future.

Historical Perspective on the Development of the US Transportation System – 19th century

Canals, bridges, riverboats, and road construction paved the interconnectivity of the eastern United States before and during the first third of the 19th century. The advent of steam locomotives, however, changed that. "America's first steam locomotive made its debut in 1830, and over the next two decades, railroad tracks linked many cities along the East Coast. By 1850, some 9,000 miles of track had been laid as far west as the Missouri River" (History.com Editors, 2018).

The first half of the 1800's witnessed dramatic expansion of the U.S. territory through outright purchase, or war and its ensuing treaties. The Louisiana purchase in 1803 added land from

Louisiana through Montana including Missouri, Kansas, Nebraska, and the Dakotas. Florida was annexed in 1819 followed by Oregon in 1842 and Texas in 1845. Finally, California, Arizona, Colorado, New Mexico, Nevada, Utah, and Wyoming in 1848 following the Mexican American war. Spawned by a righteous belief in Manifest Destiny – the fulfillment to overspread the continent allotted by Providence – presidents, business leaders, capitalists and entrepreneurs of every stripe saw expansion and development of the United States as their right guided by Manifest Destiny and as an investment well worth the riches that would rightfully follow (History.com Editors, 2018).

Despite success in the acquisition of large swaths of land, the challenges to develop such enormous territory remained. To reach San Francisco or other west coast destinations from the eastern seaboard, travelers confronted three hazardous and time-consuming options: sea voyage around South America's Cape of Horn, sea and land travel over the Isthmus of Panama or trek the uncharted prairie, mountains, and rivers of the vast western United States. Transportation successes witnessed in the east assured entrepreneurs the same victories could be had in the west. Thus, steam locomotives powered the vision and provided the spirit to connect the United States from coast to coast by constructing a network of transcontinental railways (History.com Editors, 2018).

The first transcontinental railroad ran from Omaha, Nebraska to Sacramento, California. Completed in 1869, it effectively connected the U.S. from ocean to ocean. Railway travel cut the 3,000-mile journey east to west from months to days. Moreover, success demonstrated, a network of transcontinental railroad lines grew to link the west border to border during the late 19th century. The Great Northern, Northern Pacific, Union Pacific, Central Pacific, Southern Pacific, and many others, networked the eastern United States from Chicago, St. Louis, New Orleans and Houston to Denver, Seattle, San Francisco, Los Angeles, Albuquerque and back again (UShistory.org, 2019).

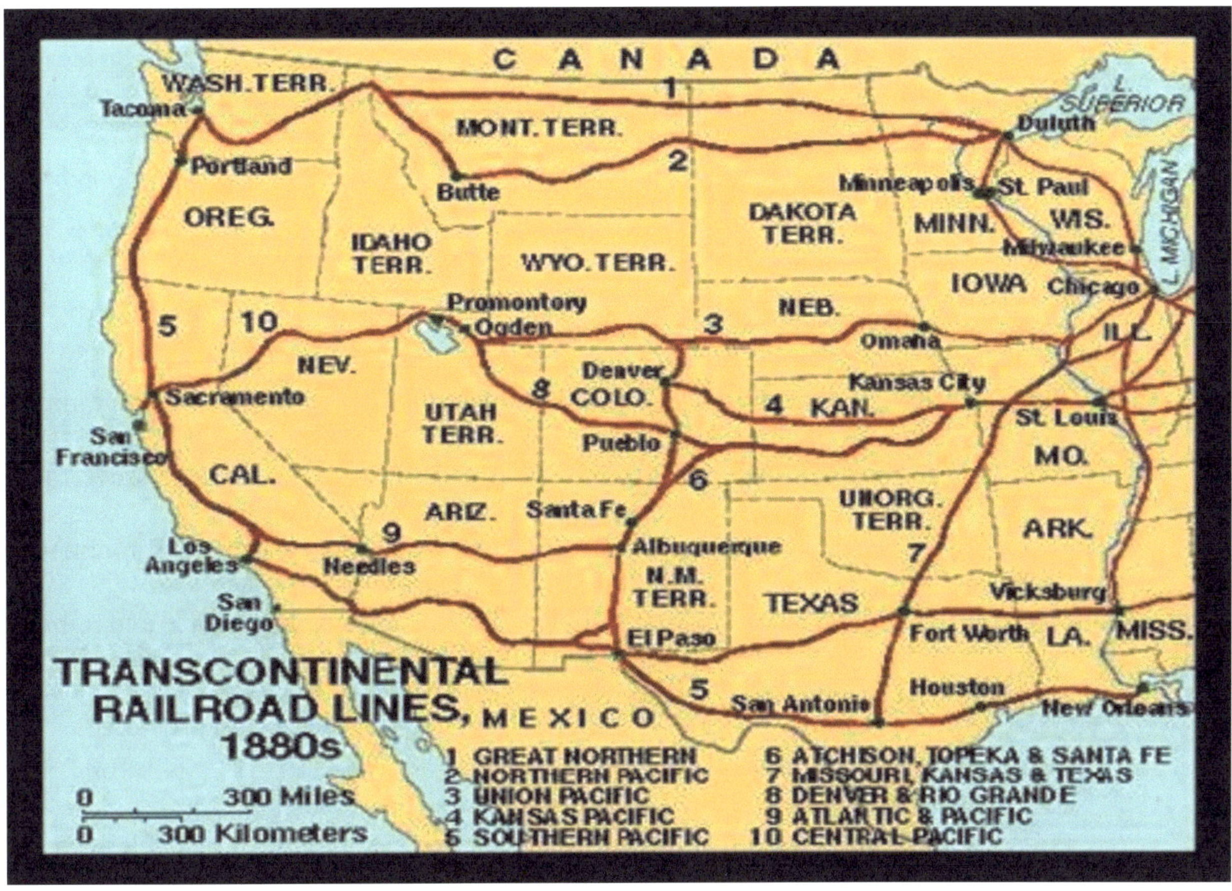

UShistory.org. (2019). Binding the Nation by Rail [ushistory.org]. [online] Available at: https://www.ushistory.org/us/36a.asp.

Westward expansion and the railroad tycoon's quest for fortune, succeeded beyond the wildest expectations – commercial opportunities expanded, cities grew, towns dotted the landscape, jobs were created, enterprising spirit blossomed – but it came with significant and lasting social and public health consequences.

The extraordinary commercial success of railroad building in the United States during the 19th century served as a template for future U.S. transportation development, the entrepreneurial strategies to ensure its success, and the disregard for the social implications to carry it out in the 20th century. Hallmarks included:

- Leveraging the doctrine of Manifest Destiny to assert and validate dominion as allotted by Providence – enterprise as a God given right (History.com Editors, 2010).
- Embracing the pillars of capitalism, exerting influence by which people act in pursuit of their own good, without regard for sociopolitical pressure and with disdain for government regulation (Jahan and Mahmud, 2023).
- Land taking – utilizing the power of eminent domain to enhance business opportunities. Eminent domain refers to power of government to take private property and convert it to public use (LII/Legal Information Institute, n.d.). In the instance of the transcontinental railroad construction, this meant taking Native American lands by brute force and military intervention, if necessary, further disrupting their way of life and marginalizing Native American heritage (Gandhi, 2021).
- Exploitation of labor – backbreaking work and hazardous conditions characterized the work of railroad building. Construction supervisors recruited disenfranchised groups – Chinese, but many African Americans – to do the grueling work at a fraction of the wages paid to white counterparts (Gandhi, 2021).

Historical Perspective on the Development of the US Transportation System – 20th century

World War I, the Great Depression and World War II consumed the American spirit during the first half of the twentieth century in the United States. Although Roosevelt's New Deal set the table for a prosperous, modern America, the Second World War torpedoed its momentum.

Apart from Route 66 – a stretch of highway connecting Chicago to Los Angeles as it meandered through Missouri, Oklahoma, Texas, New Mexico, and Arizona – America's highway system was a mix of paved and unpaved roads, old bridges, and narrow passages (Longfellow, 2022). That chapter in America's transportation history ended in 1956 when President Dwight D. Eisenhower signed the *Federal-Aid Highway Act of 1956* to create the Interstate Highway System (Lacy, 2018).

When Congress approved the Federal-Aid Highway Act of 1956, it authorized what was then the largest public works program in U.S. history (Evans, 2023). "The law promised to construct 41,000 miles of an ambitious interstate highway system that would crisscross the nation, dramatically expanding America's roadways and connecting 42 state capital cities and 90 percent of all American cities with populations over 50,000. Its goal was to eliminate unsafe roads, inefficient routes and traffic jams that impede fast and safe cross-country travel" (Evans, 2023). According to the Federal Highway Administration (www.fhwa.dot.gov, 2022), since its inception the Interstate System has been a part of our culture and is integral to the American way of life. Nevertheless, "its construction came at a huge cost to America's urban communities of color" (Evans, 2023).

The architects of the Interstate System borrowed from the playbook of 19th century railroad tycoons – especially eminent domain, disregard for sociopolitical pressure, and marginalization of disenfranchised minorities – to achieve the means to their ends.

Transportation as a Social Determinant of Health

In the context of Community Cohesion

The Federal Highway Act of 1956 came as a stimulus package to create 40,000 miles of roadways that make up the Interstate Highway System. State and local governments invoked eminent domain, the legal authority to seize private property for public use, to make room for the new highways. In cities, this practice often meant the forced displacement of low-income and Black neighborhoods where land was cheaper and there was less organized political resistance.

The construction of highways physically divided neighborhoods, disrupting community, social and economic fabric. Businesses were destroyed and communities were fragmented, making it difficult for residents to access essential services and economic opportunities. The Civil Rights movement challenged race-based discrimination in the law, but simultaneous events in modern America's nascent transportation system contributed to sub-legal, de facto race-based segregation. This de facto segregation has lasting impacts to this day (Blas, 2010).

According to Evans (2023), the U.S. Department of Transportation estimates that more than 475,000 households and over a million people were displaced nationwide due to Interstate Highway construction. Hulking roadways cut through neighborhoods; darkened and disrupted the pedestrian landscape; worsened air quality and torpedoed property values. Communities lost churches, green space, and whole swaths of homes. They also lost small businesses that provided jobs and kept money circulating locally – crucial middle-class footholds in areas already struggling from racist zoning policies, disinvestment, and white flight.

"Racial and economic segregation in urban communities is often understood as a natural consequence of poor choices by individuals. In reality, racially and economically segregated cities are the result of many factors, including the nation's interstate highway system. In states around the country, highway construction displaced Black households and cut the heart and soul out of thriving Black communities as homes, churches, schools, and businesses were destroyed. In other communities, the highway system was a tool of a segregationist agenda, erecting a wall that separated White and Black communities and protected White people from Black migration. In these ways, construction of the interstate highway system contributed to the residential concentration of race and poverty and created physical, economic, and psychological barriers that persist" (Archer, 2020).

The neighborhood of Jackson Ward in Richmond, Virginia exemplifies how discriminatory transportation planning fragmented communities. Once known as "Black Wallstreet" and the "Harlem of the South," Jackson Ward developed into a bustling cultural and economic center by the end of the 19th century. Black-owned banks and professional offices lined 2nd street, as did historic brownstone mansions owned by Black doctors and businessmen. Due to gerrymandering, however, the Richmond city council had just one Black representative in the 1950s. After fending

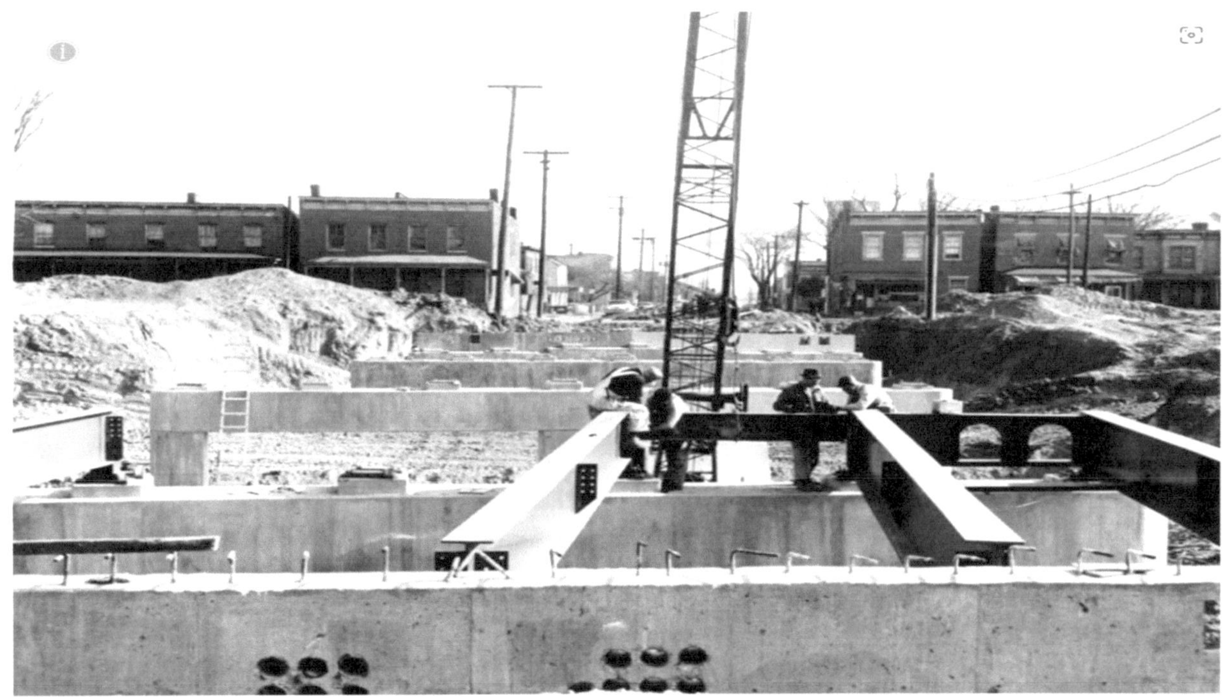

Construction of the Richmond-Petersburg Turnpike in Jackson Ward (1955)

Davis, B.C. (2023). *Under the Highway: North Jackson Ward.* [online] ArcGIS StoryMaps. [online] Available at: https://storymaps.arcgis.com/stories/0ca5d5523fa7435199aeaa00a43f14b4 [Accessed 22 October 2023].

off several attempts to raze Jackson Ward for highway construction, the city council ultimately approved the Richmond turnpike project with the highway plowing through historic 2nd street

(Davis, 2023; Campbell, 2016). According to Davis (2023), "as much as Richmonders were able to delay the project, in the end their resistance was ruthlessly sidestepped by City Council."

The highway devastated Jackson Ward. Between January 1955 and August 1957, more than seven thousand Richmonders were displaced to make room for the Richmond-Petersburg Expressway – ten percent of Richmond's Black population had to relocate. Today, Jackson Ward is one of the most impoverished areas in the city of Richmond, never recovering from the strategies and impact of Interstate Highway building (Davis, 2023).

Map 1.

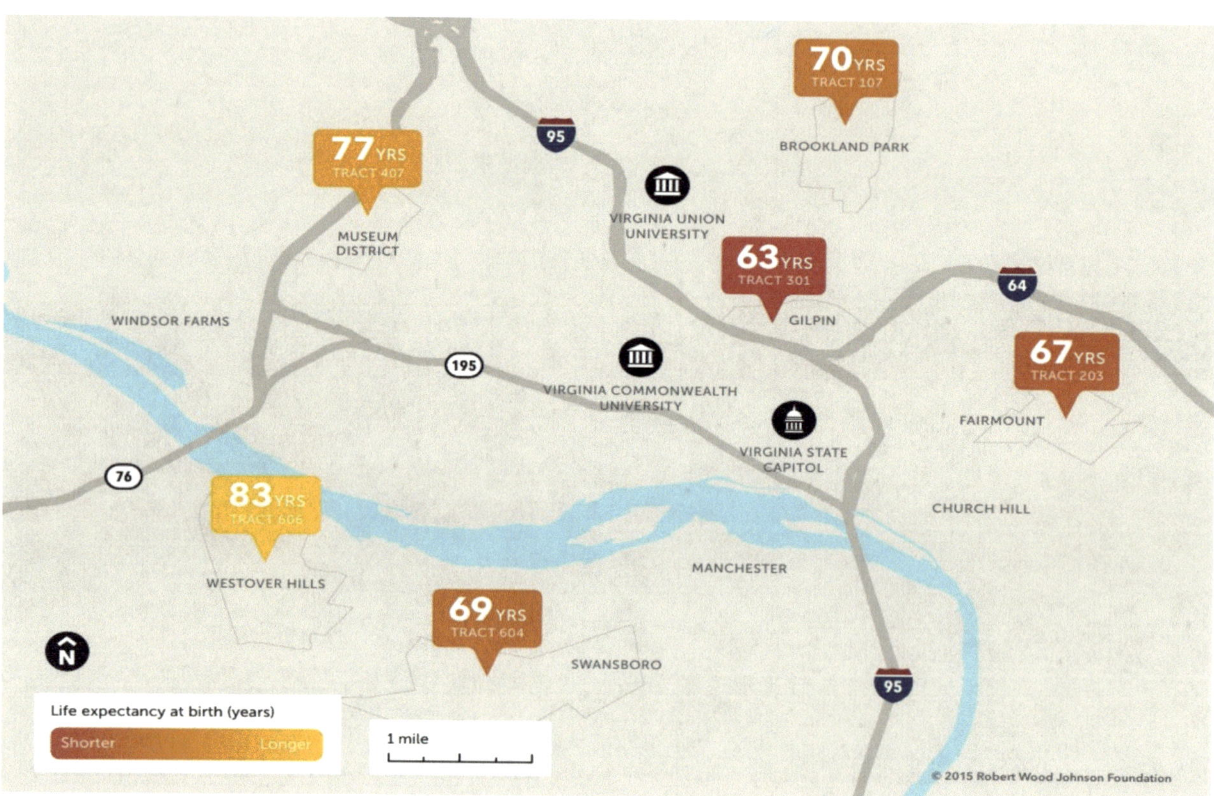

societyhealth.vcu.edu. (2015). *Center on Society and Health.* [online] Available at: https://societyhealth.vcu.edu/work/the-projects/mapsrichmond.html#gsc.tab=0

To further illustrate its perpetual and lasting impact, the Center on Society and Health of the Virginia Commonwealth University estimates "babies born within five miles of downtown Richmond face up to a 20-year difference in life expectancy" (societyhealth.vcu.edu, 2015).

Contemplate as well Interstate 95's effect on longevity by examining **Map 1**, which lays witness to the disparate life expectancy consequences fostered by construction of Interstate 95 and Interstate 64 nearly seventy-five years ago (societyhealth.vcu.edu, 2015).

History hails New York City's construction coordinator Robert Moses as the urban planner most influential in establishing urban Interstate Highway construction schemes. According to Evans (2023), Moses held the opinion that constructing highways through urban centers served the dual purpose of improving traffic and clearing slums, "go right through the cities and not around them" legacy documents his mindset.

What took place in Richmond's Jackson Ward proved to be the rule rather than the exception. Driven by Robert Moses' strategies, cities across the country replicated his tactics from the Bronx to Buffalo, Chicago, Pittsburgh, San Diego, Miami, Atlanta and back – the Interstate System established a trek of "white men's roads through Black men's homes" (Archer, 2020) utilizing 19th century transcontinental railroad strategies – eminent domain, disregard for sociopolitical pressure, and marginalization of disenfranchised minorities – to achieve objectives.

"The pattern was repeated over and over across the nation: White leaders used the specter of urban deterioration to justify construction through low-income neighborhoods of color. Homes and businesses were razed. Logan Heights, the bastion of San Diego's Latino community, was severed in two by Interstate 5; Black Bottom, Detroit's majority-Black neighborhood, was bulldozed to make way for Interstate 375; in Montgomery, Ala., the state's highway director, a member of the Ku Klux Klan, ignored swaths of empty land in favor of a route that displaced Black civil rights leaders" (Blakemore, 2021). In Miami, Florida Interstate 95 "tore through the center of Overtown, a large and vibrant Black community considered to be the center of economic and cultural life for Black people living in Miami," (Archer, 2020). Miami's interchange consumed forty square miles, devoured the Black business district, and displaced the homes of 10,000 people (Archer, 2020).

President Eisenhower's address to the Congress February 22, 1955 appealed the construction of the Interstate Highway System and stated thus:

President Eisenhower's address to the Congress February 22, 1955

"To the Congress of the United States: our unity as a nation is sustained by free communication of thought and by easy transportation of people and goods. The ceaseless flow of information throughout the Republic is matched by individual and commercial movement over a vast system of interconnected highways crisscrossing the country and joining it at our national borders with friendly neighbors to the north and the south. Together, the uniting forces of our communication and transportation systems are dynamic elements and the very name we bear -- United States. Without them, we would be a mere alliance of many separate parts," (The White House, 1955).

The White House (1955). *To the Congress of the United States*. [online] Available at: https://www.eisenhowerlibrary.gov/sites/default/files/research/online-documents/interstate-highway-system/1955-02-22-message-to-congress.pdf

Eisenhower appointed General Lucious Clay as his point person for the Interstate Highway Plan development, which the President used extensively in his February 22 address to Congress. Regarding urban routes, Clay made the following statement in testimony to Congress February 21, 1955, "While it is very true, we want traffic to be able to go around the cities, also we want to have expressways connecting the cities themselves with this expressway, so that you can have instant access to and egress from the city," (Weingroff, 2017).

To be certain, the Interstate Highway system propagated the vast array of amenities identified as modern America in the 21st century. Eisenhower's appeal and the activities leading up to the signing of the Federal Aid Highway Act on June 29, 1956 in no way reflect deliberate intent to promote segregation across the United States. However, confluent with white flight to the suburbs, redlining, restrictive covenants, marginalized political influence, diminished tax base, and disenfranchised voice, Interstate Highway construction evolved into strategies that segregated and decimated Black communities in every viable way. A horrific storm left them behind culturally, socially, and economically without access to essential social determinants of health – access to food, healthcare, education, jobs, infrastructure services, and housing. Urban planners, legislative leaders, and state governors throughout the United States leveraged transportation – a vital social determinant of health – to deprive disenfranchised populations access to essential health determinants.

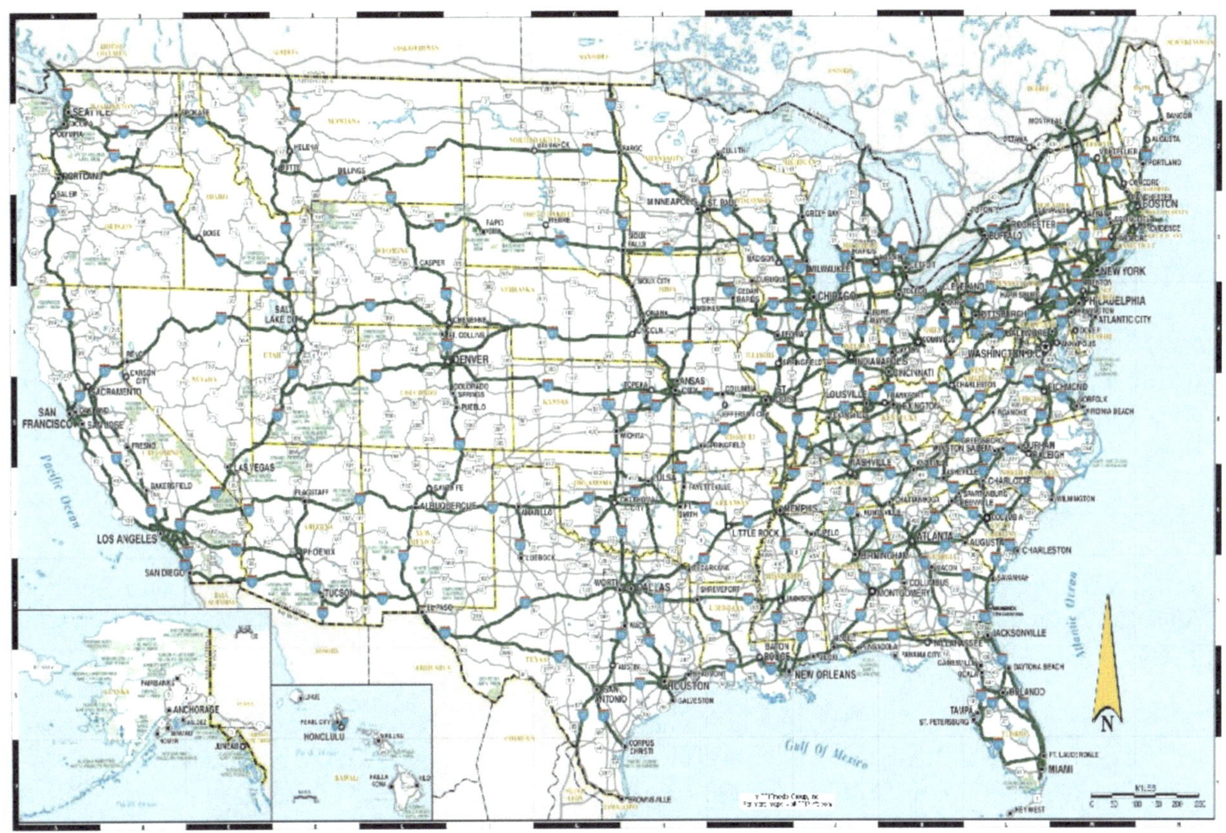

United States Highway Map February 2018

Best (2018). *United States Highways Map | Usa Map 2018.* [online] United States Highways Map | Usa Map 2018. Available at: https://usamapnew.blogspot.com/2018/02/united-states-highways-map.html

Transportation as a Social Determinant of Health

In the context of Rebuilding Community Cohesion – Point ~ Counterpoint

The extraordinary history and the damage done in the build of the Interstate System reflects devastation 75 years in the making. The *Reconnecting Communities* program offers hope for racially divided communities.

> ## Pete Buttigieg launches $1B pilot to build racial equity in America's roads
>
> June 30, 2022 5:55 AM ET by the Associated Press
>
> WASHINGTON — Transportation Secretary Pete Buttigieg on Thursday launched a $1 billion first-of-its-kind pilot program aimed at helping reconnect cities and neighborhoods racially segregated or divided by road projects, pledging wide-ranging help to dozens of communities despite the program's limited dollars.
>
> Under the *Reconnecting Communities* program, cities and states can now apply for the federal aid over five years to rectify harm caused by roadways that were built primarily through lower-income, Black communities after the 1950s creation of the interstate highway system.
>
> New projects could include rapid bus transit lines to link disadvantaged neighborhoods to jobs; caps built on top of highways featuring green spaces, bike lanes and pedestrian walkways to allow for safe crossings over the roadways; repurposing former rail lines; and partial removal of highways.
>
> Still, the grants, being made available under President Joe Biden's bipartisan infrastructure law, are considerably less than the $20 billion the Democratic president originally envisioned. Advocacy groups say the money is not nearly enough to have a major impact on capital construction for more than 50 citizen-led efforts nationwide aimed at dismantling or redesigning highways — from Portland, Oregon, to New Orleans; St. Paul, Minnesota; Houston; Tampa, Florida; and Syracuse, New York.
>
> "Transportation can connect us to jobs, services and loved ones, but we've also seen countless cases around the country where a piece of infrastructure cuts off a neighborhood or a community because of how it was built," said Buttigieg, who was announcing the pilot program later Thursday in Birmingham, Alabama. He described *Reconnecting Communities* as a broad department "principle" — not just a program — to address the issue with many efforts underway.
>
> "This is a forward-looking vision," Buttigieg said. "Our focus isn't about assigning blame. It is not about getting caught up in guilt. It's about fixing a problem. It's about mending what has been broken, especially when the damage was done with taxpayer dollars."
>
> Press, T.A. (2022). Pete Buttigieg launches $1B pilot to build racial equity in America's roads. NPR. [online] 30 Jun. Available at: https://www.npr.org/2022/06/30/1108852884/pete-buttigieg-launches-1b-pilot-to-build-racial-equity-in-americas-roads

In March, 2023, the US Department of Transportation granted $185 million to forty-five Reconnecting Communities pilot projects (Zukowski, 2023).

Transportation as a Social Determinant of Health

In the context of Building Community Cohesion – "Kool" Routes to School

"Kool" routes to school provides a real time strategy to successfully resolve community severance by encouraging pedestrian traffic. An ongoing Chilean study called "Kool Routes to School" exemplifies the broad sweeping benefits of promoting connected communities. Initially designed to combat childhood obesity by encouraging children to walk to school - "Kool Routes to School" expanded endpoints beyond weight loss to include emotional health, social connection, and civic engagement (Sagaris and Lanfranco, 2019).

As the project progressed, researchers detected that that students and teachers involved in the program built strong bonds not just with each other, but also with the community they interacted with during their walks. These bonds served as a tool to build social support; researchers noticed fewer classroom disruptions and less frequent arguments between peers. Students were observed discussing home life, gender identities, and emotional wellbeing, and got to participate in planning bus routes and bicycle repair (Sagaris and Lanfranco, 2019). In the fourth year of the project, community advocates for "Kool Routes to School" have partnered with the local government to expand pedestrian corridors throughout the city. This initiative exemplifies how access to adequate transportation can lead to vibrant, healthy communities.

Transportation as a Social Determinant of Health

Politics, policies, and governance – Transportation Resilience

The concepts of transportation "resilience" gained urgency and impetus following the attacks of September 11 as the Congress, the Department of Homeland Security, various state agencies, and the National Academies began addressing a variety of topics around transportation security (AASHTO, 2017). According to the Committee on Transportation Resilience (2021), transportation resilience is defined as "the ability to prepare for and adapt to changing conditions and withstand and recover rapidly from disruption."

Four foundational concepts shape transportation resilience (AASHTO, 2017).

1. *Critical infrastructure* – systems and assets, whether physical or virtual, so vital to the United States that the incapacity or destruction of such systems and assets would have a debilitating impact on security, national economic security, national public health or safety, or any combination of those matters.
2. *Risk* – the potential for an unwanted outcome resulting from an incident, event, or occurrence, as determined by its likelihood and associated consequences.
3. *Protection* – to reduce the vulnerability of critical infrastructure to deter, mitigate or neutralize terrorist attack or natural disaster.
4. *Climate change* – destruction of infrastructure caused by extreme weather events.

Munich RE (2023) reports that in 2020 six of the world's ten most costly natural disasters occurred in the United States and that large-scale natural disasters wreaking havoc on the condition and functioning of transportation systems and other infrastructure are on the rise. For example, during the 1980s, billion-dollar natural disasters, when adjusted for inflation, averaged 2.9 per year, in 2020 alone the United States experienced more than 20, according to the Committee on Transportation Resilience (2021).

Beyond these disastrous events, climate change harbors slow but persistent changes in sea level. Temperature and precipitation extremes are intensifying storm damage and accelerating infrastructure deterioration. The United States experienced a record-breaking 22 billion-dollar natural disasters during 2020. To varying extents, all damaged or disrupted the operations of transportation infrastructure vital for emergency services, evacuations, and the movement of supplies (Committee on Transportation Resilience, 2021).

The United States Congress passed the Further Consolidated Appropriation Act, 2020 a component of which directed the U.S. Department of Transportation to enter into an agreement with the National Academies of Sciences, Engineering and Medicine (The National Academies) to conduct a study through the Transportation Research Board on effective ways to measure the resilience of transportation systems and services to national disasters, national hazards, and other potential disruptions (Committee on Transportation Resilience, 2021).

On November 6, 2021, the U.S. Congress passed the Bipartisan Infrastructure Investment and Jobs Act. According to the White House (2021), the Act will rebuild America's roads, bridges, and rails, expand access to clean drinking water, ensure every American has access to high-speed internet, tackle the climate crisis, advance environmental justice, and invest in communities that have too often been left behind.

The legislation will ease inflationary pressures and strengthen supply chains by making long overdue improvements in our nation's ports, airports, railways, and roads. It will drive the creation of good-paying union jobs and grow the economy sustainably and equitably so that everyone gets ahead for decades to come.

Conclusion and Future Directions

While the "Kool Routes to School" project takes place in small Chilean cities, the key findings may be applied to any community. Collaborative efforts with local partners in transportation projects enhance resilience within underserved communities by tailoring solutions unique to their needs. The success of flexible problem-solving approaches as exemplified in Washington, D.C., where Lyft's partnership with hospitals has significantly reduced emergency room utilization, underscores the effectiveness of community-focused initiatives. By providing medical transportation for patients, Lyft has reduced emergency room utilization by 40%

(www.lyft.com, 2020). Initiatives at the city and state level have begun to reverse decades of transportation inequity. For example, San Diego's long-term commitment to creating a walkable inner-city (Reynault, 2013) and Virginia's adoption of a more equitable funding allocation formula are steps toward rectifying decades of transportation inequality (Schweninger, 2021). Focusing on equity in transportation resilience at the local, state, and national level holds promise to pave the way for healthy, connected communities. When fully realized, the Bipartisan Infrastructure Investment and Jobs Act stands to modernize, if not revolutionize, national transportation and communication infrastructure.

Questions for Further Consideration:

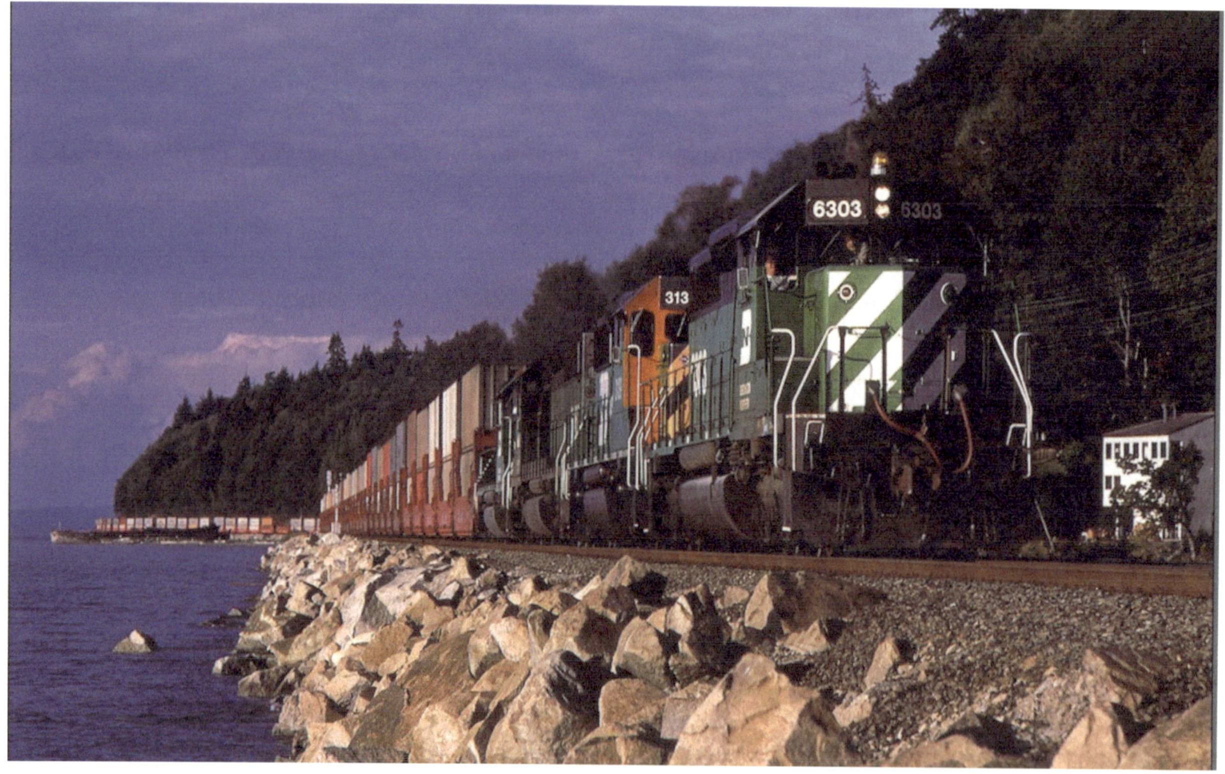

Repp, M. (2012). RailPictures.net Photo: BN 6303 Burlington Northern Railroad EMD SD40 at Along Puget Sound, Washington by M. S. Repp. [online] railpictures.net. Available at: https://railpictures.net/viewphoto.php?id=413530

1. A Burlington Northern Stack train rolls west along Puget Sound en-route to the Seattle area on a summer day. What elements of natural disasters and climate change challenge this railroad? How will melting in West Antarctica affect sea level rise? Reference this URL:

   Ramirez, R. (2023). *Rapid melting in West Antarctica is 'unavoidable,' with potentially disastrous consequences for sea level rise, study finds*. [online] CNN. Available at: https://www.cnn.com/2023/10/23/world/west-antarctic-ice-melt-climate/index.html.

2. How does the historical legacy of discriminatory transportation policies, such as redlining and the development of automobile-centric infrastructure, continue to shape transportation disparities and health outcomes in marginalized communities today?
3. In what ways can transportation be both a barrier to accessing healthcare and a determinant of health? How might addressing transportation disparities lead to improved overall public health?
4. What if any, are the downsides to a revitalized transportation infrastructure? Come up with several ways to prevent adverse effects of gentrification of urban areas. Is the DOT *Reconnecting Communities* initiative too little too late?
5. As cities strive for more sustainable and equitable transportation systems, what strategies and policies can be implemented to promote both transportation justice and public health, especially in underserved and vulnerable communities?

Sentinel Readings for a Deeper Dive

Campbell, A. (2016). *The Rise and Fall of Black Wall Street*. [online] The Atlantic. Available at: https://www.theatlantic.com/business/archive/2016/08/the-end-of-black-wall-street/498074/

Davis, B. (2023). *Under the Highway: North Jackson Ward*. [online] ArcGIS StoryMaps. [online] Available at: https://storymaps.arcgis.com/stories/0ca5d5523fa7435199aeaa00a43f14b4

Schweninger, E., Edmunds, M. and Atherton, E. (2020). *Transportation A COMMUNITY DRIVER OF HEALTH*. [online] Available at: https://iomc.org/resources/Documents/Transportation_Health_Community_Driver.pdf

Spieler, C. (2020). *Racism has shaped public transit, and it's riddled with inequities | Kinder Institute for Urban Research*. [online] Kinder Institute for Urban Research | Rice University. Available at: https://kinder.rice.edu/urbanedge/racism-has-shaped-public-transit-and-its-riddled-inequities

Wolfe, M., McDonald, N. and Holmes, G. (2020). Transportation Barriers to Health Care in the United States: Findings from the National Health Interview Survey, 1997–2017. *American Journal of Public Health*, 110(6), pp.815–822. [online] Available at: https://ajph.aphapublications.org/doi/abs/10.2105/AJPH.2020.305579?journalCode=ajphdoi:https://doi.org/10.2105/ajph.2020.305579

Urban Institute (2020). *Access to Opportunity through Equitable Transportation | Urban Institute*. [online] www.urban.org. Available at: https://www.urban.org/research/publication/access-opportunity-through-equitable-transportation

Evans, F. (2023). How Interstate Highways Gutted Communities—and Reinforced Segregation. [online] HISTORY. Available at: https://www.history.com/news/interstate-highway-system-infrastructure-construction-segregation.

The White House (2021). *Fact Sheet: The Bipartisan Infrastructure Deal*. [online] The White House. Available at: https://www.whitehouse.gov/briefing-room/statements-releases/2021/11/06/fact-sheet-the-bipartisan-infrastructure-deal/

References

AASHTO (2017). *Understanding Transportation Resilience: A 2016 - 2018 Roadmap*. [online] Available at: https://transportation.org/ctssr/wp-content/uploads/sites/37/2023/01/UTR-1-book-vers-5.pdf [Accessed 7 Nov. 2023].

Archer, D. (2020). *'White Men's Roads Through Black Men's Homes': Advancing Racial Equity Through Highway Reconstruction*. [online] Vanderbilt Law Review. Available at: https://wp0.vanderbilt.edu/lawreview/2020/10/white-mens-roads-through-black-mens-homes-advancing-racial-equity-through-highway-reconstruction/ [Accessed 6 November 2023].

Best (2018). *United States Highways Map | Usa Map 2018*. [online] United States Highways Map | Usa Map 2018. Available at: https://usamapnew.blogspot.com/2018/02/united-states-highways-map.html [Accessed 5 Nov. 2023].

Blakemore, E. (2021). Interstate highways were touted as modern marvels. Racial injustice was part of the plan. *Washington Post*. [online] 17 Aug. Available at: https://www.washingtonpost.com/history/2021/08/16/interstate-highways-were-touted-modern-marvels-racial-injustice-was-part-plan/ [Accessed 27 Sept. 2023].

Blas, E. (2010). The Dwight D. Eisenhower National System of Interstate and Defense Highways: The Road to Success? *The History Teacher*, [online] Available at: https://www.jstor.org/stable/25799401 [Accessed 27 Sept. 2023].

BTS (2017). *National Household Travel Survey Daily Travel Quick Facts | Bureau of Transportation Statistics*. [online] Available at: https://www.bts.gov/statistical-products/surveys/national-household-travel-survey-daily-travel-quick-facts [Accessed 27 Sept. 2023].

Campbell, A. (2016). *The Rise and Fall of Black Wall Street*. [online] The Atlantic. Available at: https://www.theatlantic.com/business/archive/2016/08/the-end-of-black-wall-street/498074/ [Accessed 28 Sept. 2023].

Committee on Transportation Resilience Metrics, Policy Studies, Transportation Research Board and National Academies of Sciences, Engineering, and Medicine (2021). *Investing in Transportation Resilience: A Framework for Informed Choices*. [online] *National Academies Press*. Washington, D.C.: Transportation Research Board. Available at: https://nap.nationalacademies.org/catalog/26292/investing-in-transportation-resilience-a-framework-for-informed-choices [Accessed 7 Nov. 2023].

Davis, B. (2023). *Under the Highway: North Jackson Ward*. [online] ArcGIS StoryMaps. [online] Available at: https://storymaps.arcgis.com/stories/0ca5d5523fa7435199aeaa00a43f14b4 [Accessed 27 Sept. 2023].

Evans, F. (2023). *How Interstate Highways Gutted Communities—and Reinforced Segregation*. [online] HISTORY. Available at: https://www.history.com/news/interstate-highway-system-infrastructure-construction-segregation [Accessed 6 Nov. 2023].

Gandhi, L. (2021). *The Transcontinental Railroad's Dark Costs: Exploited Labor, Stolen Lands*. [online] HISTORY. Available at: https://www.history.com/news/transcontinental-railroad-workers-impact [Accessed 6 Nov. 2023].

Hinton, E. and Artiga, S. (2018). *Beyond Health Care: The Role of Social Determinants in Promoting Health and Health Equity*. [online] KAISER FAMILY FOUNDATION. [online] Available at: https://www.kff.org/racial-equity-and-health-policy/issue-brief/beyond-health-care-the-role-of-social-determinants-in-promoting-health-and-health-equity/ [Accessed 27 Sept. 2023].

History.com Editors (2010). *Manifest Destiny*. [online] HISTORY. [online] Available at: https://www.history.com/topics/19th-century/manifest-destiny [Accessed 6 Nov. 2023].

History.com Editors (2018). *Transcontinental Railroad*. [online] HISTORY. [online] Available at: https://www.history.com/topics/inventions/transcontinental-railroad [Accessed 6 Nov. 2023].

Huxley-Reicher, B. (2022). *Fact file: Americans Drive the Most*. [online] Frontier Group. [online] Available at: https://frontiergroup.org/resources/fact-file-americans-drive-most/ [Accessed 26 Sept. 2023].

Jahan, S., and Mahmud, A. (2023). *What Is Capitalism?* [online] International Monetary Fund. [online] Available at: https://www.imf.org/en/Publications/fandd/issues/Series/Back-to-Basics/Capitalism [Accessed 6 Nov. 2023].

Lacy, L. (2018). *Dwight D. Eisenhower and the birth of the Interstate Highway System.* [online] www.army.mil. Available at: https://www.army.mil/article/198095/dwight_d_eisenhower_and_the_birth_of_the_interstate_highway_system [Accessed 6 Nov. 2023].

LII / Legal Information Institute. (n.d.). *Eminent Domain.* [online] Available at: https://www.law.cornell.edu/wex/eminent_domain#:~:text=Eminent%20domain%20refers%20to%20the [Accessed 6 Nov. 2023].

Longfellow, R. (2022). *Route '66' The Mother Road - Back in Time - General Highway History - Highway History - Federal Highway Administration.* [online] Available at: https://www.fhwa.dot.gov/infrastructure/back0303.cfm [Accessed 6 Nov. 2023].

Meyer, M. and Elrahman, O. (2019). *Transportation and public health : an integrated approach to policy, planning, and implementation.* [online] Available at: https://www.sciencedirect.com/book/9780128167748/transportation-and-public-health [Accessed 27 Sept. 2023].

Munich RE (2023). *Climate change and its consequences | Munich Re.* [online] www.munichre.com. Available at: https://www.munichre.com/en/risks/climate-change.html [Accessed 7 Nov. 2023].

Press, T.A. (2022). Pete Buttigieg launches $1B pilot to build racial equity in America's roads. *NPR.* [online] Available at: https://www.npr.org/2022/06/30/1108852884/pete-buttigieg-launches-1b-pilot-to-build-racial-equity-in-americas-roads [Accessed 6 Nov. 2023].

Ramirez, R. (2023). *Rapid melting in West Antarctica is 'unavoidable,' with potentially disastrous consequences for sea level rise, study finds.* [online] CNN. Available at: https://www.cnn.com/2023/10/23/world/west-antarctic-ice-melt-climate/index.html [Accessed 6 Nov. 2023].

Repp, M. (2012). *RailPictures.net Photo: BN 6303 Burlington Northern Railroad EMD SD40 at Along Puget Sound, Washington by M. S. Repp.* [online] railpictures.net. Available at: https://railpictures.net/viewphoto.php?id=413530 [Accessed 7 Nov. 2023].

Reynault, E. (2013). *How Does Transportation Affect Public Health? | FHWA.* [online] Available at: https://highways.dot.gov/public-roads/mayjune-2013/how-does-transportation-affect-public-health [Accessed 27 Sept.. 2023].

Sagaris, L. and Lanfranco, D. (2019). Beyond 'safe': Chilean 'Kool' routes to school address social determinants of health. *Journal of Transport & Health*, 15, p.100665. [online] https://www.sciencedirect.com/science/article/abs/pii/S2214140519301070 [Accessed 27 Sept. 2023].

Schweninger, E., Edmunds, M. and Atherton, E. (2020). *Transportation A COMMUNITY DRIVER OF HEALTH*. [online] Available at: https://iomc.org/resources/Documents/Transportation_Health_Community_Driver.pdf [Accessed 26 Sept. 2023].

societyhealth.vcu.edu. (2015). *Center on Society and Health*. [online] Available at: https://societyhealth.vcu.edu/work/the-projects/mapsrichmond.html#gsc.tab=0 [Accessed 26 Sept. 2023].

The White House (1955). *To the Congress of the United States*. [online] Available at: https://www.eisenhowerlibrary.gov/sites/default/files/research/online-documents/interstate-highway-system/1955-02-22-message-to-congress.pdf [Accessed 6 Nov. 2023].

The White House (2021). *Fact Sheet: The Bipartisan Infrastructure Deal*. [online] The White House. Available at: https://www.whitehouse.gov/briefing-room/statements-releases/2021/11/06/fact-sheet-the-bipartisan-infrastructure-deal/.[Accessed 6 Nov. 2023].

US EPA (2017). *Basic Information about the Built Environment | US EPA*. [online] US EPA. Available at: https://www.epa.gov/smm/basic-information-about-built-environment [Accessed 27 Sept. 2023].

UShistory.org. (2019). *Binding the Nation by Rail [ushistory.org]*. [online] Available at: https://www.ushistory.org/us/36a.asp {Accessed 5 Nov. 2023].

Weingroff, R. (2017). *General Lucius D. Clay - The President's Man - Interstate System - Highway History - Federal Highway Administration*. [online] www.fhwa.dot.gov. Available at: https://www.fhwa.dot.gov/infrastructure/clay.cfm [Accessed 5 Nov. 2023].

www.fhwa.dot.gov. (2022). *History of the Interstate Highway System - 50th Anniversary - Interstate System - Highway History - Federal Highway Administration*. [online] Available at: https://www.fhwa.dot.gov/interstate/history.cfm#:~:text=The%20Interstate%20System%20has%20been%20called%20the%20Greatest [Accessed 6 Nov. 2023].

www.lyft.com. (2020). *New data shows Lyft is improving access to care for millions of Medicaid recipients*. [online] Available at: https://www.lyft.com/blog/posts/research-improving-access-to-care-medicaid [Accessed 27 Sept. 2023].

Zukowski, D. (2023). *45 projects receive first Reconnecting Communities grants from US DOT.* [online] Smart Cities Dive. [online] Available at: https://www.smartcitiesdive.com/news/first-reconnecting-communities-grants-45-projects-us-dot/643759/ [Accessed 8 Nov. 2023].

Lexicon of Listed Terms and Agencies

- **AASHTO** The American Association of State Highway and Transportation Officials (AASHTO) is a standards setting body which publishes specifications, test protocols, and guidelines that are used in highway design and construction throughout the United States.

- **Dwight D. Eisenhower** was an American military officer and statesman who became the **34th president of the United States** from 1953 to 1961. During World War II, he served as Supreme Commander of the Allied Expeditionary Force in Europe and achieved the five-star rank as General of the Army. The crowning achievement of his presidency was establishment of the Interstate Highway System.

- **Federal-Aid Highway Act of 1956** Popularly known as the National Interstate and Defense Highways Act of 1956, the Federal-Aid Highway Act of 1956 established an interstate highway system in the United States.

- **Kaiser Family Foundation** KFF is the independent source for health policy research, polling, and journalism. Our mission is to serve as a nonpartisan source of information for policymakers, the media, the health policy community, and the public.

- **National Academies** The National Academies of Sciences, Engineering, and Medicine (NASEM), also known as the **National Academies**, is a congressionally chartered organization that serves as the collective scientific national academy of the United States.

- **Roosevelt's New Deal** The New Deal established a broad series of programs, public work projects, financial reforms, and regulations enacted by President Franklin D. Roosevelt in the United States between 1933 and 1938 to address the Great Depression

- **Transportation Research Board** The Transportation Research Board (TRB) is a division of the National Academy of Sciences, Engineering, and Medicine, formerly the National Research Council of the United States, which serves as an independent adviser to the President of the United States, the Congress and federal agencies on scientific and technical questions of national importance. It is jointly administered by the National Academy of Sciences, the National Academy of Engineering, and the National Academy of Medicine.

- **U.S. Department of Transportation** The goal of the U.S. Department of Transportation is to deliver the world's leading transportation system serving the American people and economy through the safe, efficient, sustainable, and equitable movement of people and goods.

- **US EPA** The mission of Environmental Protection Agency (EPA) is to protect human health and the environment. The EPA works to ensure that Americans have clean air, land, and water.

AUTHOR'S BIO SKETCH

James Pecsok, MD
Dr. Pecsok is originally from Virginia Beach, Virginia, and received his undergraduate degree in neuroscience from The College of William and Mary. He completed medical school at Virginia Commonwealth University and residence in Family Medicine at University of Washington affiliated Community Healthcare Family Medicine Residency in Tacoma. He is enthusiastic about working in underserved communities and will remain at Community Health Care as an attending physician. When he is not working you can find Dr. Pecsok rock climbing, mountain biking, kayaking, or playing frisbee with his wife.

Chapter 14

Housing as a Social Determinant of Health

Laura Whitehill MD, MSc. Author
Laila Siddiqui, MD Editor

"Everyone has the right to a standard of living adequate for the health and well-being of himself and of his family, including food, clothing, housing and medical care and necessary social services, and the right to security in the event of unemployment, sickness, disability, widowhood, old age or other lack of livelihood in circumstances beyond his control."

- The Universal Declaration of Human Rights, Article 25 1. The United Nations,1948

Housing as a Social Determinant of Health

The Facts of Homelessness in the U.S.

The U.S. Department of Housing and Urban Development (USHUD) annually commissions a report on homelessness in the U.S. utilizing point in time (PIT) estimates. PIT counts estimate the number of Americans, including Veterans, without safe, stable housing. In 2022, the PIT count revealed the following:

- People experiencing homelessness (PEH), exist on a spectrum from doubling up due to housing cost, sleeping in a car, or sleeping in a shelter or on the street.
- Approximately 500,000 (~0.0014%) people were homeless.
- Sixty percent of these people were in emergency or transition housing while 40% were on the street (~200,000).
- Twelve percent of the U.S. population was Black or African American but made up 37% of the homeless population.
- Eighteen percent of the population was Hispanic or Latinx but made up 24% of those people experiencing homelessness.

- The majority of PEH were males (60%).
- Adults over twenty-five made up 90% of people who were homeless (De Sousa, et al., 2022).

While overall rates of homelessness and families experiencing homelessness in the U.S. have steadily declined since the 2010's, a deeper dive astonishes. Between 2020 and 2022 the number of people experiencing homelessness increased in more states than it decreased. Homelessness increased in twenty-seven states and decreased in twenty-three states and the District of Columbia (De Sousa, et al., 2022).

To further magnify the challenge of homelessness, the 2022 USHUD PIT survey highlighted the wide variations in distribution of PEH per state and the percentage of those homeless *and* unsheltered (**Figure 1**).

Figure 1.

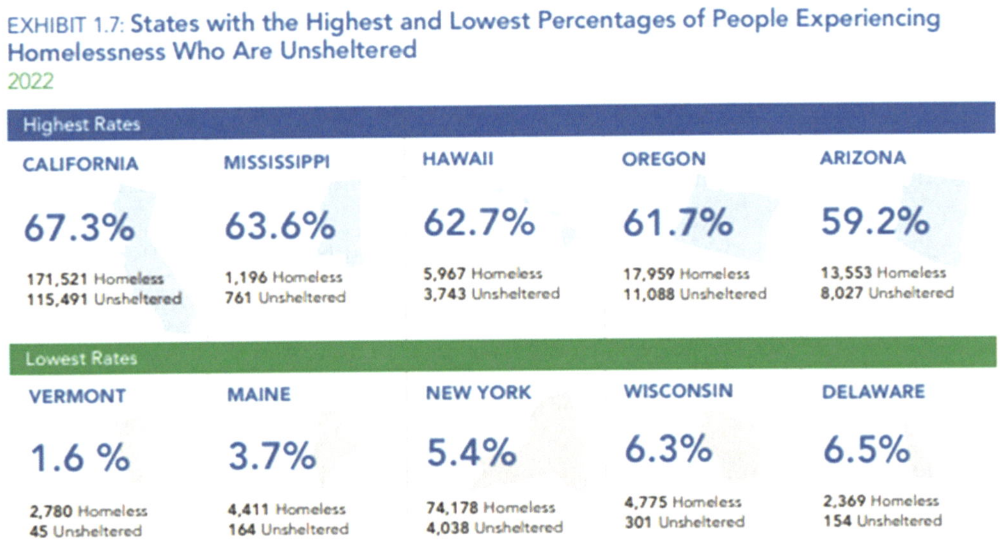

EXHIBIT 1.7: **States with the Highest and Lowest Percentages of People Experiencing Homelessness Who Are Unsheltered**
2022

Highest Rates				
CALIFORNIA	MISSISSIPPI	HAWAII	OREGON	ARIZONA
67.3%	63.6%	62.7%	61.7%	59.2%
171,521 Homeless 115,491 Unsheltered	1,196 Homeless 761 Unsheltered	5,967 Homeless 3,743 Unsheltered	17,959 Homeless 11,088 Unsheltered	13,553 Homeless 8,027 Unsheltered
Lowest Rates				
VERMONT	MAINE	NEW YORK	WISCONSIN	DELAWARE
1.6 %	3.7%	5.4%	6.3%	6.5%
2,780 Homeless 45 Unsheltered	4,411 Homeless 164 Unsheltered	74,178 Homeless 4,038 Unsheltered	4,775 Homeless 301 Unsheltered	2,369 Homeless 154 Unsheltered

The U.S. Department of Housing and Urban Development (2022). *The 2022 Annual Homelessness Assessment Report (AHAR) to Congress*. [online] Available at: https://www.huduser.gov/portal/sites/default/files/pdf/2022-AHAR-Part-1.pdf.

Homelessness permeates populations world-wide. According to Moiz (2022), this multi-dimensional crisis takes roots in poverty, unemployment, skyrocketing property costs, domestic violence, legal problems, alcohol abuse, drug use as well as physical and mental illnesses.

Housing as a Social Determinant of Health

In the context of Quality

Between the dichotomy of housed versus homeless, sit living conditions that may or may not promote physical and emotional well-being. Depending on location, environmental hazards and neighborhood ambience can vary significantly. Low-income neighborhoods situated in areas near industrial zoning, commercial activities, and increased motor vehicle traffic expose residents to noise, ingestible environmental toxins, contaminated water, and respiratory irritants. By comparison, high-income areas have communal spaces, parks, regulated water and sanitation systems and reduced housing density as well as minimal industrial and commercial activity (Shroyer, 2023).

Low-income housing exhibits deteriorating living conditions from age related disrepair, obsolete building codes, and maintenance neglect. Living in a home with inadequate heating and ventilating is linked with high blood pressure and depression (Healthy People 2030, n.d.). Inferior housing quality exposes occupants to the threats of mold, lead, rodents, pests, and asbestos. Molds cause respiratory infections in children and adults (Healthy People 2030, n.d.). According to the CDC, any level of lead in children may adversely impact intelligence, ability to concentrate, and academic potential (CDC, 2022). The Environmental Protection Agency (EPA) strictly regulates asbestos due to its carcinogenic properties, especially lung cancers (US EPA, 2023). Rodents and pests carry infectious disease.

To complicate housing challenges, historical policies and structural racism restrict minority groups access to adequate housing relegating them to low-income housing in neighborhoods with increased adverse environmental exposures, safety, and health outcomes (Healthy People 2030, n.d.).

Housing as a Social Determinant of Health

In the context of Stability

While faced with the challenges of accessing quality housing, people may simultaneously confront the dual threat of housing insecurity (**Figure 2**). Rent burden, or the percentage of income used to meet rent expense, defines housing insecurity. Stated another way, families that make less money per year spend a higher proportion of their income on housing compared with those making over $100,000 per year. The higher the rent burden, the less money available for families to spend on necessities like food, healthcare, transportation, medications, and school supplies. Put this into perspective: "Nowhere in the U.S. can a worker earning the federal or prevailing state minimum wage rent a two-bedroom apartment without having to pay more than 30% of their income. In fact, a minimum wage worker must clock 127 hours per week, more than three full-time jobs, to afford a two-bedroom rental" (Habitat for Humanity, 2023).

Healthy People 2030 advocates the reduction in the proportion of families spending more than 30% of their income on housing. In 2021, 35% of all families were housing cost burdened. When broken down by race, 44% of Latinx families were spending over 30% of their income on housing Healthy People 2030, (2020). In OECD country comparisons, the U.S. ranked second to the UK with over 45% of low-income tenants spending more than 40% of income on rent (OECD, 2021).

High rent burden encourages overcrowding or "doubling up" where multiple families may live in the same property to reduce cost (Healthy People 2030, n.d.). Overcrowding fosters adverse health effects, including communicable disease spread, which the U.S. witnessed during the COVID-19 pandemic. Overcrowding translates into lack of quiet, personal space to receive restful sleep, complete homework, or conduct private conversations impairing the quality of adult relationships and academic performance in children (Healthy People 2030, n.d.).

Figure 2.

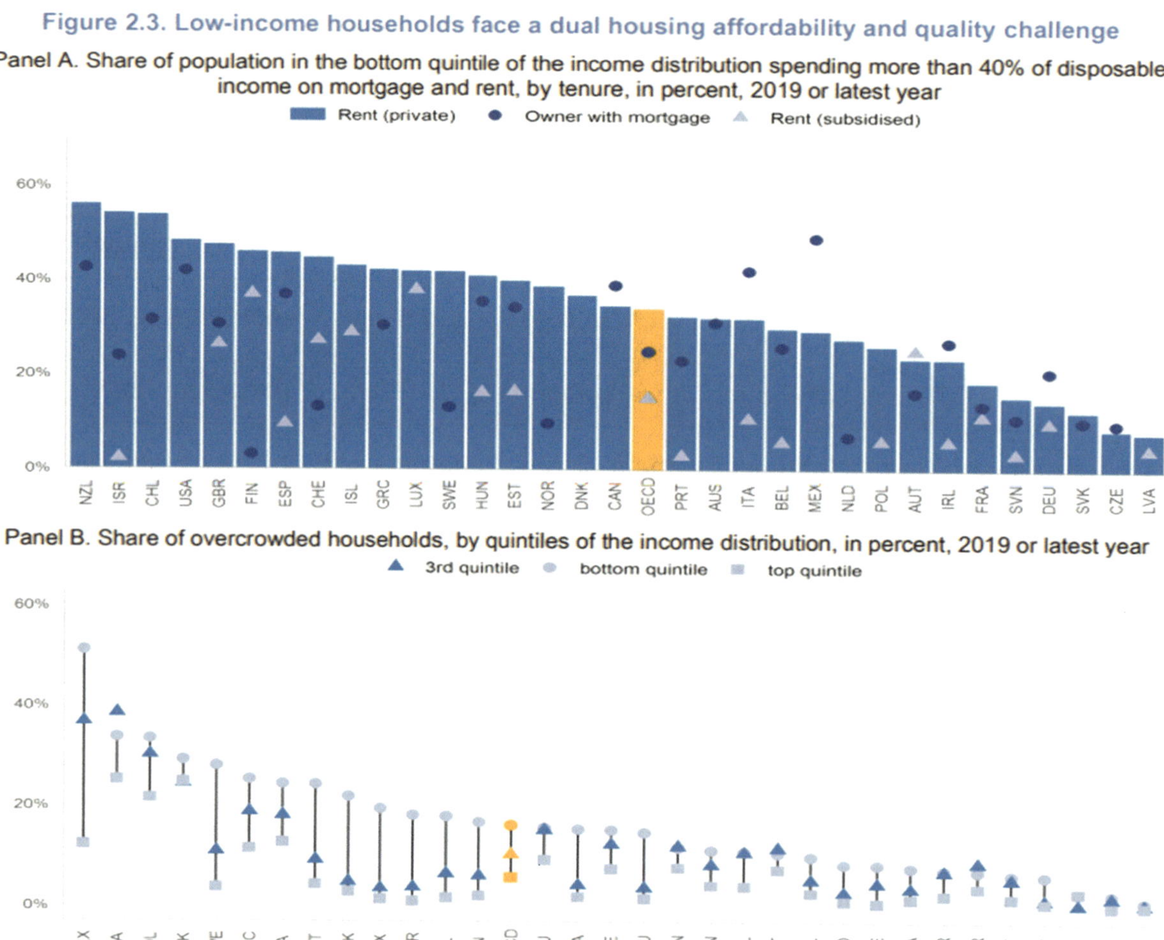

Note: See section "Data and comparability issues" of Indicator HC2.1 on limits to comparability across countries due to the definition of rooms.
Source: OECD Affordable Housing Database (http://www.oecd.org/housing/data/affordable-housing-database/housing-conditions.htm), indicators HC1.2 and HC2.1.

Figure 1. Comparing OECD countries and the percentage of low-income households that are cost burdened and cost burden across countries OECD Housing Policy Toolkit – Synthesis Report.pdf

The burden of housing costs positions people at risk for eviction due to inability to meet rent expense, also known as "forced displacement." Low-income families are at substantial risk for being forcibly displaced. According to Brown, Shinn and Khadduri (2017), this creates a "knock-on" effect as obtaining new housing can be more difficult if one has a history of eviction, which leads to poorer quality housing by default. For children, evictions and displacement impact school performance and development. Children domiciled in emergency housing demonstrate significantly more behavioral problems a year later than those in more stable living conditions.

More recently the intersection of urban "gentrification" complicates low-income access to housing. According to USHUD (2018), gentrification is a form of neighborhood change that occurs when higher-income groups move into low-income areas, potentially altering the cultural and financial landscape of the original neighborhood as well as displacement of long-term low-income residents, long-run resegregation of neighborhoods, and heightened barriers to entry for new low-income residents looking for places to move (USHUD, 2018).

Housing as a Social Determinant of Health

In the context of Physical and Emotional Health

People experiencing homelessness have higher rates of chronic disease, communicable disease, trauma, and victimization. Inferior quality housing promotes exposure to environmental toxins, lead, rodents, pests, and mold. Homeless people often do not have safe storage for medications, which worsens chronic conditions like diabetes and hypertension (National Health Care for Homeless Council, 2019). Unstable housing and high-cost burden leads to increased stress and anxiety for families (HUD USER, n.d.).

PEH exhibit increased rates of substance use disorder and mental health diagnoses. One study found that among people with opioid use disorder, those experiencing homelessness had almost double (48% compared to 26%) rates of bipolar disorder. The same study found that those experiencing homelessness were less likely to utilize psychotherapy as treatment for mental health conditions and naloxone to mitigate the consequences of opioid overdose (Ali, Sutherland and Rosenoff, 2021). According to Sutherland, PEH are more likely to seek treatment in emergency department settings rather than primary care facilities, increasing cost of care and disrupting the healthcare advantages of continuity care.

The increased rates of alcohol and opioid use, higher rates of traumatic injuries and amplified rates of viral hepatitis in those with a history for homelessness underscore the lasting consequences of housing instability (Sutherland, Ali and Rosenoff, 2021). Thus, taken in context, it comes as no surprise, people experiencing homelessness endure mortality rates significantly higher than the general population (Healthy People 2030, n.d.).

Finally, violence often rules the day in homeless camps. Frequent gun violence, stabbings and beatings result in high rates of homicide. To further complicate the crisis, "the misperception that people without homes are perpetrators, rather than victims, of violence contributes to both criminalizing homelessness and dehumanizing people without housing" (Kushel, 2022).

Housing as a Social Determinant of Health

In the context of Poverty & Standard of Living

Having sufficient financial resources to access housing, food, transportation, clothing, and healthcare – the overall ability to make ends meet – measures standard of living. The gross domestic product (GDP) per capita provides a dollar-for-dollar assessment in the U.S. and it naturally follows those areas with higher GDP, support higher wages and higher standards of living. According to USA Facts (2022), the GDP per capita in the U.S. stood at $78,347. States like New York, Massachusetts, Washington, and California boasted GDPs of more than $95,000 per capita, while South Carolina, Alabama, Arkansas, West Virginia, and Mississippi reported levels below $55,000.

Consider the gap – the cost of goods and services does not vary up and down with regional U.S. GDP differences. International, national, and regional manufacturing, raw materials expense, agricultural production, cost of transportation and global supply chain factors establish the price of goods like toothpaste, light bulbs, Toyotas, lettuce, shoes, water heaters, construction materials, and smart phones.

Affordability of suitable housing – construction, repair, and maintenance – is no less tied to market dynamics. It simply takes a greater percentage of income to access the goods and services necessary to provide safe, secure, healthy housing where local GDP falls far short of national GDP per capita. Compounding matters, regional GDP plays directly into the tax base that funds infrastructure for schools, roads, sanitation, water, and utilities which promote local livability including access to housing and other necessary goods and services that define standard of living.

Poverty aligns across minority groups. In the U.S., the 2020 Census Bureau pegged the poverty rate across the U.S. at ~12%, however, American Indians & Alaskan Natives (24%), Black people (20%), and Hispanics (17%) shouldered a disproportionate share of the poverty burden. By comparison, White, not Hispanic stood at just 8% (Bureau, U.C., 2021).

This data partially explains the phenomenon that people living in poverty, cluster with coincident minority groups. Poor neighborhoods have less safe outdoor space such as parks and sidewalks and worse public transportation (Healthy People 2030, n.d.). People living in rampant poverty have worse housing, worse crime rates, more adverse health conditions and less access to healthy foods and education for their children (USDA, 2022). According to HUD, low-income neighborhoods are more likely to be food deserts, meaning increased fast food consumption and fewer supermarkets to provide healthy food options (HUD USER, n.d.).

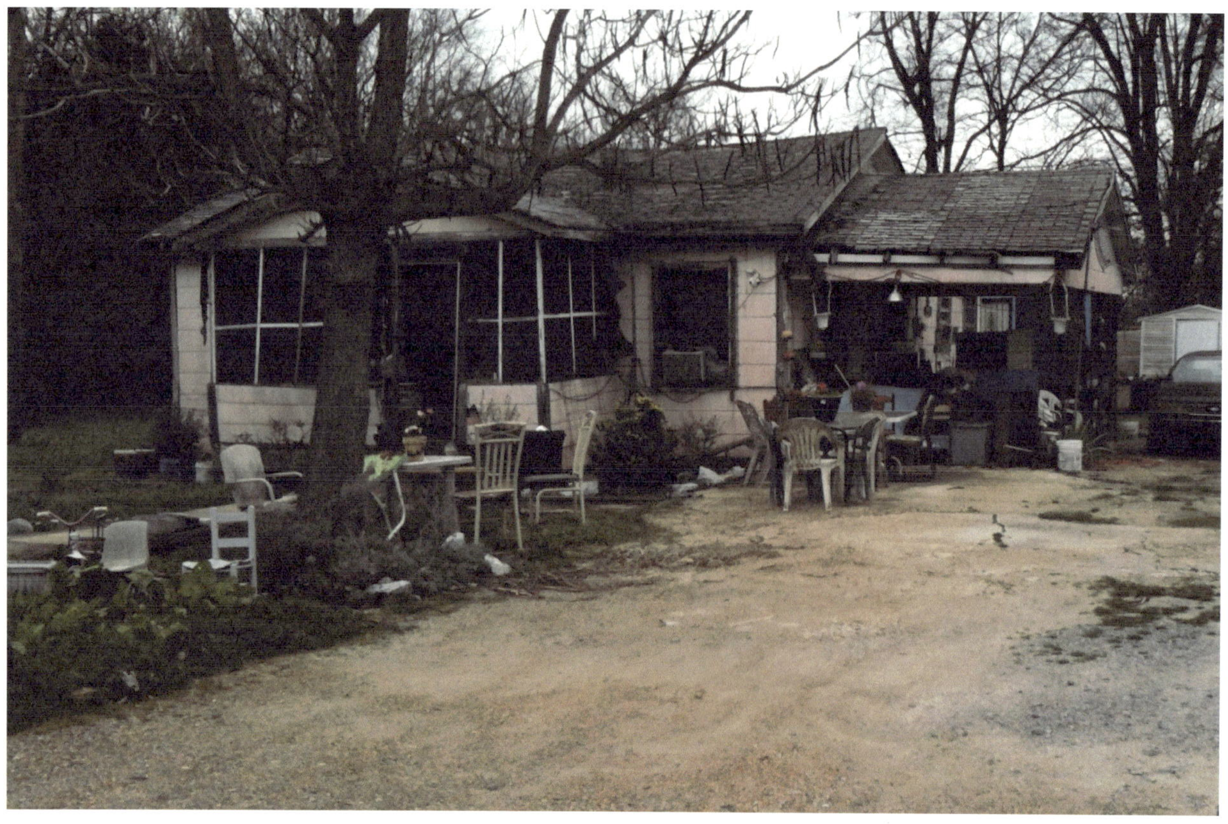

A typical home situated in the heart of the Mississippi Delta; an area of the United States stretched by poverty to the bones.

Housing as a Social Determinant of health

In the context of International Strategies and Outcomes

The Office of Economic Co-operation and Development (OCED, 2021), espouses the triple pronged dimensions of inclusiveness, efficiency, and sustainability to define the linkages between polices and outcomes (**Figure 3**). Inclusiveness relates to the possibility for low-income households and other vulnerable groups to live in decent quality dwellings that serve their needs. Efficiency describes the capacity of the sector to supply housing that matches demand. Sustainability refers to the compatibility of residential construction with high local eenvironmental quality and climate objectives (OECD, 2021).

Figure 3.

Box 1.3. Housing reforms pursue multiple objectives: Inclusiveness, efficiency and sustainability

Three key dimensions underpin the OECD Horizontal Project on Housing: inclusiveness, efficiency and sustainability (Figure 1.17). Inclusiveness relates to the possibility for low-income households and other vulnerable groups, such as people with unstable jobs, to live in good-quality dwellings that serve their needs, including access to labour markets, schools and amenities. Efficiency describes the capacity of the sector to supply housing that matches demand both quantitatively and qualitatively without unnecessary costs. Sustainability refers to the compatibility of residential construction and housing use with high local environmental quality and climate objectives.

Figure 1.17. Housing affects inclusiveness, efficiency and sustainability

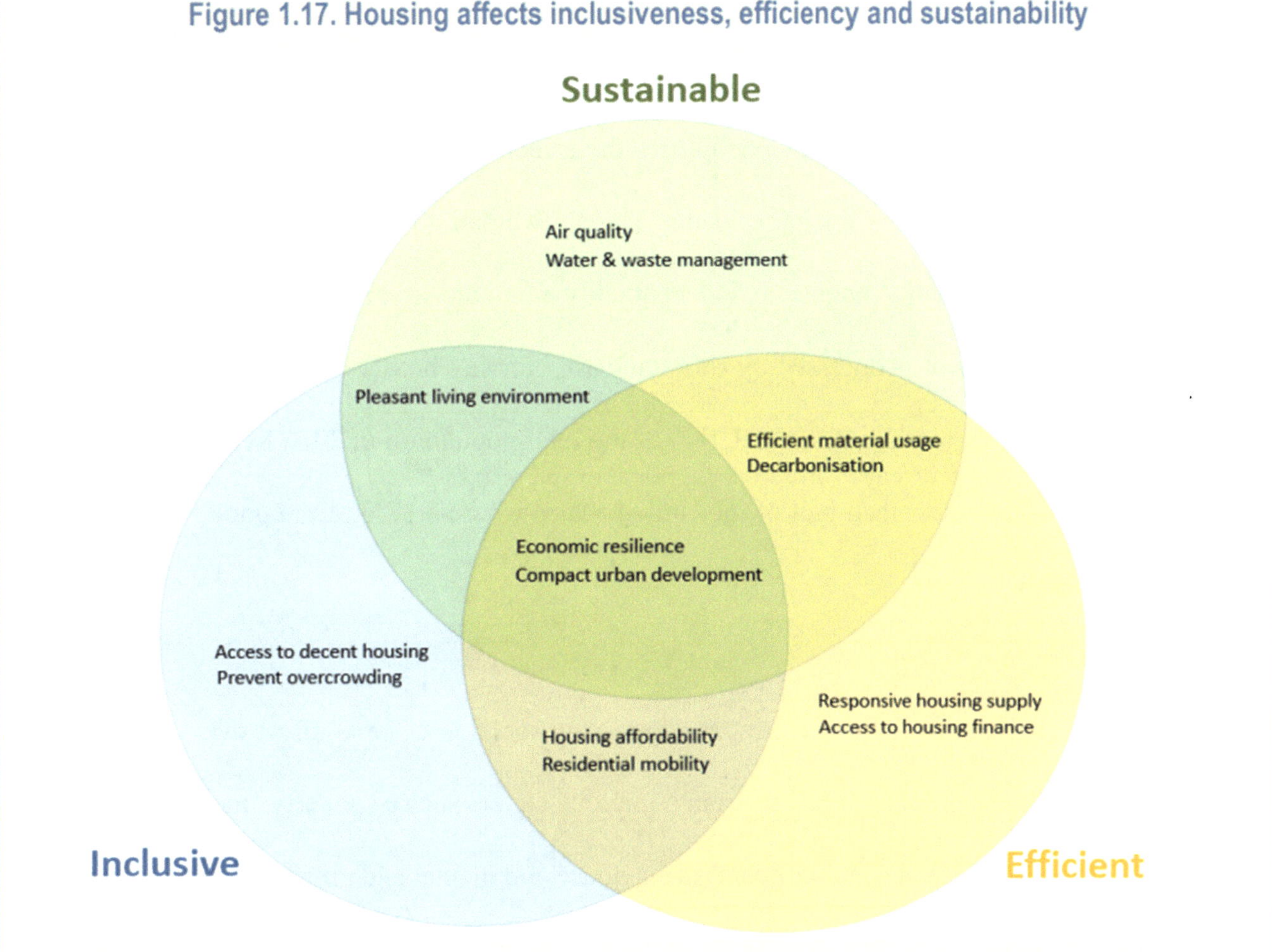

OECD Housing Policy Toolkit- Synthesis Report. (2021). [online] Meeting of the Council at Ministerial Level, 31 May-1 June 2021: Organisation for Economic Co-operation and Development. Available at: https://www.oecd.org/mcm/OECD%20Housing%20Policy%20Toolkit%20%E2%80%93%20Synthesis%20Report.pdf

Internationally reflected, Canada, Norway, and France wrestle with the challenges of homelessness uutilizing unique, albeit differing strategies.

Canada

Accurate data on PEH, high-cost burden and housing insecurity assists policy makers to analyze and understand ways these factors intertwine with social and healthcare systems. Canada has developed a *Homeless Individuals and Families Information System* which allows real time data collection. Utilization of the data helps service providers facilitate assistance for PEH (OECD, 2020). The U.S. lacks a comparable data collection system to address homelessness.

Norway

Nordic countries historically embrace social security to promote high living standards. The rate of homelessness in Norway exemplifies the effectiveness of the Norwegian welfare state in providing livable housing for its residents. The Norwegian government defines homelessness as an individual or family unable to independently maintain a safe, consistent, and appropriate housing arrangement. Addressed by this standard, Norway boasts one of the smallest homeless populations in the world with only 0.07% of the total population in 2016 living in homelessness. This proportion is less than half of the United States where 0.17% of the population is homeless (Jones, 2020).

France

Homelessness in France presents significant social issues that affect over 200,000 people, including 30,000 children. It results from numerous factors such as poverty, unemployment, rising rent, domestic violence, legal problems, drug abuse and mental and physical illness (Moiz, 2022). Homeless people in France face harsh living conditions, such as shantytowns, lack of running water, and high mortality rates.

French law embraces an enforceable right to housing for residents who cannot find decent accommodations and meet the financial conditions required to access social housing (San Martin,

2022) that aligns with the United Nations Universal Declaration of Human Rights. The French are most likely to view homelessness as the result of financial crisis, unemployment, and housing crises and the least likely to blame the individual for personal reasons such as drugs or alcohol (Filter, 2018).

"Rough sleepers" in Paris.

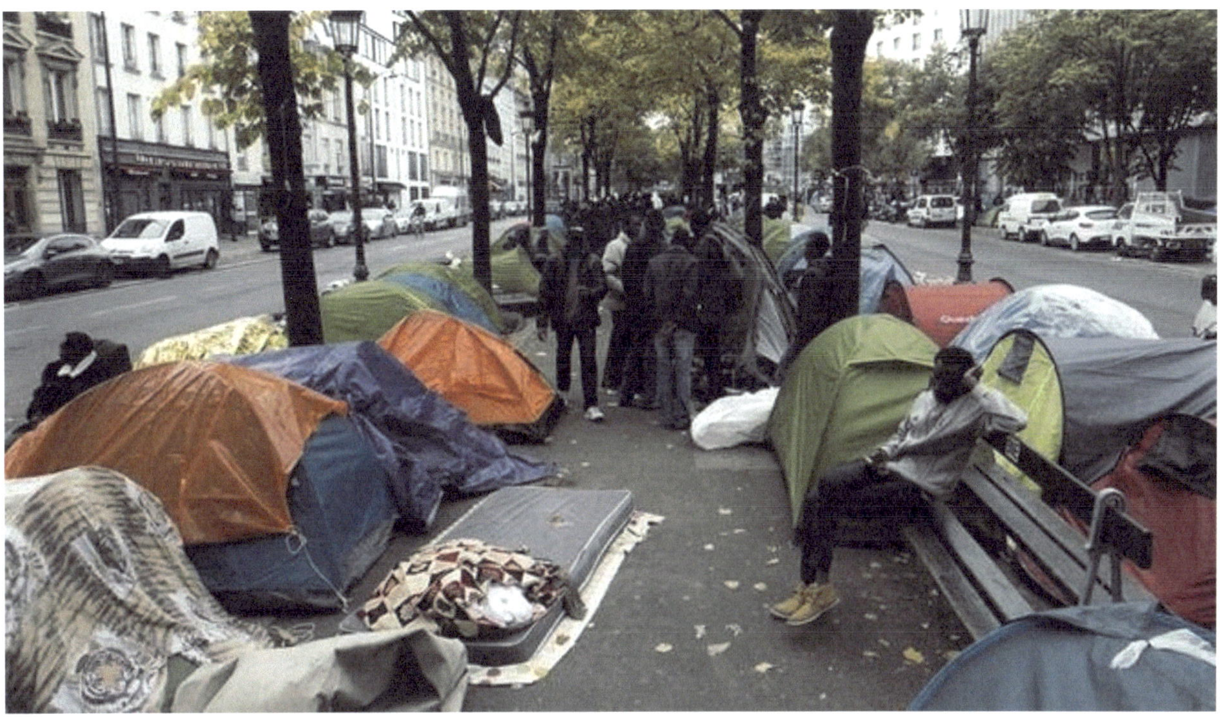

Filter, G. (2018). Rough Sleepers: Homelessness in France. Mercy Pedalers [online] Available at: https://mercypedalers.com/rough-sleepers-homelessness-france/.

Housing as a Social Determinant of Health

Politics, policies, and governance

Throughout the last century in the United States, legislative acts aimed to solve the challenges of homeownership, housing segregation, and environmentally healthy neighborhoods have been passed by Congress. The National Housing Act of 1934 and the Fair Housing Act of 1968 and its Amendments in 1974 and 1988 serve as important examples.

The National Housing Act of 1934

The National Housing Act of 1934 intended to strengthen the residential real estate market and promote homeownership. A cornerstone of FDR's New Deal, the act established the Federal Housing Administration (FHA) which, by creating a federally guaranteed mortgage insurance program, allowed banks to issue lower-cost loans and make them more accessible to more people (Hayes and Brock, 2022).

The FHA was tasked with insuring "economically sound" loans, as part of an overhaul of the system of residential mortgage finance that had been decimated by the Depression. The FHA began redlining (refusing to finance individuals living in an area deemed to be poor financial risk) at the very beginning of its operations in 1934. For example, FHA staff concluded that no loan could be economically sound if the property were in a neighborhood that was or could become populated by Black people, as property values might decline over the life of the 15 to 20-year loans. Therefore, the FHA's 1938 Underwriting Manual emphasized the negative impact of "infiltration of inharmonious racial groups" on credit risk (Federal Reserve History, 2023). *This bias and its integration into lending policy promoted the blight of neighborhood segregation for over 30 years until the Fair Housing Act was passed in 1968.*

The Fair Housing Act of 1968

The Fair Housing Act of 1968 prevented discrimination based on race, religion, and national origin in the selling and renting of housing. However, the provisions did not apply to individuals selling or renting three or less houses and apartments. In application, the Act prevented discrimination not just in the sale or renting of housing, but also in advertisement, terms, and other discrete ways of discriminating. Congress amended the Fair Housing Act in 1974 to include discrimination based on sex, and again in 1988 to prohibit discrimination based on familial status and disabilities (LII/Legal Information Institute, n.d.)

The Fair Housing Act of 1968

The Fair Housing Act of 1968

On April 11, 1968, President Lyndon Johnson signed the Civil Rights Act of 1968, which was meant as a follow-up to the Civil Rights Act of 1964. The 1968 Act expanded on previous acts and prohibited discrimination concerning the sale, rental, and financing of housing based on race, religion, national origin, sex, (and as amended) handicap and family status. Title VIII of the Act is also known as the Fair Housing Act (of 1968).

The enactment of the federal Fair Housing Act on April 11, 1968 came only after a long and difficult journey. From 1966-1967, Congress regularly considered the fair housing bill, but failed to garner a strong enough majority for its passage. However, when the Rev. Dr. Martin Luther King, Jr. was assassinated on April 4, 1968, President Lyndon Johnson utilized this national tragedy to urge for the bill's speedy Congressional approval. Since the 1966 open housing marches in Chicago, Dr. King's name had been strongly associated with the fair housing legislation. President Johnson viewed the Act as a fitting memorial to the man's life work and wished to have the Act passed prior to Dr. King's funeral in Atlanta (USHUD, n.d.)

USHUD (n.d.) History of Fair Housing [online] Available at: https://www.hud.gov/program_offices/fair_housing_equal_opp/aboutfheo/history [Accessed 17 September 2023].

The Civil Rights Division of the U.S. Department of Justice (DOJ) overseas and enforces violations of the Federal Housing Act. Despite the well-known regulations pertaining to discrimination based on race, religion, national origin, sex, familial status, and disabilities, *redlining* continues to this day. Here are three recent examples:

United States v. Evolve Bank and Trust

On October 17, 2022, the court entered a consent order* in United States v. Evolve Bank and Trust (W.D. Tenn.). The complaint, which was filed on September 29, 2022, alleges that from at least 2014 through 2019, the bank engaged in lending discrimination based on race, sex, and national origin in the pricing of its residential mortgage loans. The consent order requires the bank to amend its pricing policies, employ a fair lending officer who will work closely with the bank's leadership, and have employees undergo fair lending training. The consent order also includes a $1.3 million settlement fund to remediate borrowers harmed by this pricing discrimination and a $50,000 civil penalty.

United States v. Park National Bank

On March 2, 2023, the court entered a consent order* United States v. Park National Bank (S.D. Ohio). The complaint, which was filed on February 28, 2023, alleges that, from at least 2015 to 2021, Park National Bank (Park National) violated the Fair Housing Act and the Equal Credit Opportunity Act on the basis of race, color, and national origin by engaging in unlawful redlining of Black and Hispanic neighborhoods within the Columbus, Ohio metropolitan area. The consent order requires Park National to invest at least $7.75 million in a loan subsidy fund to increase access to credit in majority-Black and Hispanic neighborhoods in the Columbus area; $750,000 in outreach, advertising, consumer financial education, and credit counseling initiatives; and $500,000 in developing community partnerships to provide services that expand access to residential mortgage credit.

United States v. ESSA Bank & Trust

On June 9, 2023, the court entered a consent order* United States v. ESSA Bank & Trust (E.D. Pa.). The complaint, which was filed on May 31, 2023, alleges that ESSA violated the Equal Credit Opportunity Act (ECOA) and the Fair Housing Act (FHA) by engaging in unlawful redlining in the Philadelphia Metropolitan Statistical Area by avoiding providing mortgage services to majority-Black and Hispanic neighborhoods and discouraging prospective applicants from those neighborhoods from applying for credit. The consent order requires ESSA to: (1) invest at least $2.92 million in a loan subsidy fund to increase access to credit in majority-Black and Hispanic neighborhoods; (2) spend an additional $125,000 on community partnerships and $250,000 on advertising, outreach, consumer financial education, and credit counseling in majority-Black and Hispanic communities; (3) hire two new mortgage loan officers to serve its existing branches in West Philadelphia; and (4) conduct a research-based market study to help identify the needs for financial services in communities of color.

Department of Justice (2023). Recent Accomplishments of The Housing And Civil Enforcement Section. [online] Available at: https://www.justice.gov/crt/recent-accomplishments-housing-and-civil-enforcement-section

* A consent order is a decree made by a judge with the consent of all parties. It is not strictly a judgement, but rather a settlement agreement approved by the court. The agreement is submitted to the court in writing after the parties have reached a settlement, and once approved by the judge, the agreement is binding and enforceable on both parties.

LII/Legal Information Institute (n.d.) Consent Order. [online] Available at: https://www.law.cornell.edu/wex/consent_order

HOPE VI

HOPE VI: a Severely Distressed Public Housing solution with demonstrated success but many detractors.

According to the (USHUD About HOPE, n.d.), the HOPE VI Program, originally known as the Urban Revitalization Demonstration (URD), grew out of recommendations by the National

Commission on Severely Distressed Public Housing, which was charged with proposing a National Action Plan to eradicate distressed public housing.

The HOPE VI program served a vital role for over a decade in the Department of Housing and Urban Development's efforts to transform Public Housing (USHUD About HOPE, n.d.).

HOPE VI

The specific elements of public housing transformation that proved key to HOPE VI included:

- Changing the physical shape of public housing.
- Establishing positive incentives for resident self-sufficiency and comprehensive services that empower residents.
- Lessening concentrations of poverty by placing public housing in nonpoverty neighborhoods and promoting mixed-income communities.
- Forging partnerships with other agencies, local governments, nonprofit organizations, and private businesses to leverage support and resources.

In October of 2000, HOPE VI was honored with national recognition as a recipient of an Innovations in American Government Award. HOPE VI was among ten winners chosen by the Innovations in American Government Program, one of the nation's most prestigious public service awards programs. HOPE VI was recognized for its Mixed-Finance Public Housing program, "an innovative approach that is transforming some of the nation's most severely distressed public housing from sources of urban blight to engines of neighborhood renewal" (USHUD About HOPE VI, n.d.).

Over time, HOPE VI grantees used inadequate planning methodologies and mismanaged funds thus, combined with delays in grant awards and completion of projects, President George W. Bush proposed eliminating the Program in 2004. Eventually, Congress defunded it at lower levels effectively ending the promise of HOPE VI (A DECADE of HOPE VI, 2004).

Nobody to Care

People experiencing homelessness often endure longer hospital stays due to discharge planning complicated by unsafe or unsuitable housing – simply put, discharging back to the streets or shelters constitutes a recipe for re-admission, medical complications layered over existing conditions, and even death. Creative non-profits and some hospitals have developed low cost, short-term facilities for patients to complete recovery and reduce the risk for re-admission (McCarthy, 2021). In California, this model assists transition to stable housing by providing wrap-around services like care navigators and social workers that traditional post-acute care might not offer (McCarthy, 2021).

Gentrification Tacoma, Washington

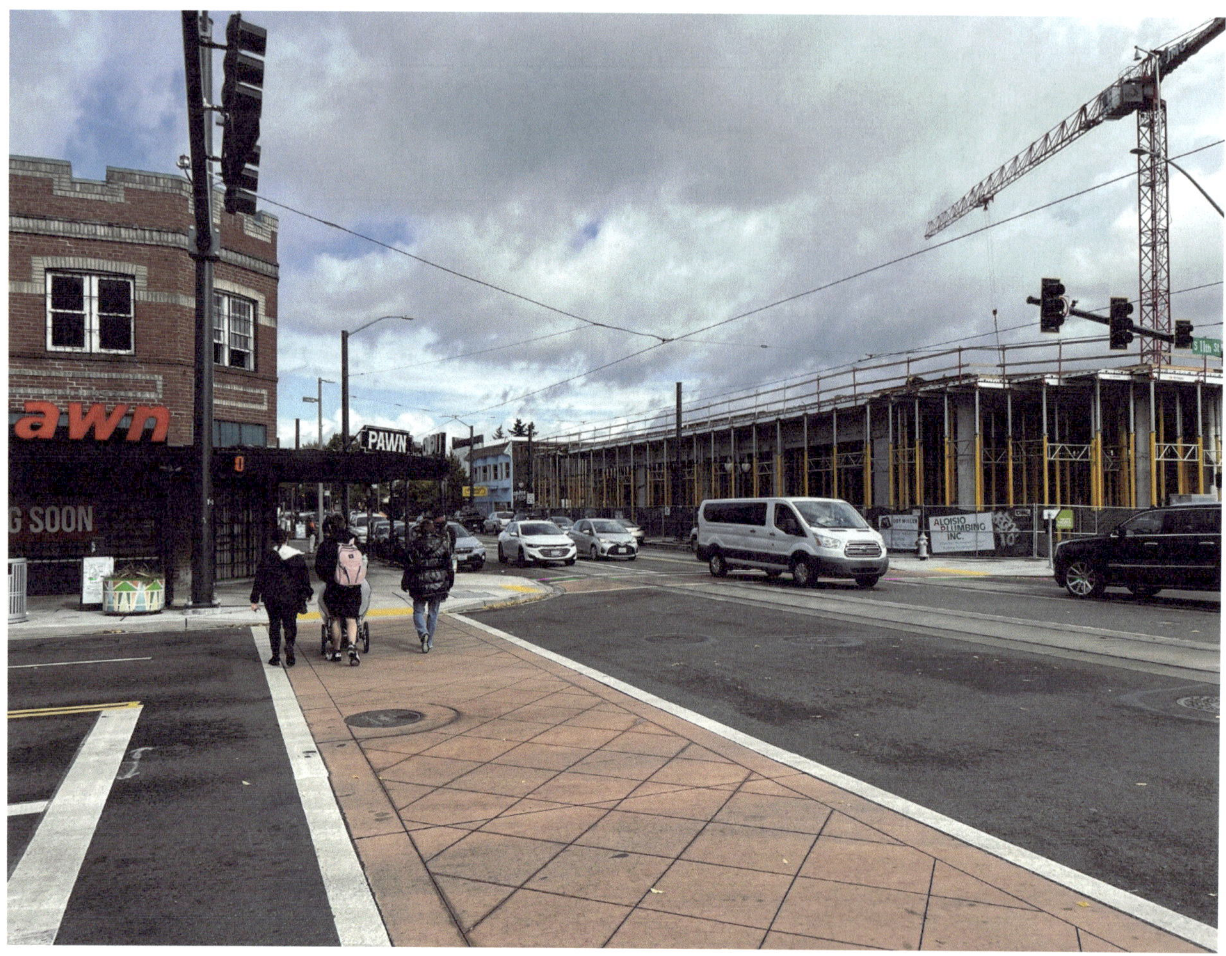

Like many U.S. cities, Tacoma, Washington gentrification replaces aged commercial and residential structures in prime real estate sectors with modern high-rise condominiums that displace former residents into homelessness unable to the afford sky high rents.

Housing as a Social Determinant of Health

Summary

Homelessness exists throughout the world. The many facets leading to inadequate housing and homelessness – unemployment and underemployment, poverty, domestic violence, housing costs, drug use, alcoholism, mental and physical illness defy one size fits all solutions to this crisis. The downward spiral that marks homelessness places the victims of this epidemic in a cyclical, if not perpetual swirl of exposure to infectious diseases, trauma, malnutrition, limited access to healthcare, disrupted family relationships, increasing drug and alcohol use and deteriorating health due to its many manifestations. The result is significantly decreased healthy life expectancy and life expectancy. Simply put housing is a social determinant of health.

Questions for Further Consideration

1. Name two specific policies that have immediate impact on housing quality and who should enforce them?
2. How does stable housing impact employment opportunities and economic mobility for low-income families?
3. How can healthcare providers be most helpful in combating the detrimental effects of homelessness?
4. Describe the dynamic between housing as a social determinant of health and the COVID-19 pandemic.

Sentinel Readings for a Deeper Dive

Organization for Economic Co-operation and Development: OCED Housing Policy Toolkit (2021). [online] Available at: OECD Housing Policy Toolkit – Synthesis Report.pdf

Habitat for Humanity (2023). 7 things you should know about poverty and housing. *Habitat for Humanity* [online] Available at: https://www.habitat.org/stories/7-things-you-should-know-about-poverty-and-housing

Displacement of Lower-Income Families in Urban Areas Report, 2018. [online] Available at: Displacement of Lower-Income Families in Urban Areas Report (huduser.gov)

Jones, L. (2020). *Everything you need to know about Homelessness in Norway.* The Borgen Project [online] Available at: https://borgenproject.org/homelessness-in-norway/#How%20Norway%20Defines%20%E2%80%9CHomelessness%E2%80%9D

Policy Brief on Affordable Housing: Better data and policies to fight homelessness in the OECD [online] Available at:
homelessness-policy-brief-2020.pdf (oecd.org)

References

A DECADE OF HOPE VI: Research Findings and Policy Challenges. (2004). [online] Available at: https://www.urban.org/sites/default/files/publication/43756/411002_HOPEVI.pdf. [Accessed 17 September 2023]

Ali, M., Sutherland, H. and Rosenoff, E. (2021). Comorbid Health Conditions and Treatment Utilization among Individuals with Opioid Use Disorder Experiencing Homelessness. *Substance Use & Misuse*, [online] Available at: https://doi.org/10.1080/10826084.2021.1884723 [Accessed May-June 2023].

Brown, S., Shinn, M. and Khadduri, J. (2017). *Well-Being of Young Children after Experiencing Homelessness*. [online] Available at https://aspe.hhs.gov/sites/default/files/migrated_legacy_files//173366/homefambrief.pdf [Accessed May-June 2023].

Bureau, U.C. (2021). *Income and Poverty in the United States: 2020.* [online] Census.gov. Available at: https://www.census.gov/library/publications/2021/demo/p60-273.html#:~:text=The%20official%20poverty%20rate%20in%202020%20was%2011.4 [Accessed May-June 2023].

CDC (2022) *Childhood Lead Poisoning Prevention.* [online] Available at: https://www.cdc.gov/nceh/lead/default.htm [Accessed May-June 2023].

Department of Justice (2023). Recent Accomplishments of The Housing And Civil Enforcement Section. [online] Available at: https://www.justice.gov/crt/recent-accomplishments-housing-and-civil-enforcement-section [Accessed 17 September 2023].

De Sousa, T., Andrichik, A., Cuellar, M., Marson, J., Prestera, E., and Rush, K. (2022). *The 2022 Annual Homelessness Assessment Report (AHAR) to Congress DECEMBER 2022.* [online] Available at: https://www.huduser.gov/portal/sites/default/files/pdf/2022-AHAR-Part-1.pdf [Accessed May-June 2023].

Federal Reserve History (2023). *Redlining | Federal Reserve History*. [online] www.federalreservehistory.org Available at: https://www.federalreservehistory.org/essays/redlining. [Accessed 26 august 2023].

Filter, G. (2018). *Rough Sleepers: Homelessness in France.* Mercy Pedalers [online] Available at: https://mercypedalers.com/rough-sleepers-homelessness-france/ [Accessed May-June 2023].

Goplerud, D. and Pollack, C. (2021). *Prevalence and Impact of Evictions | HUD USER*. [online] Available at: https://www.huduser.gov/portal/periodicals/em/Summer21/highlight2.html [Accessed May-June 2023].

Habitat for Humanity (2023). 7 things you should know about poverty and housing. *Habitat for Humanity* [online] Available at: https://www.habitat.org/stories/7-things-you-should-know-about-poverty-and-housing [Accessed May-June 2023].

Hayes, A. and Brock, T. (2022). National Housing Act; Overview, Impact, Criticisms, *Investopedia* [online] Available at: https://www.investopedia.com/terms/n/national-housing-act.asp [Accessed 26 August 2023].

Healthy People 2030 (2020). *Poverty - Healthy People 2030 | health.gov*. [online] Healthy People 2030. Available at: https://health.gov/healthypeople/priority-areas/social-determinants-health/literature-summaries/poverty [Accessed May-June 2023].

Healthy People 2030 (n.d.). *Housing Instability - Healthy People 2030 | health.gov*. [online] Available at: https://health.gov/healthypeople/priority-areas/social-determinants-health/literature-summaries/housing-instability [Accessed May-June 2023].

Healthy People 2030 (n.d.). *Quality of Housing - Healthy People 2030 | health.gov*. [online] Available at: https://health.gov/healthypeople/priority-areas/social-determinants-health/literature-summaries/quality-housing [Accessed May-June 2023].

Healthy People 2030 (n.d.). *Reduce the proportion of people living in poverty — SDOH-01 - Healthy People 2030 | health.gov*. [online] Available at: https://health.gov/healthypeople/objectives-and-data/browse-objectives/economic-stability/reduce-proportion-people-living-poverty-sdoh-01 [Accessed May-June 2023].

HUD USER (n.d.). *Housing and Neighborhood Contexts Affect Children's Outcomes | HUD USER*. [online] Available at: https://www.huduser.gov/portal/pdredge/pdr_edge_featd_article_111714.html [Accessed 30 May 2023].

Jones, L. (2020). *Everything you need to know about Homelessness in Norway.* The Borgen Project [online] Available at: https://borgenproject.org/homelessness-in-norway/#How%20Norway%20Defines%20%E2%80%9CHomelessness%E2%80%9D [Accessed May-June 2023].

Kushel, M. (2022). *Violence Against People Who Are Homeless: The Hidden Epidemic*. [online] Benioff Homelessness and Housing Initiative. Available at: https://homelessness.ucsf.edu/blog/violence-against-people-homeless-hidden-epidemic [Accessed May-June 2023].

LII/Legal Information Institute (n.d.) Fair Housing Act & Fair Housing Amendments Act. [online] Available at: https://www.law.cornell.edu/wex/fair_housing_act_fair_housing_amendments_act [Accessed 17 September 2023].

LII/Legal Information Institute (n.d.) Consent Order. [online] Available at: https://www.law.cornell.edu/wex/consent_order [Accessed 23 September 2023].

McCarthy, D. and Waugh, L. (2021). *How a Medical Respite Care Program Offers a Pathway to Health and Housing for People Experiencing Homelessness*. [online] www.commonwealthfund.org. Available at: https://www.commonwealthfund.org/publications/case-study/2021/aug/how-medical-respite-care-program-offers-pathway-health-housing [Accessed May-June 2023].

Moiz, M. (2022). *Homelessness in France.* CAUF Society. [online] Available at; Homelessness in France - 7 great questions answered by experts (caufsociety.com) [Accessed May-June 2023].

National Health Care for the Homeless Council (2019). *Homelessness & Health: What's the Connection?* National Health Care for the Homeless Council. [online] Available at: https://nhchc.org/wp-content/uploads/2019/08/homelessness-and-health.pdf [Accessed May-June 2023].

OECD (2020). Better data and policies to fight homelessness in the OECD Policy Brief on Affordable Housing. [online] Available at: https://www.oecd.org/housing/data/affordable-housing-database/homelessness-policy-brief-2020.pdf [Accessed May-June 2023].

OECD (2021). Housing Policy Toolkit- Synthesis Report. Meeting of the Council at Ministerial Level, 31 *Organisation for Economic Co-operation and Development*. [online]: Available at: https://www.oecd.org/mcm/OECD%20Housing%20Policy%20Toolkit%20%E2%80%93%20Synthesis%20Report.pdf [Accessed May-June 2023].

San Martin, I. (2022) *Homelessness in France* Fundación Fernando Pombo A Pro Bono Project. [online] Available at: https://www.probono4homelessnesscovid19.org/france [Accessed May-June 2023].

Shroyer, A. (2023). *POLICY & PRACTICE | Pro-Housing Land Use and Zoning Reforms.* [online] Available at: https://www.huduser.gov/portal/sites/default/files/pdf/policy-and-practice-publication-2023-april.pdf [Accessed 30 May 2023].

Sutherland, H., Ali, M. and Rosenoff, E. (2021). *Disability and Aging Policy, Health Conditions Among Individuals With A History of Homelessness*. ASPE Research Brief, HHS Office of the Assistant Secretary for Planning and Evaluation of Office of Behavioral Health. [online] Available at:
https://aspe.hhs.gov/sites/default/files/migrated_legacy_files//199441/HomelessHistRB.pdf [Accessed May-June 2023].

The U.S. Department of Housing and Urban Development (2022). *The 2022 Annual Homelessness Assessment Report (AHAR) to Congress*. [online] Available at: https://www.huduser.gov/portal/sites/default/files/pdf/2022-AHAR-Part-1.pdf [Accessed May-June 2023].

USA Facts (2022). *What is the current state of the US standard of living?* USA Facts [online] Available at:
https://usafacts.org/topics/standard-of-living/ [Accessed May-June 2023].

US EPA (2023). *Asbestos.* [online] Available at: https://www.epa.gov/asbestos/asbestos-laws-and-regulations [Accessed May-June 2023].

USDA (2022). *USDA ERS - Rural Poverty & Well-Being.* [online] Available at: https://www.ers.usda.gov/topics/rural-economy-population/rural-poverty-well-being/#geography [Accessed May-June 2023].

USHUD (2018). Displacement of Lower-Income Families in Urban Areas Report [online] Available at: https://www.huduser.gov/portal/sites/default/files/pdf/DisplacementReport.pdf [Accessed May-June 2023].

USHUD (n.d.) History of Fair Housing [online] Available at: https://www.hud.gov/program_offices/fair_housing_equal_opp/aboutfheo/history [Accessed 17 September 2023].

USHUD (n.d.). About HOPE VI - Public and Indian Housing - HUD | HUD.gov / U.S. Department of Housing and Urban Development (HUD). [online] Available at: https://www.hud.gov/program_offices/public_indian_housing/programs/ph/hope6/about [Accessed 16 September 2023].

Lexicon of Listed Terms and Agencies

- **Emergency Provisions:** A facility whose primary purpose is to provide temporary shelter for those experiencing homelessness.

- **Homeless or People Experiencing Homelessness (PEH):** A person who lacks fixed, regular, and adequate nighttime residence.

- **Point in Time Estimates (PIT):** Data that is gathered at one time and used to extrapolate data over a long term.

- **Social Determinants of Health:** Aspects outside the physical and mental body that impact health outcomes.

- **The Universal Declaration of Human Rights (UDHR)** is a milestone document in the history of human rights. Drafted by representatives with different legal and cultural backgrounds from all regions of the world, the declaration was proclaimed by the United Nations General Assembly in Paris on 10 December 1948 as a common standard of achievements for all peoples and all nations. It sets out, for the first time, fundamental human rights to be universally protected and it has been translated into over five hundred languages. The UDHR is widely recognized as having inspired, and paved the way for, the adoption of more than seventy human rights treaties, applied today on a permanent basis at global and regional levels (all containing references to it in their preambles).

- **US Department of Health and Human Services (HHS):** A cabinet level agency that's goal is to promote the health and well-being of all Americans, by providing for effective health and human services and by fostering sound, sustained advances in the sciences underlying medicine, public health, and social services.

- **US Department of Housing and Urban Development (HUD):** A cabinet level agency that is responsible for policy and programs that address America's housing needs, which improve and develop the Nation's communities, and enforce fair housing laws.

AUTHOR'S BIO SKETCH

Laura Whitehill, MSc, MD

Originally from the east coast, Laura studied human biology at Georgetown University. Following graduation, she completed a Masters in Sociology at University College Dublin focusing on disability as a social determinant of health. Laura remained in Ireland to pursue a Doctor of Medicine degree after completion of master's studies, then returned to the United States as a surgical resident. During her surgery intern year, Laura recognized she desired work in a community-based setting serving a diverse patient population consistent with her passion for the manifestations of social determinants of health. She is completing a residency in Family Medicine at University of Washington affiliated Community Health Care a Federally Qualified Teaching

Health Center in Tacoma, Washington. She lives with her husband and their dog Remy, enjoying life in the Pacific Northwest.

Chapter 15

The Environment & the Social Determinants of Health

Karl Riecken, DO, MA, Author
Stephen Cook, MD, Editor

"We are the environment and how we treat each other is really how we treat the environment."
- John Francis, PhD Planetwalker

The Environment, Climate Change, and Social Determinants of Health

The World Health Organization (WHO) lists the basic prerequisites to good health, which include "clean air, stable climate, adequate water, sanitation and hygiene, safe use of chemicals, protection from radiation, healthy and safe workplaces, sound agricultural practices, health-supportive cities and built environments, and a preserved nature" (World Health Organization, 2022). The environment in which people live influences each of these factors. In a rapidly changing climate, the environment ever more so affects the social determinants of health, which are those "non-medical factors that influence health outcomes" (World Health Organization, 2023). This chapter elucidates the *environmental prerequisites* for health and their ecological impact on socioeconomic status, education, employment, working conditions, food security, housing, early childhood development, structural conflict, and access to healthcare. It closes with the larger implications for governance and policy.

Climate Change

According to Shumake-Guillemot, Villalobos-Prats and Campbell-Lendrum (2015), the evidence for global warming demands urgent attention due to the "challenges increasingly presented by climate variability and change." **Figure 1** provides a qualitative assessment for the predicted burden of ill-health due to climate change for the period 2030–2040 during which the world will inevitably experience ~1.5 °C of warming due to past and present greenhouse gas emissions.

Figure 1.

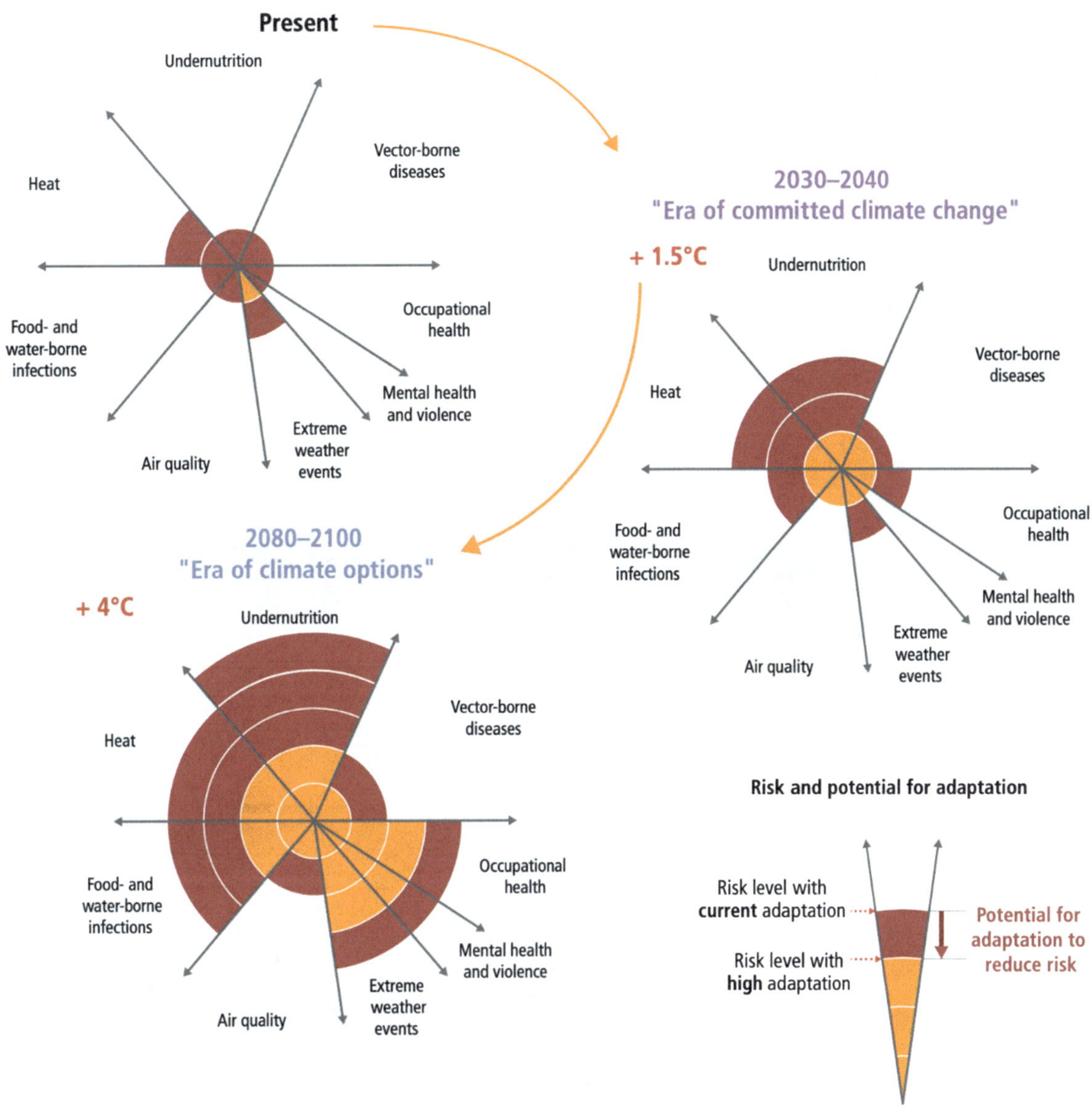

Note: The width of the slices gives a qualitative indication of the relative burden of ill health at the global level. For each timeframe, impact levels are estimated for the current state of adaptation and for a hypothetical highly adapted state, indicated by different colours.

Source: Reproduced from the health chapter, Working group II of the IPCC Fifth assessment report (*1*).

Shumake-Guillemot, J., Villalobos-Prats, E. and Campbell-Lendrum, D. (2015). *Operational Framework for Building Climate Resilient Health Systems*. [online] www.who.int. Available at: https://iris.who.int/bitstream/handle/10665/189951/9789241565073_eng.pdf?sequence=1

Figure 1 also illustrates the period 2080–2100, for which the global mean temperature is expected to increase by ~4 °C above preindustrial levels, unless vigorous mitigation efforts are undertaken. The assorted colours indicate the extent to which disease burdens could be avoided by effective adaptation measures in each period. To elucidate, even with concerted effort, undernutrition, heat, infections, extreme weather, and general assets of health will be strained over the next century (Shumake-Guillemot, Villalobos and Campbell-Lendrum, 2015).

Climate change has significant impacts on health, both directly (e.g., injury or death from extreme weather events and heat illnesses related to temperature increases) and indirectly (e.g., malnutrition, increased spread of vector-borne diseases and effects on mental health) according to Savage et al., (2021).

Figure 2.

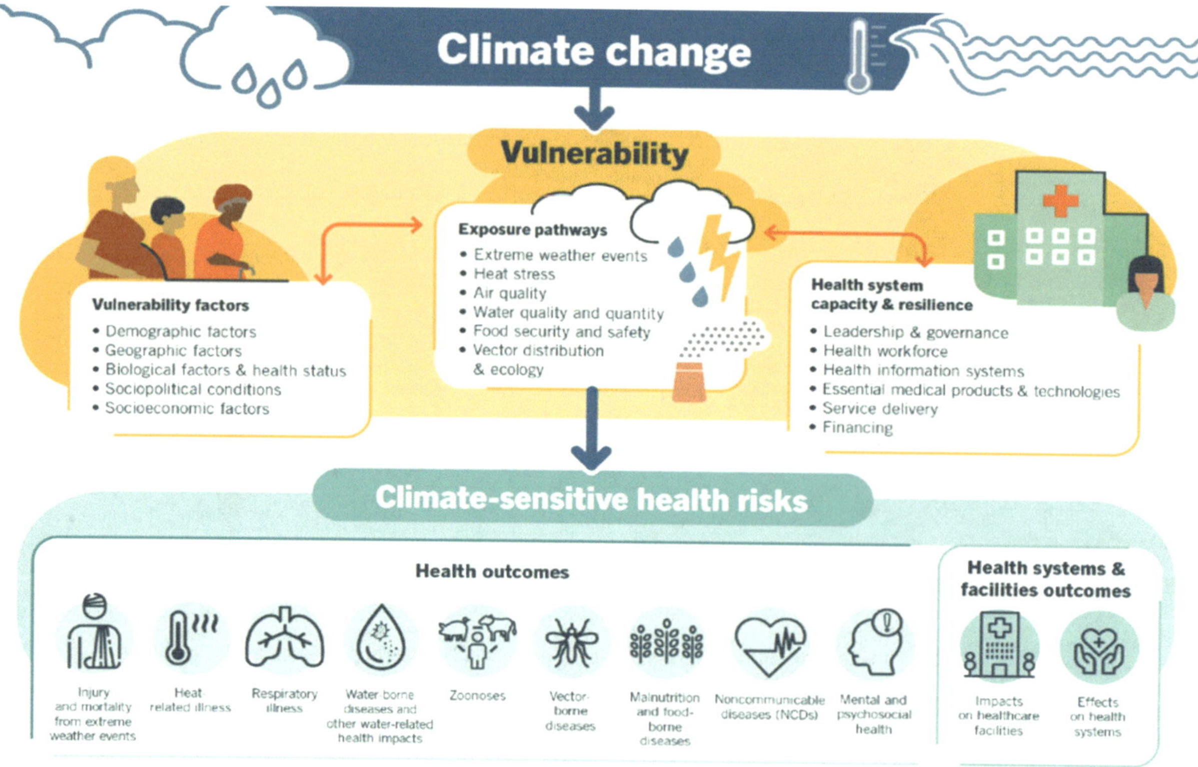

Figure 2: Climate-sensitive health risks
From: Savage, A., Villalobos, E., Campbell-Lendrum, D. and Dazé, A. (2021). *Review of Health in National Adaptation Plans*. [online] www.who.int. Available at: https://www.who.int/publications/i/item/9789240023604

The algorithm in **Figure 2** illustrates some of the major climate-sensitive health risks (CSHRs) and causal pathways. Conservative WHO (2021) estimates suggest climate change will cause an extra 250,000 deaths per year by 2030 from malnutrition, malaria, diarrhea, and heat stress. Furthermore, climate change places added pressure on health systems and facilities, with increasing burdens disproportionately affecting more vulnerable countries and communities Savage et al., (2021).

The Environment

In the context of Socioeconomic Status & Poverty

Socioeconomic status (SES) is a combined economic and social measure of an individual's economic and social position in relation to others based on income, education, and occupation. It is typically broken into three levels (high, middle, and low) to describe the hierarchy a family or an individual may be categorized in relation to other people. Socioeconomic status is an important source of health *inequity*, as there is a robust positive correlation between socioeconomic status and health (Worthy, Lavigne and Romero, 2020). Climate change directly undermines the social determinants of health, including "livelihoods, equality and access to health care and social support structures" (Bassi et al., 2023).

Stable environments promote access to the components necessary to manage personal affairs. Environmental stability fosters environmental predictability and the ability to focus on life's essentials like personal safety, housing, and food security as well as individual financial growth laying the foundation for sustainable personal, community and societal socioeconomic status (SES).

Experience shows that climate change cannot be segregated from its potential for extraordinary devastation – wildfires, hurricanes, drought, floods – on the lives of so many as well as its direct and drastic effect on those with lower socioeconomic status (see "Vulnerability Factors" in **Figure 2**).

Healthy People 2020 found predictable access to healthy food as a foundational component to SES. The Food and Agriculture Organization of the United Nations estimates that in 2020, 768 million (9.9% of the world's population) people faced hunger, unable to reliably know where their next meal would come from (Food and Agriculture Organization of the United Nations, 2021). Rising commodity prices through 2021, pushed an added thirty million people toward food insecurity (World Bank, 2022). Due to combination of environmental change and commodity price increases, climate change is projected to result in tremendous numbers of people falling below the poverty line. "Without solutions, falling crop yields, especially in the world's most food-insecure regions, will push more people into poverty – an estimated 43 million people in Africa alone could fall below the poverty line by 2030 as a result" (World Bank, 2022).

Overall, relative poverty is decreasing throughout the world, according to the World Economic Forum (Schoch, Jolliffe and Lakner, 2021). However, certain areas are likely to be heavily affected by climate change, such as sub-Saharan Africa, where the decline in poverty has stagnated in recent years and in the Middle East and Northern Africa, where relative poverty continues to increase. The overall increase in relative poverty of these areas corresponds to proportionate increases in extreme poverty in those regions.

The Environment

In the context of Education

Socioeconomic stability and upward mobility rely on the underpinnings of education. The Brookings Institute claims that a college degree offers a ticket out of poverty (Greenstone et al., 2013). A safe, non-toxic, positive environment that includes essential services for learners promotes school attendance, academic performance, and the trajectory toward graduation (National Center on Safe and Supportive Learning Environments, 2011). According to Wood (2023), climate change seriously affects the education of more than 40 million pupils every year mostly in low and low-middle income countries (Wood, 2023). Climate change affects education both directly through destruction of infrastructure, degradation of learning spaces, and with increased disease burden from vector- and water-borne disease prevalence (Wood, 2023). Indirect effects include increased migration, disruption of student physical and mental well-being, and negative impact on households. Wood (2023) argues these effects compound, worsening gender inequality, conflict, and poverty (**Figure 3**).

Figure 3.

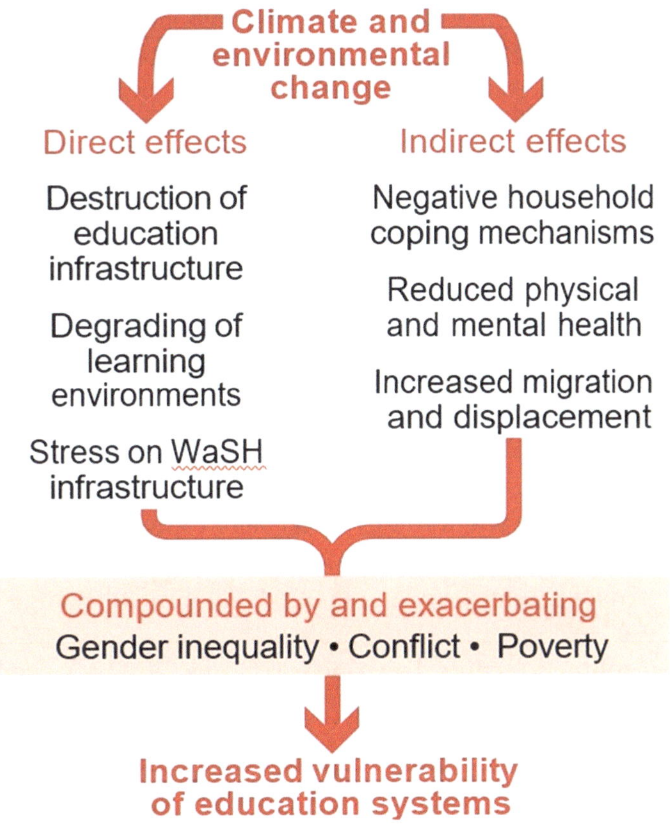

Figure 3. Wood, J. (2023). The climate crisis disrupts 40 million children's education every year. Here's how we could fix it. [online] World Economic Forum. Available at: https://www.weforum.org/agenda/2023/02/girls-education-climate-crisis-educational-disruption-resilience/

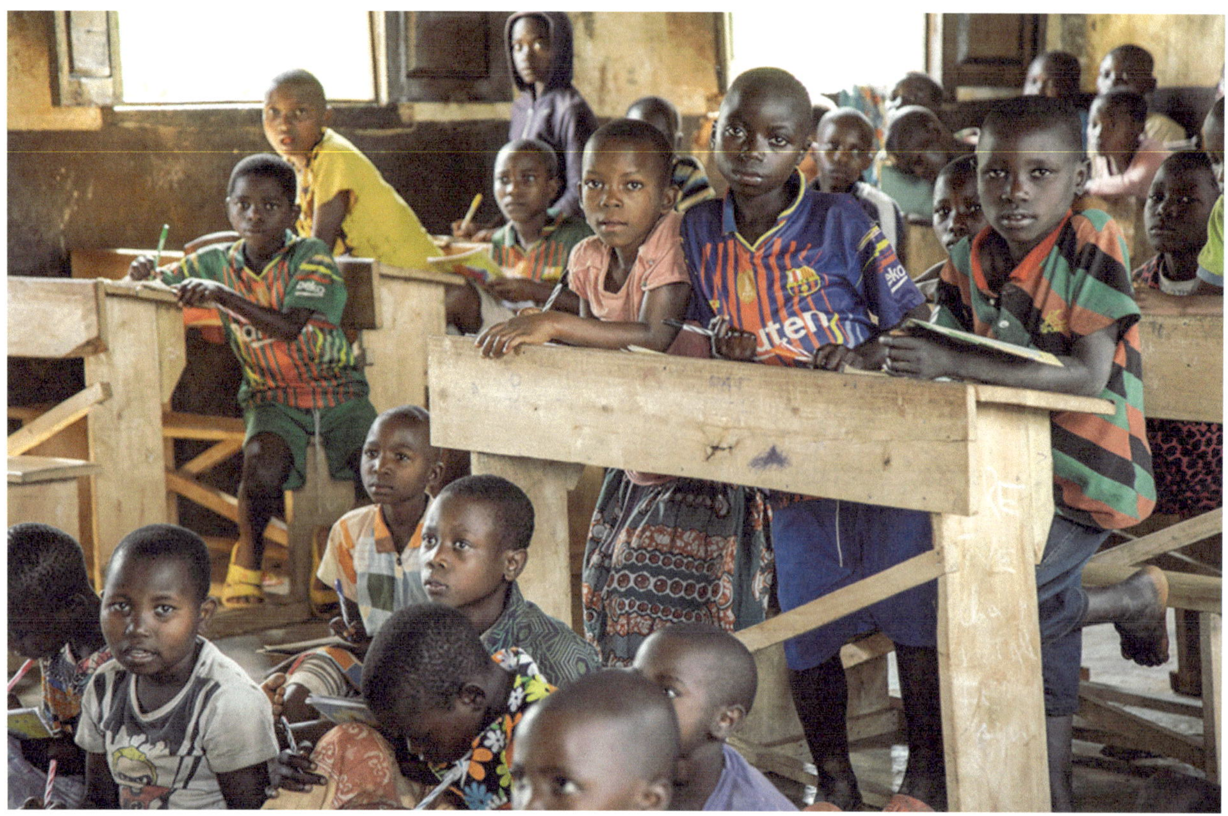

In Burundi, the influx of children into this school (after a landslide in the neighbouring village destroyed their school) means that classrooms are overcrowded, and children often must sit on the floor.

Foreign, Commonwealth and Development Office (2022). *Addressing the Climate, Environment, and Biodiversity Crisis in and Through Girls' Education* [online] Available at: https://www.gov.uk/government/publications/addressing-the-climate-environment-and-biodiversity-crises-in-and-through-girls-education/addressing-the-climate-environment-and-biodiversity-crises-in-and-through-girls-education

Leveraged correctly, education stands to have the greatest impact on the world's climate. Educating the world's young minds about the ramifications of climate change, they are better able to adapt to a changing world, and work to solve current day and future problems (Jorgensen, 2022). In more immediate terms, providing education on the effects of climate change has been shown to modify people's behavior, resulting in reduced energy use (Evans, 2022). According to UNESCO, educating the youth of our world is the single best way to change behavior in the future (UNESCO, 2022).

The Environment

In the context of Health and Well-being

Health is a state of complete physical, mental, and social well-being and not merely the absence of disease or infirmity, according to the WHO's Constitution (World Health Organization, 2023). Exposures to chemicals, particulates, pests, diseases, or negative social influences, affect health and, therefore, socioeconomic status. For instance, exposure to toxic chemicals can result in irreversible neurodevelopmental problems, congenital defects, and endocrine disruption according to the United States Environmental Protection Agency (2017). Children may be the most susceptible to environmental exposures – they drink more water and consume more food per kilogram body weight and may be exposed to pollutants during vulnerable times of development (United States Environmental Protection Agency, 2017).

Flint, Michigan Water Crisis

The impoverished city of Flint, Michigan faces a lead poisoning crisis that threatens the health and wellbeing of more than 26,000 children. Young children are particularly vulnerable; lead has significant and devastating effects on children's brains –it lowers IQ, affects learning, and decision making and negatively impacts social behaviors.

Even low levels of lead exposure in children have been linked to learning disabilities, shorter stature, and impaired hearing.

Save the Children (n.d.) *Flint Water Crisis* [online] Available at: https://www.savethechildren.org/us/what-we-do/emergency-response/flint

Children with the highest levels of lead exposure, which often comes through drinking water, have lower cortical brain volumes, and achieve poorer overall cognitive test results, changing their long-term ability to optimize socioeconomic status (Marshall et al., 2020).

The same or similar impact may occur at the other end of the age spectrum, with increasing cognitive decline seen in elderly populations in areas of higher air pollution, resulting in increased healthcare costs (Christensen et al., 2022).

The world's reliance on plastics results in substantial climate change. Plastics directly affect the environment through air and water pollution, both from their production and from their longevity (most do not readily bio degenerate).

Plastics

Plastics are complex, highly heterogeneous, synthetic chemical materials. Over 98% of plastics are produced from fossil carbon – coal, oil, and gas. Plastics are formed form a carbon-based polymer backbone and thousands of additional chemicals that are incorporated into polymers to convey specific properties such as color, flexibility, stability, water repellence, flame retardation, and ultraviolet resistance. Many of these added chemicals are highly toxic. They include carcinogens, neurotoxicants and endocrine disruptors such as phthalates, bisphenols, per - and poly-fluoroalkyl substances (PFAS), brominated flame retardants, and organophosphate flame retardants. They are integral components of plastic and are responsible for many of plastics' harms to human health and the environment.

Global plastic production has increased exponentially since World War II, and during this time more than 8,300 megatons (Mt) of plastic have been manufactured. Annual production volume has grown from under 2 Mt in 1950 to 460 Mt in 2019, a 230-fold increase, and is on track to triple by 2060. More than half of all plastic ever made has been produced since 2002. Single-use plastics account for 35–40% of current plastic production and represent the most rapidly growing segment of plastic manufacture.

Plastic manufacture is energy-intensive and contributes significantly to climate change. At present, plastic production is responsible for an estimated 3.7% of global greenhouse gas emissions. This fraction is projected to increase to 4.5% by 2060 if current trends continue unchecked.

Plastic production workers are at increased risk of leukemia, lymphoma, hepatic angiosarcoma, brain cancer, breast cancer, mesothelioma, neurotoxic injury, and decreased fertility. Workers producing plastic textiles die of bladder cancer, lung cancer, mesothelioma, and interstitial lung disease at increased rates. Plastic recycling workers have increased rates of cardiovascular disease, toxic metal poisoning, neuropathy, and lung cancer. Residents of "fenceline" communities adjacent to plastic production and waste disposal sites experience increased risks of premature birth, low birth weight, asthma, childhood leukemia, cardiovascular disease, chronic obstructive pulmonary disease, and lung cancer. The detrimental effects of plastics disproportionately affect those in poor, disempowered, and marginalized peoples.

Landrigan et al., (2023). The Minderoo-Monaco Commission on Plastics and Human Health. Annals of Global Health, 89(1). [online] Available at: https://annalsofglobalhealth.org/articles/10.5334/aogh.4056

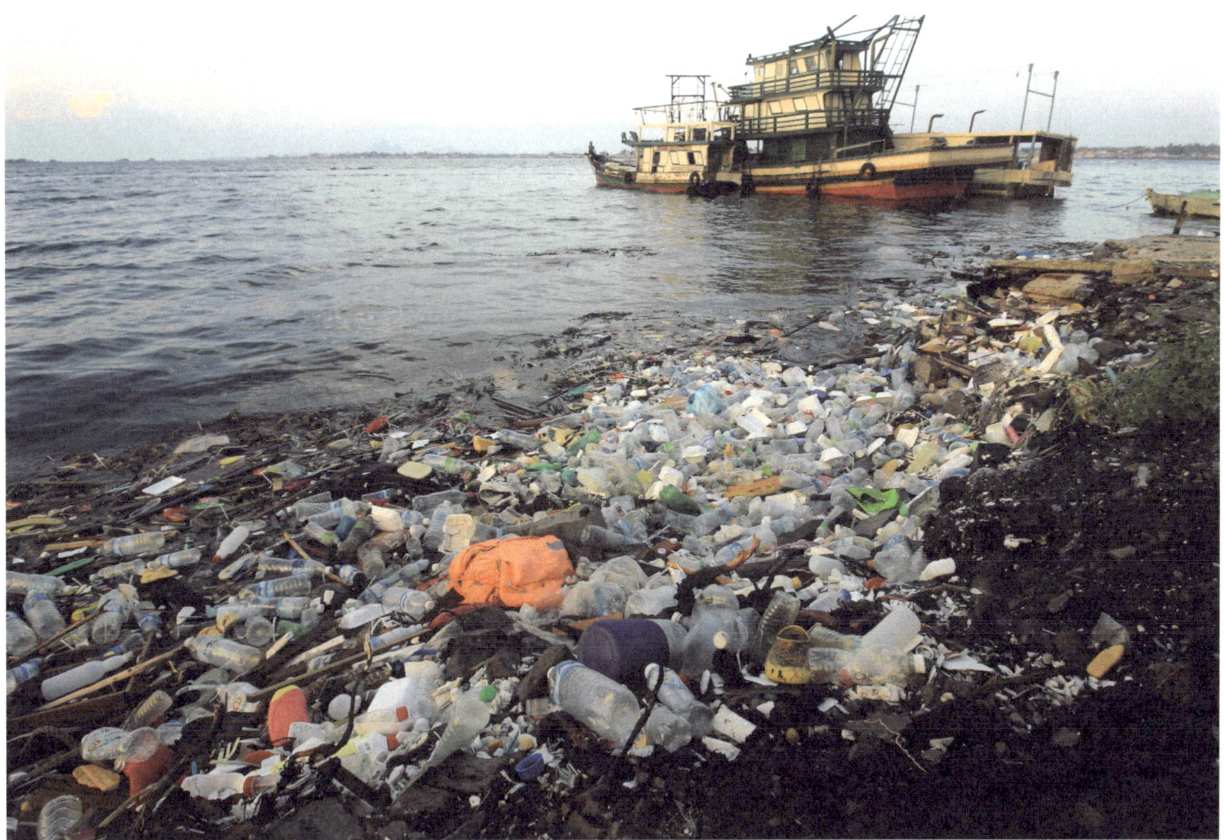

Sexton, C. (2019) Plastic pollution becoming one of the world's biggest health threats. Earth.com [online] Available at: https://www.earth.com/news/plastic-pollution-health-threats/

According to a report from the United Nations, 25 percent of global disease and mortality is caused by environmental damage, and plastic pollution is one of the biggest growing threats. The Global Environmental Outlook (GEO) warns that immediate action is needed to address the eight million tons of plastic litter that is making its way into the ocean each year (Sexton, 2019).

Finally, due to changing worldwide environmental conditions, *experts predict increased frequency and severity of pandemics and epidemics* like the COVID-19 experience in 2020 (de Oliveira and Tegally, 2023). The possibilities of previously rare or nonexistent diseases emerging from melting permafrost or novel diseases evolving due to favorable environmental conditions (e.g., rising temperatures) contribute to the overall predicted pandemic prevalence. Those of lower SES are less likely to have access to treatments as they develop, as evidenced by the lower access to the COVID-19 vaccination by those groups worldwide (Acharya, Ghimire and Subramanya, 2021).

The Environment

In the context of Working Conditions and Job Security in a Green Economy

Industrial exposures present a wide range of detrimental health risks including contacts to vector borne diseases, wildfires, and violence according to Applebaum, et al., 2016. Construction, agricultural, health care, building maintenance and transportation workers shoulder the burden of these exposures. As a correlate, this translates into missed days from work, decreased income, reduced economic stability, unemployment, reliance on income assistance and serious threats to individual health. Workers most affected by climate change include the most vulnerable – women, ethnic minorities, migrant workers, displaced persons, older populations, and those with underlying health conditions (WHO, 2021).

The transition to carbon zero industries poses new opportunities and significant threats to workers. According to the Organization for Economic Cooperation and Development (OECD, n.d.), successful transition toward a greener economy demands novel work force perspectives. Labor market and skill policies must maximize the benefits for workers and assure fair sharing of adjustment costs, while supporting green growth policies in this light speed work force evolution. This includes the need for inclusive green-specific labor market and skill policies – top-up training for mid-career workers who need to adapt to greener ways of working and ensuring that both men and women are equally well-prepared for the shift to a greener economy.

As industry transforms into a low-carbon economy, marked shifts toward green business services jobs will displace the traditional work force and traditional economies. The OECD (n.d.) predicts more than 80% of jobs by 2020 are expected to require medium to high-level skills, while low-skills jobs will continue to decline. The transformation to a green economy necessitates high level green skills. Green skills include specific abilities to modify products, services, or operations due to climate change adjustments, requirements, or regulations (OECD, n.d.). The green economy threats to persons of low socioeconomic status, limited education and low job skills suggests regrettably deeper disadvantages.

The Environment

In the context of Food Security

Figure 4. Global impacts of climate change on crop productivity

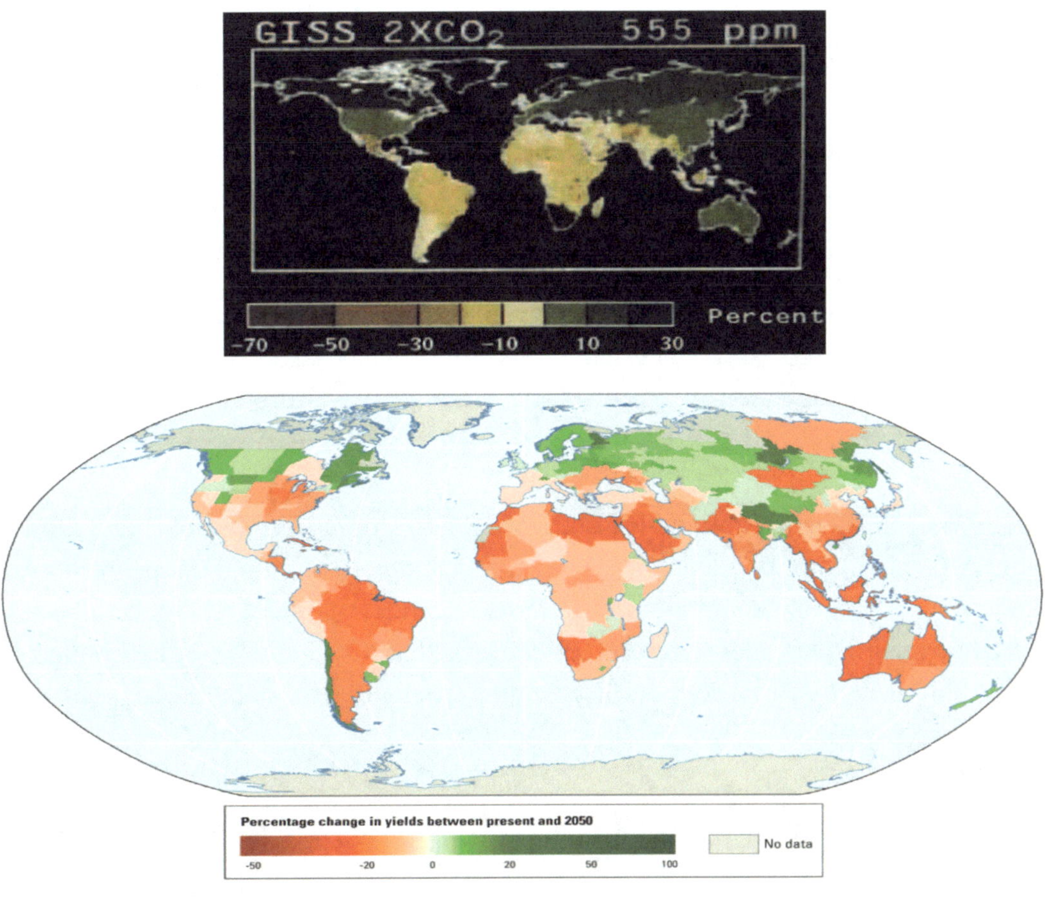

Figure 4. Global impacts of climate change on crop productivity from simulations published in 1994 and 2010.
From: Wheeler, T., Braun, J. von, 2013. Climate Change Impacts on Global Food Security. Science 341, 508–513.
https://doi.org/10.1126/science.1239402

Data published nearly a decade ago indicated that two-billion people were considered food insecure **Figure 4** (Wheeler and von Braun, 2013). Detailed in their report, nearly every region in the world experienced changes in agricultural productivity. Some regions saw increases because warming temperatures were more hospitable to food production. However, most regions saw a net negative change in the ability to produce crops. More recent data shows that the effect of climate change on food insecurity is increasing in probability and in magnitude, which according to Dasgupta and Robinson, erases some of the previously made gains in combating worldwide food insecurity (Dasgupta and Robinson, 2022).

Climate: One of Many Drivers for Food Insecurity

According to the Food and Agriculture Organization of the United Nations twelve percent of the global population was severely food insecure in 2020, representing 928 million people – 148 million more than in 2019.

It is projected that between 720 and 811 million people in the world faced hunger in 2020. Considering the middle of the projected range (768 million), around 118 million more people were facing hunger in 2020 than in 2019 – or as many as 161 million more, considering the upper bound of the range. The COVID-19 pandemic drove this startling increase.

More than half of the world's undernourished are found in Asia (418 million) and more than one-third in Africa (282 million). Compared with 2019, about 46 million more people in Africa, 57 million more in Asia, and about 14 million more in Latin America and the Caribbean were affected by hunger in 2020. New projections confirm that hunger will not be eradicated by 2030 unless bold actions are taken to accelerate progress, especially actions to address inequality in access to food.

Conflict, *climate variability and extremes*, as well as economic slowdowns and downturns (worsened by COVID-19 pandemic) are major drivers of food insecurity and malnutrition that continue to increase in both frequency and intensity and are occurring more frequently in combination.

Food and Agriculture Organization of the United Nations (2021). *The State of Food Security and Nutrition in the World 2021.* [online] Available at: https://www.fao.org/3/cb4474en/cb4474en.pdf

The Environment

In the context of Housing

In a 2021 meta-analysis of review articles, Bezgrebelna, et al., (2021) showed an increased risk of homelessness for vulnerably housed and lower socio-economic populations. Their research highlighted energy insecurity (costs associated with heating and colling) and climate change as contributing factors and showed that these populations are disproportionately exposed to climatic events (temperature extremes and natural disasters). The physical and mental health of homeless/vulnerably housed populations is excessively impacted by weather extremes and climate change, adding to the cumulative downside effects on their fragile social determinants of health profile (Bezgrebelna et al., 2021). Wild fires, floods, and hurricanes ravage communities throughout the world leaving destruction behind and sparing no one irrespective of economic means – including the quaint 200-year-old whaling village tourist destination Lahaina, Maui, HI.

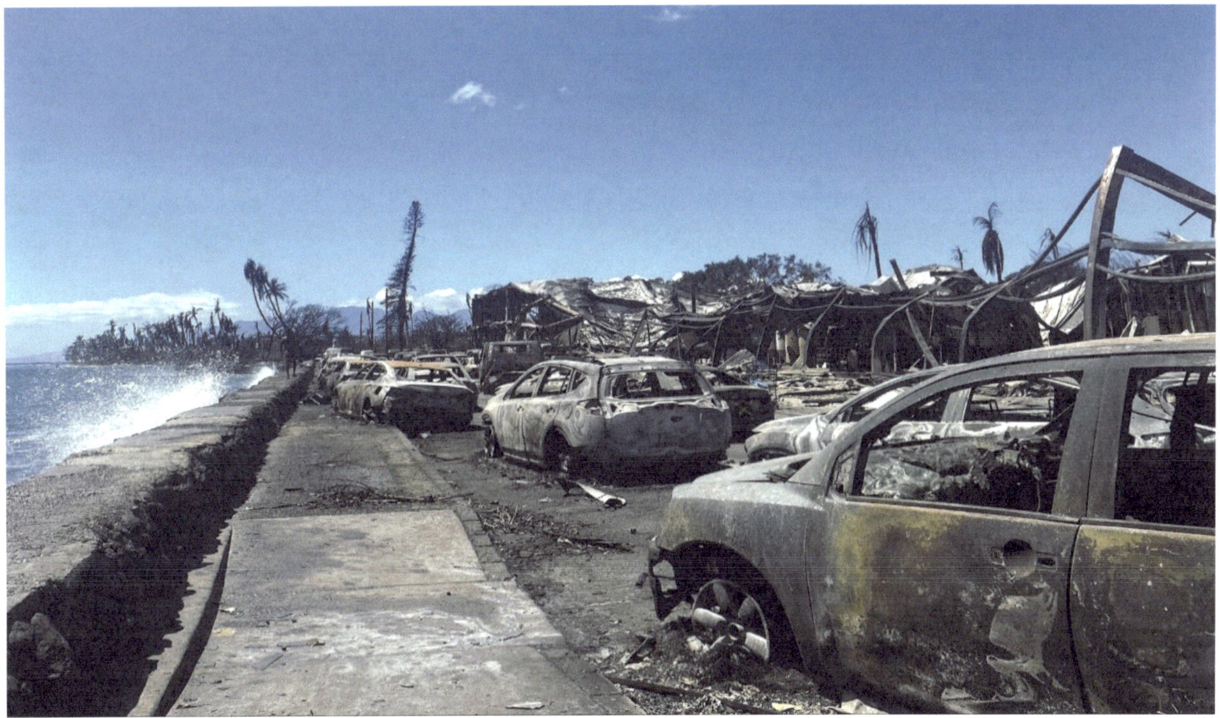

Bickerton, J. (2023) Maui fire Update: Death toll Rises as Efforts to Fight Blaze Continues *Newsweek 90.* [online] Available at: https://www.newsweek.com/maui-fire-update-death-toll-rises-efforts-fight-blazes-continue-1819307

Climate and Housing

On September 22, 2022, HUD's Office of Policy Development and Research (PD&R) held its quarterly event which focused on climate and housing as well as HUD's role in climate change mitigation and adaptation.

The housing sector in the United States accounts for a significant percentage of the greenhouse gas emissions that contribute to climate change. The environmental impact of producing and operating housing depends on the construction materials and methods employed and the energy consumption of the resulting dwelling. The location of new construction also can contribute to climate change, particularly when homes are built in *suburban or rural areas that encourage car-dependent lifestyles.* Meanwhile, climate change has already increased the frequency and severity of natural disasters, putting more U.S. homes at risk of damage or destruction. The panelists explained how natural disasters and other climate-related events have threatened housing in their communities.
For example:

- In Iowa, stronger storms have caused massive floods that have destroyed thousands of homes.
- Melting permafrost has lowered the foundations of some homes in northern Alaska.
- Low-income communities of color are disproportionately burdened by several environmental and climate hazards.

HUD has a significant interest in addressing climate change. The 4.5 million public and HUD-assisted housing units produce about 13.6 million tons of carbon emissions annually. HUD also spends billions of dollars to help families recover from climate-induced natural disasters. A recent HUD study associated natural disasters with an additional $800 million to $2 billion in Federal Housing Administration claims between 2004 and 2019 — an amount that will increase as such disasters become more frequent.

HUD USER (2022). PD&R Quarterly Update: Climate and Housing [online] Available at: https://bit.ly/3ZEhc1C

The Environment

In the context of Early Childhood Development

Youth, especially those just born or yet-to-be born, represent important national assets. The environment in which a child is raised—especially the first 1000 days—is critical to the long-term health of every child. A report from the East Asia and Pacific Office of UNICEF provides insight into the severity of a crisis within the climate crisis (UNICEF East Asia and Pacific Regional Office (EAPRO) (2022). The report outlines several intersecting factors. First, mothers exposed to excessive amounts of air pollution are more likely to experience premature birth – a significant risk factor for cognitive delay and poorer long-term neurodevelopmental outcomes. Exposure to excessive ambient heat during pregnancy results in poorer birth outcomes – neural tube defects, premature rupture of membranes, heat stroke, hypertension, and preeclampsia (EAPRO) (2022) and (CDC, 2022). Young children have immature thermoregulatory mechanisms as compared to adults (Notley et al., 2020), with the potential inability to sufficiently thermoregulate should the prospect of extreme 4+ centigrade global warming be realized.

Worldwide investment in early childhood development represents a critical neurocognitive strategy, according to the UNICEF report (EAPRO, 2022). Climate change is likely to affect the vulnerable populations proportionately more than those with higher SES. Investing in resources to mitigate environmental risks for children intuitively seems more efficient than waiting for the impact of adult of neurocognitive delay to manifest. According to the UNICEF report, a $1USD investment in early childhood development has a long-term economic return of roughly $17 USD (Heckman et al., 2010). Children born and yet unborn are powerful agents of change (Simmons, 2021). Even if activists are not able to solve the climate challenges immediately, our current and future youth may be able to create real solutions. However, if early childhood development across the world is not a focus of systemic investment, youths may never gain the ability or opportunity to contribute.

Environment

In the context of Healthcare Access

Disruption of healthcare services secondary to extreme weather events affects healthcare systems worldwide; systems that serve the most vulnerable have serious challenges bringing services back to pre-disaster levels, especially in poorer and developing countries (Savage et al., 2021). The World Health Organization has set objectives for bolstering the health systems that are most vulnerable, but this requires worldwide economic and resource investment (Shumake-Guillemot, Villalobos-Prats and Campbell-Lendrum, 2015). The principal components of the WHO recommendations are in the six categories of leadership and governance, health workforce, health information systems, emerging medical products and technologies, service delivery, and financing.

The Environment

Politics, policies, and governance

A call to action

The social determinants of health have an upward-cascading effect on global stability. The United Nations envisions, "Ending poverty in all its forms everywhere" as its number one sustainable development goal, stating that, "as human beings, our well-being is linked to each other. Growing inequality is detrimental to economic growth and undermines social cohesion, increasing political and social tensions and, in some circumstances, driving instability and conflicts" (United Nations, 2022). The International Institute for Sustainable Development highlights that "ecosystem collapse" will make everyone poorer and thus we all have a personal stake in correcting this trajectory (Paul, 2021).

To illustrate the UN's point, *violence and conflict* increase directly with surges in global temperature or more extreme rainfall with interpersonal violence rising 4% with each standard deviation rise in temperature or rainfall and proportionate intergroup conflict rising 14% (Hsiang, Burke, and Miguel, 2013). The impact of this conflict will affect the entire world, but it is likely to have its most profound impacts of those least economically able to absorb the resultant instability. According to de Oliviera and Tegally, climate change will increase the number and the severity of epidemics and pandemics further illustrating the need for a pressing call to action (de Oliveira and Tegally, 2023).

United Nations Secretary General António Guterres presented a unifying strategy to address the broad needs of the world to combat climate change. Specifically, his strategy argued that one of the goals was to "leave no one behind," showing that by helping the world's most vulnerable, we can "breakthrough" instead of "breakdown" (United Nations, 2021). Another of the UN's Sustainable Development Goals calls for a renewed contract between governments and their people, ensuring comprehensive human rights: "universal social protection, health coverage, skills, decent work and housing, as well as universal access to the Internet by 2030." Each of these is inseparable from, and essential to, the universal recognition and application of the social determinants of health to steer meaningful public policy.

Climate change threatens the world order creating an urgent call to action for healthcare professionals to educate patients and the public about climate change and the environment (Tan Ngo, 2021). Our voices must be loud and clear as we advocate on local and national levels in support of public policy that embraces the devastating consequences of climate change. Healthcare professionals and major medical organizations represent trusted sources of information – duty neglected; we violate that trust.

Evidence suggests we must amp up the call. A 2022 analysis of front-facing websites from major medical organizations showed that 55% of those organizations made no mention of climate change (Bush, Jensen, and Katsumoto, 2022). The American College of Physicians in 2020 put forth a vision for the future of the American healthcare system that specifically addresses social determinants of health (Butkus et al., 2020). Yet, during boots on the ground patient care, selecting evidence based medical therapies trumps addressing the social determinants that led to the maladies every time.

Climate change advocates argue the need for a comprehensive and unified approach to address the social determinants of health impacted by the environment and climate change. The Paris Agreement 2015 leads in that direction.

The Paris Agreement

The Paris Agreement constitutes a landmark international accord that was adopted by nearly every nation in 2015 to address climate change and its negative impacts. The agreement aims to substantially reduce global greenhouse gas emissions to limit the global temperature increase in this century to 2 degrees Celsius above preindustrial levels, while pursuing the means to limit the increase to 1.5 degrees. The agreement includes commitments from all major emitting nations to cut their climate pollution and to strengthen those commitments over time. The pact provides a pathway for developed nations to assist developing nations in their climate mitigation and adaptation efforts, and it creates a framework for the transparent monitoring, reporting, and ratcheting up of countries' individual and collective climate goals (National Resources Defense Council, 2021).

According to the National Resources Defense Council (NRDC), U.S. President Barrack Obama announced in December 2015 that the United States, along with nearly 200 other countries, had committed to the Paris Climate Agreement, an ambitious global action plan to fight climate change. Obama envisioned that the accord would leave today's children, "A world that is safer and more secure, more prosperous, and more free."

However, less than two years later, then-president Donald Trump put that future in jeopardy by announcing his plan to withdraw the United States from the accord—a step that became official on November 4, 2020—as part of a larger plan to dismantle decades of U.S. environmental policy. Fortunately, American voters also got their say in November 2020, ousting Trump and sending Joe Biden and Kamala Harris to the White House.

Following President Biden's day one executive order, the United States officially rejoined the landmark Paris Agreement on February 19, 2021, positioning the country to once again be part of the global climate solution (National Resources Defense Council, 2021).

National Resources Defense Council (NRDC) (2021). Paris Climate Agreement: Everything You Need to Know [online] Available at:
https://www.nrdc.org/stories/paris-climate-agreement-everything-you-need-know#sec-whatis

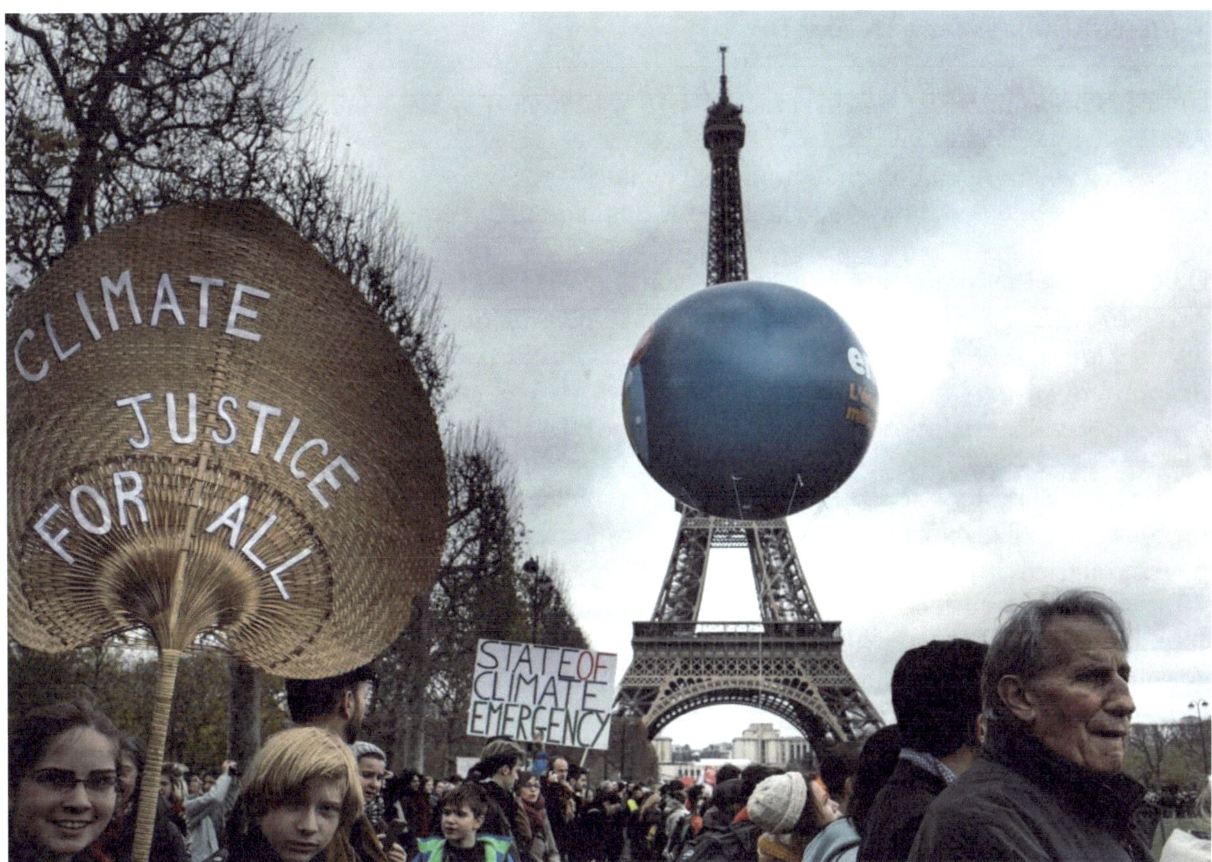

Protesters gather near the Eiffel Tower in Paris, France during the 2015 UN Climate Conference. *Credit Clement Martin/Sipa USA via Associated Press*

National Resources Defense Council (NRDC) (2021). Paris Climate Agreement: Everything You Need to Know [online] Available at: https://www.nrdc.org/stories/paris-climate-agreement-everything-you-need-know#sec-whatis

Questions for Further Consideration:

1. Given that the environment and changes to it result in potentially drastic effects on the health and well-being of all people, what is the role of healthcare professionals in protecting patient health from environmental insults? What is the role of the healthcare professionals and lawmakers in working toward systemic change?

2. This chapter selects several environmental impacts on health and well-being. Name another environmental impact not mentioned in this chapter. Outline how it may affect you or the patients you care for. See if you can find evidence for your claim in extant research. If you are unable to find support for your assertion, how might you propose studying its effects?

Sentinel Readings for a Deeper Dive

United Nations (2021). *OUR COMMON AGENDA Report of the Secretary-General*. [online] Available at:
https://www.un.org/en/content/common-agenda-report/assets/pdf/Common_Agenda_Report_English.pdf

United States Environmental Protection Agency (2021). *CLIMATE CHANGE AND SOCIAL VULNERABILITY IN THE UNITED STATES A Focus on Six Impacts 2 Climate Change and Social Vulnerability in the United States: A Focus on Six Impacts FRONT MATTER Acknowledgments*. [online] Available at: https://www.epa.gov/system/files/documents/2021-09/climate-vulnerability_september-2021_508.pdf [Accessed 12 Sep. 2023].

Paul, D. (2021). Merging the Poverty and Environment Agendas. [online] International Institute for Sustainable Development. Available at: https://www.iisd.org/articles/deep-dive/merging-poverty-and-environment-agendas [Accessed 22 Sep. 2023].

John Francis, PhD *Planetwalker* author, traveler, student, and teacher, has traveled from coast to coast across the United States, visited Antarctica, and sailed through the Caribbean. He has done this all without the use of motorized travel. National Geographic (n.d.) Planetwalker: Dr. John Francis [online] Available at: https://education.nationalgeographic.org/resource/real-world-geography-dr-john-francis/ [Accessed 24 September 2023].

References

Acharya, K., Ghimire, T. and Subramanya, S. (2021). Access to and equitable distribution of COVID-19 vaccine in low-income countries. *Npj Vaccines*, [online] https://doi.org/10.1038/s41541-021-00323-6 [Accessed 11 September 2023].

Applebaum, K., Graham, J., Gray, G., LaPuma, P., McCormick, S., Northcross, A., and Perry, M. (2016). An Overview of Occupational Risks from Climate Change. *Current Environmental Health Reports*, https://pubmed.ncbi.nlm.nih.gov/26842343/ [Accessed 12 September 2023].

Bassi, A., Sanchez, L., Campbell-Lendrum, D., Egorova, A., Maiero, M., Nevillle, T., Pega, F. and Schweizer, C. (2023). *A Framework for the Quantification and Economic Valuation of Health Outcomes Originating from Health and non-health Climate Change Mitigation and Adaptation Action*. [online] www.who.int. Available at: https://iris.who.int/bitstream/handle/10665/367385/9789240057906-eng.pdf?sequence=1 [Accessed 15 Sep. 2023].

Bezgrebelna, M., McKenzie, K., Wells, S., Ravindran, A., Kral, M., Christensen, J., Sotiropoulos, V., Gaetz, S. and Kidd, S.A. (2021). Climate Change, Weather, Housing Precarity, and Homelessness: A Systematic Review of Reviews. *International Journal of Environmental Research and Public Health*, https://www.mdpi.com/1660-4601/18/11/5812 [Accessed 15 Sep. 2023].

Bickerton, J. (2023) Maui Fire Update: Death toll Rises as Efforts to Fight Blaze Continues *Newsweek 90.* [online] Available at: https://www.newsweek.com/maui-fire-update-death-toll-rises-efforts-fight-blazes-continue-1819307 [Accessed 26 September 2023].

Bush, T., Jensen, W., and Katsumoto, T. (2022). U.S. medical organizations and climate change advocacy: a review of public facing websites. *BMC Public Health*, [online] Available at: https://bmcpublichealth.biomedcentral.com/articles/10.1186/s12889-022-14339-7 [Accessed 13 September 2023].

Butkus, R., Rapp, K., Cooney, T., and Engel, L. (2020). Envisioning a Better U.S. Health Care System for All: Reducing Barriers to Care and Addressing Social Determinants of Health. *Annals of Internal Medicine*, [online] Availabel at: https://pubmed.ncbi.nlm.nih.gov/31958803/ [Accessed 14 September 2023].

CDC (2022). Heat and Pregnant Women. *CDC: Natural Disasters and Sever Weather* [online] Available at: https://www.cdc.gov/disasters/extremeheat/heat_and_pregnant_women.html [Accessed 26 September 2023].

Christensen, G., Li, Z., Pearce, J., Marcus, M., Lah, J., Waller, L., Ebelt, S., and Hüls, A. (2022). The complex relationship of air pollution and neighborhood socioeconomic status and their association with cognitive decline. *Environment International*, [online] Available at: https://pubmed.ncbi.nlm.nih.gov/35868076/ [Accessed 13 September 2023].

Dasgupta, S., and Robinson, E. (2022). Attributing changes in food insecurity to a changing climate. *Scientific Reports*, 12(1) [online] Available at: https://www.nature.com/articles/s41598-022-08696-x [Accessed 13 September 2023].

de Oliveira, T. and Tegally, H. (2023). Will climate change amplify epidemics and give rise to pandemics? *Science (New York, N.Y.)*, [online] Available at: https://www.science.org/doi/10.1126/science.adk4500 [Accessed 15 September 2023]

Evans, V. (2022). *Why is education important in tackling climate change?* Cambridge University Press & Assessment. Available at: https://www.cambridge.org/news-and-insights/insights/why-is-education-important-in-tackling-climate-change [Accessed 12 Sep. 2023].

Food and Agriculture Organization of the United Nations (2021). *The State of Food Security and Nutrition in the World 2021*. [online] Available at: https://www.fao.org/3/cb4474en/online/cb4474en.html [Accessed 14 September 2023].

Foreign, Commonwealth and Development Office (2022). *Addressing the Climate, Environment, and Biodiversity Crisis in and Through Girls' Education* [online] Available at: https://www.gov.uk/government/publications/addressing-the-climate-environment-and-biodiversity-crises-in-and-through-girls-education/addressing-the-climate-environment-and-biodiversity-crises-in-and-through-girls-education [Accessed 25 September 2023].

Greenstone, M., Looney, A., Patashnik, J. and Yu, M. (2013). *Thirteen Economic Facts about Social Mobility and the Role of Education*. [online] Brookings. Available at: https://www.brookings.edu/articles/thirteen-economic-facts-about-social-mobility-and-the-role-of-education/ [Accessed 12 Sep. 2023].

Heckman, J., Moon, S., Pinto, R., Savelyev, P., and Yavitz, A. (2010). The Rate of Return to the High/Scope Perry Preschool Program. *Journal of Public Economics*, [online] Available at: https://www.ncbi.nlm.nih.gov/pmc/articles/PMC3145373/ [Accessed 14 September 2023].

HUD USER (2022). PD&R Quarterly Update: Climate and Housing [online] Available at: https://bit.ly/3ZEhc1C [Accessed 26 September 2023].

Hsiang, S., Burke, M., and Miguel, E. (2013). Quantifying the Influence of Climate on Human Conflict. *Science* [online] Available at: https://www.science.org/doi/10.1126/science.1235367 [Accessed 13 September 2023].

Jorgensen, M. (2022). *Education and Climate Change | Harvard Graduate School of Education*. [online] Available at: https://www.gse.harvard.edu/ideas/askwith-education-forum/22/10/education-and-climate-action [Accessed 12 Sep. 2023].

Landrigan, P., Raps, H., Cropper, M., Bald, C., Brunner, M., Canonizado, E., Charles, D., Chiles, T., Donohue, M., Enck, J., Fenichel, P., Fleming, L., Ferrier-Pages, C., Fordham, R., Gozt, A., Griffin, C., Hahn, M., Haryanto, B., Hixson, R. and Ianelli, H. (2023). The Minderoo-Monaco Commission on Plastics and Human Health. *Annals of Global Health*, [online] Available at: https://annalsofglobalhealth.org/articles/10.5334/aogh.4056 [Accessed 14 September 2023].

Marshall, A., Betts, S., Kan, E., McConnell, R., Lanphear, B. and Sowell, E. (2020). Association of lead-exposure risk and family income with childhood brain outcomes. *Nature Medicine*, [online] Available at: https://pubmed.ncbi.nlm.nih.gov/31932788/ [Accessed 16 September 2023].

National Center on Safe and Supportive Learning Environments (2011). *Environment | Safe Supportive Learning*. [online] Ed.gov. Available at: https://safesupportivelearning.ed.gov/topic-research/environment [Accessed 11 Sep. 2023].

National Geographic (n.d.) Planetwalker: Dr. John Francis [online] Available at: https://education.nationalgeographic.org/resource/real-world-geography-dr-john-francis/ [Accessed 24 September 2023].

National Resources Defense Council (NRDC) (2021). Paris Climate Agreement: Everything You Need to Know [online] Available at: https://www.nrdc.org/stories/paris-climate-agreement-everything-you-need-know#sec-whatis [Accessed 27 September 2023].

Notley, S., Akerman, A., Meade, R., McGarr, G., and Kenny, G. (2020). Exercise Thermoregulation in Prepubertal Children: A Brief Methodological Review. *Medicine & Science in Sports & Exercise* [online] Available at: https://pubmed.ncbi.nlm.nih.gov/32366798/ [Accessed 14 September 20203].

OECD (n.d.). *Greening jobs and skills*. [online] Available at: https://web-archive.oecd.org/2012-07-13/57773-greeningjobsandskills.htm [Accessed 26 September 2023].

Paul, D. (2021). Merging the Poverty and Environment Agendas. [online] International Institute for Sustainable Development. Available at: https://www.iisd.org/articles/deep-dive/merging-poverty-and-environment-agendas [Accessed 22 Sep. 2023].

Savage, A., Villalobos, E., Campbell-Lendrum, D. and Dazé, A. (2021). *Review of Health in National Adaptation Plans*. [online] www.who.int. Available at: https://iris.who.int/bitstream/handle/10665/340915/9789240023604-eng.pdf?sequence=1 [Accessed 13 Sep. 2023].

Save the Children (n.d.) *Flint Water Crisis* [online] Available at: https://www.savethechildren.org/us/what-we-do/emergency-response/flint [Accessed 25 September 2023].

Schoch, M., Jolliffe, D.M. and Lakner, C. (2021). *A quarter of the world lives in 'societal poverty' – here's what that means*. [online] World Economic Forum. [online] Available at: https://www.weforum.org/agenda/2021/01/societal-poverty-economics-development-finance-sdgs/ [Accessed 16 September 2023].

Sexton, C. (2019) Plastic pollution becoming one of the world's biggest health threats. Earth.com [online] Available at: https://www.earth.com/news/plastic-pollution-health-threats/ [Accessed 25 September 2023].

Shumake-Guillemot, J., Villalobos-Prats, E. and Campbell-Lendrum, D. (2015). *Operational Framework for Building Climate Resilient Health Systems*. [online] www.who.int. Available at: https://iris.who.int/bitstream/handle/10665/189951/9789241565073_eng.pdf?sequence=1 [Accessed 15 September 2023].

Simmons, S. (2021). *How to Address the Climate crisis? 5 Young People Share Their Solutions*. [online] World Economic Forum. [online] Available at: https://www.weforum.org/agenda/2021/11/how-to-address-the-climate-crisis-5-young-people-share-their-solutions/ [Accessed 16 September 2023].

Tan Ngo, N. (2021). Climate Change and Health Equity. *AMA Journal of Ethics*, [online] Available at: https://journalofethics.ama-assn.org/article/climate-change-and-health-equity/2021-02 [Accessed 15 September 2023].

UNESCO (2022). *Why climate change education for social transformation?* [online] Unesco.org. Available at: https://www.unesco.org/en/articles/why-climate-change-education-social-transformation [Accessed 12 Sep. 2023].

UNICEF East Asia and Pacific Regional Office (EAPRO) (2022). *Early Childhood Development and Climate Change*. [online] Available at: https://www.unicef.org/eap/media/12801/file/UNICEF%20EAPRO%20ECD%20and%20Climate%20Change%20Advocacy%20Brief%20doc.pdf [Accessed 15 Sep. 2023].

United Nations (2021). *OUR COMMON AGENDA Report of the Secretary-General*. [online] Available at: https://www.un.org/en/content/common-agenda-report/assets/pdf/Common_Agenda_Report_English.pdf [Accessed 15 September 2023].

United Nations (2022). Goal1: End Poverty in All Its Forms Everywhere. [online] United Nations Sustainable Development. Available at: https://www.un.org/sustainabledevelopment/poverty/ [Accessed 15 September 2023].

United States Environmental Protection Agency (2017). *Exposure to Environmental Contaminants*. [online] US EPA. Available at: https://www.epa.gov/report-environment/exposure-environmental-contaminants [Accessed 12 Sep. 2023].

United States Environmental Protection Agency (2021). *CLIMATE CHANGE AND SOCIAL VULNERABILITY IN THE UNITED STATES A Focus on Six Impacts 2 Climate Change and Social Vulnerability in the United States: A Focus on Six Impacts FRONT MATTER Acknowledgments*. [online] Available at: https://www.epa.gov/system/files/documents/2021-09/climate-vulnerability_september-2021_508.pdf [Accessed 12 Sep. 2023].

Wheeler, T. and von Braun, J. (2013). Climate Change Impacts on Global Food Security. *Science*, [online] 341(6145), pp.508–513. https://www.science.org/doi/10.1126/science.1239402 [Accessed 12 September 2023].

WHO (2021). *Climate change and health*. [online] World Health organization. Available at: https://www.who.int/news-room/fact-sheets/detail/climate-change-and-health [Accessed 12 September 2023].

Wood, J. (2023). *The climate crisis disrupts 40 million children's education every year. Here's how we could fix it*. [online] World Economic Forum. Available at: https://www.weforum.org/agenda/2023/02/girls-education-climate-crisis-educational-disruption-resilience/ [Accessed 12 Sep. 2023].

World Health Organization (2022). *Environmental health*. [online] www.who.int. Available at: https://www.who.int/health-topics/environmental-health#tab=tab_1 [Accessed 12 September 2023].

World Health Organization (2023). *Constitution of the World Health Organization*. [online] World Health Organization. Available at: https://www.who.int/about/governance/constitution [Accessed 12 Sep. 2023].

World Bank (2022). What You Need to Know About Food Security and Climate Change [online] *World Bank*. Available at: https://www.worldbank.org/en/news/feature/2022/10/17/what-you-need-to-know-about-food-security-and-climate-change [Accessed 12 Sep. 2023].

Worthy, L., Lavigne, T., and Romero, F. (2020) *Culture and Psychology* [online] Available at: https://open.maricopa.edu/culturepsychology/chapter/socioeconomic-status-ses/ [Accessed 25 September 2023].

Lexicon of Listed Terms and Agencies

- **John Francis, PhD** National Geographic Education Fellow, is nicknamed "the Planetwalker." For 22 years, he did not use motorized transportation. He is the program director for Planetwalk, a nonprofit environmental awareness organization, which aims to educate people not only about the physical environment, but the human environment as well. *Planetwalker: 22 Years of Walking. 17 Years of Silence* frames his autobiography and travels without the use of motorized vehicles for 22 years.

- **National Resources Defense Council** NRDC (the Natural Resources Defense Council) combines the power of more than 3 million members and online activists with the expertise of some 700 scientists, lawyers, and other environmental specialists to confront the climate crisis, protect the planet's wildlife and wild places, and to ensure the rights of all people to clean air, clean water, and healthy communities.

- **The Environmental Protection Agency (EPA)** is an American governmental organization that ensures Americans have access to clean air, water, and land; ensure scientific evidence shapes environmental policy; federal laws protect human health and the environment; environmental stewardship is factored into US environmental policy; Americans have access to accurate information; contamination is cleaned up; and chemicals in the marketplace are reviewed for safety.

- **The United Nations (UN)** is an intergovernmental organization whose stated purposes are to support international peace and security, develop friendly relations among nations, achieve international cooperation, and serve as a centre for harmonizing the actions of nations.

- **The United Nations Educational, Scientific and Cultural Organization (UNESCO)** is a specialized agency of the United Nations aimed at promoting world peace and security through international cooperation in education, arts, sciences and culture.

- **The World Economic Forum (WEF)** is an independent international organization committed to improving the state of the world by engaging business, political, academic and other leaders of society to shape global, regional and industry agendas.

- **The World Health Organization (WHO)** is the United Nations agency that connects nations, partners and people to promote health, keep the world safe and serve the vulnerable with the goal that everyone, everywhere can attain the highest level of health.

- **UNICEF**, originally called the United Nations International Children's Emergency Fund in full, now officially **United Nations Children's Fund**, is an agency of the United Nations responsible for supplying humanitarian and developmental aid to children worldwide.

AUTHOR'S BIO SKETCH

Karl Riecken, DO, MA

Dr. Riecken holds bachelor's degrees in Anthropology and Music Performance, a master's degree in Exercise Physiology, and earned his Doctor of Osteopathic Medicine degree at Rocky Vista University in 2021. He has additional credentials in strength and conditioning, sports nutrition, functional medicine, and for coaching several Olympic sports. He has been involved in the health and human performance to varied populations from patients seen during his Family Medicine residency at the University of Washington affiliated FQHC Community Health Care in Tacoma, WA to Olympic athletes during work at the USOPC in Colorado Springs, CO and the National Training Center in Clermont, FL. He has particular interest in uncovering root causes of health so that all populations can find and create the best in themselves. He runs the independent functional, human performance medicine and consulting company, Complete Concept Athletics, LLC.

Chapter 16

The Exposome, Microbiome & the Social Determinants of Health

David Greco, MD, Author
Gary Reichard, MD, Editor

"It really boils down to this: that all life is interrelated. We are all caught in an inescapable network of mutuality, tied into a single garment of destiny. Whatever affects one destiny, affects all indirectly."

- Dr. Martin Luther King, Jr., Civil Rights Leader, 1967

"All illnesses have some hereditary contribution. Genetics loads the gun and environment pulls the trigger"

- Francis Collins, Director of the National Human Genome Research Institute, 2006

The Exposome and the Microbiome

Social Determinant of Health Drivers

Biological discoveries to unlock the fundamental nature of human health evolved over the course of the 20th century. Breakthroughs in biochemistry and molecular biology forged paths forward. The Human Genome Project – an effort to map the genes that comprise the human genome – accelerated this research in the 1990's. Scientist declared the Human Genome Project complete in 2003, and while it allowed scientists to better understand the biological nature of the human body, it spawned further inquiry, leading to a new realm of science called "exposomics."

The genesis of the term exposomics, comes from the word exposome. Coined in 2005, scientists define the term exposome as "the measure of all of the exposures an individual has in a lifetime and how those exposures relate to health. The exposome represents the totality of exogenous (external) and endogenous (internal) exposures from conception onwards" (Juárez, 2018). The interplay between the array of lifetime exposures and individual health (or population health) defined a new area of research that continues to develop and be utilized in many ways. Francis Collins, who led the Human Genome Project, has been a leader in the field of exposomics and a proponent of the importance in which the interplay of the genome and exposome impacts health.

Figure 1 visually illustrates the exposome-genome relationship as a Venn diagram with health and disease the commonality between them.

Figure 1.

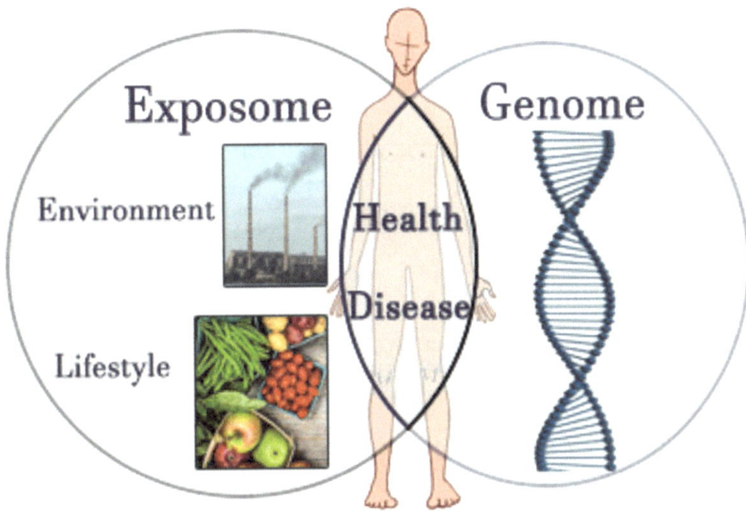

From the Genome to the Exposome: Mapping Causal Associations between Environmental Factors and Population Health | Blogs | CDC [online] Available at: https://blogs.cdc.gov/genomics/2022/09/06/from-the-genome-to-the-exposome/

From the Genome to the Exposome: Mapping Causal Associations Between Environmental Factors and Population Health

Environmental factors such as lifestyle, diet, and exposure to toxins and chemical agents, play a significant role in health. Complementary to the *genome*, which is the complete set of an individual's genetic information, the *exposome* represents an individual's complete set of environmental exposures throughout their lifetime. Coined in 2005, the exposome captures the variable and dynamic environmental exposures from the prenatal period onwards.

From the Genome to the Exposome: Mapping Causal Associations between Environmental Factors and Population Health | Blogs | CDC [online] Available at: https://blogs.cdc.gov/genomics/2022/09/06/from-the-genome-to-the-exposome/

This interaction is complicated by the social determinants of health, which lead to significant differences in the health of individuals, communities, and populations with low-income levels, limited educational access, minority race representation, food insecurity, and other factors leading to disparities in health. To clarify, the exposome of low-income individuals and populations forms differently than groups in a higher socioeconomic status (SES) with ready access to education, health care, transportation, food, internet communication, water, and similar social determinant experiences.

The Flint Water Crisis represents an example. Starting in 2014 and continuing through 2017, an environmental exposure in Flint, Michigan – in this case lead contamination in resident drinking water – impacted an African American low socioeconomic status community. The lead exposure resulted in Legionnaire's disease, childhood developmental delay, learning disabilities, and seizure disorders among many others (Masten, et al., 2016). Based on this illustration, advancing exposomal knowledge represents critically important methodologies for measuring and understanding the several ways SES and other social determinants of health couple with environmental exposures to modify health outcomes among individuals, communities, and entire populations.

Exposomics

Exposomics studies the exposome (the totality of environmental exposers that individuals encounter throughout life and how these exposures affect health). Researchers' break them down into internal and external exposures.

Internal exposure fields include genomics, lipidomics, and transcriptomics, among many others. Internal exposure exposomics involves all the processes that occur *inside the human body* that lead to specific health outcomes. For example, higher or lower cholesterol levels or predispositions for myocardial infarction or not. The fields of internal exposomics include utilization of biomarkers to determine the interrelationship between exposure, effect, disease progression, and susceptibility; utilization of technology that result in enormous quantities of data; and use of data mining to find statistical associations between exposure, effect, and other factors (DeBord, et al., 2016).

External exposure exposomics includes measuring *environmental stressors*. Methods of studying external exposure include the use of direct reading instruments, laboratory-based analysis, and/or survey instruments (McDermott, et al., 2012). Effective use of this data leads to discovering and implementing primary and secondary prevention methods for disease as well as more effective treatment at the individual level that may be scalable to entire populations.

The Human Genome Project, a multibillion-dollar initiative, launched in 1990 as a coordinated effort by the U.S. Department of Energy and the National Institutes of Health. The project was originally planned to last 15 years, but rapid technological advances accelerated the completion in 2003 (National Human Genome Research Institute, 2020). Although scientists sought to map the human genome as central to the Project, additional goals included furthering scientific knowledge pertaining to the cause, prevention and cure of disease based on genetics.

Through time and extensive research, scientific evidence now shows that genetics accounts for just 10% of disease (National Human Genome Research Institute, 2020). In other words, the majority of diseases stem from environmental exposures and to fully understand disease science must discover how environmental exposures contribute to acute and chronic conditions and delineation of the differential manifestations among individuals of similar background and socioeconomic status.

Exposomic research can be performed in several diverse ways. Mapping causal relationships between environmental factors and population health is essential to the effectiveness of exposomic research. A common study design in exposomics is the Epigenome-Wide

Association Study (EWAS), which found its origin in the genome variant called GWAS (Genome-Wide Association Study). The EWAS consists of two primary methodological steps: 1) utilizing a large subset of unique environmental assays, or environmental loci measured across cases and controls, yielding environmental factors with significantly high association with a disease and 2) validating associations by taking advantage of data from large cohort databases to theorize new affiliations with the disease (Patel, Bhattacharya, and Butte, 2010).

Figure 2 presents a diagrammatic representation of exposomics research relating to health and disease management.

Figure 2. Exposome-informed epidemiologic research.

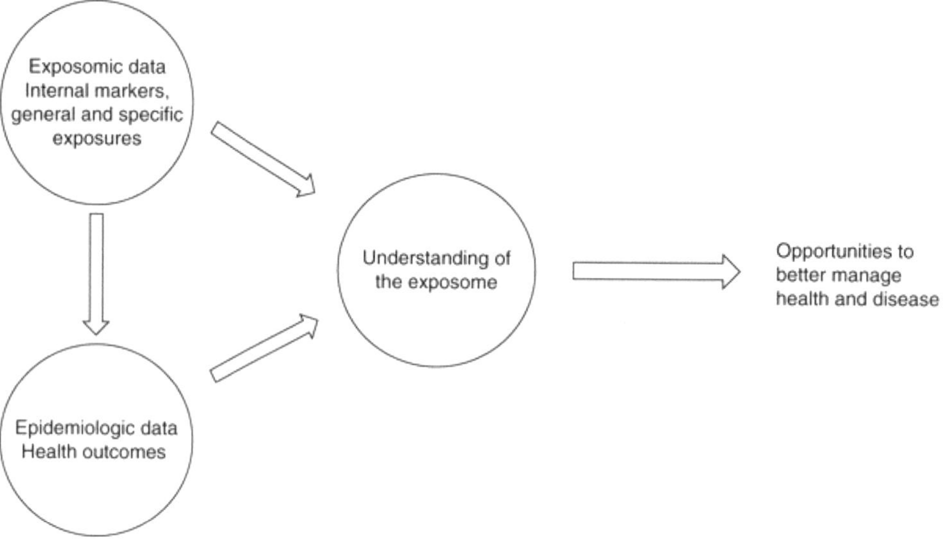

DeBord, D. et al 2016. Use of the "Exposome" in the Practice of Epidemiology: A Primer on -Omic Technologies." American Journal of Epidemiology, [online] Available at: https://academic.oup.com/aje/article/184/4/302/2236658

The Social Determinants of Health - Exposome

As alluded, exposures and genetics taken in concert, influence disease processes. This occurs through gene-environment interactions and begs the question how exposures differ between individuals with different genotypes. For example, specific genetic variants that modify the risk of developing Parkinson disease after exposure to organophosphate pesticides or studies that examine active and passive cigarette smoking exposure among individuals homozygous for delta F508 mutations for cystic fibrosis, illustrate how individuals with the same genotype, but various levels of environmental exposure, result in different health outcomes (Rasooly, D., et al., 2021).

Additionally, epigenetics, which is "the process of altering gene expression without changing the DNA Sequence," shows how a dynamic interaction between modifiable and non-modifiable risks and exposures, such as smoking and air pollution, increase lung cancer risk. Finally, "epigenetic dysregulation" contributes to certain diseases, such as Angelman syndrome, Alzheimer's disease, autism, and certain cancers, and can be used as a marker for biological aging (Drzymalla, Rasooly and Khoury, 2023).

These examples are deeply related to social determinants of health. For example, rates of people living near polluting factories or rates of smoking due to targeted advertising in low-income communities, can significantly alter the exposomics of an individual, thereby leading to different health outcomes. Groups livings in areas with high rates of poverty, housing crises, racial injustice, unemployment, educational inequities, and poor access to healthcare acquire a much different exposomal profile than those not experiencing these health challenges.

According to Emeny, et.al., (2022), the most common health related social determinants of health (SDH) exposures are food and housing insecurity, financial instability, transportation needs, low levels of education, and psychosocial stress. These domains describe risks that impact health outcomes more than health care. Epidemiologic and translational research demonstrates that SDH factors represent exposures that predict harm and impact the health of individuals. International and national guidelines urge health professionals to address social determinants of health in clinical practice and public health (Emeny, et al., 2022).

The "SDH-exposome" describes the interplay between the social determinants of health and the exposome. For example, a study on the intracellular changes of oxidative and reductive stress in communities of need showed that SDH impacted rates of asthma significantly and was further impacted by factors like air and noise pollution, smoking exposure, and household income (Emeny, et al., 2022). **Figure 3** conceptualizes this interplay.

Figure 3.

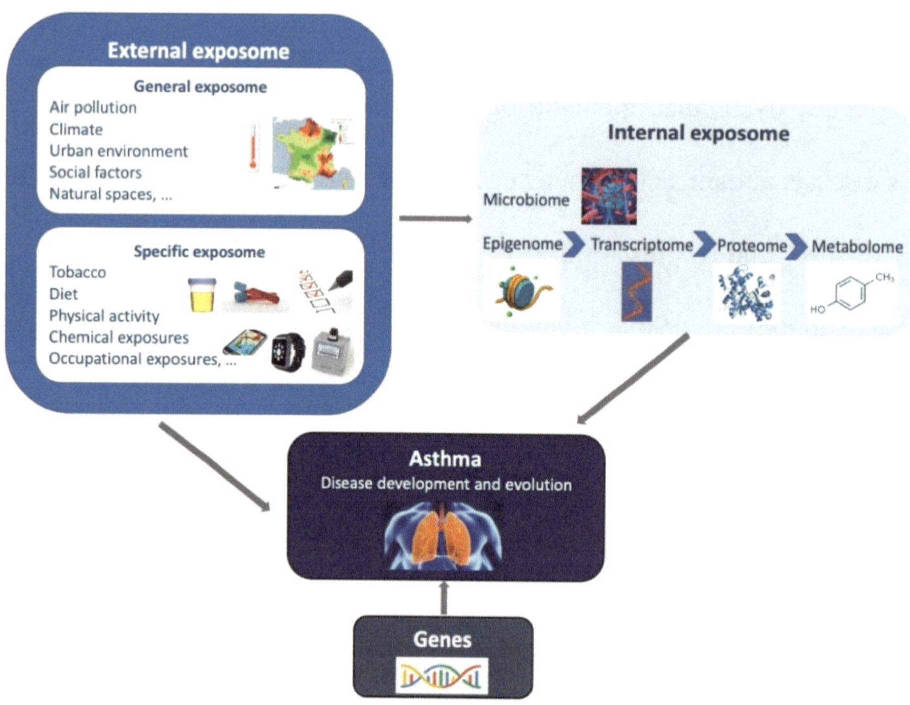

Guillien, Alicia, et al. "Profile of Exposures and Lung Function in Adults with Asthma: An Exposome Approach in the EGEA Study." *Environmental Research*, vol. 196, May 2021, https://www.sciencedirect.com/science/article/abs/pii/S0013935120313190?via%3Dihub

The Social Determinants of Health - Microbiome

The entire genome of microbial communities that *live in and on the human body (microbiota)*, including skin, respiratory, urinary, reproductive, and digestive tracts define the microbiome. These microbial communities work symbiotically on and within the body to prevent illness and maintain homeostasis. Changes in the composition and diversity of the gut microbiota, for example, can have consequences ranging from risks for infection to gastrointestinal disease.

Microbial ecology is the study of relationships between germ communities in humans, plants, and other animals to understand their impact on health (Ogunrinola, et al., 2020). The microbiome develops as a composition of all experiences of an individual throughout lifetime. Researchers implicate the gut microbiome as influential in the health and well-being of individuals in multiple ways – antibiotic resistance, *Clostridium difficile* recurrence, digestive and metabolic functions, bioavailability of vitamins B12 & K as well as cancer prevention (Kho, 2018).

Figure 4 graphically illustrates gut microbiome concepts.

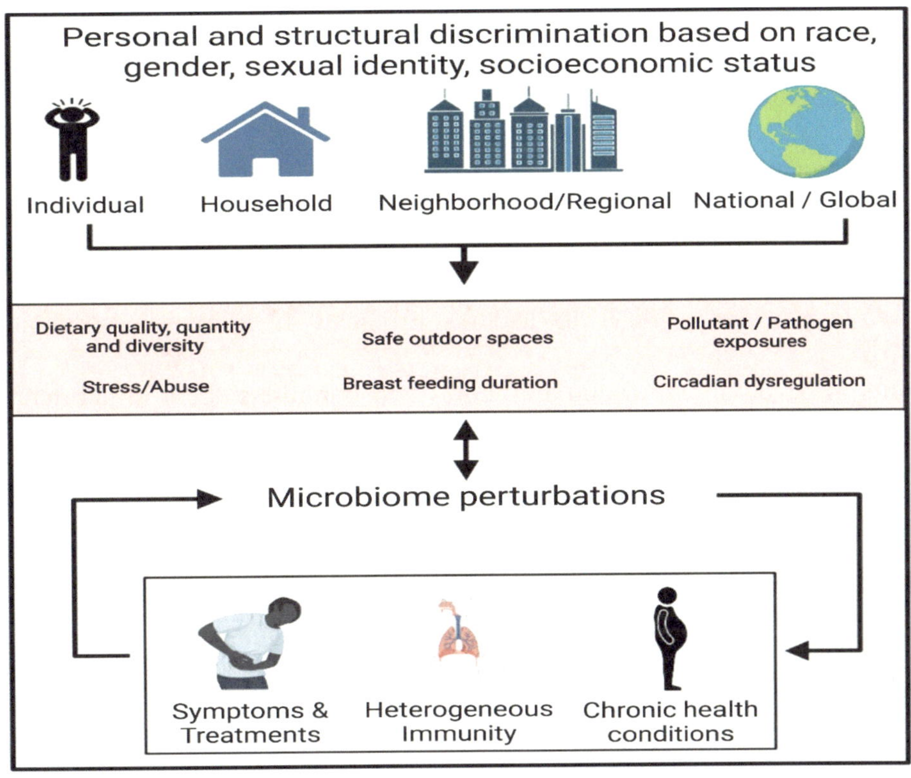

Figure 4. Amato, et al., (2021). The human gut microbiome and health inequities. *Proceedings of the National Academy of Sciences*, [online] Available at: https://doi.org/10.1073/pnas.2017947118

The experience of vaginal birth further elucidates these important constructs. According to research by Coelho, et al., (2021), vaginal birth confers newborns with a greater number and variety of colonizing microorganisms in contrast to newborns birthed through Cesarean section.

Vaginal birth jumpstarts immune system development and, according to Coelho, et al., (2021) is the ideal route for birth – C-sections should only be performed when there are medical indications.

Making Sense of the Relationship of Social Determinants of Health, Exposome and Microbiome

Periodontal disease provides a practical opportunity to pull together concepts of the interposition between the social determinants of health, the exposome and the microbiome.

Thornton-Evans, G. et al., (2013) describe periodontal disease as a *chronic infection* of the hard and soft tissue supporting the teeth, which leads to tooth loss in older adults. Tooth loss impairs dental function, impacts access to nutritional foods, and disrupts quality of life. The severity of periodontal disease is categorized as mild, moderate, or severe based on multiple measurements of dental plaque, periodontal pocket depth, evidence of infection, attachment loss, and gingival inflammation around teeth. Loesche (2017), implicates the bacteria *Treponema denticola* and *Porphyromonas gingivalis* as most frequent infecting microorganisms. Chronic infection results in development of autoantibodies and immune system inflammatory responses that lead to association with increased risk for several diseases (**Table 1.**)

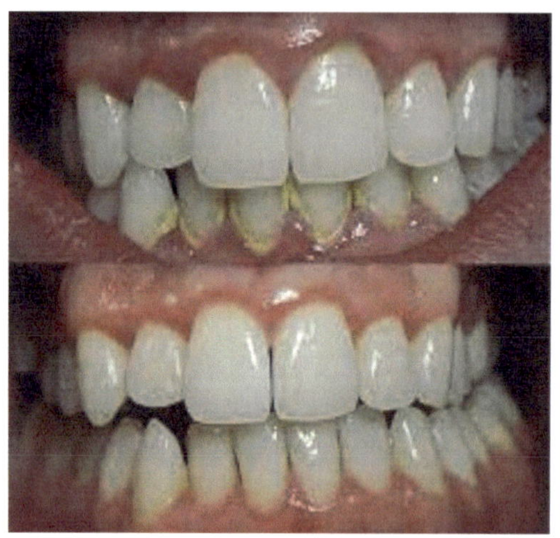

Periodontitis: gum inflammation (gingivitis), extensive plaque accumulation, gum retraction

Gingivitis: reduced plaque, gum erythema, and inflammation of gingival tissues following hygiene

Source of photo not available

Approximately 47% of adults aged ≥30 years in the United States (65 million adults) have periodontitis, 8.5% with severe periodontitis (Thornton-Evans, G. et al., (2013).

Table 1. Illustrates the exposomic relationship between the SDH, exposures and microbiota.

SOCIAL DETERMINANTS of HEALTH : EXPOSOME : MICROBIOME
SDH EXPOSURES LEADING TO PERIODONTAL DISEASE
EDUCATION The prevalence of periodontitis is associated with a low level of educational attainment. Thornton-Evans, G. et al; (2013). Available at: https://bit.ly/46TyqKv
POVERTY The prevalence of periodontitis is associated with poverty. Thornton-Evans, G. et al; (2013). https://bit.ly/46TyqKv Low-income whites residing in disadvantaged neighborhoods had 1.8-fold higher odds of having severe periodontitis than high-income whites residing in advantaged neighborhoods. Borrell, L., Beck, J. and Heiss, G. (2006). Available at: https://doi.org/10.2105/AJPH.2004.055277
RACE The prevalence of periodontitis was significantly higher in non-Hispanic Black people (58.6%) and Mexican Americans (59.7%) compared with non-Hispanic whites (42.6%). Thornton-Evans, G. et al; (2013). Available at: https://bit.ly/46TyqKv
GENDER The prevalence of periodontitis was significantly higher among men (56.4%) than women (38.4%) overall, and this finding was consistent among racial/ethnic groups. Thornton-Evans, G. et al; (2013). Available at: https://bit.ly/46TyqKv
HOMELESSNESS Homelessness presents extraordinary barriers oral health – access to dental care, clean water, toothbrush, toothpaste, dental floss, nutritious foods. Oral Health and Diabetes in Patients Experiencing Homelessness (2019). Available at: https://bit.ly/3tC58lt
MICROBIATA of PERIODONTAL DISEASE
CARDIOVASCULAR DISEASE There is now a significant body of evidence to support independent associations between severe periodontitis and several non-communicable diseases, in particular CVD. Sanz, M., et al., (2020). Available at: https://www.ncbi.nlm.nih.gov/pmc/articles/PMC7027895/
DEMENTIA In this meta-analysis, there was an association between periodontitis and cognitive impairment, and moderate or severe periodontitis was a risk factor for dementia. Guo, H., et al., (2021). Available at: https://www.ncbi.nlm.nih.gov/pmc/articles/PMC8297088/
CANCERS Advanced periodontitis was associated with a 2.5-fold increase in smoking-related cancers among never smokers. Periodontitis may impact cancer risk via system immune dysregulation. Michaud, D., et al., (2016). Available at: https://pubmed.ncbi.nlm.nih.gov/26811350/
SPONTANEOUS PRETERM BIRTH Periodontal disease is common in adults. Two systematic reviews have reported an association between periodontal disease and adverse pregnancy outcome, such as spontaneous pre-term birth (sPTB); more research necessary to prove conclusively. Robinson, J. (2023). Available at: https://bit.ly/3FjQp1a
RHEUMATOID ARTHRITIS Evidence emerging from numerous clinical and epidemiological studies suggest an association between rheumatoid arthritis and periodontal disease. Koziel, J., Mydel, P., and Potempa, J. (2014). Available at: https://www.ncbi.nlm.nih.gov/pmc/articles/PMC3930831/

To further exemplify, a young, single parent of African American descent living on the edge of poverty gives birth to Josiah, a vigorous infant male weighing in the 20th percentile. By circumstance, low socioeconomic status prevails and at times leads to periods of homelessness, and food insecurity throughout Josiah's early and adolescent life. Transportation challenges interfere with access to medical and dental care. Overtime, Josiah's school performance declines. He drops out of school during his senior year, taking a job at a local pizza store to supplement mom's income. By age thirty he has moderate to severe periodontal disease.

Josiah's exposome is riddled by adverse social determinants of health – poverty, homelessness, minority race, low educational attainment, food insecurity and fragile access to health care, especially dental care. His microbiome concurrently plays out through the lens of chronic infection, the development of autoantibodies to the microbiota of periodontal disease and immune system inflammatory responses. As detailed in **Table 1**, although the mechanisms are not entirely understood, periodontal disease is associated with an increased incidence of cardiovascular disease, dementia, certain cancers, preterm birth, and rheumatoid arthritis.

Policies, politics, and governance

How might advance social spending – aka remodeling public policy – impact the value of exposomics and microbiomics at population levels, especially in communities with low SES, homelessness, food insecurity and transportation challenges? The social determinants of health implications abound with guiding lights for health professionals, lawmakers, social advocates, and educators in identifying areas through which public policy changes influence population health.

Exposomics and microbiomics make *and take* the understanding of well-being from a macro level to a micro level. As an example, this essay makes the case for the importance of gut microbiota interposed with well-being. The gut microbiome is negatively impacted by foods of low nutritious value. Low SES neighborhoods are often "food deserts" where individuals do not live within a reasonable distance to grocery stores with fresh fruits and vegetables. Efforts directed to improve access to community markets in low-income areas has significant implications for improving gut microbiota, vastly magnifying the meaning of well-being in the array of exposomic manifestations as described in the foregoing, not just the insult as viewed through the simplistic lens of anorexia or obesity.

Conclusions

This chapter shines important light on how poverty, homelessness, pollution, food security, employment, the environment, education, water and sanitation, and transportation impact health and well-being at a molecular level. The science of exposomics and microbiomics coupled with the expansion of artificial intelligence stand to dramatically revolutionize the delivery health care and the understanding of what it means to be healthy, also known as precision health.

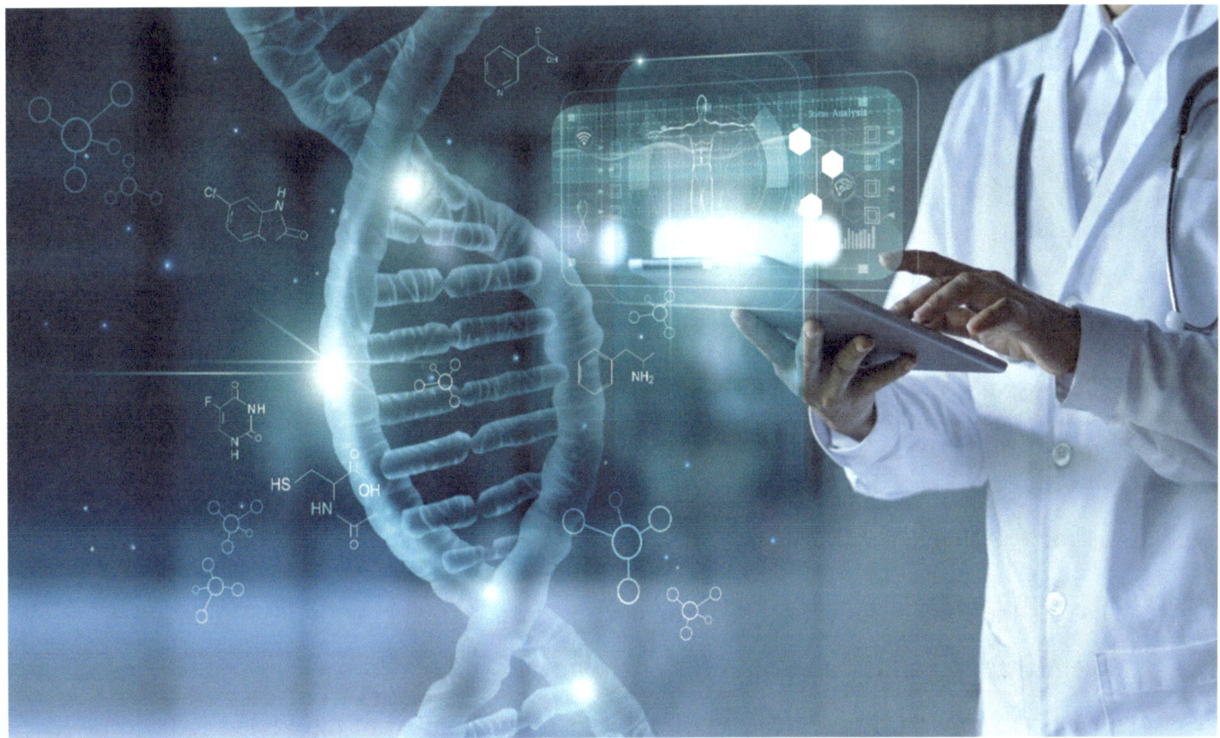

Source: Johns Hopkins Medicine (2023)

Exposomics and the future of Precision Health

In January 2015, when President Barak Obama launched the Precision Medicine Initiative, it was the first time that the general population was exposed to the greater concept of precision medicine as a bold new effort to revolutionize how to improve health care and "help people live longer, happier, and healthier lives."

In "precision medicine" the focus is on identifying optimal care based on a unique personal profile (i.e., individual differences in genetics, exposures, lifestyle, and health factors) to determine disease susceptibility, understand the clinical course of the disease and prescribe appropriate drugs or other therapies in defined subpopulations of patients, rather than on the average population.

The expansion of precision medicine is based on using multiple sources from genomics, biological data, transcriptomics, and proteomics crucial for prediction, to be more precise and accurate in diagnoses, definitions, and treatments of disease subtypes. Precision medicine is a new medical strategy that defines a disease at a higher resolution to enable the more precise targeting of subgroups of disease with new therapies; prominent examples include cystic fibrosis and cancer.

The discovery of biomarkers that can be identified before the emergence of overt clinical symptoms, together with technological development, have paved the way for rapid genomic discovery, thereby transforming the current healthcare approach from one centered on precision medicine to a more comprehensive focus on precision health, offering the possibility of preventing disease altogether.

The future of precision medicine will enable health care providers to tailor treatment and prevention strategies to people's unique characteristics, including their genome sequence, microbiome composition, health history, lifestyle, and diet.

Strianese, et al., (2020. "Precision and Personalized Medicine: How Genomic Approach Improves the Management of Cardiovascular and Neurodegenerative Disease." Genes, https://doi.org/10.3390/genes11070747

Questions for Further Consideration:

1. Discuss the current trajectory of precision and personalized medicine. What is the potential for expanded inequities in healthcare?
2. Discuss the onset and progression of diabetes in the context of the SDH : Exposome : Microbiome interface.

3. You decide you would like to know your genome. What are the pros and cons, risks, and benefits? What companies provide genome testing and what is the cost?

Sentinel Readings for a Deeper Dive

Amato, K., et al., (2021). The human gut microbiome and health inequities. *Proceedings of the National Academy of Sciences*, [online] Available at: https://www.pnas.org/doi/full/10.1073/pnas.2017947118

Wharton, K. and Birsner, M. (2022). Vaginal Seeding. *ACOG Clinical* [online] www.acog.org. Available at: https://www.acog.org/clinical/clinical-guidance/committee-opinion/articles/2017/11/vaginal-seeding

National Human Genome Research Institute (2020). The Human Genome Project. [online] Genome.gov. Available at: https://www.genome.gov/human-genome-project

Strianese, O., et al., (2020). Precision and Personalized Medicine: How Genomic Approach Improves the Management of Cardiovascular and Neurodegenerative Disease. Genes, [online] Available at: https://www.mdpi.com/2073-4425/11/7/747

Thornton-Evans, G. et al; (2013). Periodontitis Among Adults Aged ≥30 Years — United States, 2009–2010. Morbidity and Mortality Weekly [online] Available at: https://bit.ly/46TyqKv

References

Amato, K., et al., (2021). The human gut microbiome and health inequities. *Proceedings of the National Academy of Sciences*, [online] Available at: https://www.pnas.org/doi/full/10.1073/pnas.2017947118 [Accessed 5 October 2023].

Beck, J. and Offenbacher, S. (2001). The Association Between Periodontal Diseases and Cardiovascular Diseases: A State-of-the-Science Review. *Annals of Periodontology*, [online] Available at: https://aap.onlinelibrary.wiley.com/doi/abs/10.1902/annals.2001.6.1.9 [Accessed 4 October 2023].

Borrell, L.N., Beck, J.D. and Heiss, G. (2006). Socioeconomic Disadvantage and Periodontal Disease: The Dental Atherosclerosis Risk in Communities Study. *American Journal of Public* Health [online] https://ajph.aphapublications.org/doi/full/10.2105/AJPH.2004.055277 [Accessed 15 October 2023].

Coelho, G., et al., (2021). Acquisition of microbiota according to the type of birth: an integrative review. *Revista Latino-Americana de Enfermagem*, [online] Available at: https://www.scielo.br/j/rlae/a/r959F4dwG98qnXMgf3Y8wBb/?lang=en [Accessed 5 October 2023].

DeBord, D., et al., (2016). Use of the 'Exposome' in the Practice of Epidemiology: A Primer on -Omic Technologies. *American Journal of Epidemiology*, [online] https://academic.oup.com/aje/article/184/4/302/2236658 [Accessed 6 October 2023].

Drzymalla, E., Rasooly, D. and Khoury, M. (2023). *Interplay Between the Exposome and the Genome in Health and Disease | Blogs | CDC.* [online] CDC. Available at: https://blogs.cdc.gov/genomics/2023/02/17/interplay-between-the-exposome/#Epigenetics [Accessed 22 Jan. 2024].

Emeny, R., Carpenter, D., and Lawrence, D., (2021). Health disparities: Intracellular consequences of social determinants of health. *Toxicology and Applied Pharmacology* [online] Available at: https://www.sciencedirect.com/science/article/abs/pii/S0041008X2100051X?via%3Dihub [Accessed 8 October 2023].

Guillien, A., (2021). Profile of exposures and lung function in adults with asthma: An exposome approach in the EGEA study. *Environmental Research* [online] Available at: https://www.sciencedirect.com/science/article/abs/pii/S0013935120313190?via%3Dihub [Accessed 8 October 2023].

Guo, H., et al., (2021). The Effect of Periodontitis on Dementia and Cognitive Impairment: A Meta-Analysis. *International Journal of Environmental Research and Public Health*, [online] Available at: https://www.ncbi.nlm.nih.gov/pmc/articles/PMC8297088/ [Accessed 15 October 2023].

Kho, Z.Y. and Lal, S.K. (2018). The Human Gut Microbiome – A Potential Controller of Wellness and Disease. *Frontiers in Microbiology*, [online] Available at: https://pubmed.ncbi.nlm.nih.gov/30154767/ [Accessed 8 October 2023].

Koziel, J., Mydel, P., and Potempa, J. (2014). The Link Between Periodontal Disease and Rheumatoid Arthritis: An Updated Review. Current Rheumatology Reports, [online] https://www.ncbi.nlm.nih.gov/pmc/articles/PMC3930831/ [Accessed 15 October 2023].

Juárez, P. (2018). The Public Health Exposome. *Springer eBooks* [online] Available at: https://doi.org/10.1007/978-3-319-89321-1_2 [Accessed 22 January 2024].

Loesche, W.J. (2017). *Microbiology of Dental Decay and Periodontal Disease*. [online] National Library of Medicine [online] Available at: https://www.ncbi.nlm.nih.gov/books/NBK8259/ [Accessed 15 October 2023].

Masten, S., Davies, S. and McElmurry, S. (2016). Flint Water Crisis: What Happened and Why? *Journal - American Water Works Association*, [online] Available at: https://awwa.onlinelibrary.wiley.com/doi/abs/10.5942/jawwa.2016.108.0195 [Accessed 5 October 2023].

McDermott, J., et al., (2012). Challenges in biomarker discovery: combining expert insights with statistical analysis of complex omics data. *Expert Opinion on Medical Diagnostics* [online] Available at: https://www.tandfonline.com/doi/abs/10.1517/17530059.2012.718329 [Accessed 6 October 2023].

Michaud, D., et al., (2016). Periodontal disease and risk of all cancers among male never smokers: an updated analysis of the Health Professionals Follow-up Study. *Annals of Oncology: Official Journal of the European Society for Medical Oncology*, [online] Available at: https://pubmed.ncbi.nlm.nih.gov/26811350/ [Accessed 15 October 2023].

National Human Genome Research Institute (2020). *The Human Genome Project*. [online] Genome.gov. Available at: https://www.genome.gov/human-genome-project [Accessed 4 October 2023].

Ogunrinola, G., et al., (2020). The Human Microbiome and Its Impacts on Health. *International Journal of Microbiology*, [online] Available at: https://pubmed.ncbi.nlm.nih.gov/32612660/ [Accessed 3 October 2023].

Oral Health and Diabetes in Patients Experiencing Homelessness. (2019). [online] Available at: https://nhchc.org/wp-content/uploads/2019/08/nhchc-nnoha-faq_final3.pdf [Accessed 15 October 2023].

Patel, C., Bhattacharya, J. and Butte, A. (2010). An Environment-Wide Association Study (EWAS) on Type 2 Diabetes Mellitus. *PLoS ONE*, 5(5). [online] Available at: https://journals.plos.org/plosone/article?id=10.1371/journal.pone.0010746 [Accessed 5 October 2023].

Rasooly, D., Drzymalla, E. and Khoury, M. (2021). *From the Genome to the Exposome: Mapping Causal Associations Between Environmental Factors and Population Health | Blogs | CDC*. [online] Available at: https://blogs.cdc.gov/genomics/2022/09/06/from-the-genome-to-the-exposome/ [Accessed 4 October 2023].

Robinson, J. (2023). Spontaneous preterm birth: Overview of risk factors and prognosis UpToDate. [online] Available at: https://bit.ly/3FjQp1a [Accessed 15 Oct. 2023].

Sanz, M., et al., (2020). Periodontitis and cardiovascular diseases: Consensus report. *Journal of Clinical Periodontology*, [online] Available at: https://www.ncbi.nlm.nih.gov/pmc/articles/PMC7027895/ [Accessed 15 October 2023].

Strianese, O., et al., (2020). Precision and Personalized Medicine: How Genomic Approach Improves the Management of Cardiovascular and Neurodegenerative Disease. *Genes*, [online] Available at: https://www.mdpi.com/2073-4425/11/7/747 [Accessed 6 October 2023].

Thornton-Evans, G. et al; (2013). *Periodontitis Among Adults Aged ≥30 Years — United States, 2009–2010*. Morbidity and Mortality Weekly [online] Available at: https://bit.ly/46TyqKv [Accessed 5 Oct. 2023].

Lexicon of Listed Terms and Agencies

- **Exposome** describes the environmental exposures encountered throughout life and the way in which they impact health and well-being.
- **Genome** all the genetic information (DNA and RNA) of an organism.
- **Human Genome Project** the Human Genome Project (HGP) is one of the greatest scientific feats in history. The project was a voyage of biological discovery led by an international group of researchers looking to comprehensively study all the DNA (known as a genome) of a select set of organisms.
- **Microbiome** the collection of all microbes, such as bacteria, fungi, viruses, and their genes, that naturally live on our bodies and inside us collectively known as microbiota.

AUTHOR'S BIO SKETCH

David Greco, MD

Dr. Greco is a Family Medicine resident physician in Washington state at the University of Washington affiliated Community Health Care – a Federally Qualified Health Center. Originally from the Midwest where he split his time between multiple states with very cold winters, he made the move to the Pacific Northwest with the goal of learning how to provide equitable healthcare to underserved patient populations. Before medicine, he served as a high school teacher and continues to have a passion for education. When he is not in clinic, you can find Dr. Greco enjoying a good book or film, out for a jog, or drinking a local cup of coffee.

Chapter 17

The Obesity Pandemic and Social Determinants of Health

David Estroff MD, FAAP, Author
Clinical Professor Emeritus of Pediatrics, University of Washington
Janell Harro, MD, Editor

"The physical and emotional health of an entire generation and the economic health and security of our nation is at stake."

- First Lady Michelle Obama, Let's Move!

Obesity in the context of Prevalence

An epidemic of overweight and obesity and its health consequences began in the mid-1970's in the United States of America and has spread widely in the rest of the world, meeting the definition of a pandemic. While the problem is present in both developed and developing countries, the focus in this review is on the United States of America.

The latest CDC National Health and Nutrition Examination Survey (Stierman, et al., 2021) showed that among children and adolescents aged 2–19 years, the prevalence of obesity [BMI ≥95%ile] has increased since 1976 from approximately 6% to 19.7% (**Figure 1**). Among adults aged 20 and over, the age-adjusted prevalence of obesity [BMI ≥30 kg/m^2] has increased over the same interval from 15% to 41.9%, and severe obesity [BMI ≥40 kg/m^2] from 1% to 9.2% (**Figure 2**).

Obesity in both adults and children is not distributed uniformly in the U.S. population but is significantly more prevalent in some states and is disproportionately prevalent in different ethnic groups. For example, 3 states (Louisiana, Oklahoma, and West Virginia) have adult obesity rates ≥40%, and 6 states have rates between 25% and 30%. Nationally, obesity is most prevalent among non-Hispanic Black adults at 49.9%, in Hispanics at 45.6%, in non-Hispanic whites at 41.4%, and in non-Hispanic Asians at 16.1%. (Stierman, et al., 2021). Explore Maps **Figures 3, 4, 5, 6 & 7.**

Figure 1 Prevalence of Obesity in Children 2 - 19 years 1963 – 2018 (Fryar, Carrol, and Afful, 2021b)

Figure. Trends in obesity among children and adolescents aged 2–19 years, by age: United States, 1963–1965 through 2017–2018

Percent

25

20

15

10

5

0

12–19 years

All ages

2–5 years

6–11 years

1963–1965 | 1966–1967 | 1971–1974 | 1976–1980 | 1988–1994 | 1999–2000 | 2001–2002 | 2003–2004 | 2005–2006 | 2007–2008 | 2009–2010 | 2011–2012 | 2013–2014 | 2015–2016 | 2017–2018

NOTE: Obesity is body mass index (BMI) at or above the 95th percentile from the sex-specific BMI-for-age 2000 CDC Growth Charts.
SOURCES: National Center for Health Statistics, National Health Examination Surveys II (ages 6–11), III (ages 12–17); and National Health and Nutrition Examination Surveys (NHANES) I–III, and NHANES 1999–2000, 2001–2002, 2003–2004, 2005–2006, 2007–2008, 2009–2010, 2011–2012, 2013–2014, 2015–2016, and 2017–2018.

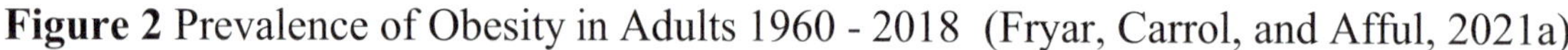

Figure 2 Prevalence of Obesity in Adults 1960 - 2018 (Fryar, Carrol, and Afful, 2021a)

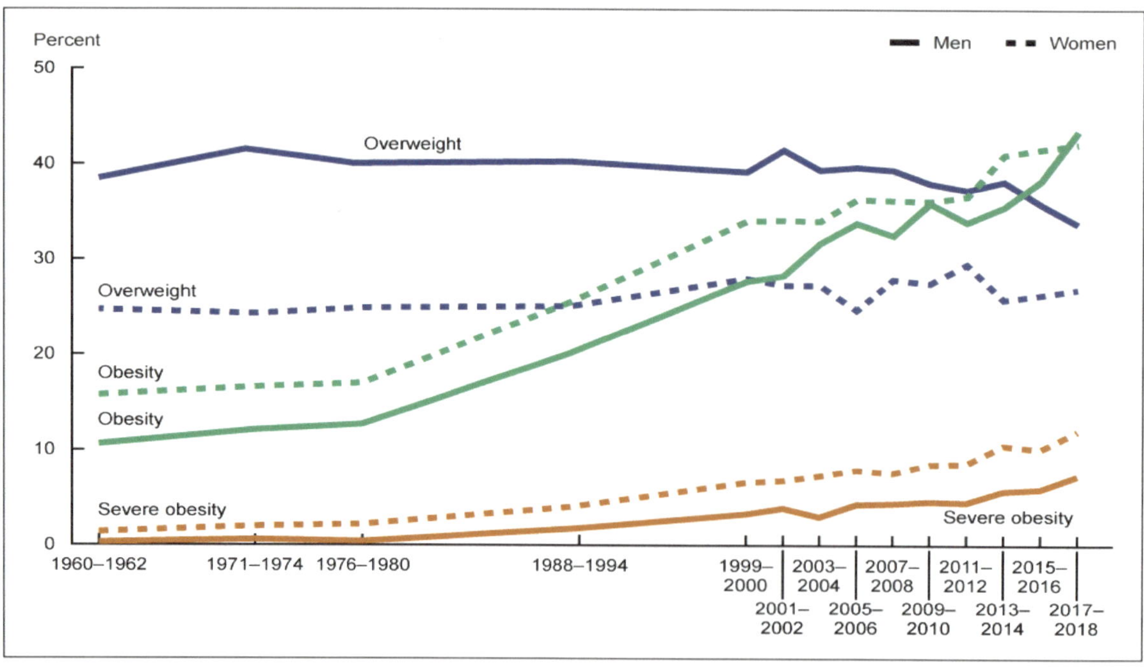

NOTES: Data are age adjusted by the direct method to U.S. Census 2000 estimates using age groups 20–39, 40–59, and 60–74. Overweight is body mass index (BMI) of 25.0–29.9 kg/m². Obesity is BMI at or above 30.0 kg/m². Severe obesity is BMI at or above 40.0 kg/m². Pregnant women are excluded from the analysis.
SOURCES: National Center for Health Statistics, National Health Examination Survey and National Health and Nutrition Examination Surveys.

Figure 3 Prevalence of Obesity Based on Self-Reported Weight and Height Among U.S. Adults by State and Territory, BRFSS, 2022 (CDC, 2023)

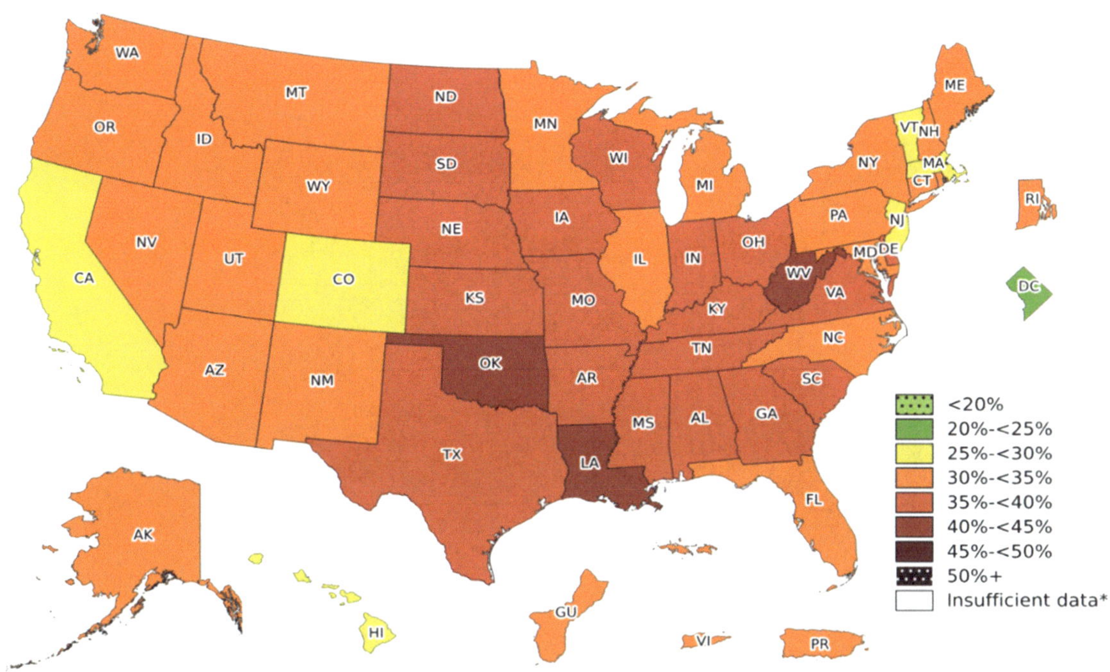

Figure 4 Prevalence of Obesity Based on Self-Reported Weight and Height Among Non-Hispanic Black Adults by State and Territory, BRFSS, 2020–2022 (CDC, 2023)

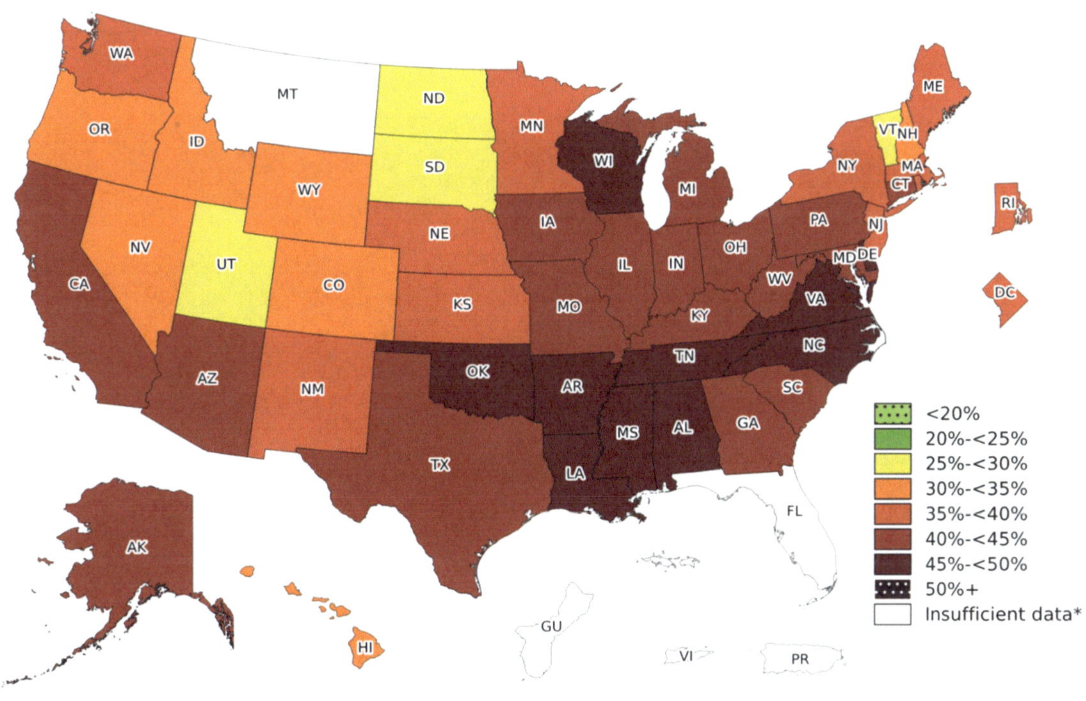

Figure 5 Prevalence of Obesity Based on Self-Reported Weight and Height Among Hispanic Adults by State and Territory, BRFSS, 2020–2022 (CDC, 2023)

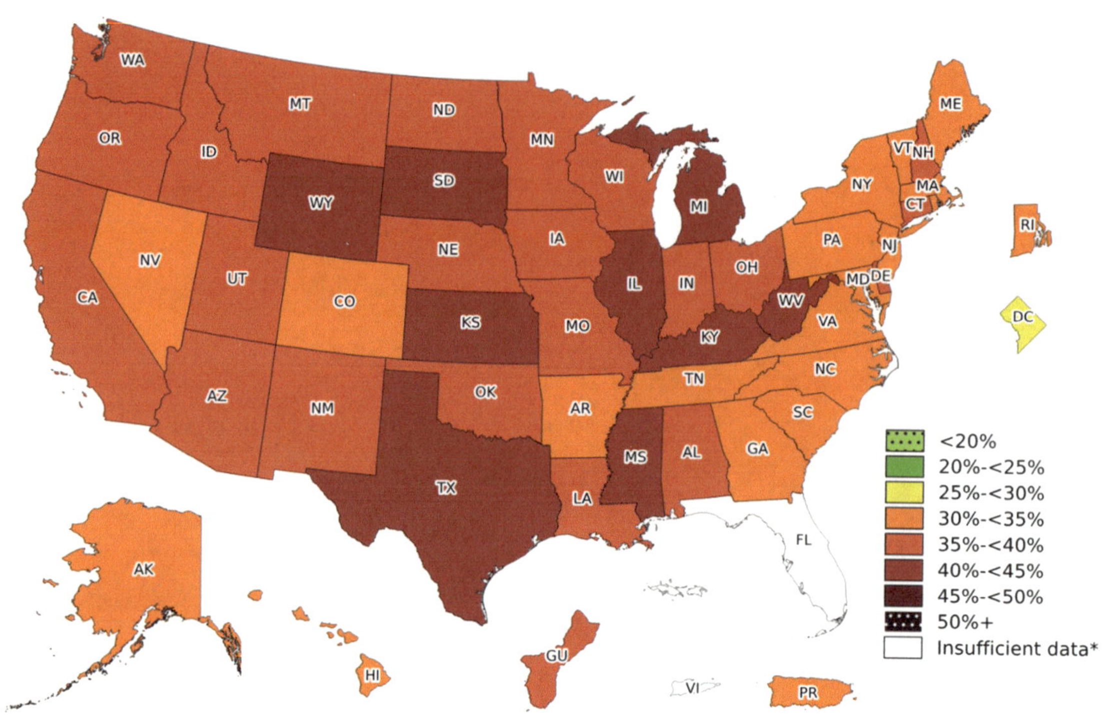

Figure 6 Prevalence of Obesity Based on Self-Reported Weight and Height Among Non-Hispanic White Adults by State and Territory, BRFSS, 2020–2022 (CDC, 2023)

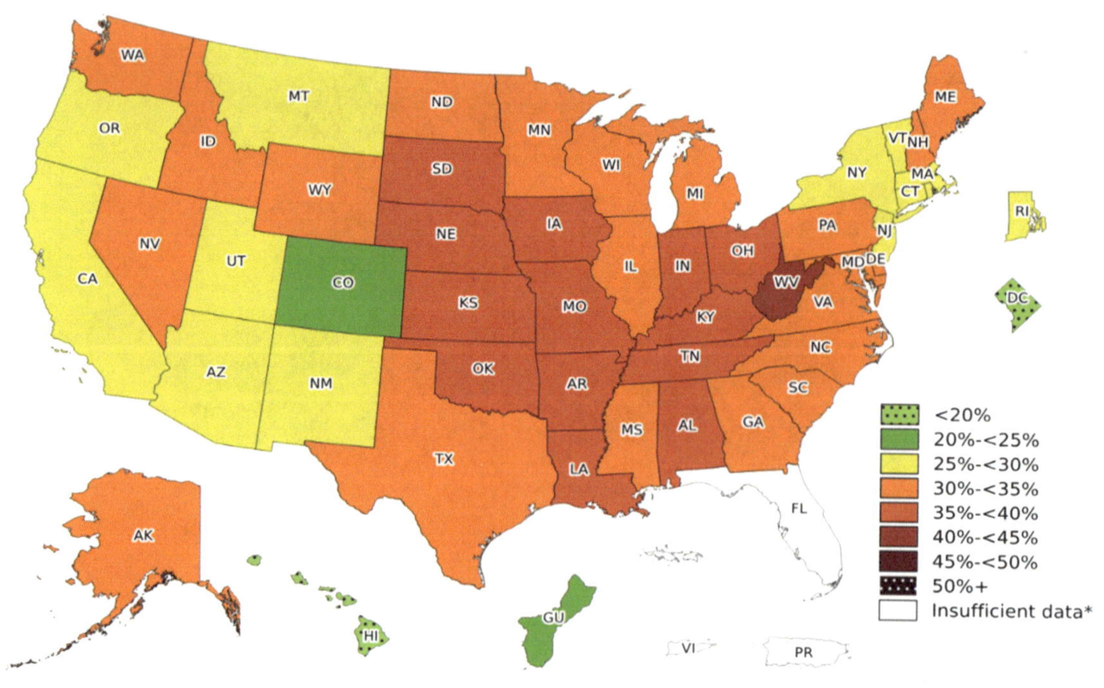

Figure 7 Estimated proportion of children aged 10 – 17 years experiencing overweight or obesity, county level United States, 2016 (Zgodic, et al., 2021)

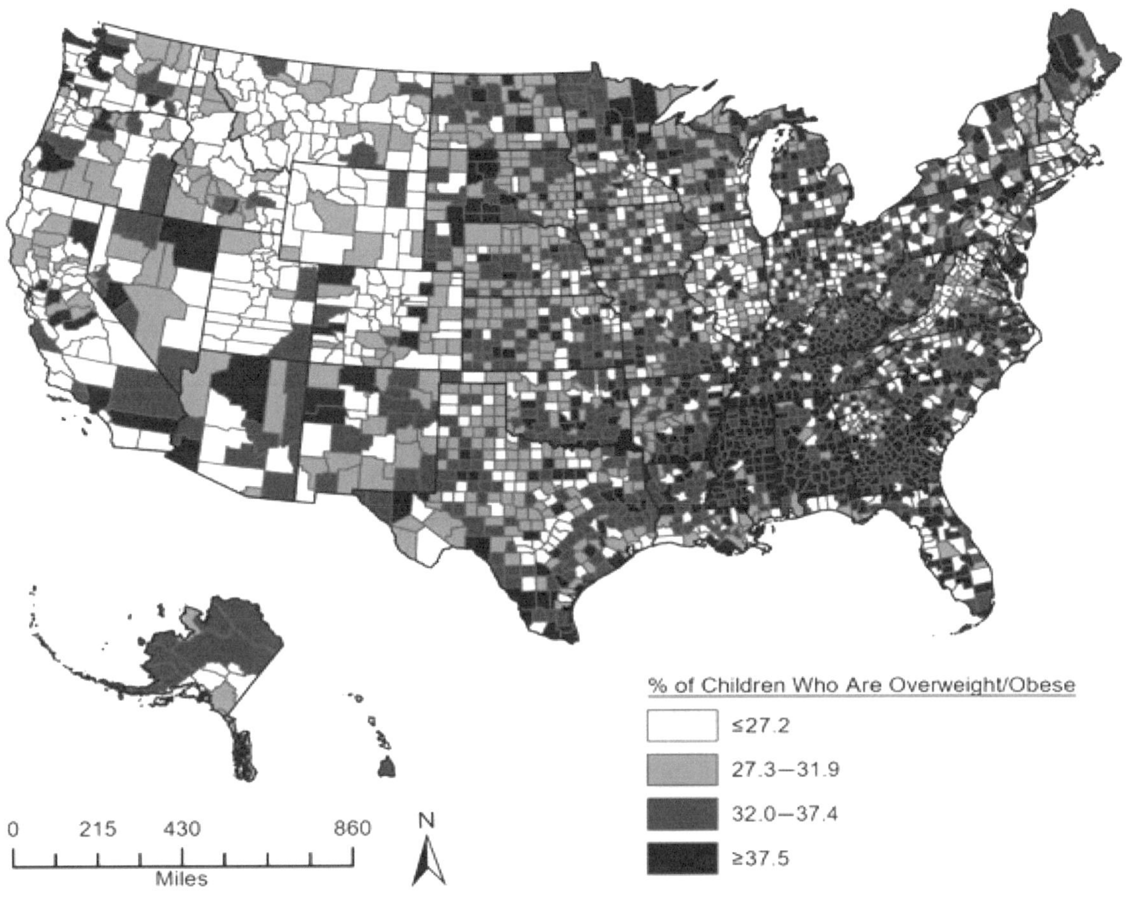

Obesity in the context of Consequences

Obesity in adults increases the risk for many acute and chronic health conditions: (CDC, 2022a)

- High blood pressure and high cholesterol – risk factors for heart disease and stroke.
- Type 2 diabetes: The current estimate is that 11.3% of the adult population has this chronic disease. (CDC, 2022b). In the United States, life expectancy for women and men with diabetes at age ≥50 years was 8.2 and 7.5 years less, respectively, than for comparable individuals without diabetes. (Rosenquist and Fox, 2018).
- Breathing problems, such as asthma and sleep apnea.
- Joint problems – osteoarthritis and musculoskeletal discomfort.
- Non-alcoholic fatty liver disease, gallstones, and gallbladder disease.
- Significant increased risk of severe outcomes and death from COVID-19.

- Higher risks for many types of cancer: 4–8% of all cancers are attributed to obesity, including post-menopausal breast, colorectal, endometrial, kidney, esophageal, pancreatic, liver, and gallbladder cancer. Excess body fat results in an approximately 17% increased risk of cancer-specific mortality. (Pati, et al., 2023). Obesity is poised to overtake tobacco as the No. 1 preventable cause of cancer (Achenbach, et al., 2023).
- Mental illness such as clinical depression and anxiety.

Childhood obesity is associated with:

- Triple the risk of hospitalization from COVID-19 (Kompaniyets, et al., 2021).
- Psychological problems such as anxiety and depression.
- Low self-esteem and lower self-reported quality of life.
- Social problems such as bullying and stigma.
- Obesity as adults. Obese children and adolescents are five times more likely to be obese in adulthood than those who were not obese. 55% of obese children go on to be obese in adolescence, 80% of obese adolescents will still be obese in adulthood and 70% will be obese over age 30. (Simmonds, et al., 2016)

Obesity associated comorbidities have had a profound effect on the health and life expectancy of the American population. Severe obesity results in an estimated 5 to 20 years shortening of life expectancy. (Olshansky, et al., 2005). The rate of obesity related deaths for adults aged 35 to 64 doubled from 1979 to 2000, then doubled again from 2000 to 2019. Obesity is one reason progress against heart disease, after accelerating between 1980 and 2000, has slowed.

A modeling study estimated that excess weight associated disease in the U.S. was responsible for over 1300 deaths per day (nearly 500,000 per year) in 2016, contributing to higher excess mortality than smoking, with large disparities by state and subgroup. Relative excess mortality rates were twice as high for women compared to men in 2016 (21.9% vs 13.9%) and were higher for Black non-Hispanic adults. Overall state-level losses in life expectancy due to excess weight ranged from 1.75 years in Colorado to 3.18 years in Mississippi. (Ward, et al., 2022).

Figure 8. Comorbidities associated with obesity (Upadhyay, et al., 2018).

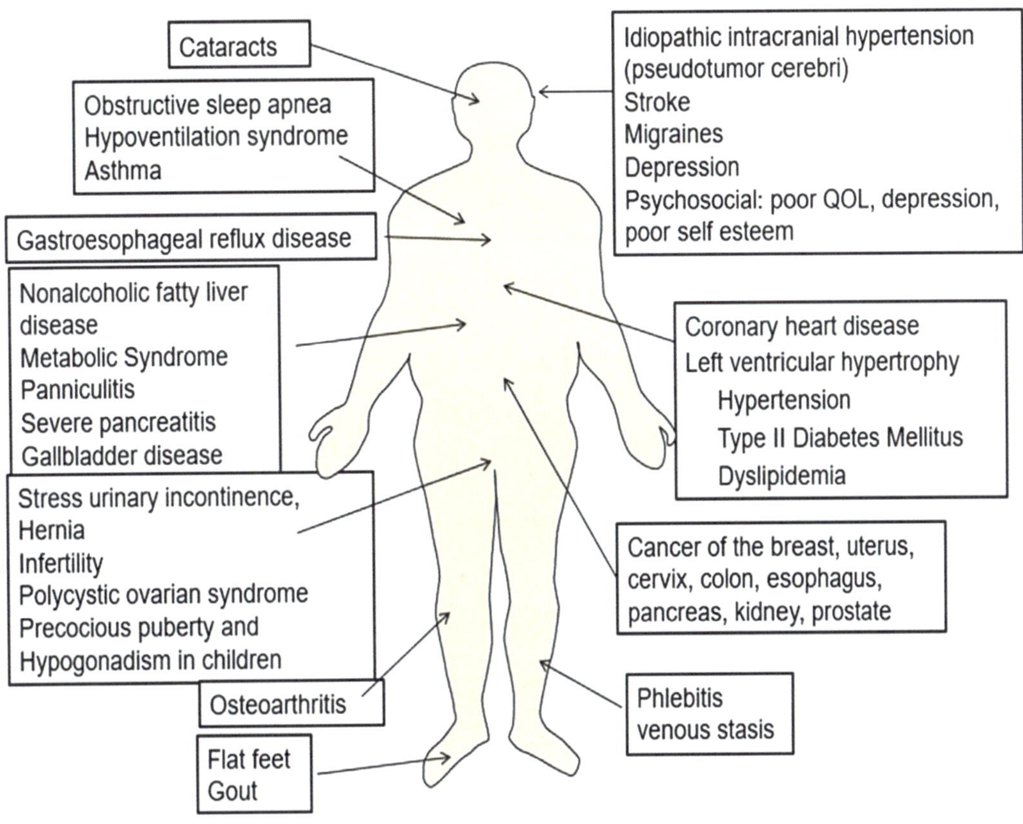

Upadhyay, J., Farr, O., Perakakis, N., Ghaly, W. and Mantzoros, C. (2018). Obesity as a Disease. *Medical Clinics of North America*, [online] Available at: https://doi.org/10.1016/j.mcna.2017.08.004

Obesity in the context of Economic Burden

"In 2016, chronic diseases driven by the risk factor of obesity and overweight accounted for $480.7 billion in direct health care costs in the U.S. (14.4% of total 2016 U.S. health care expenditure) (Rama, 2018), with an additional $1.24 trillion in indirect costs due to lost economic productivity. The total cost of chronic diseases due to obesity and overweight was $1.72 trillion, equivalent to 9.3 percent of the U.S. gross domestic product (GDP). Obesity as a risk factor is by far the greatest contributor to the burden of chronic diseases in the U.S. accounting for 47.1 percent of the total cost of chronic diseases nationwide in 2016" (Waters and Graf, 2018).

Obesity in the context of Causation

A 2023 National Library of Medicine PubMed search using "obesity AND cause" as terms, produced over 231,000 results, which speaks to the alarm, perplexity and complexity surrounding the obesity pandemic. **Figure 9** conceptualizes the vast array of factors influencing the epidemiology of obesity from a population perspective.

Figure 9.

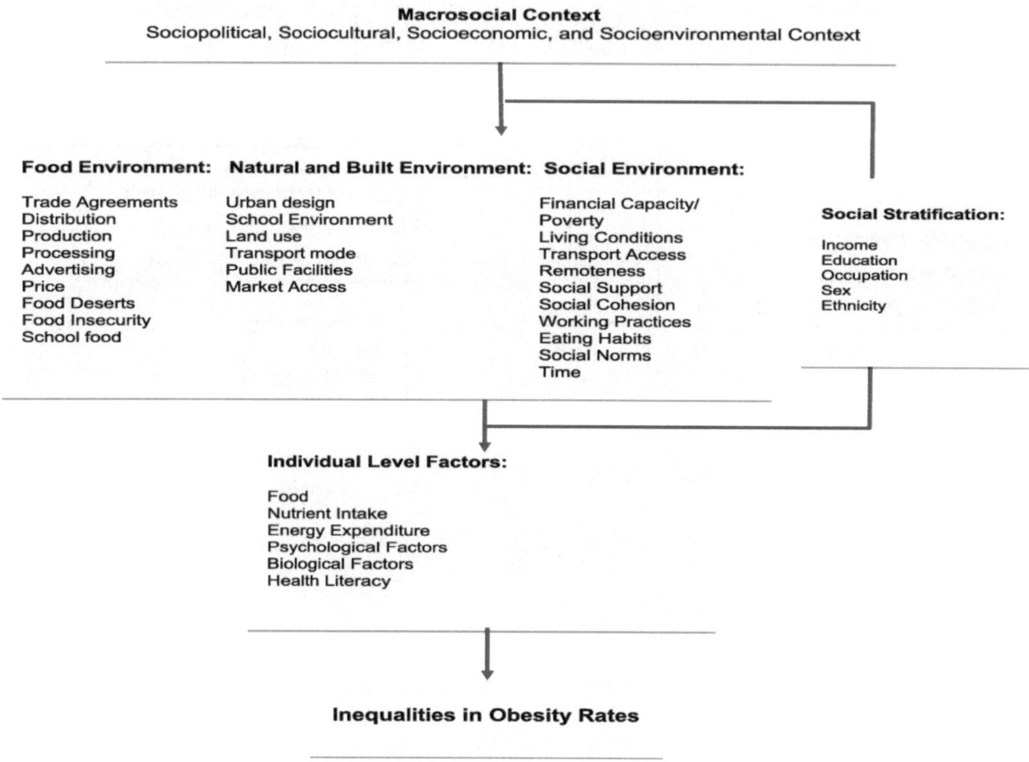

Vargas, C., Stines, E. and Granado, H. (2017). Health-equity issues related to childhood obesity: a scoping review. *Journal of Public Health Dentistry*, [online] Available at: https://doi.org/10.1111/jphd.12233

Obesity - Causation in the context of Food & Food Insecurity

On an individual level, qualifying and quantifying the array of risk factors implicated in the development of obesity defies analysis. We do know that poverty, food insecurity, food choices, physical inactivity, sedentary activity, dietary trends and habits, genetic and antenatal factors, stress, adverse life experiences, gender, social injustice, built environment, racism, and health behaviors are all risk factors (Hassink, 2023 and Ranjani, et al., 2014).

Weight gain is a critical and normal part of growth, required for development of healthy infants, children, and adults. To accomplish this, calorie and nutrient intake must exceed all of the metabolic demands required to maintain homeostasis and support physical activity, and to supply the substrates needed to build new tissues. When total food energy intake exceeds the metabolic demands needed for normal growth and/or maintenance of weight and physical activity in the fetus, infant, child or adult, our “thrifty” metabolism stores the surplus nutrients for future need should nutrient supplies decrease or cease.

The body stores all of the surplus energy it consumes from food in 2 forms, fats, and proteins, with a small amount as glycogen, a glucose polymer carbohydrate. Fats store more than twice the calories per gram than protein or glycogen. Excess ingested carbohydrates induce the formation of triglycerides by glycolysis, driven by increased insulin levels, which then are stored in adipose tissue and the liver. “Because the storage capacity for carbohydrate is extremely limited, any excess carbohydrate must be oxidized promptly. Thus, when people overeat, they oxidize carbohydrate and store [it as] fat” (Bray, 2004). Fructose, found as a sweetener in many foods and sugar sweetened beverages (often as high fructose corn syrup) is metabolized differently than glucose. It enters cells without depending on insulin and rapidly enters pathways that synthesize triglycerides (fat equivalent) and stored. (Bray, 2004).

“At a population level, changes in obesity prevalence can only be explained by broad environmental change, given the stasis in human biology over the same time frame” (Brierley, 2021). Access to processed foods accounts for a significant component of this shift. Changes in diet contribute significantly to the obesity pandemic across the socioeconomic spectrum. “The past few decades have seen enormous shifts in the global food system, with billions of people now routinely exposed to high-energy processed food and drinks, marketed with increasing sophistication by multinational corporations" (Brierley, 2021). Furthermore, changes in diet and eating habits, shaped by the economic, cultural, social, and physical environments of modern life exaggerate the adverse physiologic effects of life stress caused by multiple economic and social inequities.

Many of the agricultural staples used to make ultra-processed foods (UPFs) are subsidized by government policy. Do, et al., (2020) argue that "Agricultural subsidies from the U.S. Farm Bill, which primarily support the production of corn, soybeans, wheat, rice, sorghum, dairy, and livestock feed, may be playing a role in unhealthy food consumption patterns and, subsequently, in the development of obesity and diet-related chronic diseases. For example, corn represents one of the most widely produced and federally subsidized crops in the U.S. with the majority of its product ending up in animal and livestock feed or heavily processed foods as high fructose corn syrup, including sugar-sweetened beverages (SSBs), cereals, and alcohol."

Ultra-processed foods are "typically prepared from mostly cheap sources of dietary energy and nutrients plus additives. They are mostly high in calories, salt, sugar, and fat but contain minimal amounts of whole foods. As a result, they have a low content of dietary fiber, phytochemicals (for example, lutein, lycopene, and anthrocyanins), and of various micronutrients, such as potassium, magnesium, and vitamin C" (Temple, 2022). The spectrum of processing foods based on the NOVA classification (a framework for grouping edible substances based on the extent and purpose of processing) **Figure 10** provides examples of foods and types of processing methods within each NOVA classification group (Crimarco, Landry, and Gardner (2022).

Figure 10.

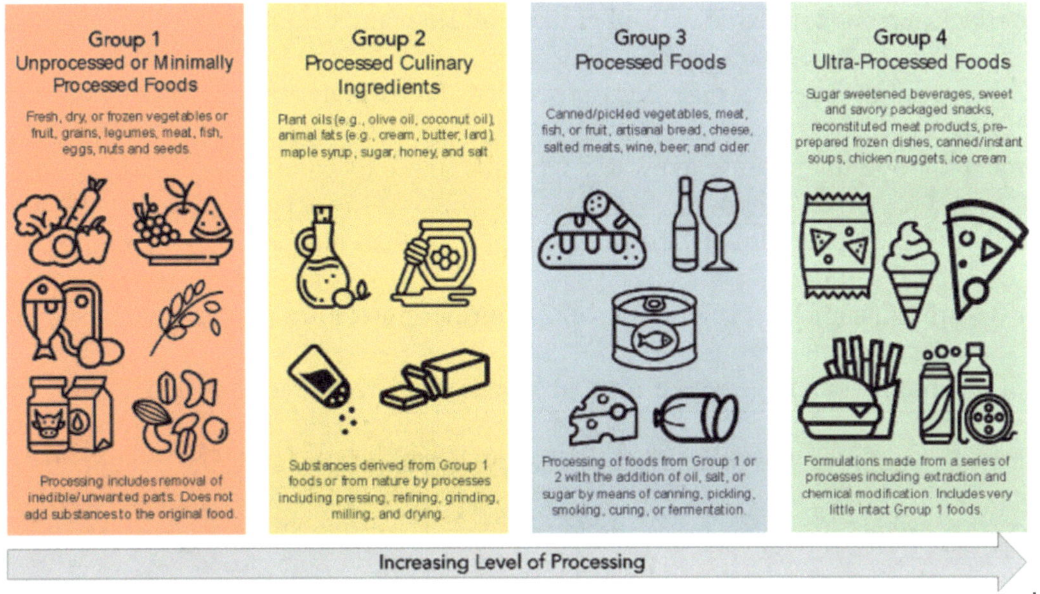

Crimarco, A., Landry, M. and Gardner, C. (2022). *Ultra-processed Foods, Weight Gain, and Comorbidity Risk*. [online] Available at: https://pubmed.ncbi.nlm.nih.gov/34677812/ Definitions adapted from Monteiro, et al (2018).

Food consumption studies lend support for the association with the parallel rise in obesity and UPF consumption as etiologic to the obesity pandemic. The majority of energy intake among individuals in high-income countries comes from ultra-processed foods and beverages. UPFs contributed 61-62% of calories in packaged food and beverage purchases from retail food stores by households in the U.S. between 2000 and 2012 (Poti, Braga, and Qin, 2017) and according to Temple (2022) estimates conclude that UPF's now provide 57% of all calories consumed while minimally processed foods only supply 27.4%.

Eating ultra-processed food at fast food restaurants now constitutes a sizable proportion of the American diet for children, adolescents, and adults. "In the 1970s, an average U.S. adult (aged 18–65 y) consumed fast food on <10% of days, but this had risen to 40.7% of days in 2017–2018. Among U.S. survey participants aged 12–39 y in 2017–2018, 45.7% consumed fast food daily for 40.6% of their daily energy intake" (Popkin, 2022). "The overall percentage of adults who consumed fast food decreased with age, increased with income, and was higher among non-Hispanic Black persons compared with other race and Hispanic-origin groups" (Fryar, et al., 2020).

Other studies suggest that ultra-processed foods may facilitate overeating and the development of obesity because they are typically high in calories, salt, sugar, and fat and engineered to have supernormal *appetitive* properties that may result in pathological eating behavior (Gearhardt and DiFeliceantonio, 2022). Furthermore, ultra-processed foods are theorized to disrupt gut-brain signaling, which may influence food reinforcement and overall intake via mechanisms distinct from the palatability or energy density of the food (Hall, et al., 2019).

During a two-week inpatient study conducted at the NIH (**Figure 11**), researchers investigated whether people ate more calories when provided with a diet composed of ultra-processed foods or a diet composed of unprocessed foods and could consume as much or as little as they wanted. Despite ultra-processed and unprocessed diets being matched for daily available

Figure 11.

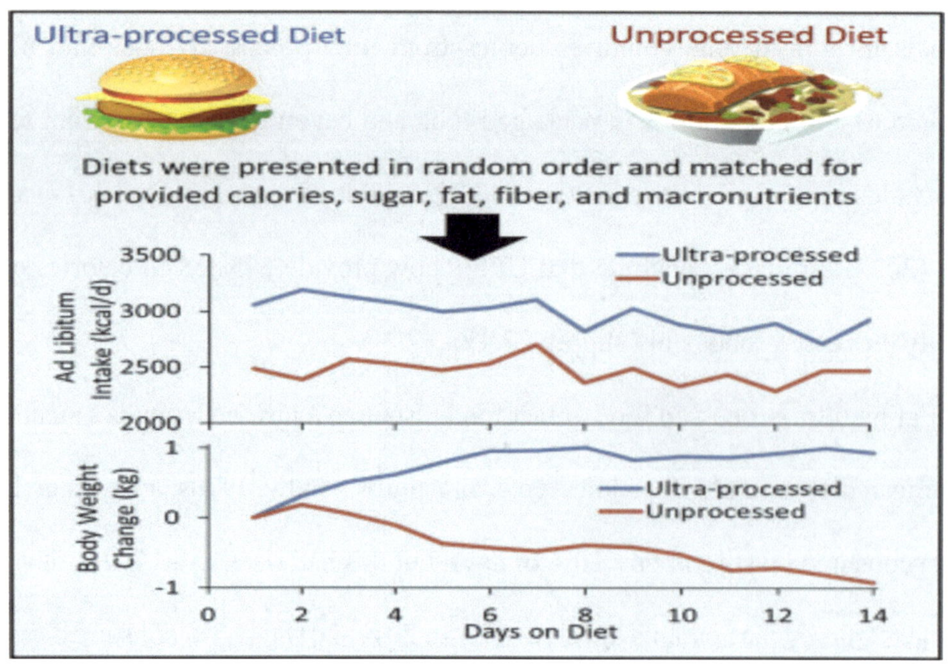

Hall, K., et al., (2019). Ultra-Processed Diets Cause Excess Calorie Intake and Weight Gain: An Inpatient Randomized Controlled Trial of Ad Libitum Food Intake. *Cell Metabolism*, [online] https://doi.org/10.1016/j.cmet.2019.05.008

calories, sugar, fat, fiber, and macronutrients, people consumed 508 kcal/day more when eating the ultra-processed diet as compared to the unprocessed diet. Furthermore, people gained weight (0.9 ±0.3 kg) on the ultra-processed diet and lost weight (0.9 ±0.3kg) on the unprocessed diet. (Hall, et al., 2019).

Ultra-processed Foods in the context of Life-Expectancy and Disease

In a 15-year cohort study of almost 20,000 Spanish university graduates, "A higher consumption of ultra-processed foods (>4 servings daily) was independently associated with a 62% increased hazard for all-cause mortality. For each additional serving of ultra-processed food, all-cause mortality increased by 18%." (Rico-Campà, et al., 2019).

In the 25-year Coronary Artery Risk Development in Young Adults (CARDIA) study, researchers analyzed fast-food disease relationships, "Increased fast food intake significantly affected every measure, ranging from visceral fat to fatty liver, waist circumference, and BMI. The results showed clinically meaningful increases such as 3.9 units of BMI and 9.4 centimeters of waist circumference in the fully controlled models but the odds for increased risk of associated metabolic factor fatty liver disease were quite substantial, rising from a risk of 2.03 to 5.18 from the lowest to the highest measure of fast-food consumption" (Lloyd-Jones, et al., 2021).

Obesity - Causation in the context of Poverty

Leung, et al., (2022) define food insecurity as "the limited or uncertain availability of nutritionally adequate and safe foods or the limited or uncertain ability to acquire acceptable foods in socially acceptable ways." Food insecurity is a critical social determinant of health. In 2019, the estimated prevalence of food insecurity was 10.5% (or 13.7 million) U.S. households.

The social determinant of health domain that most directly correlates with and predicts obesity in the United States is poverty and economic instability. Panel A in **Figure 12** shows the correlation between low income and the prevalence of obesity in over 3000 U.S. counties. Counties with poverty rates of >35% have obesity rates 145% greater than wealthy counties **Figure 12** (Levine, 2011).

Figure 12.

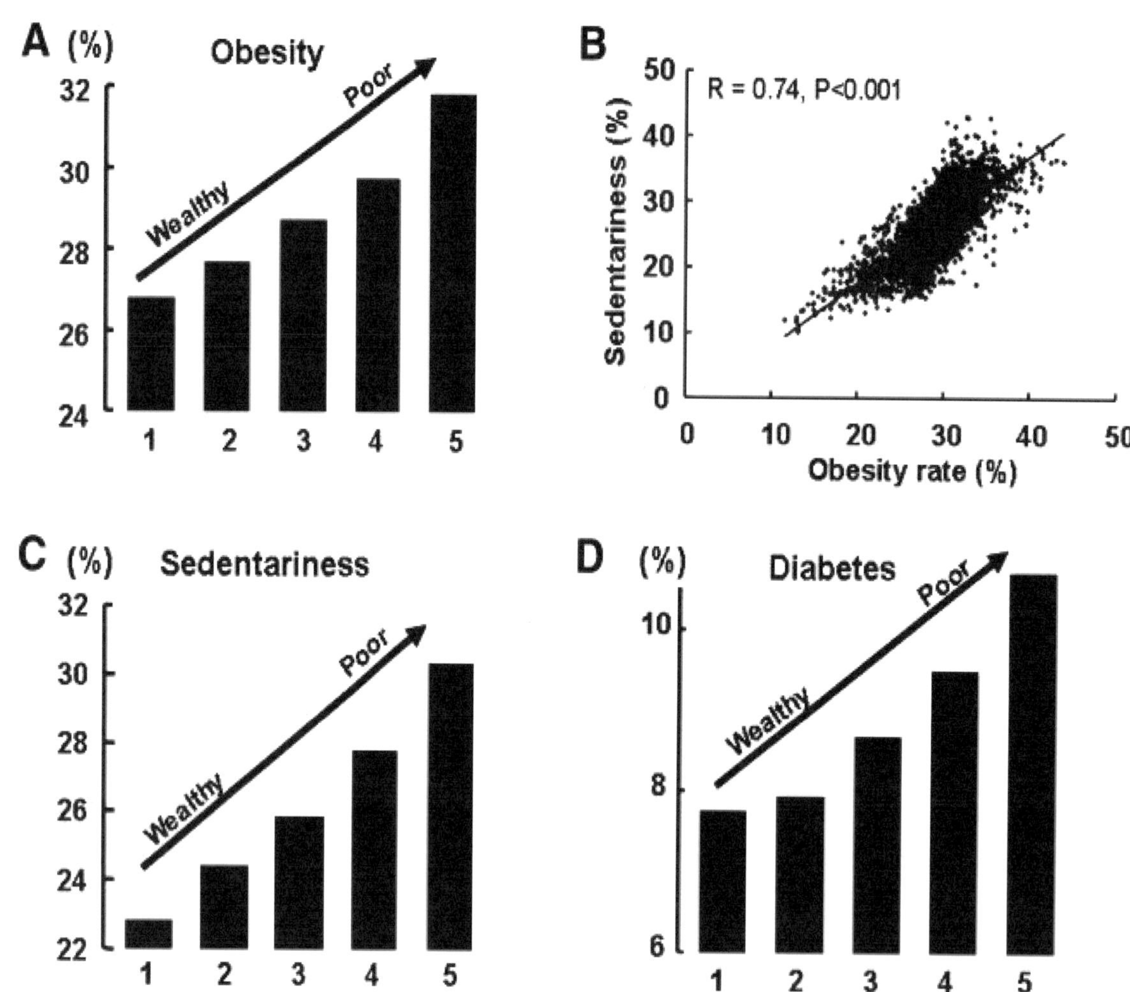

Data from 3,139 counties in the U.S. Quintiles are cohorts of counties ranked by the percentage of people living with poverty. Quintile 1, the wealthiest quintile, includes 630 U.S. counties with a mean county poverty rate of 8.2% (median household income, $56,259). Quintile 5, the poorest quintile, includes 629 counties with a mean poverty rate of 25% (median household income, $32,679). A: County age-adjusted obesity rates by poverty quintile. B: County obesity rates vs. county leisure-time sedentary rates (sedentary adults are those who report no physical activity or exercise other than at their regular job). C: County sedentary rates. D: Age-adjusted diabetes rate by poverty quintile.

Levine, J. (2011). Poverty and Obesity in the U.S. *Diabetes*, [online] Available at: https://doi.org/10.2337/db11-1118 [Accessed 24 November 2023].

Magnifying the influence of food insecurity, extreme poverty neighborhoods promote sedentary behaviors through epidemic community violence that reduces the safety for out of doors activities and neighborhood environments that lack accessible parks and sport facilities. **Figure 12** Panel B highlights the meaningful relationship between sedentariness and obesity. Panel C demonstrates the relationship between income and sedentariness, and panel D reveals the risk of diabetes increasing with poverty (Levine, 2011).

Obesity disproportionally affects low-income individuals. According to (Bentley, Ormerod and Ruck, 2018), a 2015 study revealed that in states where the median income was less than $45,000, 35% of the population were obese. This compared to states where the median income exceeded $65,000, where less than 25% of population were obese.

The proportion of obese individuals in industrialized nations correlates inversely with median household income and has been described as the "poverty-obesity paradox" according to Hruschka and Han (2017). In the simplest view, obesity in developed economies is a result of over-abundance of inexpensive food calories combined with decreases in daily physical activity in the industrialized world and its built environment (Mattson, et al., 2014).

This observation is linked to limited access to nutritious food and reduced opportunities for physical activity. Approximately 6.1 percent of the U.S. population resides in a "food desert" where the nearest supermarket is 1 to 10 miles away making access to affordable, nutritious foods challenging (Rhone, 2022). The correlation between poverty and decreased minutes of weekly exercise is well-documented. For example, a Colorado survey investigating factors influencing reduced exercise in children found that common responses from parents included a lack of affordable exercise options and concerns about the safety of the environment for physical activity (Finkelstein, Peterson, and Schottenfeld, 2017).

Obesity - Causation in the context of Life Stressors

Figure 13 depicts a complex interplay between multiple stressors and physiologic, biochemical, neurologic, and pathologic feedback loops that perpetuate an obesity cycle. According to Hassink (2023) *major life events* (death of a family member, homelessness, and violence), *adverse social determinants of health* (racism, poverty, and food insecurity), *adverse childhood experiences* (see **Table 1** below), *weight stigma and bias* (bullying, body slamming) and *chronic disease* stand out.

Figure 13.

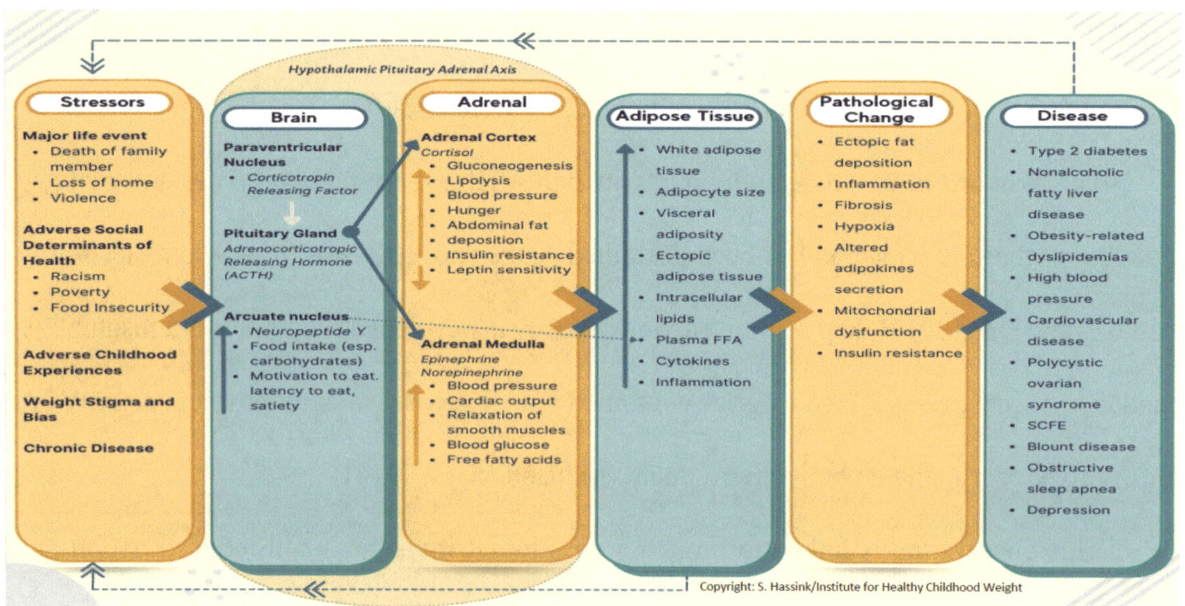

Hassink, S. (2023). *Physiologic Impact of the Social Determinants of Health. [PowerPoint] Evaluation and Treatment of Children and Adolescents with Obesity Continued… Getting the Guidelines to Work for You, Your Patients and Families in Practice.* Presentation at 'Pediatric Pearls for Office Practice' 46th Annual Day of Pediatrics. MultiCare Department of CME, Tacoma, WA. 30 September 2023.

The dramatic rise in obesity witnessed in children ages 2 – 19 years – from 6 % to 19.7% since 1976 and the surge in adult obesity over the same period from 15% to 41.9% (Fryar, Carrol, and Afful, 2021a & 2021b) confirms the extent of the obesity crisis in the U.S. A discussion on stressors, especially adverse childhood experiences, seems imperative.

The Centers for Disease Control (CDC) in conjunction with Kaiser Permanente researched health outcomes in children experiencing adverse childhood experiences in 1995-1997. According to Healthwise (2023), Kaiser defines Adverse Childhood Experiences (ACEs) as follows (**Table 1**):

Table 1.

Commonly Cited Adverse Childhood Experiences Include:

- Emotional abuse. An adult insults, puts down, or swears at a child. Or an adult acts in a way that makes the child afraid they will be hurt.
- Physical abuse. An adult hits, kicks, or physically hurts a child.
- Sexual abuse. An adult (or older child) touches a child in a sexual way, makes a child touch them in a sexual way, or has sex (or tries to have sex) with a child.
- Violence in the home. A child sees adults in the home physically harming each other.
- Substance use problems in the home. A household member has problems with drinking, drug use, or misusing prescription medicines.
- Mental health problems in the home. A household member is depressed, has mental health issues, or has attempted or died by suicide.
- Emotional neglect. An adult in the home doesn't make a child feel safe, protected, and cared for.
- Physical neglect. An adult in the home doesn't make sure that a child's basic needs are met.
- Divorce or separation of parents.
- Having a household member go to prison.

Healthwise, S. (2023). *Understanding Adverse Childhood Experiences (ACEs) | Kaiser Permanente.* [online] healthy.kaiserpermanente.org. Available at: https://healthy.kaiserpermanente.org/health-wellness/health-encyclopedia/he.understanding-adverse-childhood-experiences-aces.acm1444

"Multiple biological, psychological, and social mechanisms may operate together to link childhood psychosocial challenges to adult obesity. For example, childhood maltreatment may lead to obesity via both direct physiologic impacts of HPA-axis regulation [**Figure 14**], through disruption of normal development of executive function, which in turn may result in truncated educational attainment, or through increased sexual risk taking which can result in early childrearing. Our findings suggest a possible etiologic role of childhood exposure to maltreatment in both males and females that is not explained or mediated by other related psychosocial challenges and appears to have a particularly strong role for extreme obesity in women. Our findings also highlight the elevated risk for obesity among those experiencing childhood poverty, low educational attainment, and early childrearing. Populations with these risk patterns should be considered in obesity prevention and treatment strategies. At the same time, traditional weight management interventions may be less effective for these populations." (Wall, et al., 2019). The multiple complex factors proposed by Wall are diagrammed in **Figure 14.**

Figure 14.

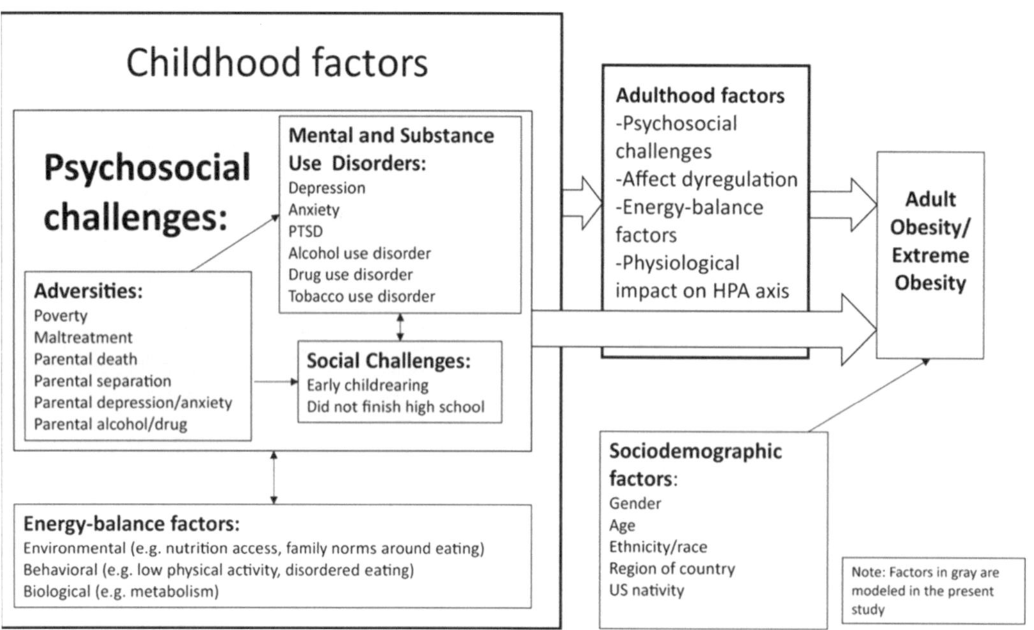

Wall, M., Mason, S., Liu, J., Olfson, M., Neumark-Sztainer, D. and Blanco, C. (2019). Childhood psychosocial challenges and risk for obesity in U.S. men and women. *Translational Psychiatry*, [online] Available at: https://doi.org/10.1038/s41398-018-0341-1.

Felitti, et al., (1998) conducted the original CDC-Kaiser research on ACEs. Their research concluded statistically significant adverse adult health outcomes, e.g., alcoholism, depression, suicide, smoking, drug abuse, sexually transmitted infections, and obesity in children who experienced 4 or more categories of childhood exposure to ACEs. In Felitti's study, adults meeting the criteria experienced a 1.4- to1.6- fold increase in incidence of obesity.

A systematic review of plausible mechanisms leading to obesity corroborated Felitti's research (Wiss and Brewerton 2020). In children, social disruption, health behaviors and chronic stress were most commonly cited exhibiting a positive association between ACEs and adult obesity with a pooled odds ratio of 1.46 (CI = 1.2 – 1.64).

A cross-sectional study of children who participated in the 2018 National Survey of Children's Health (NSCH) were investigated for associations between adverse childhood experiences and obesity (Kyler, et al., 2021). Weighted NSCH data included 29,696,808 children aged 10 to 17 years of which 15% were obese. According to the researchers, "Obesity was associated with having more ACEs compared to other children ($P < 0.01$). In adjusted analysis, children with obesity were more likely than other children to report most ACEs, including food/housing insecurity, parental divorce, witnessing physical violence, being a victim of violence, or live with a person with drug/alcohol abuse. Children with obesity were also more likely to report equal to or greater than 4 ACEs compared to other children ($P < 0.001$)."

On further reflection, many of the stressors etiologic for obesity articulated by Hassink and Wall **Figure 13** and **Figure 14** correlate with ACEs: poverty, food insecurity, violence, and homelessness. These experiences are intensified by childhood emotional, physical, and sexual abuse, childhood emotional and physical neglect and mental health problems that affect caregivers.

Concluding Remarks

This chapter reviewed that "the conditions within which people trade, live, and work affect health, partly through their influence on behavior and weight. The epidemiological pattern of obesity implies that … structures in society affect the unequal distribution of weight." (Friel,

Chopra, and Satcher, 2007) It also reviewed the serious health and economic consequences of the obesity pandemic, and the environmental, sociocultural, political, economic, adverse life experiences and behavioral factors that have led to the global obesity pandemic.

These societal structures can be understood in the social determinants of health framework, by identifying and studying the inequities in each of the social determinants of health domains – economic stability, health care access and quality, education access and quality, social and community context, and neighborhood and built environments. **Figure 9** displays details of how these factors interconnect and create the inequalities in obesity rates that are a characteristic of this unprecedented pandemic and lead to disproportionate health effects on poor and marginalized ethnic populations (Vargas, Stines, and Granado, 2017).

What Can Be Done About the Obesity Pandemic?

Unlike infectious disease pandemics such as influenza or SARS-CoV-2, the obesity pandemic does not require major scientific breakthroughs to identify a pathogen or to create a vaccine and/or effective treatments. We understand that important precipitating factors and causes of obesity are driven by poverty, food insecurity, adverse life experiences and stress, government funded food subsidies, ultra-processed foods, and "grab 'n go" life styles.

"The large racial/ethnic differences in the prevalence of overweight and obesity suggest that culturally sensitive and appropriate approaches are needed in promoting healthful eating in fighting the obesity epidemic. It is crucial to tailor treatment and prevention efforts to each particular ethnicity group's specific situation and needs. Policy makers and public health workers need to be aware of racial/ethnic differences that may affect one's health behaviors and body weight status, such as the differences in their local communities, perceptions of body weight, food preparation, eating practices, physical activity and inactivity patterns, and child-feeding practices." (Wang and Beydoun, 2007).

"This isn't like a disease where we're still waiting for the cure to be discovered – we know the cure for this. This isn't like putting a man on the moon or inventing the Internet – it doesn't take some stroke of genius or feat of technology. We have everything we need, right now, to help our kids lead healthy lives. Rarely in the history of this country have we encountered a problem of such magnitude and consequence that is so eminently solvable. So, let's move to solve it." Michelle Obama, Feb 9, 2010 (James, 2010).

Questions for Further Consideration

1. "Food, beverage, and restaurant companies spend almost $14 billion per year on food advertisements in the United States. More than 80% of this food advertising promotes fast food, sugary drinks, candy, and unhealthy snacks, dwarfing the entire $1 billion budget for all chronic disease prevention and health promotion at the U.S. Centers for Disease Control and Prevention. Furthermore, these food companies often engage in "targeted marketing" to reach children, teens, and communities of color with marketing for their least healthy products" (UConn Rudd Center, 2017).
   Given the massive advertising campaign that appears continually in all media, how can adults and children be helped to make healthier food choices, given the social and economic pressures that currently influence buying choices?

2. Should health care providers bring up the issue of overweight or obesity to patients who do not express concern about this during their visit?
3. If a patient or parent expresses concern over their weight or their child's weight, what is the recommended technique for counseling them about their concerns?
4. Given the significant role that government policies and subsidies play in the availability and costs of food, how can health care providers advocate for changes that can benefit all populations in an equitable way?

Sentinel Readings for a Deeper Dive

Salt Sugar Fat: How the Food Giants Hooked Us
Michael Moss
Random House 2013
ISBN 9781400069804

Felitti, V., Anda, R., Nordenberg, D., Williamson, D., Spitz, A., Edwards, V., Koss, M. and Marks, J. (1998). Relationship of Childhood Abuse and Household Dysfunction to Many of the Leading Causes of Death in Adults. *American Journal of Preventive Medicine*, [online] Available at: https://doi.org/10.1016/s0749-3797(98)00017-8

The end of overeating -Taking control of the insatiable American appetite
David A. Kessler
Rodale Books. Emmaus, Pennsylvania, USA. 2009.
ISBN: 978-1-60529-785-9 (hardcover)

The Omnivore's Dilemma - A natural history of 4 meals
Michael Pollan
Penguin Random House 2007
ISBN 9780143038580

References

Achenbach, J., Keating, D., McGinley, L., Johnson, A. and Chikwendiu, J. (2023). *America's epidemic of chronic illness is killing us too soon*. [online] Available at: https://www.washingtonpost.com/health/interactive/2023/american-life-expectancy-dropping/?itid=hp-top-table-main_p001_f004 [Accessed 18 November 2023].

Bentley, R., Ormerod, P. and Ruck, D. (2018). Recent origin and evolution of obesity-income correlation across the United States. *Palgrave Communications*, [online] Available at: https://doi.org/10.1057/s41599-018-0201-x [Accessed 24 November 2023].

Bray, G. (2004). The epidemic of obesity and changes in food intake: the Fluoride Hypothesis. *Physiology & Behavior* [online] Available at: https://doi.org/10.1016/j.physbeh.2004.04.033 [Accessed 20 November 2023].

Brierley, R. (2021). Obesity: another ongoing pandemic. *The Lancet Gastroenterology & Hepatology* [online] Available at: https://doi.org/10.1016/S2468-1253(21)00143-6 [Accessed 20 November 2023].

CDC (2023). *Adult Obesity Prevalence Maps*. [online] Centers for Disease Control and Prevention [online] Available at: https://www.cdc.gov/obesity/data/prevalence-maps.html [Accessed 18 November 2023].

CDC (2022a). *Consequences of Obesity*. Centers for Disease Control and Prevention. [online] Available at: https://www.cdc.gov/obesity/basics/consequences.html [Accessed 18 November 2023].

CDC (2022b). *Prevalence of Diagnosed Diabetes | Diabetes | CDC*. [online] Available at: https://www.cdc.gov/diabetes/data/statistics-report/diagnosed-diabetes.html [Accessed 18 November 2023].

Crimarco, A., Landry, M. and Gardner, C. (2022). *Ultra-processed Foods, Weight Gain, and Comorbidity Risk*. [online] Available at: https://pubmed.ncbi.nlm.nih.gov/34677812/ [Accessed 20 November 2023].

Do, W., Bullard, K., Stein, A., Mohammed, A., Venkat Narayan, K. and Siegel, K. (2020). *Consumption of Foods Derived from Subsidized Crops Remains Associated with Cardiometabolic Risk: An Update on the Evidence Using the National Health and Nutrition Examination Survey 2009–2014*. [online] Available at: https://www.ncbi.nlm.nih.gov/pmc/articles/PMC7690710/ [Accessed 20 November 2023].

Felitti, V., Anda, R., Nordenberg, D., Williamson, D., Spitz, A., Edwards, V., Koss, M. and Marks, J. (1998). Relationship of Childhood Abuse and Household Dysfunction to Many of the Leading Causes of Death in Adults. *American Journal of Preventive Medicine*, [online] Available at: https://doi.org/10.1016/s0749-3797(98)00017-8 [Accessed 6 January 2024].

Finkelstein, D., Petersen, D. and Schottenfeld, L. (2017). Promoting Children's Physical Activity in Low-Income Communities in Colorado: What Are the Barriers and Opportunities? *Preventing Chronic Disease*, [online] Available at: https://doi.org/10.5888/pcd14.170111 [Accessed 6 January 2024].

Friel, S., Chopra, M. and Satcher, D. (2007). Unequal weight: equity-oriented policy responses to the global obesity epidemic. *BMJ* [online] Available at: https://doi.org/10.1136/bmj.39377.622882.47 [Accessed 18 November 2023].

Fryar, C., Carroll, M. and Afful, J. (2021a). *Products - Health E Stats - Prevalence of Overweight, Obesity, and Extreme Obesity Among Adults Aged 20 and Over: United States, 1960–1962 Through 2017–2018*. [online] Available at: https://www.cdc.gov/nchs/data/hestat/obesity-adult-17-18/obesity-adult.htm [Accessed 18 November 2023].

Fryar, C., Carroll, M. and Afful, J. (2021b). *Products - Health E Stats - Prevalence of Overweight, Obesity, and Severe Obesity Among Children and Adolescents Aged 2–19 Years: United States, 1963–1965 Through 2017–2018*. [online] Available at: https://www.cdc.gov/nchs/data/hestat/obesity-child-17-18/obesity-child.htm [Accessed 18 Nov. 2023].

Fryar, C., Carroll, M., Ahluwalia, N. and Ogden, C. (2020). *Products - data briefs - number 375- August 2020.* [online] Available at: https://www.cdc.gov/nchs/products/databriefs/db375.htm [Accessed 21 November 2023].

Gearhardt, A. and DiFeliceantonio, A. (2022). Highly processed foods can be considered addictive substances based on established scientific criteria. *Addiction* [online] Available at: https://doi.org/10.1111/add.16065 [Accessed 21 November 2023].

Hall, K., Ayuketah, A., Brychta, R., Cai, H., Cassimatis, T., Chen, K., Chung, S., Costa, E., Courville, A., Darcey, V., Fletcher, L., Forde, C., Gharib, A., Guo, J., Howard, R., Joseph, P., McGehee, S., Ouwerkerk, R., Raisinger, K. and Rozga, I. (2019). Ultra-Processed Diets Cause Excess Calorie Intake and Weight Gain: An Inpatient Randomized Controlled Trial of Ad Libitum Food Intake. *Cell Metabolism* [online] Available at: https://doi.org/10.1016/j.cmet.2019.05.008 [Accessed 21 November 2023].

Hassink, S. (2023). *Physiologic Impact of the Social Determinants of Health. [PowerPoint] Evaluation and Treatment of Children and Adolescents with Obesity Continued... Getting the Guidelines to Work for You, Your Patients and Families in Practice*. Presentation at 'Pediatric Pearls for Office Practice' 46th Annual Day of Pediatrics. MultiCare Department of CME, Tacoma, WA. 30 September 2023.

Hruschka, D. and Han, S. (2017). Anti-fat discrimination in marriage more clearly explains the poverty–obesity paradox. *Behavioral and Brain Sciences*, 40. [online} Available at: https://doi.org/10.1017/s0140525x1600145x [Accessed 6 January 2024].

James, F. (2010). *Michelle Obama Escalates War on Childhood Obesity*. NPR.org. [online] Available at: https://www.npr.org/sections/thetwo-way/2010/02/michelle_obama_making_childhoo.html [Accessed 18 November 2023].

Kompaniyets, L., Agathis, N., Nelson, J., Preston, L., Ko, J., Belay, B., Pennington, A., Danielson, M., DeSisto, C., Chevinsky, J., Schieber, L., Yusuf, H., Baggs, J., Mac Kenzie, W., Wong, K., Boehmer, T., Gundlapalli, A. and Goodman, A. (2021). Underlying Medical Conditions Associated with Severe COVID-19 Illness Among Children. *JAMA Network Open* [online] Available at: https://doi.org/10.1001/jamanetworkopen.2021.11182 [Accessed 18 November 2023].

Kyler, K., Hall, M., Halvorson, E. and Davis, A. (2021). Associations between Obesity and Adverse Childhood Experiences in the United States. *Childhood Obesity*. [online] Available at https://doi.org/10.1089/chi.2020.0261 [Accessed 6 January 2024].

Let's Move (2010). *Learn The Facts | Let's Move!* [online] Archives.gov. Available at: https://letsmove.obamawhitehouse.archives.gov/learn-facts/epidemic-childhood-obesity [Accessed 18 November 2023].

Leung, C., Fulay, A., Parnarouskis, L., Martinez-Steele, E., Gearhardt, A. and Wolfson, J. (2022). Food insecurity and ultra-processed food consumption: the modifying role of participation in the Supplemental Nutrition Assistance Program (SNAP). *The American Journal of Clinical Nutrition* [online] Available at: https://doi.org/10.1093/ajcn/nqac049 [Accessed 24 November 2023].

Levine, J. (2011). Poverty and Obesity in the U.S. *Diabetes* [online] Available at: https://doi.org/10.2337/db11-1118 [Accessed 24 November 2023].

Lloyd-Jones, D., Lewis, C., Schreiner, P., Shikany, J., Sidney, S. and Reis, J. (2021). The Coronary Artery Risk Development in Young Adults (CARDIA) Study. *Journal of the American College of Cardiology*,[online] Available at: https://doi.org/10.1016/j.jacc.2021.05.022 [Accessed 21 November 2023].

Mattson, M., Allison, D., Fontana, L., Harvie, M., Longo, V., Malaisse, W., Mosley, M., Notterpek, L., Ravussin, E., Scheer, F., Seyfried, T., Varady, K. and Panda, S. (2014). Meal frequency and timing in health and disease. *Proceedings of the National Academy of Sciences* [online] Available at: https://doi.org/10.1073/pnas.1413965111 [Accessed 6 January 2024].

Olshansky, S., Passaro, D., Hershow, R., Layden, J., Carnes, B., Brody, J., Hayflick, L., Butler, R., Allison, D. and Ludwig, D. (2005). A Potential Decline in Life Expectancy in the United States in the 21st Century. *New England Journal of Medicine*, [online] Available at: https://doi.org/10.1056/nejmsr043743 [Accessed 18 November 2023].

Pati, S., Irfan, W., Jameel, A., Ahmed, S., and Shahid, R.K. (2023). Obesity and Cancer: A Current Overview of Epidemiology, Pathogenesis, Outcomes, and Management. *Cancers*, [online] Available at: https://doi.org/10.3390/cancers15020485 [Accessed 18 November 2023].

Popkin, B. (2022). Does excessive fast-food consumption impair our health? *The American Journal of Clinical Nutrition*. [online] Available at: https://doi.org/10.1093/ajcn/nqac110 [Accessed 21 November 2023]

Poti, J., Braga, B. and Qin, B. (2017). Ultra-processed Food Intake and Obesity: What Really Matters for Health—Processing or Nutrient Content? *Current Obesity Reports* [online] Available at: https://doi.org/10.1007/s13679-017-0285-4 [Accessed 21 November 2023].

Rama, A. (2018). *Policy Research Perspectives National Health Expenditures, 2016: Annual Spending Growth on the Downswing*. [online] Available at: https://www.ama-assn.org/sites/ama-assn.org/files/corp/media-browser/member/health-policy/prp-annual-spending-2016.pdf [Accessed 19 November 2023].

Ranjani, H., Pradeepa, R., Mehreen, T., Anjana, R., Anand, K., Garg, R. and Mohan, V. (2014). Determinants, consequences and prevention of childhood overweight and obesity: An Indian context. *Indian Journal of Endocrinology and Metabolism* [online] Available at: doi:https://doi.org/10.4103/2230-8210.145049 [Accessed 20 November 2023].

Rhone, A. (2018). *USDA ERS - Documentation.* [online] Available at: https://www.ers.usda.gov/data-products/food-access-research-atlas/documentation/ [Accessed 6 January 2024].

Rico-Campà, A., Martínez-González, M., Alvarez-Alvarez, I., Mendonça, R. de D., de la Fuente-Arrillaga, C., Gómez-Donoso, C. and Bes-Rastrollo, M. (2019). Association between consumption of ultra-processed foods and all-cause mortality: SUN prospective cohort study. *BMJ* [online] Available at: https://doi.org/10.1136/bmj.l1949 [Accessed 21 November 2023].

Rosenquist, K. and Fox, C. (2018). *Mortality Trends in Type 2 Diabetes*. 3rd ed. [online] Available at: https://www.ncbi.nlm.nih.gov/books/NBK568010/ [Accessed 18 November 2023].

UConn Rudd Center for Food Policy and Health (2017). *Food Marketing* [online] Available at: https://uconnruddcenter.org/research/food-marketing/ [Accessed 6 January 2024].

Simmonds, M., Llewellyn, A., Owen, C. and Woolacott, N. (2016). Predicting Adult Obesity from Childhood Obesity: A Systematic Review and Meta-Analysis. *Obesity Reviews* [online] Available at: https://doi.org/10.1111/obr.12334 [Accessed 18 November 2023].

Stierman, B., Afful, J., Carroll, M., Te-Ching, C., Orlando, D., Fink, S. and Fryar, C. (2021). NHSR 158. National Health and Nutrition Examination Survey 2017–March 2020 Pre-pandemic Data Files. *National Health Statistics Reports*, [online] Available at: https://doi.org/10.15620/cdc:106273 [Accessed 20 November 2023].

Temple, N. (2022). The Origins of the Obesity Epidemic in the USA–Lessons for Today. *Nutrients* [online] Available at: https://doi.org/10.3390/nu14204253 [Accessed 20 November 2023].

Upadhyay, J., Farr, O., Perakakis, N., Ghaly, W. and Mantzoros, C. (2018). Obesity as a Disease. *Medical Clinics of North America*, [online] Available at: https://doi.org/10.1016/j.mcna.2017.08.004 [Accessed 18 November 2023].

Vargas, C., Stines, E. and Granado, H. (2017). Health-equity issues related to childhood obesity: a scoping review. *Journal of Public Health Dentistry*, 77, [online] Available at: https://doi.org/10.1111/jphd.12233 [Accessed 20 November 2023].

Wang, Y. and Beydoun, M. (2007). The Obesity Epidemic in the United States Gender, Age, Socioeconomic, Racial/Ethnic, and Geographic Characteristics: A Systematic Review and Meta-Regression Analysis. *Epidemiologic Reviews* [online] https://doi.org/10.1093/epirev/mxm007 [Accessed 18 November 2023].

Wall, M., Mason, S., Liu, J., Olfson, M., Neumark-Sztainer, D. and Blanco, C. (2019). Childhood psychosocial challenges and risk for obesity in U.S. men and women. *Translational Psychiatry*, [online] Available at: https://doi.org/10.1038/s41398-018-0341-1 [Accessed 27 January 2024.

Ward, Z., Willett, W., Hu, F., Pacheco, L., Long, M. and Gortmaker, S. (2022). Excess mortality associated with elevated body weight in the USA by state and demographic subgroup: A modelling study. *eClinicalMedicine* [online] Available at: https://doi.org/10.1016/j.eclinm.2022.101429 [Accessed 18 November 2023].

Waters, H. and Graf, M. (2018). *AMERICA'S OBESITY CRISIS THE HEALTH AND ECONOMIC COSTS OF EXCESS WEIGHT*. [online] Available at: https://milkeninstitute.org/sites/default/files/reports-pdf/Mi-Americas-Obesity-Crisis-WEB_2.pdf [Accessed 19 November 2023].

Wiss, D. and Brewerton, T. (2020). Adverse Childhood Experiences and Adult Obesity: A Systematic Review of Plausible Mechanisms and Meta-Analysis of Cross-Sectional Studies. *Physiology & Behavior* [online] Available at: https://doi.org/10.1016/j.physbeh.2020.112964 [Accessed 6 January 2024].

Zgodic, A., Eberth, J., Breneman, C., Wende, M., Kaczynski, A., Liese, A. and McLain, A. (2021). Estimates of Childhood Overweight and Obesity at the Region, State, and County Levels: A Multilevel Small-Area Estimation Approach. *American Journal of Epidemiology*, [online] Available at: https://doi.org/10.1093/aje/kwab176 [Accessed 18 November 2023].

Lexicon of Listed Terms and Agencies

- **Adverse Childhood Experiences (ACEs)** Adverse Childhood Experiences (ACEs) are traumatic experiences that children experience before the age of 18 that have lasting impacts on their mental health, physical health, and general well-being.

- **Behavioral Risk Factor Surveillance System (BRFSS)** is the nation's premier system of health-related telephone surveys that collect state data about U.S. residents regarding their health-related risk behaviors, chronic health conditions, and use of preventive services. Established in 1984 with 15 states, BRFSS now collects data in all 50 states as well as the District of Columbia and three U.S. territories.

- **Kaiser Family Foundation (KFF)** publishes analysis, polling and journalism about health-care issues, and states that much of its work especially concerns persons with low income or those who are otherwise especially vulnerable to health-care cost, such as the uninsured, those with chronic illnesses, or Medicaid/Medicare recipients.

- **National Health and Nutrition Examination Survey (NHANES)** as an arm of the CDC The National Health and Nutrition Examination Survey is a program of studies designed to assess the health and nutritional status of adults and children in the United States. The survey is unique in that it combines interviews and physical examinations.

- **National Institutes of Health (NIH)** The National Institutes of Health (NIH), a part of the U.S. Department of Health and Human Services, is the nation's medical research agency — making important discoveries that improve health and save lives.

- **National Survey of Children's Health** The National Survey of Children's Health (NSCH) provides rich data on multiple, intersecting aspects of children's lives—including physical and mental health, access to and quality of health care, and the child's family, neighborhood, school, and social context. The National Survey of Children's Health is funded and directed by the Health Resources and Services Administration (HRSA) Maternal and Child Health Bureau.

AUTHOR'S BIO SKETCH

David Estroff MD, FAAP
Clinical Professor Emeritus of Pediatrics, University of Washington
Dr. Estroff graduated from Antioch College (1972) and attended Hahnemann Medical College in Philadelphia (1976). After a "flexible" pediatric internship at Emory University/Grady Memorial Hospital in Atlanta, he served in the Indian Health Service in Bethel, Alaska for 2 years, providing primary care and obstetrics for the Alaska Native population following which he completed a pediatrics residency at OHSU in Portland, OR.

He joined the faculty of the Tacoma Family Medicine Residency in 1991 and completed a faculty development fellowship at the University of Washington. Switching venues, in 2000 he entered active duty in the U.S. Army. Following military retirement, in 2014 he joined the Community Health Care Family Medicine Residency as Director of Pediatrics education.

Dr. Estroff's interest in obesity led him to study obesity prevalence in children and developing clinical practice guideline for pediatric obesity. He has worked extensively in creating pediatric curriculum for family medicine residents with the American Academy of Family Practice and the Academic Pediatric Association.

He now holds the distinction of Clinical Professor Emeritus of Pediatrics at the University of Washington.

Chapter 18

Social Determinants and Health Behaviors

Sonya Chen, MD, Author
James Lenhart, MD, MPH, Editor

"In the real world there is no nature vs. nurture argument, only an infinitely complex and moment-by-moment interaction between genetic and environmental effects"

- Gabor Maté, *In the Realm of Hungry Ghosts: Close Encounters with Addiction,* January 2019.

Lifestyles, Behaviors, and Substance Use

In the context of the Social Determinants of Health

This chapter aims to scrutinize specific lifestyles and behaviors associated with substance use while dissecting the underlying social-economic, cultural, and environmental conditions propelling these behaviors. We know that there are genetic and heritable predispositions to substance use, as evidenced by early adoption and twin studies showing a heightened risk among those with positive biological family histories. In this chapter, we discuss how, in addition to nature, there is a large proponent of *nurture* that leads to these behaviors. Besides genetics, other underlying health issues, namely mental health disorders such as ADHD, depression, PTSD, and anxiety, emerge as significant contributors to substance use (Couwenbergh, et al., 2006). The question arises: Is it the mental health issue that precipitates the substance use disorder, or does the underlying issue serve as a dual catalyst for both mental health disorders and substance use disorders? Alternatively, could the mental health issue manifest because of substance use?

According to Ewald, Strack, and Michael (2019), genetic predispositions play a significant role in determining an individual's susceptibility to social and environmental stressors, interacting with their personality traits and concurrent psychiatric conditions. These genetic influences also shape the trajectory of addiction across various stages such as acquisition, maintenance, and relapse. Epidemiological research suggests that between 30% to 60% of addiction predisposition can be attributed to hereditary factors. However, it is essential to note that genetic vulnerability interacts closely with environmental influences and drug accessibility, and it alone cannot reliably predict substance use or addiction.

The relationship between genes and the environment is complex, characterized by reciprocal determinism where both factors influence each other. Researchers aim to understand the extent to which these factors co-occur and their respective impacts. Environmental factors tend to exert a more substantial influence during early development, while genetic factors become more prominent later in life. As individuals age and gain more exposure to the environment, genetic influences gradually strengthen. Thus, both genetic predispositions and environmental factors are integral in shaping addiction susceptibility and progression (Ewald, Strack, and Michael, 2019).

Predispositions can be framed in the construct of exposomics discussed in chapter 16, known as the environmental exposures encountered throughout life including the social factors which influence human health gradually increasing their effect as individuals age (**Figure 1**).

Figure 1.

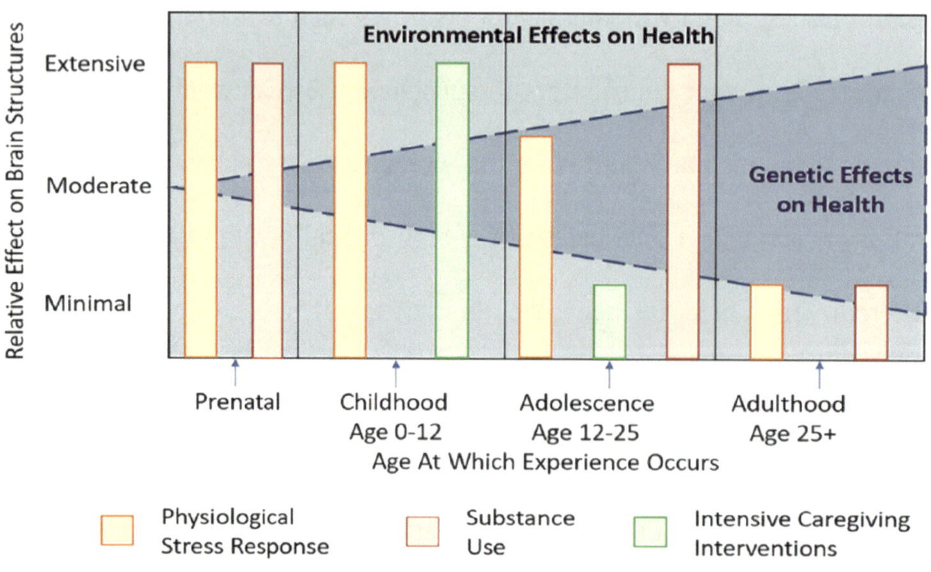

Ewald, D., Strack, R. and Orsini, M. (2019). Rethinking Addiction. Global Pediatric Health, [online] Available at: https://www.ncbi.nlm.nih.gov/pmc/articles/PMC6348542/ [Accessed 29 Feb. 2024].

According to Richesson, et al., (2022) substance use begins at early ages. In their study, "among individuals aged 12 or older in 2021, a staggering 57.8% engaged in tobacco, alcohol, or illicit drug use in the past month. Breaking down the statistics, 47.5% indulged in alcohol, 19.5% used tobacco products, and 14.3% experimented with illicit drugs."

Alcohol

In the context of the Social Determinants of Health

Alcohol drinkers cluster in networks, with social network characteristics serving as predictors of changes in substance use behaviors over time. For example, religious beliefs significantly influence drinking levels, with certain religions proscribing alcohol and contributing to lower drinking rates in regions where they prevail (MacKillop, et al., 2022). Policy strategies, such as licensing, government monopolies, and pricing, exert considerable influence on alcohol consumption patterns (Xu, et al., 2022). Additionally, the availability and affordability of evidence-based treatment across healthcare systems play a pivotal role in determining the population-level burden of substance-related health issues. Broadly encompassing social determinants of health, factors like income, housing, early childhood development, social inclusion, non-discrimination, and access to quality health services collectively contribute to an increased risk of hazardous drinking and Alcohol Use Disorders (AUDs), highlighting the interplay of diverse influences on alcohol-related behaviors and outcomes (Xu, et al., 2022).

In exploring the patterns of lifetime alcohol abstention, distinct gender and ethnic dynamics become known. Women, particularly those from non-White and Latina backgrounds, emerge as more likely to embrace lifetime abstention (Kerr, et al., 2016). Factors such as the influence of religion, with an inclination toward abstention among those whose faith discourages drinking and for whom religion holds significant importance, play a significant role, underscoring the nuanced intersections of belief systems and lifestyle choices. Higher education levels among women are associated with reduced rates of lifetime abstention, yet family dynamics, specifically problem drinking, present a paradox as it correlates with lower abstention rates in this demographic (Kerr, et al., 2016).

Smoking

In the context of the Social Determinants of Health

According to Das, et al., (2011) celebrity, peer and familial influences provoke smoking initiation among adolescents. In an Indian study involving 2535 students, with 1465 males and 1070 females, the overall prevalence of smoking was 21.58%. Notably, among boys the prevalence was higher at 34.95%, with 5.8% being experimenters, 3.9% former smokers, 59.2% heavy smokers, and 31% light smokers. In contrast, among females the prevalence was lower at 3.27%, with 77.14% being experimenters and 22.86% light smokers. The average age of smoking initiation was found to be 14.7 ± 1.4 years. The study identified influential factors for smoking initiation, revealing that students were over six times more likely to smoke if their best friend smoked (odds ratio = 6.6). Additionally, adolescents who had seen their fathers smoking were four times more likely to be smokers compared to those whose fathers did not smoke (odds ratio = 4.7). Significantly, 64% of smokers reported having seen their favorite movie stars smoke in films, while 38.3% of non-smokers reported seeing their favorite celebrities smoke on screen.

Muttarak, et al. (2013) posed the question, "Why do smokers start?" in an Italian study conducted examining the behaviors of 7469 adolescents aged 18 and under. 59.9% of individuals who had ever smoked initiated smoking before the age of 18, and 33.6% started smoking before turning 16. Among ever smokers, 61.1% reported starting smoking due to the influence of friends, 15.6% for enjoyment and satisfaction, 9.0% to feel mature and independent, 6.6% due to the influence of partners or family, 2.5% because of stress, 1.9% to feel more secure, and 1.8% out of curiosity. The study emphasized the significant role of social influence, particularly from friends, in smoking initiation among Italian men and women, especially those who began smoking at an early age. The investigators further argued the importance for anti-smoking campaigns to address social dynamics, resistance factors, and self-esteem dimensions to effectively target and discourage smoking initiation, particularly among the youth (Muttarak, et al. 2013).

Substance Use Disorder Spectrum

In the context of the Social Determinants of Health

Substance use disorders, including alcohol consumption and smoking, are significantly influenced by social networks, cultural norms, and neighborhood dynamics. Neighborhoods burdened by poverty and socioeconomic disparities experience higher rates of substance use, reflecting environmental factors impacting individual behaviors. These communities may lack access to resources and face social norms that normalize substance use, exacerbating the prevalence of substance use disorders. Research reveals that living in a neighborhood with an alcohol retailer is associated with higher risk of developing alcohol use disorder. (Karriker-Jaffe, et al., 2018).

Adverse childhood experiences, including abuse or neglect, pose a significant risk factor in the development of substance use disorder and often intertwine with prenatal alcohol exposure to amplify their impact (MacKillop, et al., 2022). Childhood economic difficulty is a predictor of lower abstention, particularly among White women, while childhood sexual abuse is notably linked to lower lifetime abstention, specifically among Black women. These patterns exhibit gender-specific nuances, with ethnic minority women displaying a higher likelihood of lifetime abstention compared to White women. Generational differences, though more pronounced among women, show an increased likelihood of being a lifetime abstainer for older cohorts across genders. Notably, the influence of family dynamics on offspring becomes evident as problem drinking within the family exerts an impact on the drinking patterns of the next generation, highlighting the interplay between genetic predispositions and environmental factors (Kerr, et al., 2016).

Low socioeconomic status impacts the prevalence of substance use disorder. According to Settipani, et al., (2018), in a study involving 188 adolescents and adults from white Canadian backgrounds seeking mental health assistance for substance use disorder, 80% of participants expressed concerns about at least one aspect of social determinants of health (SDH). Financial difficulties for families affect childhood mental well-being several ways – insufficient access to nutritious food, cramped living conditions, and inadequate housing. These conditions, in turn, lead to additional risk factors for mental health issues, including exposure to domestic violence, abuse, neglect, and parental alcohol misuse, which circle back to increased prevalence of substance use disorder and substantial impact on treatment. **Table 1** illustrates the prevalence of four SDH domains and impact on treatment.

Table 1.

Social determinant of health domain	Concerns identified	Substantial problems	Substantial treatment impact
	Yes	Yes	Yes
Finances – n (%)	131 (69.3%)	115 (60.8%)	42 (22.2%)
Living situation – n (%)	58 (30.7%)	49 (25.9%)	32 (16.9%)
Food security – n (%)	42 (22.2%)	33 (17.5%)	13 (6.9%)
Treatment access – n (%)	42 (22.2%)	32 (16.9%)	27 (14.3%)

Settipani, C., Hawke, L., Virdo, G., Yorke, E., Mehra, K. and Henderson, J. (2018). Social Determinants of Health among Youth Seeking Substance Use and Mental Health Treatment. Journal of the Canadian Academy of Child and Adolescent Psychiatry, [online] 27(4), pp.213–221. Available at: https://www.ncbi.nlm.nih.gov/pmc/articles/PMC6254257/

A Stockholm University study (Room, 2005), revealed that hospitalization rates for alcohol-specific causes were significantly higher among manual workers, being 3.6 times as high for men and 2.5 times as high for women compared to higher-level non-manual workers. A systematic review and meta-analysis including 336,287 participants across 55 countries indicates that socioeconomic inequalities in alcohol-attributable mortality are 1.5 to 2.0 times larger than those in all-cause mortality. The prevalence of current drinking was positively associated with socioeconomic status, while heavy episodic drinking (HED) showed a negative association. Interestingly, in upper-middle-income countries, individuals with low socioeconomic status were more likely to engage in HED, while the opposite was true in low-income countries, with no socioeconomic differences observed in lower-middle-income countries (Xu, et al., 2022).

There is a parallel in tobacco use across various socioeconomic distributions. Prevalence is significantly higher in lower socioeconomic strata and vulnerable groups, particularly adolescents, contributing to a cycle of poverty and missed opportunities due to its highly addictive nature. This issue is especially pronounced in low- and middle-income countries where over 80% of the global smoking population resides. In these regions, poor households are estimated to allocate 10% of their disposable income to tobacco, further exacerbating economic disparities. The link between poverty and tobacco use is multifaceted, influenced by the lack of power and impact in policymaking for impoverished individuals and the unplanned, poverty-driven urbanization leading to the prevalence of tobacco use in shantytowns and informal settlements (Mentis, A. 2017).

Alcohol: National and International Comparisons

In the U.S. of the 133.1 million current alcohol users aged 12 or older in 2021, 45.1% engaged in past-month binge drinking. Young adults aged 18 to 25 exhibited the highest prevalence (29.2%), followed by adults aged 26 or older. Adolescents aged 12 to 17, while comparatively lower, still demonstrated significant numbers. Global alcohol consumption patterns vary, with over 80% of adults reporting lifetime alcohol use in high-income countries and approximately 2.3 billion adults engaging in annual alcohol consumption globally (Richesson, et al., 2023). Interestingly, although disadvantaged neighborhoods had more alcohol outlets, analysis of *advantaged* neighborhoods demonstrated young adults were more likely to drink, get drunk, and face alcohol-related issues. Despite this, people living in lower income areas were more likely to have heavy *episodic* drinking and to suffer from more significant poor health outcomes from their alcohol use (Slutske, Deutsch and Piasecki, 2016).

According to the Organization for Economic Co-operation and Development (OECD), **Table 2** provides a graphical snapshot of alcohol consumption amongst representative high-income countries in 2017. France, Germany, and the UK lead consumption. Norway, Japan and Sweden rank lowest in consumption.

Table 2.

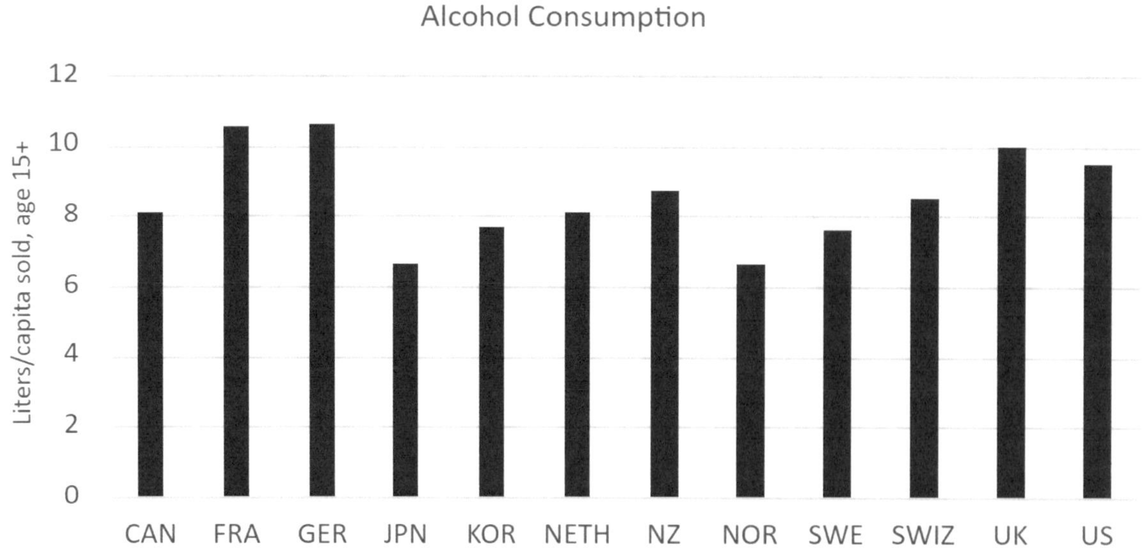

OECD. (2017b). Health risks - Alcohol consumption - OECD Data. [online] Available at: https://data.oecd.org/healthrisk/alcohol-consumption.htm

Smoking and Vaping Nicotine: National and International Comparisons

According to the Global Burden of Disease Collaborators (GBD) in 2015, smoking ranked as the second-leading health risk factor for men, contributing to 9.6% of the number of years lost due to ill-health, disability, or early death (also known as Disability-Adjusted Life Years or DALYs), which plays a significant role in male diseases related to cardiovascular and circulatory diseases, cancers, and chronic respiratory conditions (GBD Collaborators, 2016). Alcohol and drug use ranked as the fifth-leading risk for men, associated with 6.6% of disease burden primarily due to mental and substance use disorders, along with cirrhosis and other chronic liver diseases. For women, the burden attributable to alcohol and drug use was notably lower at 2.0%.

Smoking led as the primary risk for DALYs among both men and women in high-income regions like North America and the UK. However, in most of western Europe, smoking held the leading position only for men, while high systolic blood pressure emerged as the leading risk factor for women. A similar pattern was observed in east and southeast Asia, with smoking ranking as the leading risk factor for men in certain countries, while metabolic risk factors, particularly high systolic blood pressure, claimed the leading position for women (GBD Collaborators, 2016).

Daily smokers are defined as the population aged 15 years and over who report smoking every day. Smoking is a major risk factor for at least two of the leading causes of premature mortality - circulatory disease and cancer, increasing the risk of heart attack, stroke, lung cancer, and cancers of the larynx and mouth. In addition, smoking is an important contributing factor for respiratory diseases. This indicator is presented as a total and per gender and is measured as a percentage of the population considered (total, men or women) aged 15 years and over.

Table 3 reflects smoking rates for both men and women in various high-income countries (OECD, 2017a).

Table 3.

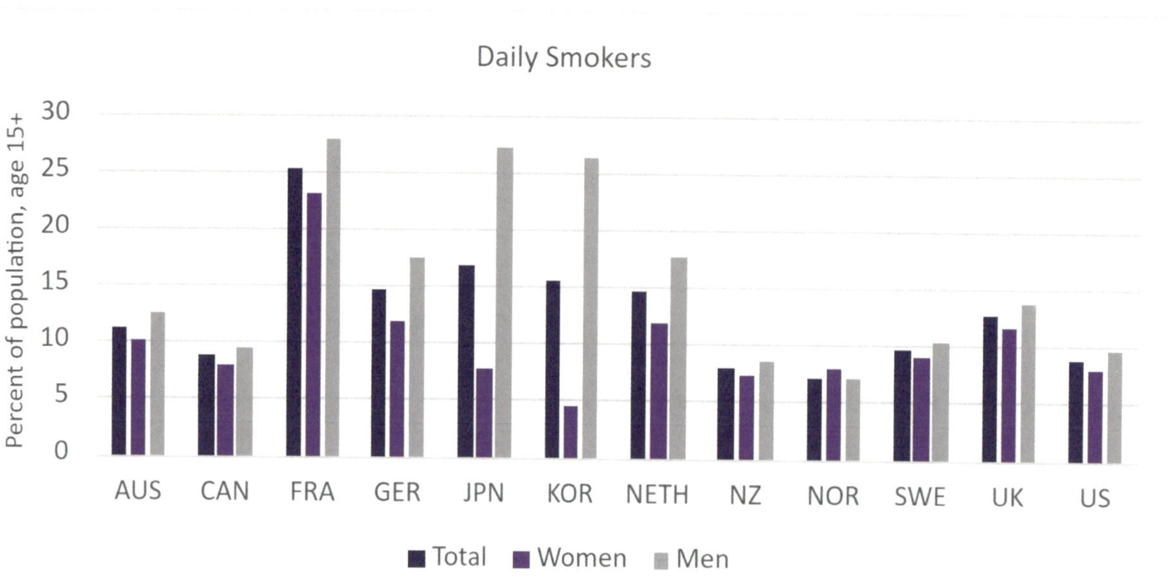

OECD (2017a). Health risks - Daily smokers - OECD Data. [online] the OECD. Available at: https://data.oecd.org/healthrisk/daily-smokers.htm

Over 25% of males in France, Japan and Korea are daily smokers. In Canada, New Zealand, Norway, Sweden and the U.S. males smoke at a rate of 10% or less.

Vaping on the Rise

The escalation of alternative nicotine consumption methods, such as vaping, reveals intriguing insights. Approximately 13.2 million individuals aged 12 or older (4.7%) used e-cigarettes or vaping devices to consume nicotine in the past month in the U.S. Notably, the highest percentage was observed among young adults aged 18 to 25, followed by adolescents and older adults (Richesson, et al., 2022).

The safety of vaping remains unknown. According to the CDC (2023), E-cigarette aerosol generally contains fewer toxic chemicals than the deadly mix of 7,000 chemicals in smoke from regular cigarettes. However, e-cigarette aerosol is not harmless. It can contain harmful substances, including nicotine, heavy metals like lead, volatile organic compounds, and cancer-causing agents.

Opioid Use Disorder

According to the 2021 National Survey on Drug Use and Health, young adults in the U.S. aged 18 to 25 exhibited the highest percentage of opioid use, with 25.6% or 8.6 million people grappling with a substance use disorder. Adults aged 26 or older followed closely, with 16.1% or 35.5 million individuals affected. Adolescents aged 12 to 17, though comparatively lower, still faced a significant burden, with 8.5% or 2.2 million people contending with a substance use disorder. Among individuals aged 12 or older in 2021, a concerning 3.3% or 9.2 million people engaged in the use of opioids, encompassing both heroin and prescription pain relievers. Of this population, 8.7 million individuals misused prescription pain relievers, while 1.1 million used heroin. Notably, 574,000 individuals demonstrated a worrisome overlap, engaging in the misuse of both prescription pain relievers and heroin in the past year (Richesson, et al., 2022).

Table 4 highlights the dramatic challenge in the U.S., which substantially leads other high-income countries in the rate of opioid deaths (OECD, 2019).

Table 4.

Opioid-related deaths

Per million populations

140
120
100
80
60
40
20
0

AUS CAN FRA GER NETH NOR SWE UK US

■ 2011 ■ 2016

OECD (2019). Addressing Problematic Opioid Use in OECD Countries - en - OECD. [online] Oecd.org. Available at: https://www.oecd.org/health/addressing-problematic-opioid-use-in-oecd-countries-a18286f0-en.htm

In 25 Organization for Economic Co-operation and Development (OECD) countries for which data are available, the average of opioid-related deaths has increased by more than 20% in 2011-2016, with the rise most pronounced in the United States, Canada, Sweden, Norway, Ireland, and England & Wales (OECD, 2019).

Canada and the United States have been experiencing an opioid crisis as a result of problematic opioid use fueled by the emergence of synthetic opioids such as fentanyl and carfentanil. Problematic opioid use is also spreading in other OECD countries, due to the upward trend of prescription opioid use and the complexities of the illegal drug supply, according to the OECD (2019).

The statistics surrounding opioid misuse and the prevalence of substance use disorders (SUD) underscore the gravity of the opioid epidemic in the United States. The substantial number of individuals misusing prescription pain relievers, coupled with the overlap of heroin use, highlights the complexity of opioid-related challenges. Additionally, the hierarchical distribution of SUD prevalence among different age groups signifies the varying vulnerabilities and susceptibility across demographics (Richesson, et al., 2022).

Public Health Challenges

Lifestyles, Behaviors, and Substance Use in the context of the Social Determinants of Health

The aforementioned data point to the specific impact of lifestyles and behaviors leading to substance use through the nuanced lens of the social determinants. Analysis implicates poverty, disruptive neighborhoods, educational opportunity, adverse childhood experiences, domestic violence, and mental health as etiologic. Substance use imposes significant reduction in life expectancy and healthy life expectancy and number of lifetime years lost due to ill-health, disability, or early death. The poultice lies not in the domain of state-of-the-art pharmaceuticals, or novel treatment programs, but public health policy that aggressively address the social determinants of health central to root causes.

Questions for Further Consideration:

1. The U.S. and Canada lead other high-income in opioid related deaths. What accounts for this significant discrepancy?
2. According to the data presented, France, Germany and the Netherlands have much lower incidence of deaths due to opioids. What strategies do those countries embrace to lower this avoidable death statistic. Answer in the frame of prevention and treatment.

Sentinel Readings for a Deeper Dive

Richesson, D., Magas, I., Brown, S. and Hoenig, J. (2023). *2021 NSDUH Annual National Report | CBHSQ Data*. [online] www.samhsa.gov. Available at: https://www.samhsa.gov/data/report/2021-nsduh-annual-national-report

Kerr, W., Ye, Y., Greenfield, T., Williams, E., Lown, E. and Lui, C. (2016). Early Life Health, Trauma and Social Determinants of Lifetime Abstention from Alcohol. *Alcohol and Alcoholism*, [online] Available at: https://www.ncbi.nlm.nih.gov/pmc/articles/PMC5004748/

CDC (2023). *Electronic Cigarettes What's the Bottom Line?* [online] Available at: https://www.cdc.gov/tobacco/basic_information/e-cigarettes/pdfs/Electronic-Cigarettes-Infographic-p.pdf

References:

CDC (2023). *Electronic Cigarettes What's the Bottom Line?* [online] Available at: https://www.cdc.gov/tobacco/basic_information/e-cigarettes/pdfs/Electronic-Cigarettes-Infographic-p.pdf [Accessed 2 Mar. 2024].

Couwenbergh, C., van den Brink, W., Zwart, K., Vreugdenhil, C., van Wijngaarden-Cremers, P. and van der Gaag, R. (2006). Comorbid psychopathology in adolescents and young adults treated for substance use disorders. *European Child & Adolescent Psychiatry* [online] Available at: https://link.springer.com/article/10.1007/s00787-006-0535-6 [Accessed 29 Feb. 2024].

Das, S., Ghosh, M., Sarkar, M., Joardar, S., Chatterjee, R. and Chatterjee, S. (2011). Adolescents Speak: Why do we Smoke? *Journal of Tropical Pediatrics* [online] Available at: https://link.springer.com/article/10.1007/s00787-006-0535-6 [Accessed 29 Feb. 2024].

Ewald, D., Strack, R. and Orsini, M. (2019). Rethinking Addiction. *Global Pediatric Health* [online] Available at: https://www.ncbi.nlm.nih.gov/pmc/articles/PMC6348542 https://www.ncbi.nlm.nih.gov/pmc/articles/PMC5004748/

GBD Collaborators (2016). *Global, regional, and national comparative risk assessment of 79 behavioural, environmental and occupational, and metabolic risks or clusters of risks, 1990–2015: a systematic analysis for the Global Burden of Disease Study 2015*. [online] Available at: https://www.ncbi.nlm.nih.gov/pmc/articles/PMC5388856/ [Accessed 2 Mar. 2024].

Karriker-Jaffe, K., Ohlsson, H., Kendler, K., Cook, W. and Sundquist, K. (2018). Alcohol Availability and Onset and Recurrence of Alcohol Use Disorder: Examination in a Longitudinal Cohort with Cosibling Analysis. *Alcoholism: Clinical and Experimental Research* [online] Available at: https://onlinelibrary.wiley.com/doi/10.1111/acer.13752 [Accessed 29 Feb. 2024].

Kerr, W., Ye, Y., Greenfield, T., Williams, E., Lown, E. and Lui, C. (2016). Early Life Health, Trauma and Social Determinants of Lifetime Abstention from Alcohol. *Alcohol and Alcoholism*, [online] Available at: https://www.ncbi.nlm.nih.gov/pmc/articles/PMC5004748/ [Accessed 29 Feb. 2024].

MacKillop, J., Agabio, R., Feldstein Ewing, S., Heilig, M., Kelly, J., Leggio, L., Lingford-Hughes, A., Palmer, A., Parry, C., Ray, L. and Rehm, J. (2022). Hazardous drinking and alcohol use disorders. *Nature Reviews Disease Primers* [online] Available at: https://www.ncbi.nlm.nih.gov/pmc/articles/PMC10284465/ [Accessed 29 Feb. 2024].

Maté, G. (2019). *In the Realm of Hungry Ghosts: Close Encounters with Addiction: MD Gabor Maté, Peter A. Levine Ph.D.* Amazon.com. [online] Available at: https://www.amazon.com/Realm-Hungry-Ghosts-Encounters-Addiction/dp/155643880X [Accessed 29 Feb. 2024].

Mentis, A. (2017). Social determinants of tobacco use: towards an equity lens approach. *Tobacco Prevention & Cessation*, [online] Available at: https://www.ncbi.nlm.nih.gov/pmc/articles/PMC7232809/ [Accessed 29 Feb. 2024].

Muttarak, R., Gallus, S., Franchi, M., Faggiano, F., Pacifici, R., Colombo, P. and La Vecchia, C. (2013). Why do smokers start? *European Journal of Cancer Prevention*, [online] Available at: https://pubmed.ncbi.nlm.nih.gov/22797676/ [Accessed 1 March 2024].

OECD (2017a). *Health risks - Daily smokers - OECD Data*. [online] Available at: https://data.oecd.org/healthrisk/daily-smokers.htm [Accessed 3 Mar. 2024].

OECD (2019). *Addressing Problematic Opioid Use in OECD Countries - en - OECD*. [online] Available at: https://www.oecd.org/health/addressing-problematic-opioid-use-in-oecd-countries-a18286f0-en.htm [Accessed 3 Mar. 2024].

OECD. (2017b). *Health risks - Alcohol consumption - OECD Data.* [online] Available at: https://data.oecd.org/healthrisk/alcohol-consumption.htm [Accessed 3 Mar. 2024].

Richesson, D., Magas, I., Brown, S. and Hoenig, J. (2023). *2021 NSDUH Annual National Report | CBHSQ Data.* [online] www.samhsa.gov. Available at: https://www.samhsa.gov/data/report/2021-nsduh-annual-national-report [Accessed 1 Mar. 2024].

Room R., (2005). Stigma, social inequality and alcohol and drug use. Drug Alcohol Rev.[online] Available at: https://pubmed.ncbi.nlm.nih.gov/16076584/ [Accessed 2 March 2024].

Settipani, C., Hawke, L., Virdo, G., Yorke, E., Mehra, K. and Henderson, J. (2018). Social Determinants of Health among Youth Seeking Substance Use and Mental Health Treatment. *Journal of the Canadian Academy of Child and Adolescent Psychiatry*, [online] Available at: https://www.ncbi.nlm.nih.gov/pmc/articles/PMC6254257/ [Accessed 2 Mar. 2024].

Slutske, W., Deutsch, A. and Piasecki, T. (2016). Neighborhood Contextual Factors, Alcohol Use, and Alcohol Problems in the United States: Evidence From a Nationally Representative Study of Young Adults. *Alcoholism: Clinical and Experimental Research* [online] https://onlinelibrary.wiley.com/doi/10.1111/acer.13033 [Accessed 2 March 2024]

Xu, Y., Geldsetzer, P., Manne-Goehler, J., Theilmann, M., Marcus, M., Zhumadilov, Z., Jaacks, L, et al. (2022). The socioeconomic gradient of alcohol use: an analysis of nationally representative survey data from 55 low-income and middle-income countries. *The Lancet Global Health*, [online] https://www.ncbi.nlm.nih.gov/pmc/articles/PMC9582994/ [Accessed 1 March 2024].

Lexicon of Listed Terms and Agencies

- **DALYs Disability-adjusted life years (DALYs)** are a measure of overall disease burden, expressed as *the number of years lost due to ill-health, disability, or early death.* Developed as a method evaluate and compare the overall health and life expectancy of different countries.

- **Global Burden of Diseases (GBD)** is a systematic, scientific effort to quantify the comparative magnitude of health loss due to diseases, injuries, and risk factors by age, sex, and geographies for specific points in time.

- **The Institute for Health Metrics and Evaluation (IHME)** at the University of Washington engages a large network of individual collaborators with specialties in various topic areas of expertise to conduct the Global Burden of Diseases, Injuries, and Risk Factors Study (GBD) and its affiliated research projects.

- **Organization for Economic Co-operation and Development (OECD)** is an international organisation that works to build better policies for better lives. Our goal is to shape policies that foster prosperity, equality, opportunity and well-being for all. We draw on 60 years of experience and insights to better prepare the world of tomorrow.

AUTHOR'S BIO SKETCH

Sonya Chen, MD

Sonya Chen, a third-year resident at the Community Health Care Family Medicine Residency, examines how healthcare intersects with social factors influencing health outcomes. With an interest in preventative care, mental health, and procedures, she advocates for fair access to healthcare. Despite limited experience, she's plans to become more involved in social reform, particularly concerning homelessness and its health implications. Leveraging her experiences with marginalized communities, Sonya aims to bridge healthcare and social justice. She urges readers to cultivate more compassion, hoping her chapter will shed light on the circumstances of those facing adverse social circumstances, fostering understanding and empathy. Beyond medicine, she enjoys exploring new destinations and cherishing quiet moments at home with her partner and their cats.

Chapter 19

Expressions for the Hope of Social Compassion

James Lenhart, MD, MPH, Author

"Art is the lie that enables us to realize the truth."
- Pablo Picasso (1881-1973) Spanish artist.

"Jazz speaks for life. The Blues tell the story of life's difficulties, and if you think for a moment, you will realize that they take the hardest realities of life and put them into music, only to come out with some new hope or sense of triumph. This is triumphant music."
- Martin Luther King (1964) Berlin Jazz Festival.

"You see, we are here, as far as I can tell, to help each other; our brothers, our sisters, our friends, our enemies. That is to help each other and not hurt each other."
- Stevie Ray Vaughan (1954-1990) American blues rock musician.

"We want to see drama told in a cathartic way, with power, with emotion, where you empathize and then you're frightened. All those feelings charge up in you and you feel for the story."
- Danny Boyle (1956) English director and producer. *Slumdog Millionaire* 2008.

Expressions for the Hope of Social Compassion

This chapter illustrates the literary, artistic, theatrical and musical expressions that over the centuries have called out human injustice and clamored for social reform.

Philosophers of the Enlightenment

"The Enlightenment, a European intellectual movement of the 17th and 18th centuries in which ideas concerning God, reason, nature, and humanity were synthesized into a worldview that gained wide assent in the West and that instigated revolutionary developments in art, philosophy, and politics. Central to Enlightenment thought were the use and celebration of reason, the power by which humans understand the universe and improve their own condition. The goals of rational humanity were considered to be knowledge, freedom, and happiness" (Britannica, 2024).

Among the several philosophers that influenced the leaders of the American and French Revolutions were Beccaria, Montesquieu and Voltaire.

Cesare Beccaria *(1738-1794),* an Italian philosopher, politician, and economist whose celebrated book *On Crimes and Punishments (Dei delitti e delle pene)* condemned the use of torture, argued for the abolition of capital punishment, and advocated many reforms for the rational and fair administration of law. Beccaria's ideas about legal and penal reforms, which influenced intellectuals and statesmen throughout Europe and in North America, inspired many significant reforms in the last decades of the 18th century and the first decades of the 19th century (Carpenter, 2010).

On Crimes and Punishments: With A Commentary of the Book of Crimes and Punishments by Voltaire (1764)

"Published in 1764 and included two years later in the Index of Forbidden Books, *On Crimes and Punishments* is the best-known work of the Italian Enlightenment. It was immediately a great success in Europe and United States, and was appreciated by characters such as Voltaire, Blackstone and Bentham. The first four U.S. Presidents were inspired by Beccaria's treatise, and America's foundational legal documents were shaped by it. In his aspiration for a more modern and just society, Beccaria demonstrates the uselessness, injustice, dangerousness and inhumanity of the death penalty and torture" (Amazon https://amzn.to/3SN8H1f).

Montesquieu (Charles-Louis de Secondat)'s *(1689-1755)* most famous book was *The Spirit of Laws*, published in 1748. Montesquieu's theory reflected his admiration for the English government. In England, Parliament made the laws. The monarch enforced the laws, and courts interpreted them. Each branch of government checked, or limited, the power of the others. When powers were not separated in this way, Montesquieu warned, liberty was soon lost. Historian's maintain that Montesquieu's ideas had a powerful impact on the men who wrote the U.S. Constitution making the separation of powers a key part of the American system of government (McIntosh, 2020).

The Spirit of Laws (1748)

"In this timeless masterpiece, Montesquieu delves into the intricate anatomy of societies, unveiling the hidden mechanics that shape their laws, customs, and destinies.

With eloquence and insight that have resonated through centuries, Montesquieu takes readers on a journey through the labyrinthine workings of political systems. He explores the delicate balance between liberty and authority, dissecting the diverse forms of government and the dynamics that propel them. Through a panoramic exploration of historical and cultural contexts, he unveils the complex tapestry of human governance, each thread woven with precision and depth.

Montesquieu's brilliance lies not only in his analytical prowess but also in his ability to question and challenge prevailing assumptions. He champions the notion of the separation of powers, a revolutionary concept that would influence the very foundations of modern democracies. With sagacious observations, he dissects the relationships between rulers and citizens, uncovering the profound influence of climate, religion, and culture on legal systems"
(Amazon https://bit.ly/3SJmIgm).

Voltaire (François-Marie Arouet) *(1694-1778)* was one of the greatest French writers of all time. His wide-ranging body of work includes plays, letters, essays, novellas, poems, and treatises that champion freedom of speech, freedom of religion, separation of church and state, and respect for the rights of man. Using wit and satire, Voltaire crusaded against all forms of tyranny, bigotry, and cruelty. A major figure of the Enlightenment, he is credited with influencing the shape of European civilization (Amazon https://bit.ly/42N73Rx)

Candide (1759)

"Voltaire's magnum opus is a matchless satirical take-down of religion, theologians, governments, armies, philosophies, and philosophers. The novella unfolds as the sheltered and privileged Candide, a young man enraptured of his facile mentor Pangloss, experiences the hardships and injustices of life, forcing him to abandon the naïve notion that "all is for the best" in favor of a practical determination that life is best lived "cultivating one's garden." Considered by many to be one of the greatest achievements of Western literature, Candide has influenced modern writers of black humor such as Céline, Joseph Heller, John Barth, Thomas Pynchon, Kurt Vonnegut, and Terry Southern" (Amazon https://bit.ly/42N73Rx)

Literary Civil Rights Leaders

Frederick Douglas *(1817-1895)* "an astonishing orator and a skillful writer, Douglass became a newspaper editor, a political activist, and an eloquent spokesperson for the civil rights of African Americans. He lived through the Civil War, the end of slavery, and the beginning of segregation. He was celebrated internationally as the leading Black intellectual of his day, and his story still resonates in ours. Born a slave circa 1818 on a plantation in Maryland, Douglass taught himself to read and write.

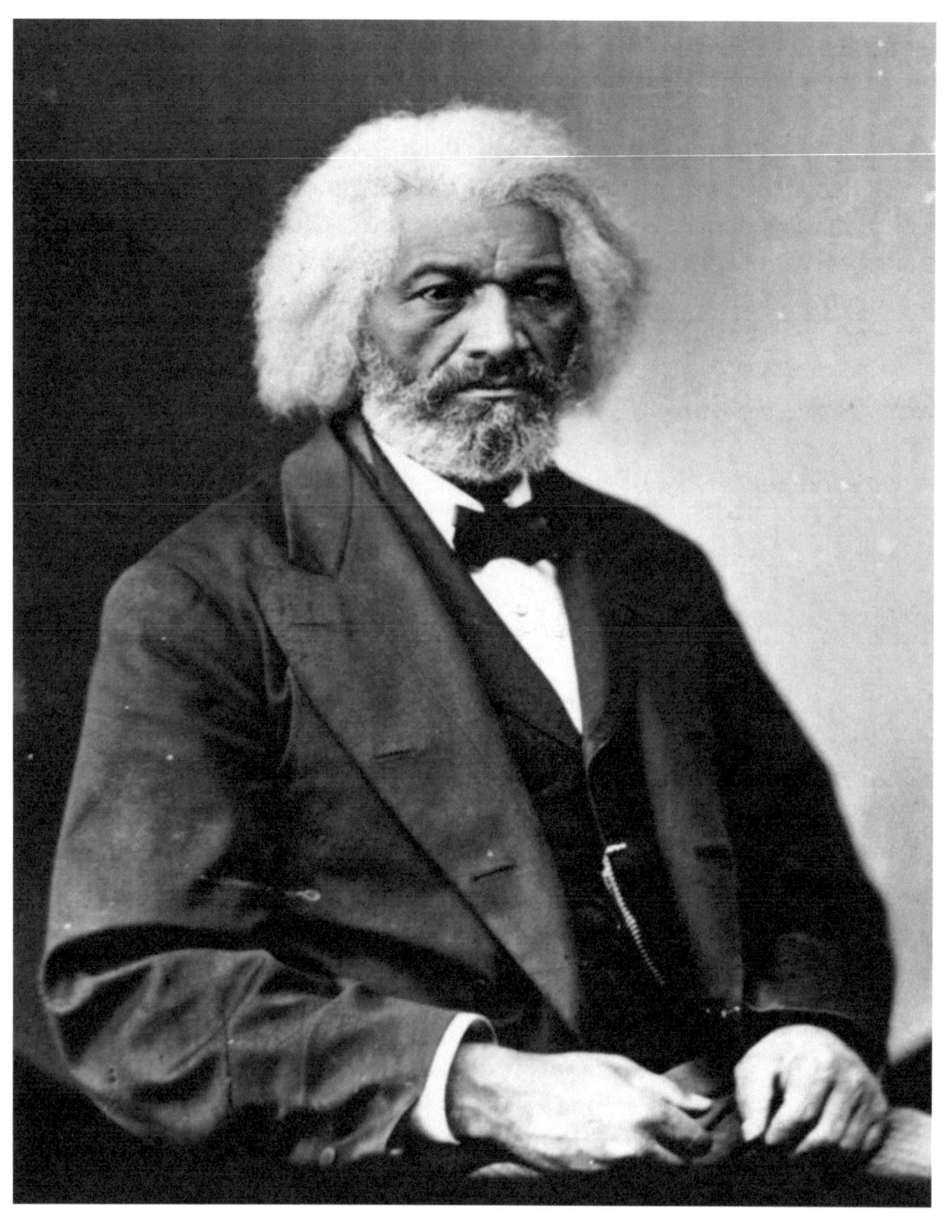

Frederick Douglas (1817-1895)
Howard, A. (2016). *The Black History Month Debate is Back.* [online] NBC News. Available at: https://www.nbcnews.com/news/nbcblk/black-history-month-debate-back-n502226

Narrative of the Life of Frederick Douglas calmly but dramatically recounts the horrors and the accomplishments of his early years—the daily, casual brutality of the white masters; his painful efforts to educate himself; his decision to find freedom or die; and his harrowing but successful escape" (Amazon https://amzn.to/3SNgBHG).

Narrative of the Life of Frederick Douglas an American Slave (1845)

"This is an Original Edition which was first Published in 1845. Narrative of the Life of Frederick Douglass is an 1845 memoir and treatise on abolition written by famous orator and former slave Frederick Douglass. It is generally held to be the most famous of a number of narratives written by former slaves during the same period"
(Amazon https://amzn.to/3SNgBHG).

John Howard Griffin *(1920-1980)*

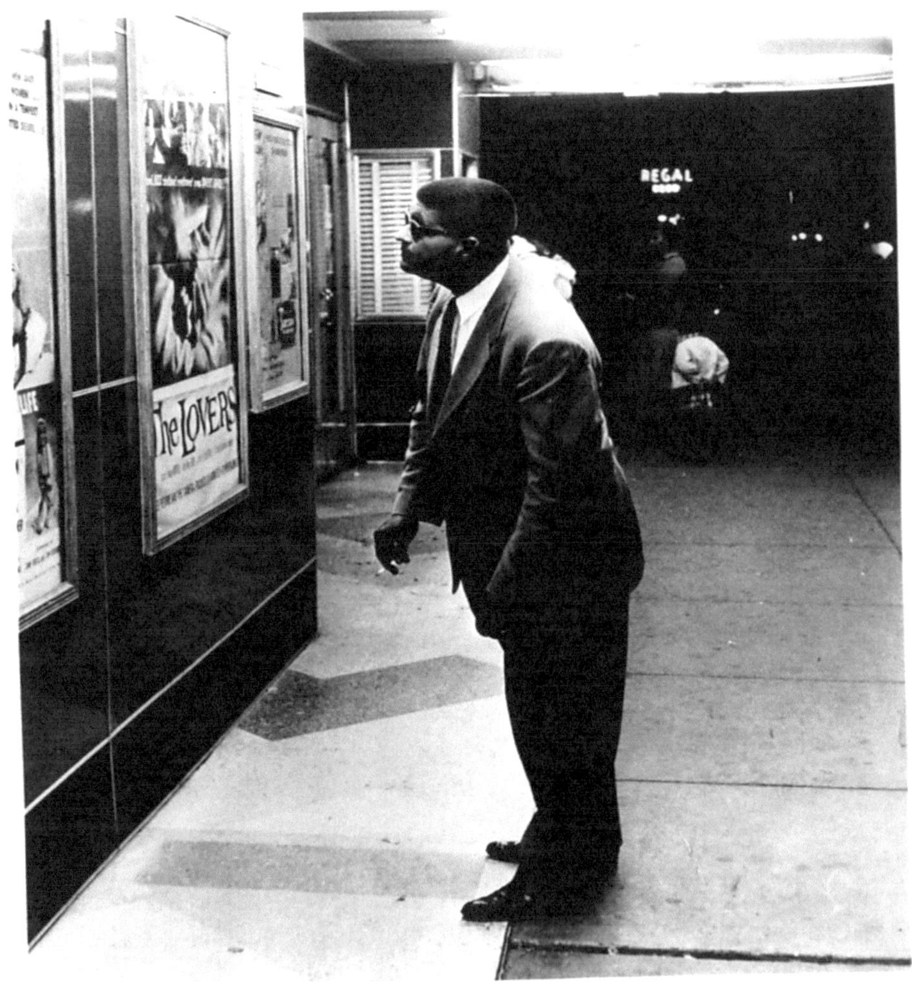

John Howard Griffin New Orleans1959
Black Like Me (1960)
Galehouse, M. (2011). John Howard Griffin's 'Black Like Me' at 50. *SFGATE*. [online] Available at: https://www.sfgate.com/entertainment/article/John-Howard-Griffin-s-Black-Like-Me-at-50-2328639.php

John Howard Griffin *(June 16, 1920 – September 9, 1980)* "was an American journalist and author from Texas who wrote about and championed racial equality. He is best known for his

1959 project to temporarily pass as a Black man and journey through the Deep South in order to see life and segregation from the other side of the color line first-hand" (Wikipedia, 2022).

Black Like Me (1959)

"In the Deep South of the 1950's, a color line was etched in blood across Louisiana, Mississippi, Alabama, and Georgia. Journalist John Howard Griffin decided to cross that line. Using medication that darkened his skin to deep brown, he exchanged his privileged life as a Southern white man for the disenfranchised world of an unemployed Black man.

What happened to John Howard Griffin—from the outside and within himself—as he made his way through the segregated Deep South is recorded in this searing work of nonfiction. His audacious, still chillingly relevant eyewitness history is a work about race and humanity every American must read" (Amazon https://bit.ly/49CYxH8).

James Baldwin *(1924-1987)* Baldwin's fiction "posed fundamental personal questions and dilemmas amid complex social and psychological pressures. Themes of masculinity, sexuality, race, and class intertwine to create intricate narratives that run parallel with some of the major political movements toward social change in mid-twentieth century America, such as the civil rights movement and the gay liberation movement. Baldwin's protagonists are often but not exclusively African American, and gay and bisexual men frequently feature prominently in his literature. These characters often face internal and external obstacles in their search for self- and social acceptance. *Time* magazine included his novel *Go Tell It on the Mountain (1953)* on the list of the 100 best English novels since 1923" (Wikipedia Contributors, 2019b).

Go Tell It on the Mountain (1953)

"Baldwin's classic novel opened new possibilities in the American language and in the way, Americans understand themselves. With lyrical precision, psychological directness, resonating symbolic power, and a rage that is at once unrelenting and compassionate, Baldwin tells the story of the stepson of the minister of a storefront Pentecostal church in Harlem one Saturday in March of 1935. Originally published in 1953, Baldwin said of his first novel, 'Mountain is the book I had to write if I was ever going to write anything else'" (Amazon https://bit.ly/48tcJRT).

Art as an Expression for Social Compassion - WWII

During the Spanish Civil War (1936-1939) two political factions fought for control of Spain's government. According to pablopicasso.org (2009), the town of Guernica located in the province of Biscay in Basque Country was regarded as the northern bastion of the Republican resistance movement and the epicenter of Basque culture, adding to its significance as a target by the opposing Nationalists. "At about 16:30 on Monday, 26 April 1937, warplanes of the German Condor Legion, commanded by Colonel Wolfram von Richthofen, bombed Guernica for about two hours. Germany, at this time led by Hitler, had lent material support to the Nationalists and were using the war as an opportunity to test out new weapons and tactics" (pablopicasso.org, 2009).

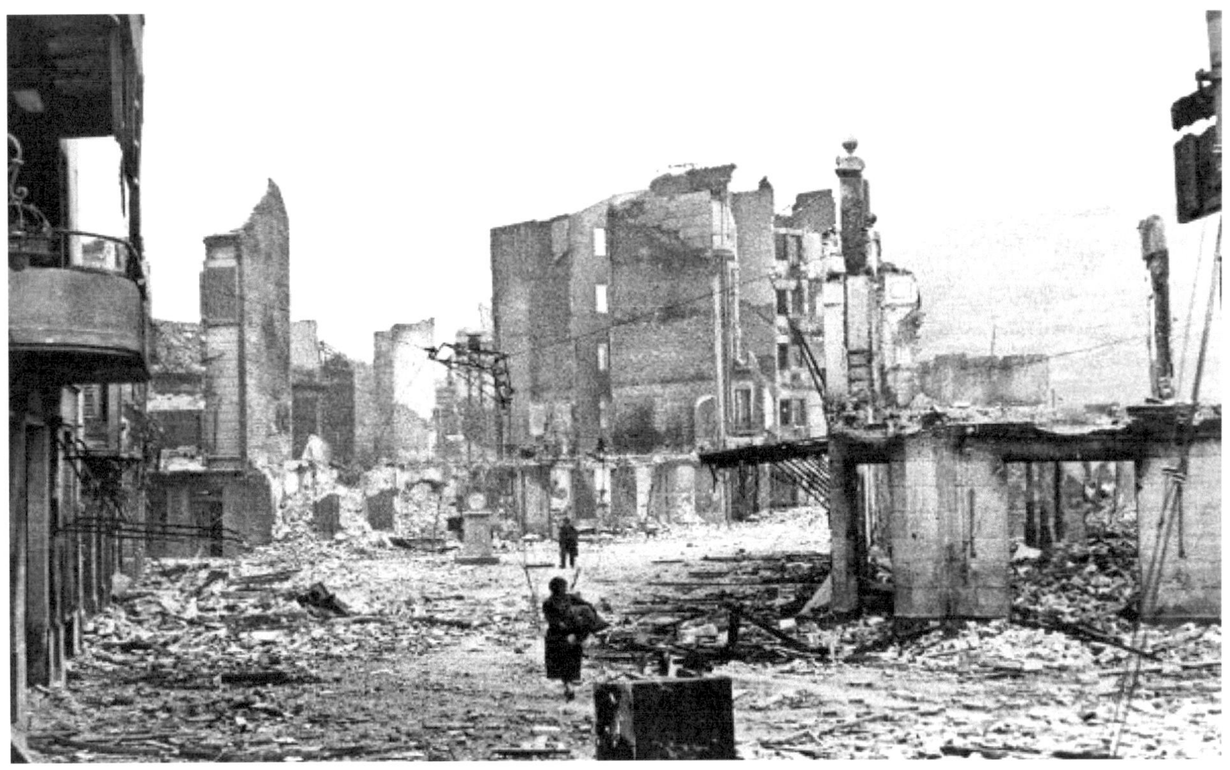

Guernica, April 1937
D'Alfonso, F. (2018). 26 aprile 1937: il bombardamento su Guernica. [online] Fanpage. Available at: https://www.fanpage.it/cultura/26-aprile-1937-il-bombardamento-su-guernica/

Although a native of Spain, Pablo Picasso took up residence in Paris early in life and was living in France at the time of Guernica's bombing. According to art historians, "Guernica should be seen as Picasso's comment on what art can actually contribute towards the self-assertion that liberates every human being and protects the individual against overwhelming forces such as political crime, war, and death" (pablopicasso.org, 2009).

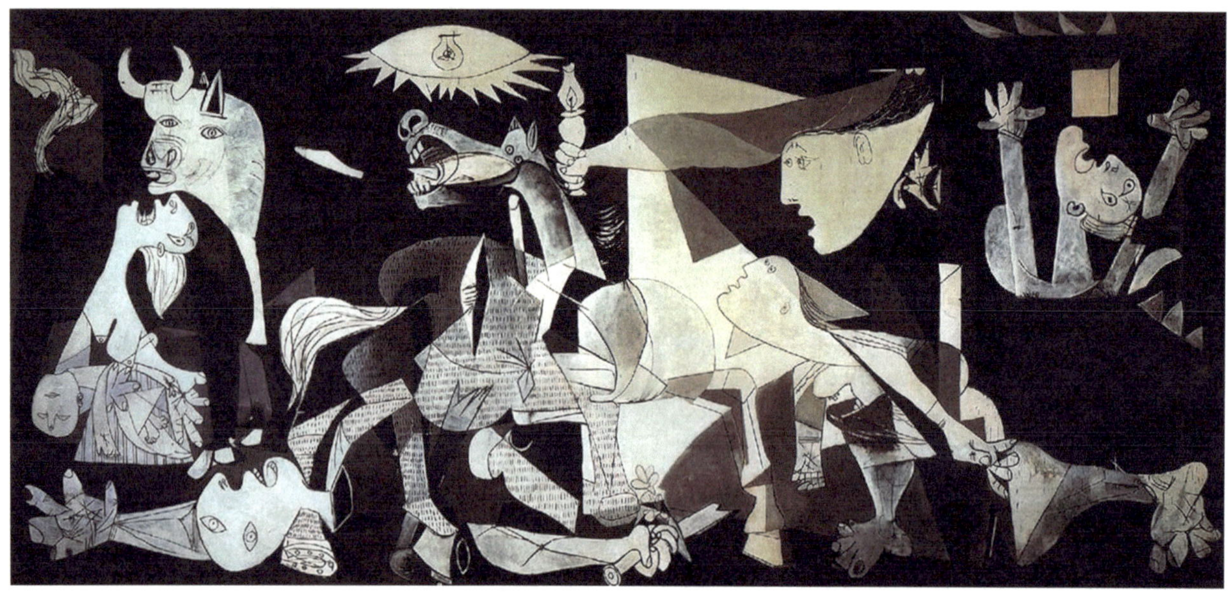

Guernica, 1937 by Pablo Picasso
Pablopicasso.org (2009). Guernica by Pablo Picasso. [online] https://www.pablopicasso.org. Available at: https://www.pablopicasso.org/guernica.jsp

Art as an Expression for Social Compassion - U.S. Civil Rights 1960's

The profound events of the 1960s civil rights movement in the U.S. culminated in an extortionary body of art works. To that end, the Brooklyn Museum celebrated the artists with an exhibition of their works March 7- July 13, 2014. According to the museum, "*Witness: Art and Civil Rights in the Sixties* offers a focused look at painting, sculpture, graphics, and photography from a decade defined by social protest and American race relations. In observance of the fiftieth anniversary of the Civil Rights Act of 1964, this exhibition considers how sixty-six of the decade's artists, including African Americans and some of their white, Latino, Asian American, Native American, and Caribbean contemporaries, used wide-ranging aesthetic approaches to address the struggle for racial justice" (Brooklyn Museum, 2014). Benny Andrew's *Witness* 1968 is one such painting.

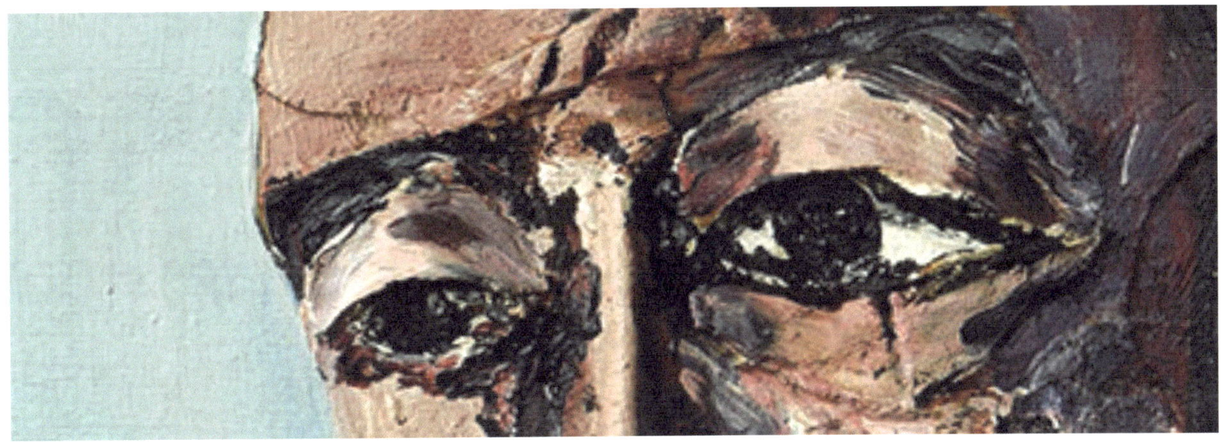

Witness (1968) Benny Andrews (1930-2006)

Brooklyn Museum (2014). *Brooklyn Museum: Witness: Art and Civil Rights in the Sixties*. [online] www.brooklynmuseum.org. Available at: https://www.brooklynmuseum.org/exhibitions/witness_civil_rights/

"The 1960s was a period of dramatic social and cultural upheaval, when artists aligned themselves with the massive campaign to end discrimination and bridged racial borders through creative work and acts of protest. Bringing activism to bear in gestural and geometric abstraction, assemblage, Minimalism, Pop imagery, and photography, these artists produced powerful works informed by the experience of inequality, conflict, and empowerment. In the process, they tested the political viability of their art, and originated subjects that spoke to resistance, self-definition, and blackness" (Brooklyn Museum, 2014).

Philip Guston (1913 -1980) was a Canadian American artist caught up in the brutality of the 1960's civil rights movement and the Vietnam war. In the late 1960s, Guston experienced an artistic crisis and is quoted as saying: "I was feeling split, schizophrenic. The war, what was happening in America, the brutality of the world. What kind of man am I, sitting at home, reading magazines, going into a frustrated fury about everything—and then going into my studio to adjust a red to a blue" (Brooklyn Museum, 2014). Many of his works portray images of the Ku Klux Klan.

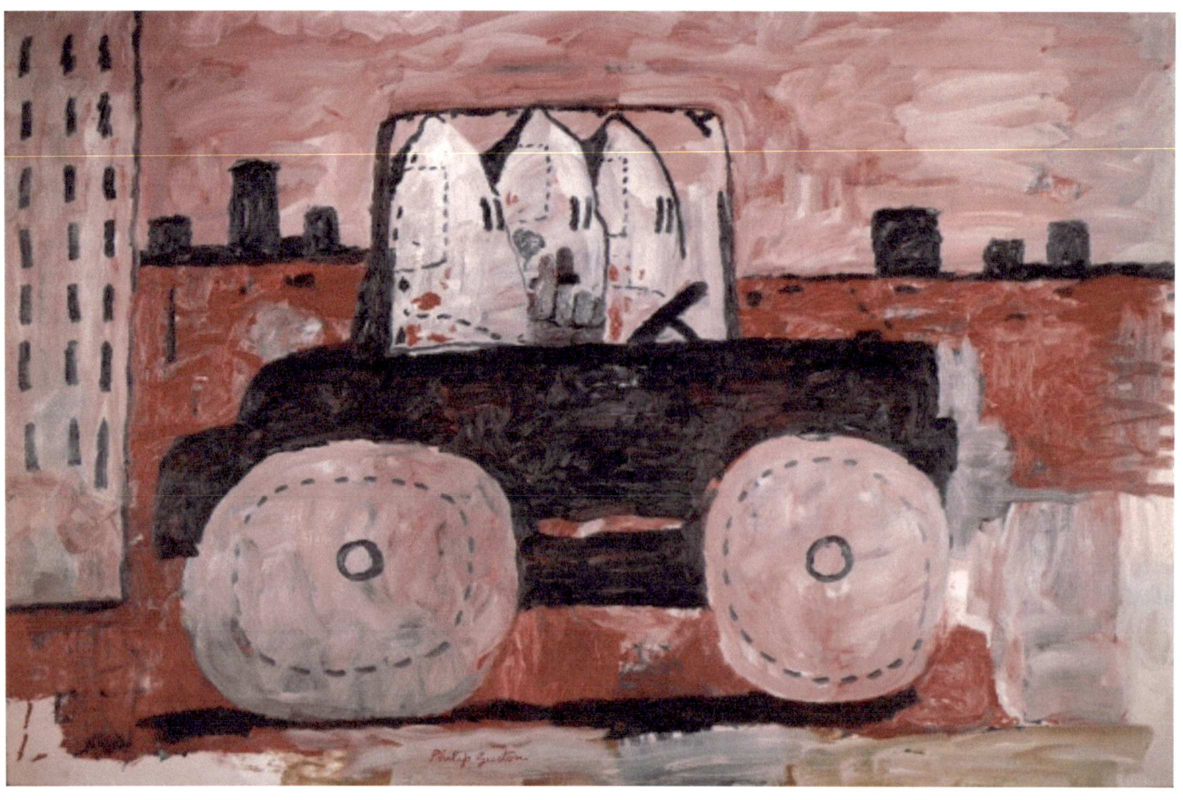

City Limits (1969) Philip Gaston (1913-1980)

Brooklyn Museum (2014). *Brooklyn Museum: Witness: Art and Civil Rights in the Sixties*. [online] www.brooklynmuseum.org. Available at: https://www.brooklynmuseum.org/exhibitions/witness_civil_rights/ [Accessed 23 Feb. 2024].

Music as an Expression for Social Compassion

The powerful voices of the civil rights movement wrought by Martin Luther King, Rosa Parks and Malcolm X "crafted the core messages of the movement and amplified our collective passion for a better world without prejudice, without violence and without racism — an ideal that our country is still fighting for today" (Feinstein, 2023). Ever present and accompanying the commanding voices of civil rights leaders rise an amazing chorus of musical genius.

Thought to be 19th Century African American song rising before, during or after the Civil War, *Oh Freedom!* has been performed by many artists including Odetta and Joan Baez.

The Odetta *Spiritual Trilogy: Oh Freedom/Come and Go with Me/I'm on My Way* can be discovered on Amazon: https://amzn.to/3wzXgSO . Here are the lyrics.

Oh Freedom!

Oh, freedom!
Oh, freedom!
Oh, freedom over me!
And before I'd be a slave
I'll be buried in my grave
And go home to my Lord and be free

No more moanin'
No more moanin'
No more moanin' over me
And before I'd be a slave
I'll be buried in my grave
And go home to my Lord and be free

There'll be singin'
There'll be singin'
There'll be singin' over me
And before I'd be a slave
I'll be buried in my grave
And go home to my Lord and be free

There'll be shoutin'
There'll be shoutin'
There'll be shoutin' over me
And before I'd be a slave
I'll be buried in my grave
And go home to my Lord and be free

Oh, freedom!
Oh, freedom!
Oh, freedom over me!
And before I'd be a slave
I'll be buried in my grave
And go home to my Lord and be free

According to Music's Voice in the American Civil Rights Movement (Feinstein, 2023), no song was more strongly associated with the Civil Rights movement than *We Shall Overcome.* Believed to be based on a 19th-century African American Gospel song it gained popularity during the 1940's labor movement and was performed by Joan Baez at the 1963 March on Washington. Legend has it that President Johnson Lyndon quoted it before Congress in proposing the Voting Rights Act in 1965 (Feinstein, 2023).

"Joan Baez was the most important artist to rise from the folk music movement that first blossomed in the late 1950s and early '60s. Baez was also the finest and most influential interpretive singer in contemporary folk; blessed with a soprano voice of uncommon clarity, her performances were emotionally compelling without resorting to histrionics" (Amazon *We Shall Overcome* Joan Baez https://amzn.to/3USvI5o).

We Shall Overcome

Reverend Charles A. Tindley 1901

We shall overcome
We shall overcome
We shall overcome, someday
Oh, deep in my heart
I know that I do believe
We shall overcome, someday

We shall be alright
We shall be alright
We shall be alright, someday

Oh, deep in my heart
I know that I do believe
We shall overcome, someday

We shall live in peace
We shall live in peace
We shall live in peace, someday

Oh, deep in my heart
I know that I do believe
We shall overcome, someday

We are not afraid (oh Lord)
We are not afraid (oh Lord)
We are not afraid, today

Oh, deep in my heart
I know that I do believe
We shall overcome, someday

We shall overcome (oh Lord)
We shall overcome (oh Lord)
We shall overcome, someday

Oh, deep in my heart
I know that I do believe
We shall overcome, someday

Give Me Some Blues

The blues reflects the heart of soul. The beginnings can be traced to the late 1860s, one of the most vicious and violent periods in the United States. Vigilante justice was at an all-time high, and by 1889, the lynching of African Americans surged dramatically. It was after all post-Civil War and the white supremacists of the south were unsettled. The bluesman and blueswoman emerged in this challenging time.

The blues did not speak of the life of the enslaved but of the experiences of freed men and women during the periods of Reconstruction and Jim Crow. It spoke of cotton bales/gins, boll weevil, juke houses, and sharecropping. Farming and sharecropping were the starting places for most of the legendary blues musicians celebrated today, including Charlie Patton, Rubin Lacey,

Son House, Howling Wolf, Muddy Waters and the most famous in recent generations, B.B. King (Pearley, 2018).

"Blues incorporated spirituals, work songs, field hollers, shouts, chants, and rhymed simple narrative ballads from the African-American culture. The blues form is ubiquitous in jazz, rhythm and blues, and rock and roll, and is characterized by the call-and-response pattern, the blues scale, and specific chord progressions, of which the twelve-bar blues is the most common" (Wikipedia contributors, 2019a).

Josh White (1914-1969) was one such bluesman. He grew up in the South during the 1920s and 1930s and became a prominent race records artist, with a prolific output of recordings in genres including Piedmont blues, country blues, gospel music, and social protest songs (Wikipedia, 2024). *One Meat Ball* Josh White (Amazon https://amzn.to/48sbYZt).

One Meat Ball

Josh White (1944)

The little man walked up and down
To find an eating place in town
He read the menu through and through
To see what 15 cents could do

One meat ball
One meat ball
He could afford but one meat ball
He told the waiter near at hand
The simple dinner he had planned
The guests were startled one and all
To hear the waiter loudly call
One meat ball everbody
One meat ball
Hey this here gent wants one meat ball

You know, the little man felt ill at ease
He said some bread sir if you please
The waiter hollered down the hall

You gets no bread with one meat ball
One meat ball
One meat ball
Well, you gets no bread with one meat ball

The little man felt very bad
One meat ball was all he had
And in his dreams he hears that call
You gets no bread with one meat ball
One meat ball and no spaghetti
One meat ball
You gets no bread with one meat ball
Let's try it one more time, now
One meat ball. A little louder
One meat ball
That one was gooey
You gets no bread with one meat ball

According to Feinstein (2023), on October 8, 1963, en route to Shreveport, Louisiana, Sam Cooke called ahead to the Holiday Inn North to make reservations for his wife, Barbara, and himself, but when he and his group arrived, the desk clerk glanced nervously and explained there were no vacancies. Outraged, and certain the absence of vacancies was race based discrimination, Cooke wrote *A Change is Gonna Come.* Cooke wrote in the genre of soul and is regarded by many the "King of Soul" (Wikipedia Contributors, 2019c).

A Change Gonna Come Sam Cooke (Amazon https://amzn.to/3IdRusE).

A Change is Gonna Come
Sam Cooke 1964

I was born by the river
In a little tent
Oh, and just like the river, I've been running
Ever since
It's been a long
A long time coming, but I know
A change gon' come
Oh yes, it will

It's been too hard living
But I'm afraid to die
'Cause I don't know what's up there
Beyond the sky

It's been a long
A long time coming, but I know
A change gon' come
Oh yes, it will

I go to the movie
And I go downtown
And somebody keep telling me
"Don't hang around"

It's been a long
A long time coming, but I know
A change gon' come
Oh yes, it will
Then, I go to my brother
And I say, "Brother, help me, please"
But he winds up knockin' me
Back down on my knees, oh

There been times that I thought
I couldn't last for long
But now, I think I'm able
To carry on

It's been a long
A long time coming, but I know
A change gon' come
Oh yes, it will

Jazz: a Synthesis

"John Coltrane's Civil Rights elegy "Alabama" first appeared on Live at Birdland (1964), though it was recorded in Van Gelder Studio, Englewood Cliffs, New Jersey on November 18,

1963 – three months after the dramatic events surrounding the 16th Street Baptist Church bombing of September 15, 1963.

On this tragic date, four members of the Ku Klux Klan planted at least fifteen sticks of dynamite attached to a timing device beneath the front steps of the Church. The explosion killed four young girls and injured many others. It was a turning point in the Civil Rights movement" (Micucci, 2016).

Alabama John Coltrane (1964) (Amazon https://amzn.to/3T9D17n).

Filmography as an Expression of Social Compassion

Over the years in the 20th and 21st centuries writers, directors, actors, actresses, and produces have created spellbinding tales through the lens of moviemaking. Listed here, just a few.

Three Billboards Outside Ebbing, Mississippi (2017)

(IMDb https://www.imdb.com/title/tt5027774/?ref_=nm_knf_t_2).

A mother personally challenges the local authorities to solve her daughter's murder.

Frances McDormand, Woody Harrelson, Sam Rockwell

Dead Man Walking (1995) (IMDb https://www.imdb.com/title/tt0112818/).

A nun comforts a convicted killer on death row.

Susan Sarandon, Sean Penn, Robert Prosky

Kiss of the Spider Woman (1985) (IMDb https://www.imdb.com/title/tt0089424/)

William Hurt, Raul Julia, Sonia Braga

A gay man and a political prisoner are together in a prison.

The Hurricane (1999) (IMDb https://www.imdb.com/title/tt0174856/).

Denzel Washington, Vicellous Shannon, Deborah Kara Unger

The story of Rubin "Hurricane" Carter, a boxer wrongly imprisoned for murder.

The Shawshank Redemption (IMDb https://www.imdb.com/title/tt0111161/)

Tim Robbins, Morgan Freeman, Bob Gunton

Over the course of several years, two convicts form a friendship, seeking consolation and, redemption through basic compassion.

Slumdog Millionaire (2008) (IMDb https://www.imdb.com/title/tt1010048/).

Dev Patel, Freida Pinto, Saurabh Shukla

A teenager from the slums of Mumbai becomes a contestant on the show 'Kaun Banege Crorepati?' when interrogated under the suspicion of cheating, he revisits his past, revealing how he had all the answers.

Killers of the Flower Moon (2023) (IMDb https://www.imdb.com/title/tt5537002/).

Leonardo DiCaprio, Robert De Niro, Lily Gladstone

When oil is discovered under Osage Nation land in Oklahoma in the 1920s, Osage people are murdered one by one – until the FBI steps in to unravel the mystery.

Questions for Further Consideration:

1. What is the evidence that literary, artistic, theatrical and musical expressions promote social compassion?
2. The judicial opinions of Supreme Court Chief Justice Earl Warren (1953 – 1969) paved an expeditious path to many of the Civil Rights achievements during the height of the Civil Rights movement. Considering all media, what literary, artistic, theatrical and/or musical expressions influenced him.

3. How do proponents of book banning reconcile their perspectives with the U.S. Constitution 1st Amendment: "Congress shall make no law respecting an establishment of religion, or prohibiting the free exercise thereof; or abridging the freedom of speech, or of the press; or the right of the people peaceably to assemble, and to petition the Government for a redress of grievances."

Sentinel Readings for a Deeper Dive

Baldwin, James (1953). Go Tell It on the Mountain (Amazon https://bit.ly/48tcJRT).
Blakemore, E. (2022). The history of book bans—and their changing targets—in the U.S. [online] National Geographic. Available at: https://www.nationalgeographic.com/culture/article/history-of-book-bans-in-the-united-states

Brooks, K. (2014). These Are The Artists Of The Civil Rights Movement. [online] HuffPost Canada. Available at: https://www.huffpost.com/entry/civil-rights-art_n_4769268

Feinstein, M. (2023). Great American Songbook Foundation: Music's Voice in the American Civil Rights Movement. [online] The Center For The Performing Arts. Available at: https://thesongbook.org/about/news-media/the-songbook-blog-items/musics-voice-in-the-american-civil-rights-movement/

Griffin, John Howard (1960). *Black Like Me (*Amazon https://bit.ly/49CYxH8).

References

Blakemore, E. (2022). *The history of book bans—and their changing targets—in the U.S.* [online] National Geographic. Available at: https://www.nationalgeographic.com/culture/article/history-of-book-bans-in-the-united-states [Accessed 24 Feb. 2024].

Britannica (2024). *Enlightenment | Definition, Summary, Ideas, Meaning, History, Philosophers, & Facts | Britannica.* [online] www.britannica.com. Available at: https://www.britannica.com/event/Enlightenment-European-history#Overview [Accessed 19 Feb. 2024].

Brooklyn Museum (2014). *Brooklyn Museum: Witness: Art and Civil Rights in the Sixties.* [online] www.brooklynmuseum.org. Available at: https://www.brooklynmuseum.org/exhibitions/witness_civil_rights/ [Accessed 23 Feb. 2024].

Brooks, K. (2014). *These Are The Artists Of The Civil Rights Movement.* [online] HuffPost Canada. Available at: https://www.huffpost.com/entry/civil-rights-art_n_4769268 [Accessed 24 Feb. 2024].

Carpenter, A. (2010). Beccaria, Cesare: Classical School. *Encyclopedia of Criminological Theory*. [online] Available at: https://study.sagepub.com/system/files/Beccaria,%20Cesare%20-%20Classical%20School.pdf [Accessed 19 Feb. 2024].

D'Alfonso, F. (2018). *26 aprile 1937: il bombardamento su Guernica*. [online] Fanpage. Available at: https://www.fanpage.it/cultura/26-aprile-1937-il-bombardamento-su-guernica/ [Accessed 22 Feb. 2024].

Feinstein, M. (2023). *Great American Songbook Foundation: Music's Voice in the American Civil Rights Movement*. [online] The Center For The Performing Arts. Available at: https://thesongbook.org/about/news-media/the-songbook-blog-items/musics-voice-in-the-american-civil-rights-movement/ [Accessed 23 Feb. 2024].

Galehouse, M. (2011). John Howard Griffin's 'Black Like Me' at 50. *SFGATE*. [online] Available at: https://www.sfgate.com/entertainment/article/John-Howard-Griffin-s-Black-Like-Me-at-50-2328639.php [Accessed 20 Feb. 2024].

Howard, A. (2016). *The Black History Month Debate is Back*. [online] NBC News. Available at: https://www.nbcnews.com/news/nbcblk/black-history-month-debate-back-n502226 [Accessed 19 Feb. 2024].

McIntosh, M. (2020). *Five Philosophers of the Enlightenment*. [online] Brewminate. Available at: https://brewminate.com/five-philosophers-of-the-enlightenment/ [Accessed 19 Feb. 2024].

Micucci, M. (2016). *Nov. 18, 1963...John Coltrane records 'Alabama'*. [online] JAZZIZ Magazine. Available at: https://www.jazziz.com/nov-18-1963-john-coltrane-records-alabama/ [Accessed 24 Feb. 2024].

Pablopicasso.org (2009). *Guernica by Pablo Picasso*. [online] https://www.pablopicasso.org. Available at: https://www.pablopicasso.org/guernica.jsp [Accessed 22 Feb. 2024].

Pearley Sr., L. (2018). *The Historical Roots of Blues Music – AAIHS*. [online] Aaihs.org. Available at: https://www.aaihs.org/the-historical-roots-of-blues-music/ [Accessed 23 Feb. 2024].

Wikipedia Contributors (2019a). *Blues*. [online] Wikipedia. Available at: https://en.wikipedia.org/wiki/Blues [Accessed 23 Feb. 2024].

Wikipedia Contributors (2019b). *James Baldwin*. [online] Wikipedia. Available at: https://en.wikipedia.org/wiki/James_Baldwin [Accessed 19 Feb. 2024].

Wikipedia Contributors (2019c). *Sam Cooke*. [online] Wikipedia. Available at: https://en.wikipedia.org/wiki/Sam_Cooke [Accessed 24 Feb. 2024].

Wikipedia. (2022). *John Howard Griffin*. [online] Available at: https://en.wikipedia.org/wiki/John_Howard_Griffin [Accessed 19 Feb. 2024].

Wikipedia. (2024). *Josh White*. [online] Available at: https://en.wikipedia.org/wiki/Josh_White#Career [Accessed 24 Feb. 2024].

AUTHOR'S BIO SKETCH

James Lenhart. MD, FAAFP, MPH

Dr. Lenhart graduated from the University of New Mexico School of Medicine and took residency in Family Medicine from Brown University Affiliated Hospitals in Pawtucket/Providence, Rhode Island. In 2010 he completed a Master of Public Health degree from the University of Liverpool. He holds the distinction of academic rank of full professor from the University of North Carolina-Chapel Hill, University of Nevada, and University of Arizona.

He now serves as an Associate Program Director for the residency in Family Medicine at Community Health Care in Tacoma, Washington, a University of Washington affiliated program. In that capacity, Dr. Lenhart leads curriculum development including research and scholarship at the residency where he holds academic rank of Associate Clinical Professor.

Chapter 20

Epilogue

James Lenhart, MD, MPH, Author and Senior Editor

"Of all the forms of inequality, injustice in health is the most shocking and inhuman."

- The Reverend Martin Luther King, Jr., in address to the Medical Committee for Human Rights, 1966. King was a prominent civil rights leader, and Nobel Peace Prize laureate. He was assassinated on April 4, 1968 in Memphis, Tennessee.

In Conclusion

In this treatise the Family Physicians and Colleagues for Health Justice emphasized recent and remote events as well as information drawn from peer reviewed academic journals to shine bright light on the social determinants of health. We aimed to keep it simple in order that the imperative for health justice can be understood for all who take time to explore these pages. We dug into sentinel historical events to illustrate how race, justice, socioeconomic status, gender, food security, access to health care, educational opportunity, water and sanitation, employment, work environments, transportation, housing, communication and access to information technology impact health outcomes. No attempt was made to create an epidemiologic deep dive, but rather bring to life meaningful historical events to demonstrate the effect of social determinants of health embraced or neglected.

The essays on Justice, Race, Gender, and Poverty stand out as crucial to the overall concepts posited here. This by no way diminishes the pages rolled out by others, but Joe Eubanks' chapter on race brings in your face recognition of the abomination of racial discrimination over four centuries in the United States. Tied together with the chapters on Justice, Gender, and Poverty, authors set a solid foundation to enhance meaning in the essays that followed.

Our efforts explored the case for declining life expectancy in the United States despite extraordinary national wealth. All this, while other high-income countries continue to enjoy increasing life expectancy. Why? In retrospect, revisit the following. A probable reason unfolds.

Figure 1. ***Life expectancy at birth*** how long, on average, a newborn can expect to live, if current death rates do not change. Japan 84.7, Norway 83.2, Korea 83.5, Canada 81.7, United States 77

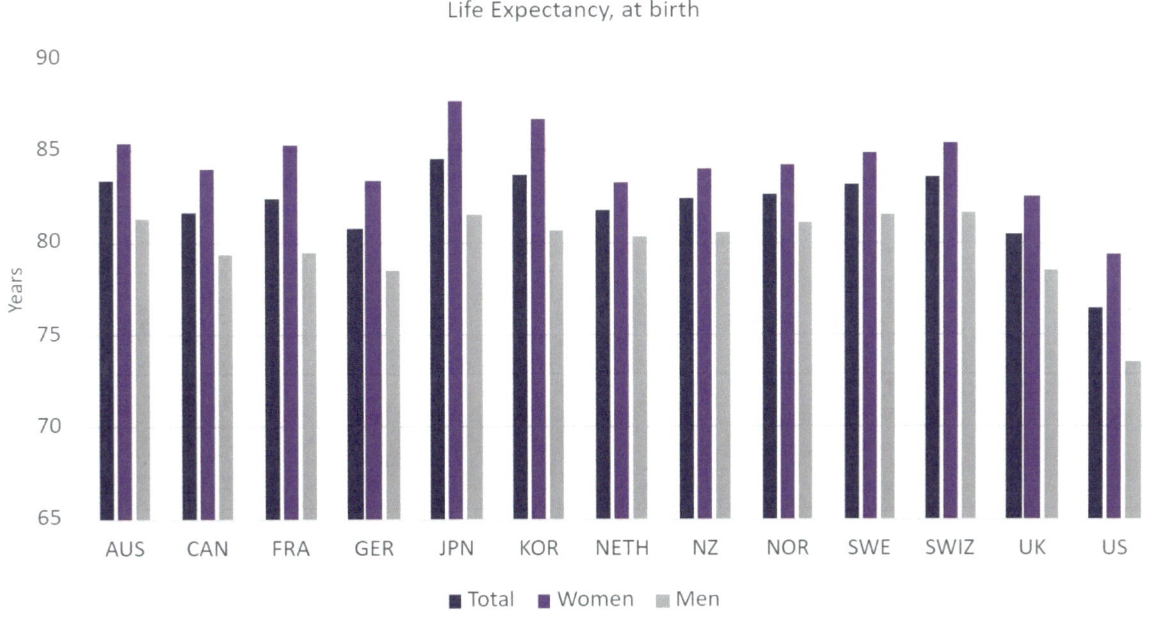

OECD (2021). *Health status - Life expectancy at birth - OECD Data.* [online] Available at: https://data.oecd.org/healthstat/life-expectancy-at-birth.htm

Figure 2. ***Life expectancy at age 65 years*** the average number of years that men & women aged 65 years can expect to live. Norway 19.8 & 21.8, Korea 19.3 & 23.8, U.S. 17 & 19.7

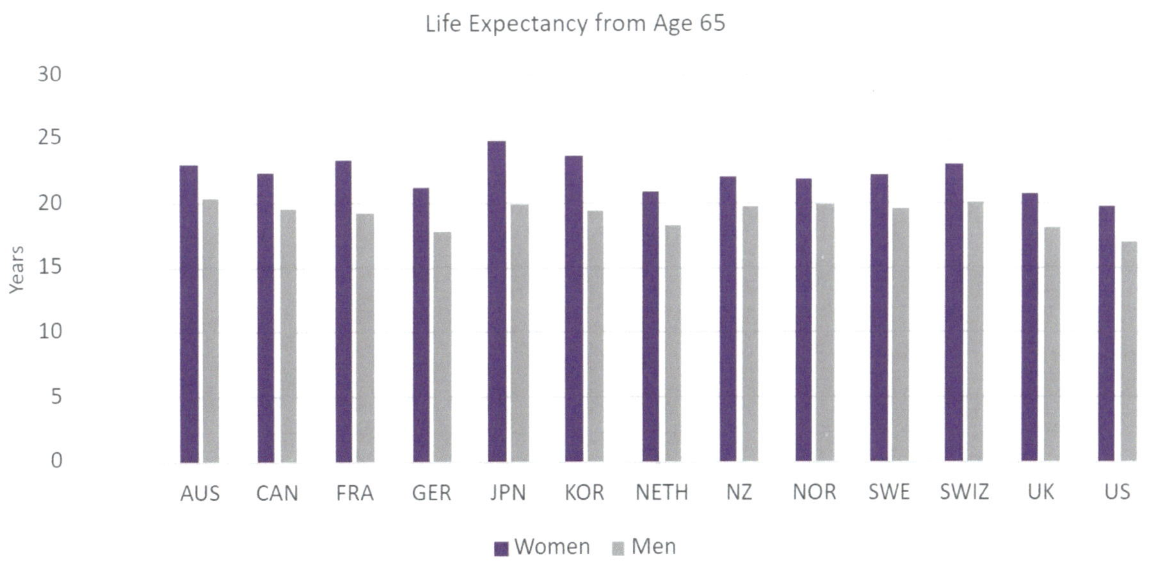

OECD (2017). *Health status - Life expectancy at 65 - OECD Data.* [online] Available at: https://data.oecd.org/healthstat/life-expectancy-at-65.htm

Figure 3. ***Infant Mortality.*** infant mortality rate is defined as the number of deaths of children under one year of age, expressed per 1 000 live births. Finland & Sweden 1.8, Norway 1.9, Korea 2.4, United States 5.4

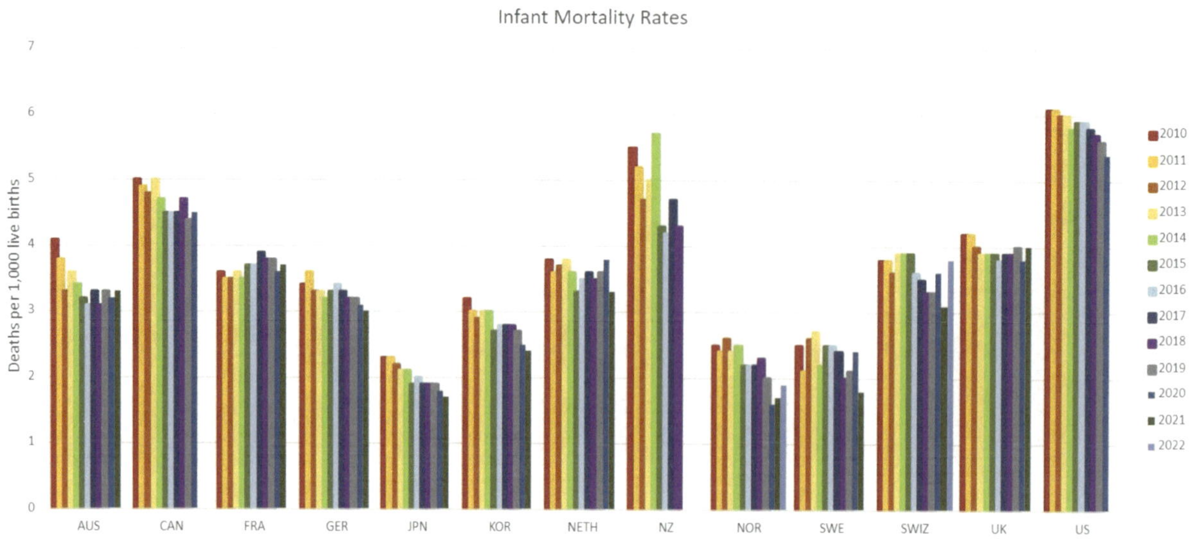

OECD (2023a). *Health status - Infant mortality rates - OECD Data.* [online] Available at: https://data.oecd.org/healthstat/infant-mortality-rates.htm

Figure 4. ***Maternal Mortality*** is defined as the death of a woman while pregnant or during childbirth or within 42 days of termination of pregnancy, irrespective of the duration and site of the pregnancy, from any cause related to or aggravated by the pregnancy or its management but not from unintentional or incidental causes. Norway 3.7, Sweden 7.0, Korea 11.8, United States 23.8

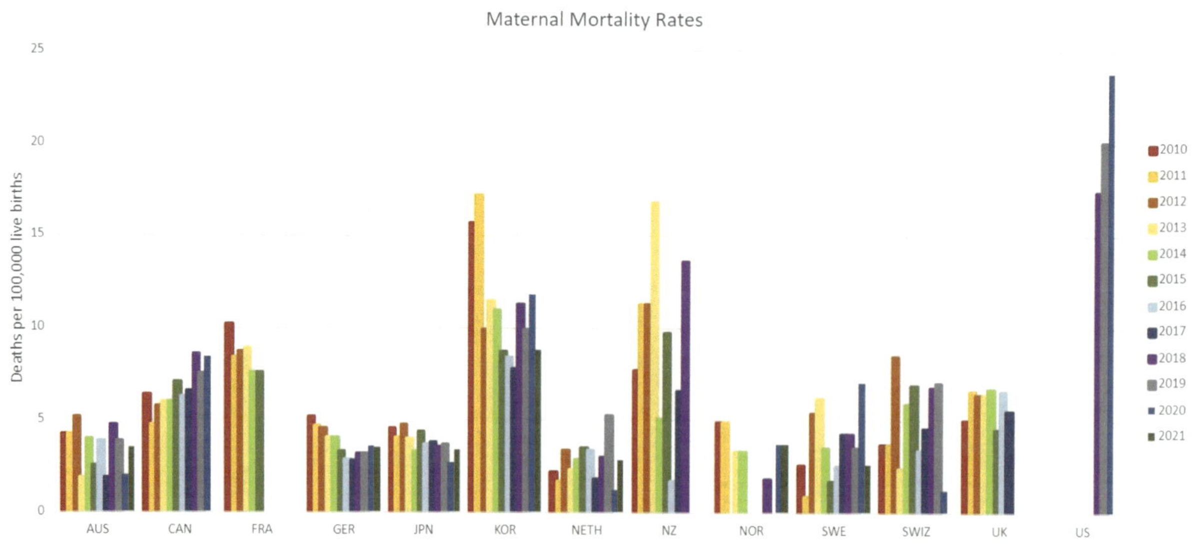

OECD (2022b). *Health Status : Maternal and infant mortality.* [online] stats.oecd.org. Available at: https://stats.oecd.org/index.aspx?queryid=30116

Figure 5. ***National Wealth:*** The total Gross Domestic Product in the U.S. leads all other countries by substantial margins.

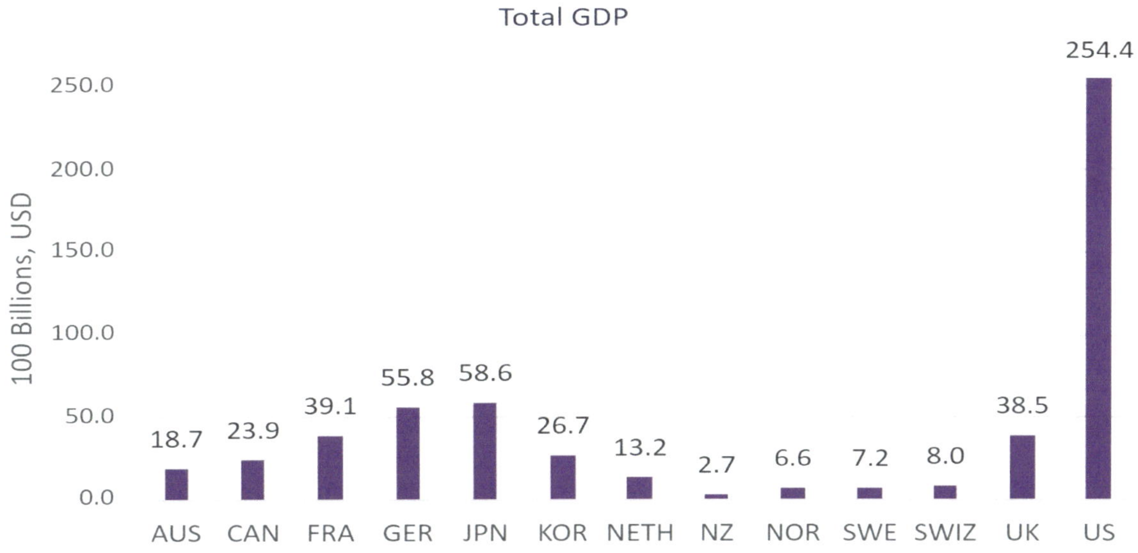

OECD (2022). *GDP and spending - Gross domestic product (GDP) - OECD Data.* [online] Available at: https://data.oecd.org/gdp/gross-domestic-product-gdp.htm

Figure 6. ***National Wealth:*** The U.S. GDP per capita is third to Norway and Switzerland.

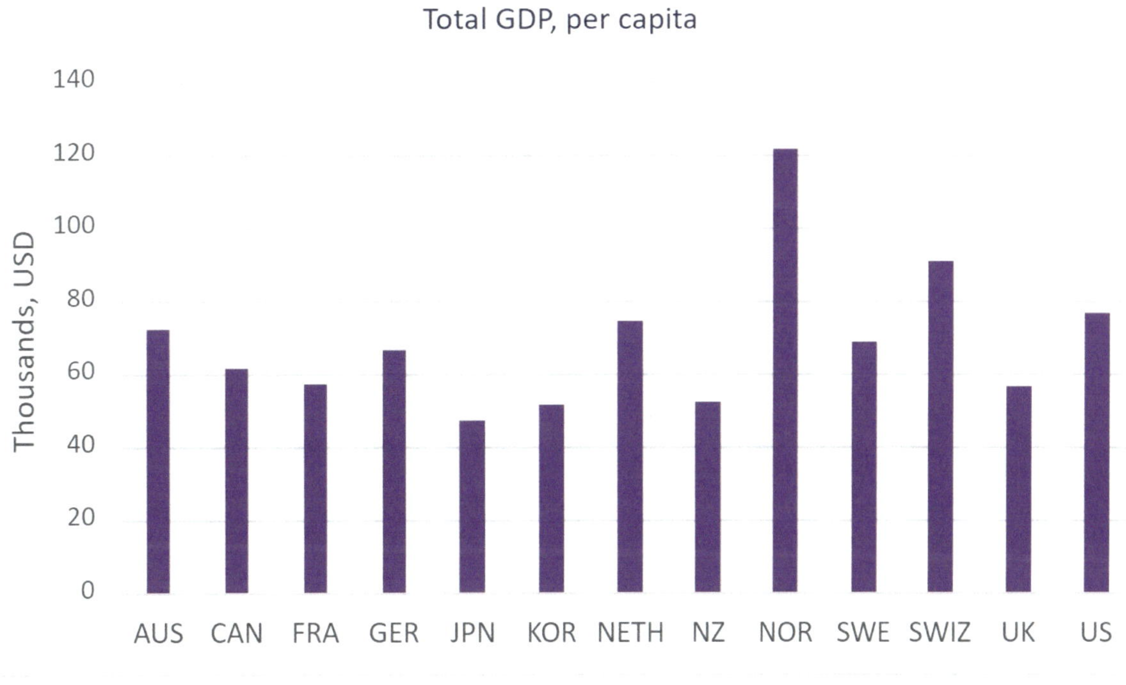

OECD (2024). *Level of GDP per capita and productivity : GDP per capita levels - most recent year.* [online] stats.oecd.org. Available at: https://stats.oecd.org/Index.aspx?QueryId=95894

Figure 7. ***The U.S. spends 17.8% of its Gross Domestic Product*** (GDP) on health care. ***Korea spends*** 8.8% of its GDP on health care.

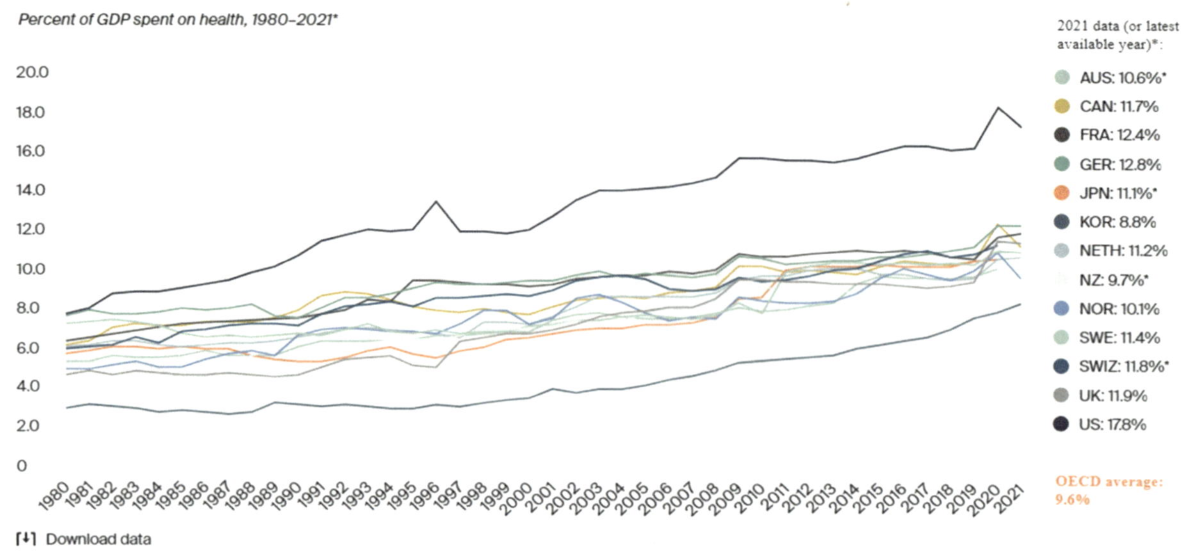

Gunja, M., Gumas, E. and Williams II, R. (2023). *U.S. Health Care from a Global Perspective, 2022: Accelerating Spending, Worsening Outcomes*. [online] The Commonwealth Fund. Available at: https://www.commonwealthfund.org/publications/issue-briefs/2023/jan/us-health-care-global-perspective-2022

Figure 8. ***U.S. Per Capita Health Spending Compared***

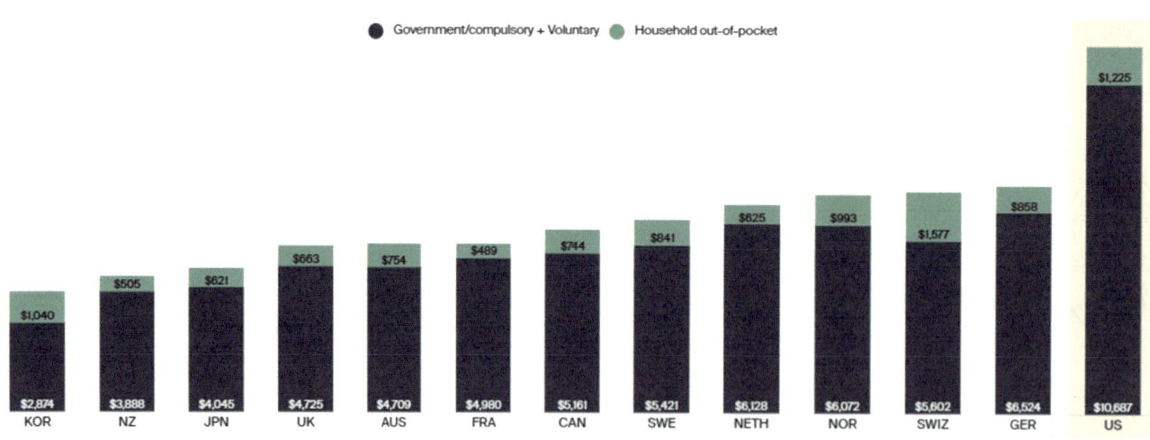

Gunja, M., Gumas, E. and Williams II, R. (2023). *U.S. Health Care from a Global Perspective, 2022: Accelerating Spending, Worsening Outcomes*. [online] The Commonwealth Fund. Available at: https://www.commonwealthfund.org/publications/issue-briefs/2023/jan/us-health-care-global-perspective-2022

Figure 9. ***Potential Years of Lost Life*** is a summary measure of premature mortality, providing an explicit way of weighting deaths occurring at younger ages, which may be preventable

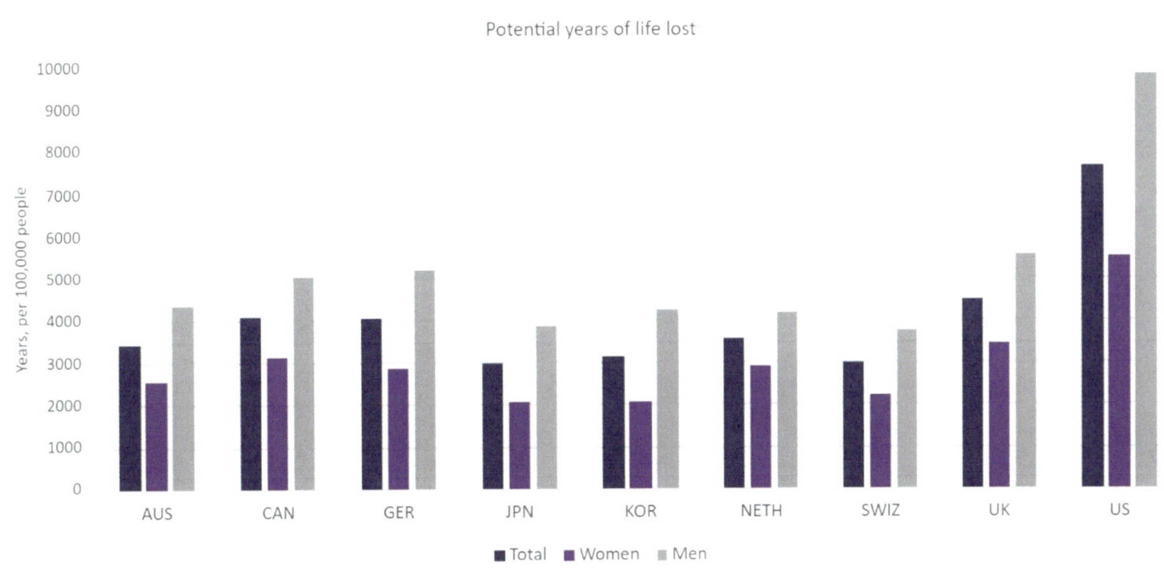

OECD (2021b). *Health Status : Potential years of life lost.* [online] stats.oecd.org. Available at: https://stats.oecd.org/index.aspx?queryid=30124

Figure 10. ***Avoidable Deaths per 100,000 Population*** preventable mortality is defined as causes of death that can be avoided through effective public health and primary prevention measures. Treatable mortality is defined as causes of death that can be avoided through timely and effective health care interventions, including secondary prevention and treatment.

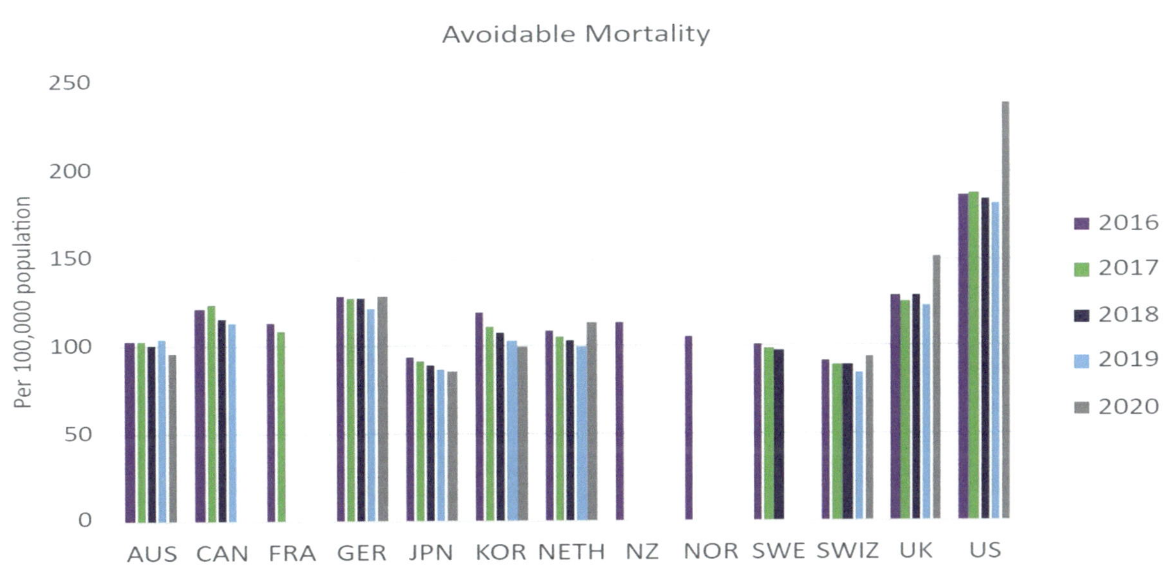

OECD (2023). *Health Status : Avoidable mortality.* [online] stats.oecd.org. Available at: https://stats.oecd.org/Index.aspx?QueryId=96018

Table 11. ***COVID-19 Death Rate***

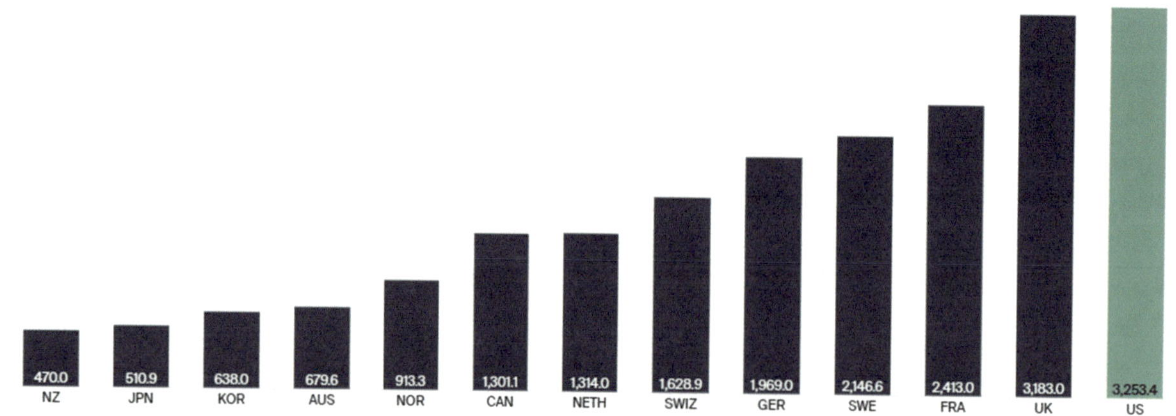

Gunja, M., Gumas, E. and Williams II, R. (2023). *U.S. Health Care from a Global Perspective, 2022: Accelerating Spending, Worsening Outcomes*. [online] The Commonwealth Fund. Available at: https://www.commonwealthfund.org/publications/issue-briefs/2023/jan/us-health-care-global-perspective-2022

Figure 12. ***Life Expectancy in the U.S. is falling:*** 1980 73.7 years; 2021 77 years. ***In Korea Life Expectancy has risen*** from 66.1 years in 1980 to 83.5 years in 2021.

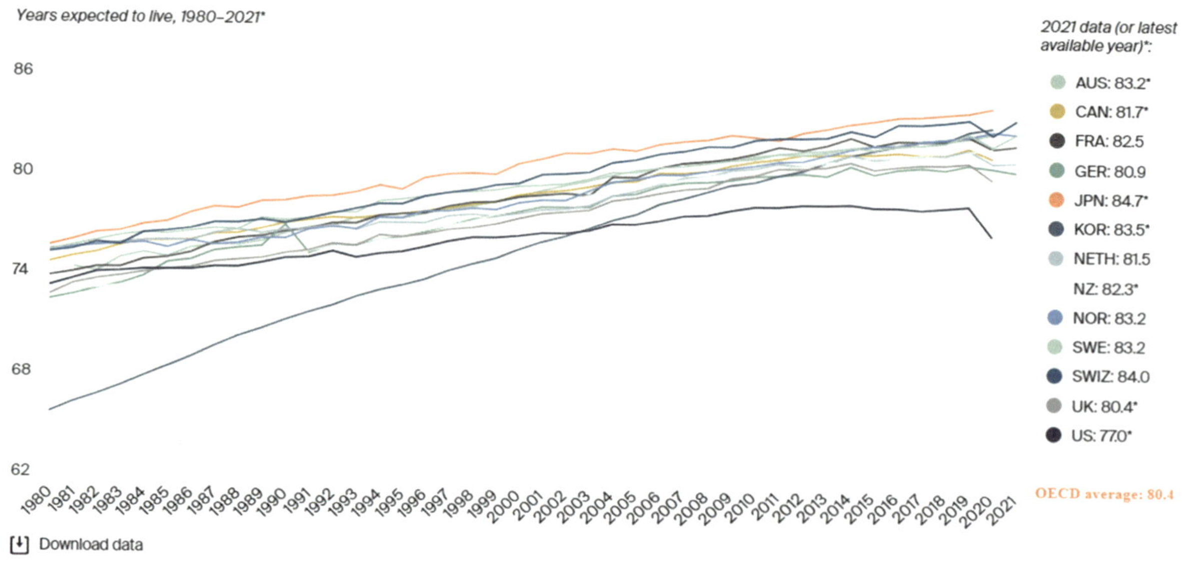

Gunja, M., Gumas, E. and Williams II, R. (2023). *U.S. Health Care from a Global Perspective, 2022: Accelerating Spending, Worsening Outcomes*. [online] The Commonwealth Fund. Available at: https://www.commonwealthfund.org/publications/issue-briefs/2023/jan/us-health-care-global-perspective-2022

Figure 13. ***Influenza Vaccination Rates 2022***

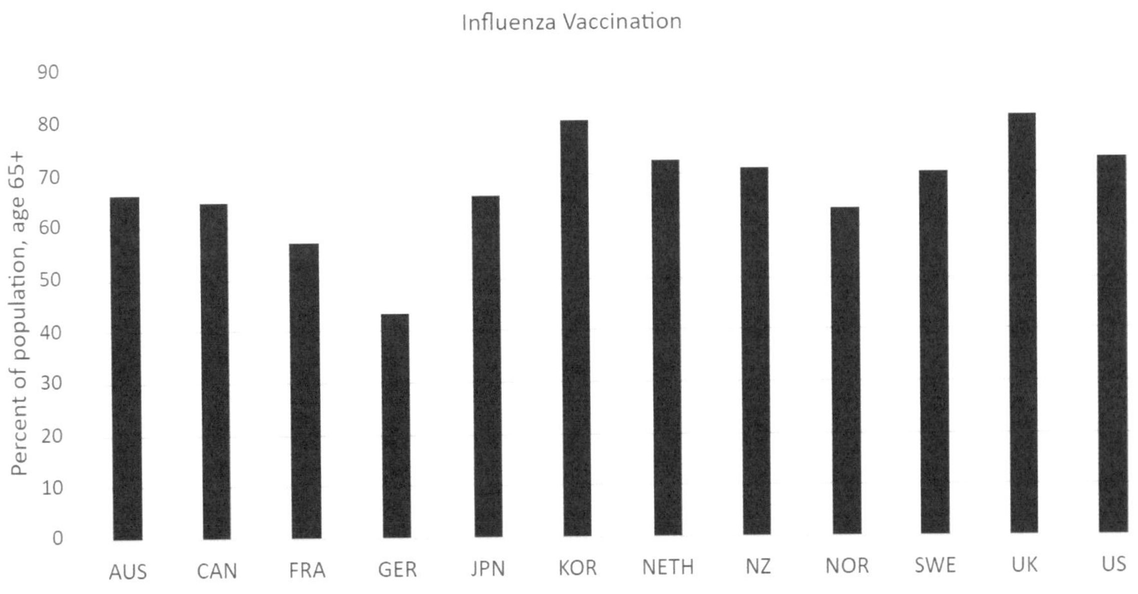

OECD (2022b). *Health care use - Influenza vaccination rates - OECD Data.* [online] Available at: https://data.oecd.org/healthcare/influenza-vaccination-rates.htm

Figure 14. ***Alcohol Consumption 2022***

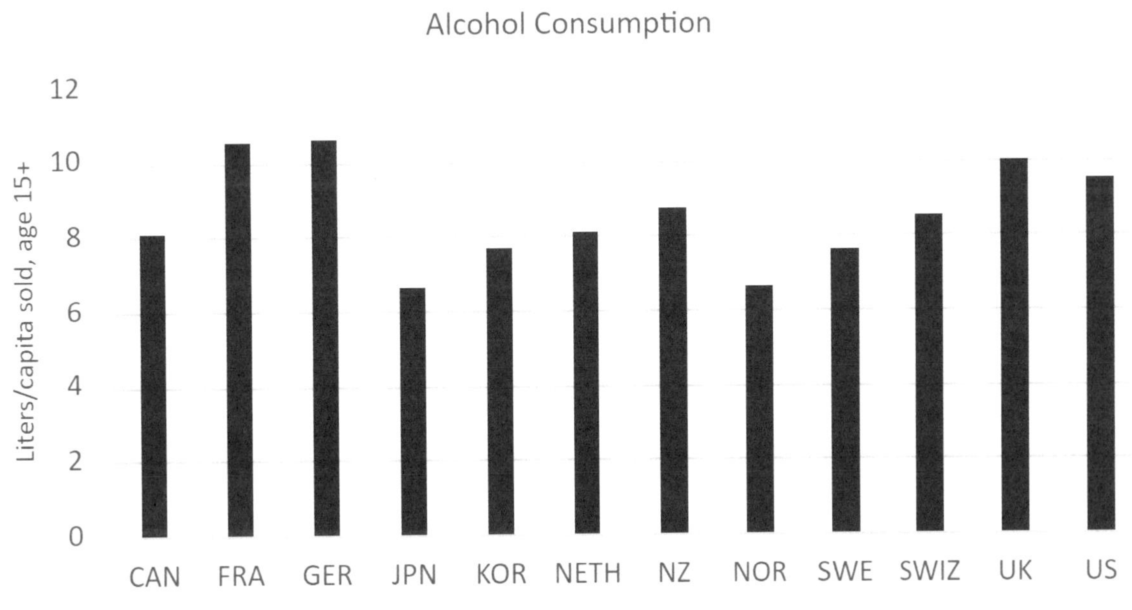

OECD (2022c). *Health risks - Alcohol consumption - OECD Data.* [online] Available at: https://data.oecd.org/healthrisk/alcohol-consumption.htm

Figure 15. ***Daily Smoking 2022***

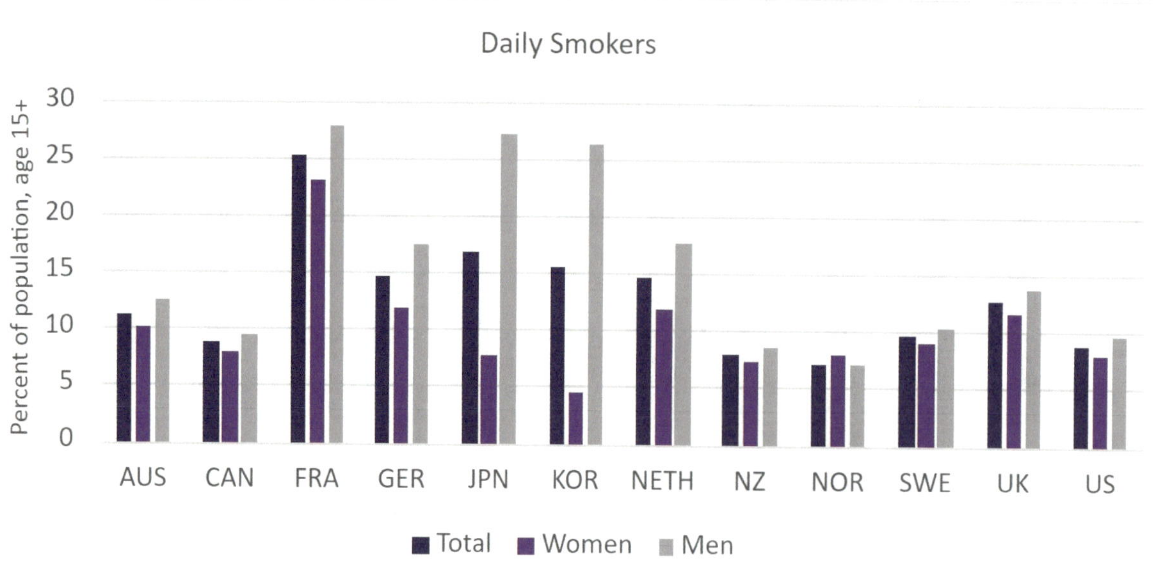

OECD (2022d). *Health risks - Daily smokers - OECD Data.* [online] Available at: https://data.oecd.org/healthrisk/daily-smokers.htm [Accessed 4 Mar. 2024].

Figure 16. ***Overweight or Obese Population*** Based on the WHO classification, adults with a BMI from 25 to 30 are defined as overweight, and those with a BMI of 30 or over as obese.

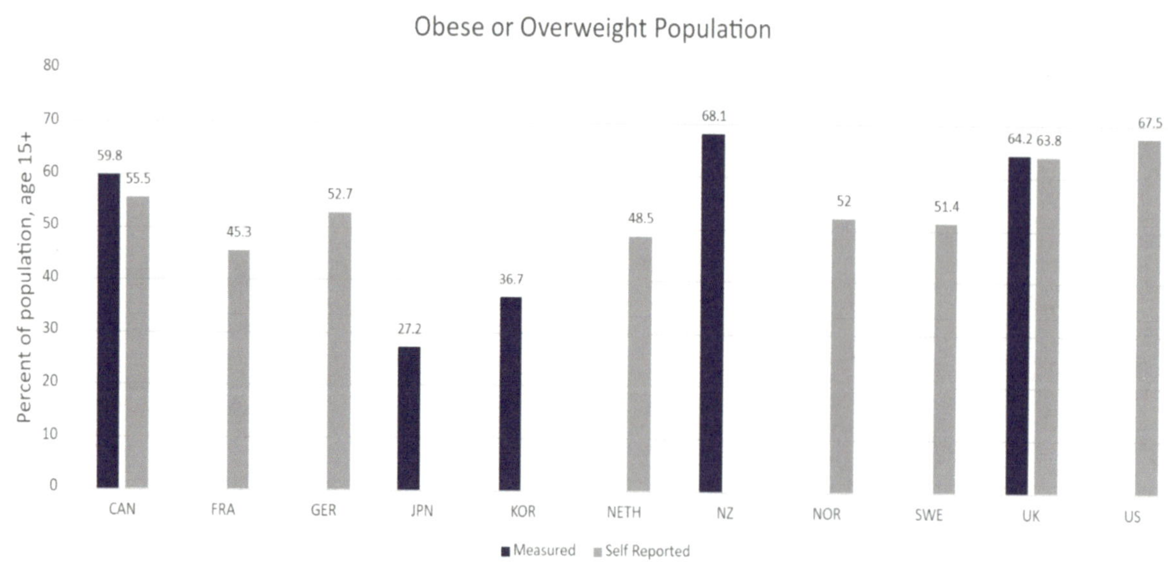

OECD (2023a). *Health Risks - Overweight or Obese Population - OECD Data.* [online] Available at: https://data.oecd.org/healthrisk/overweight-or-obese-population.htm

Figure 17. ***Happiness Ranking***

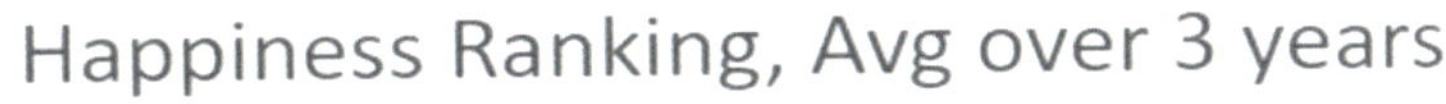

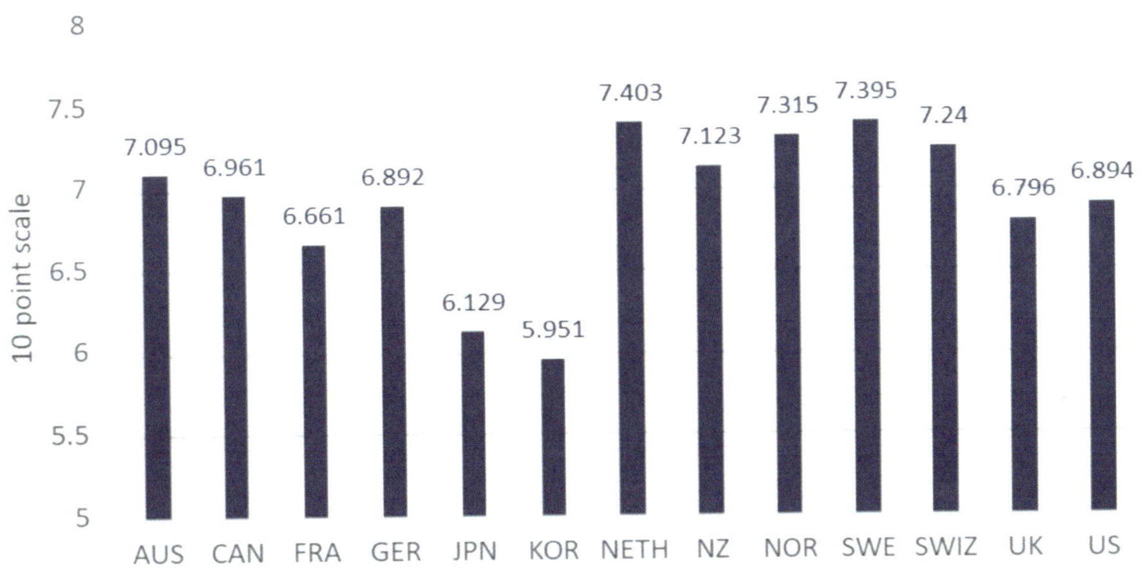

World Happiness Report (2023). *World Happiness Report*. [online] Worldhappiness.report. Available at: https://worldhappiness.report/

Figure 18. ***Suicide Rates*** Suicide rates are defined as the deaths deliberately initiated and performed by a person in the full knowledge or expectation of its fatal outcome.

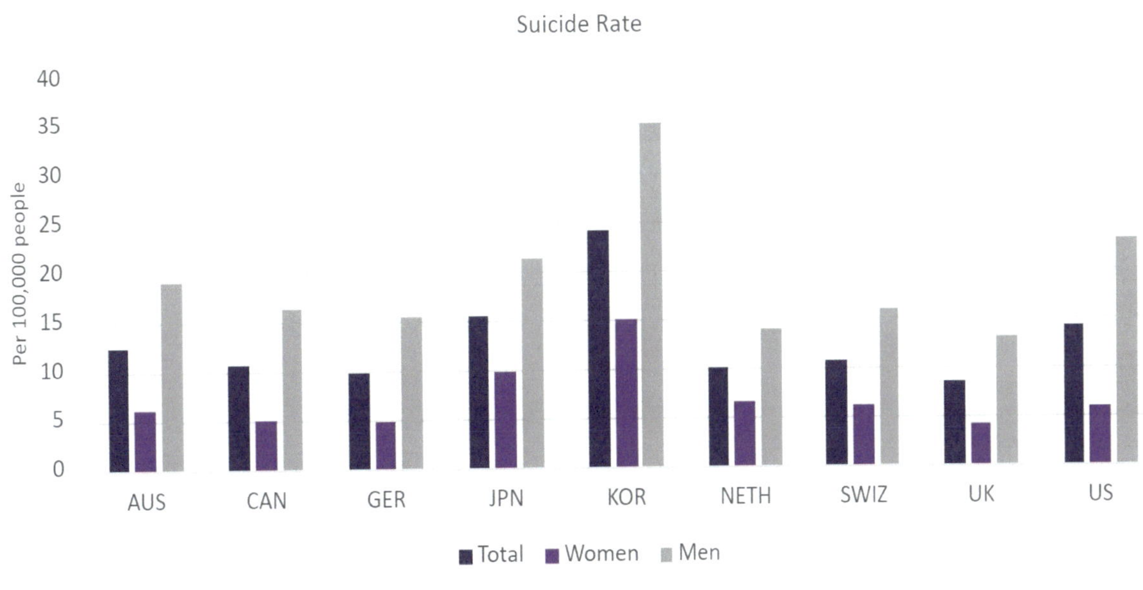

OECD (2023c). *Health Status Suicide Rates - OECD Data*. [online] Available at: https://data.oecd.org/healthstat/suicide-rates.htm

Figure 19. ***Opioid Related Deaths*** Opioid-related death data refer to deaths from opioid overdoses in adults and deaths in neonates attributed to the mother's opioid use.

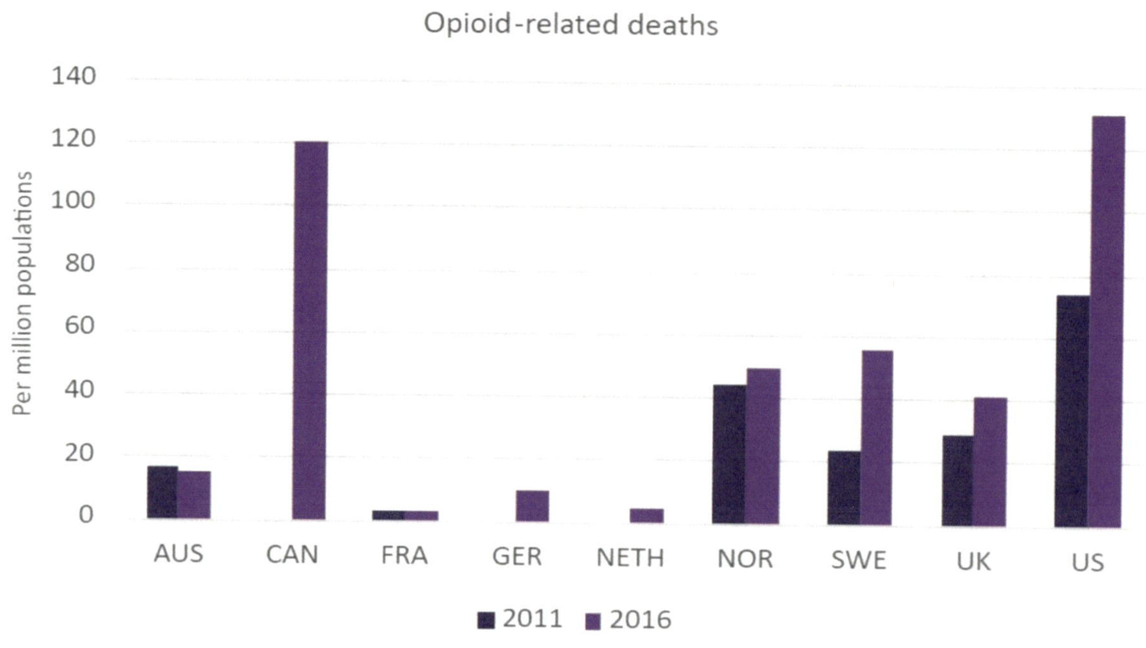

OECD (2024). *Illicit Drug Use*. [online] www.oecd-ilibrary.org. Available at: https://www.oecd-ilibrary.org/sites/3f97f180-en/index.html?itemId=/content/component/3f97f180-en

Figure 20. ***Deaths by Assault*** any death caused by injuries received in a fight, argument, quarrel, assault, or commission of a crime

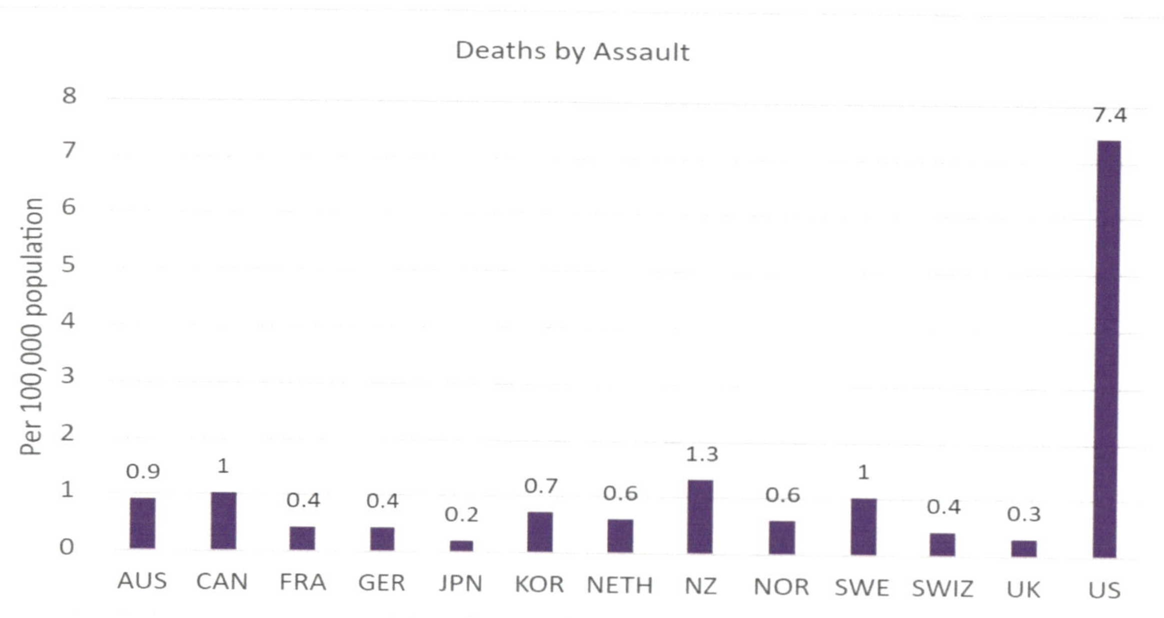

OECD (2022e). *Health Status : Causes of mortality*. [online] stats.oecd.org. Available at: https://stats.oecd.org/index.aspx?queryid=30115

Figure 21. *Social Expenditures as a % GDP* Social expenditures comprise cash benefits, direct in-kind provision of goods and services, and tax breaks with social purposes. Benefits may be targeted at low-income households, the elderly, disabled, sick, unemployed, or young persons.

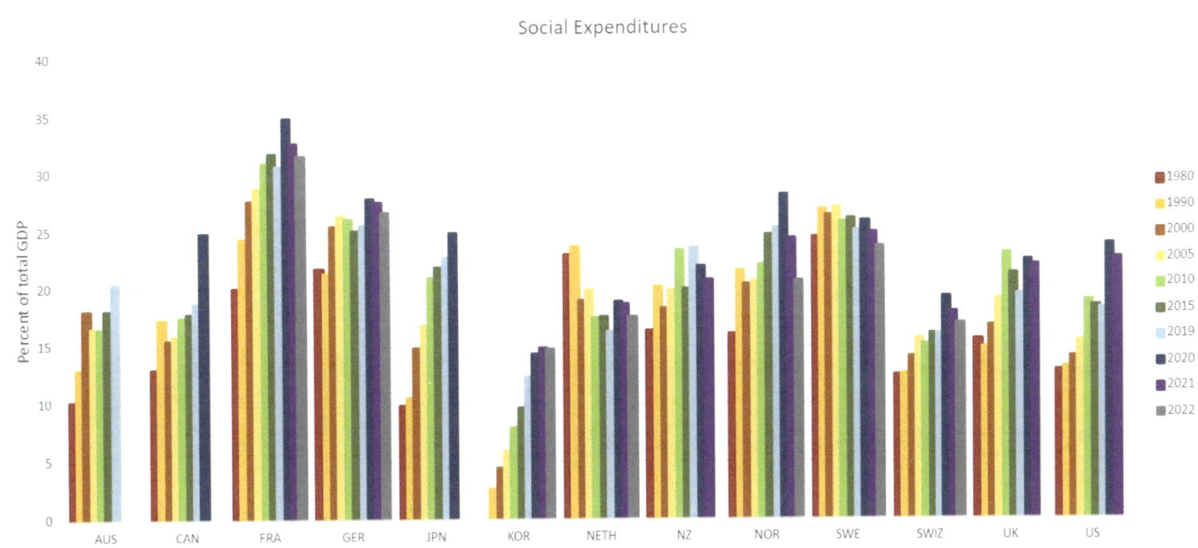

OECD (2022h). *Social protection - Social spending - OECD Data.* [online] Available at: https://data.o ecd.org/socialexp/social-spending.htm

Figure 22. *U.S. Does Not Guarantee Health Coverage*

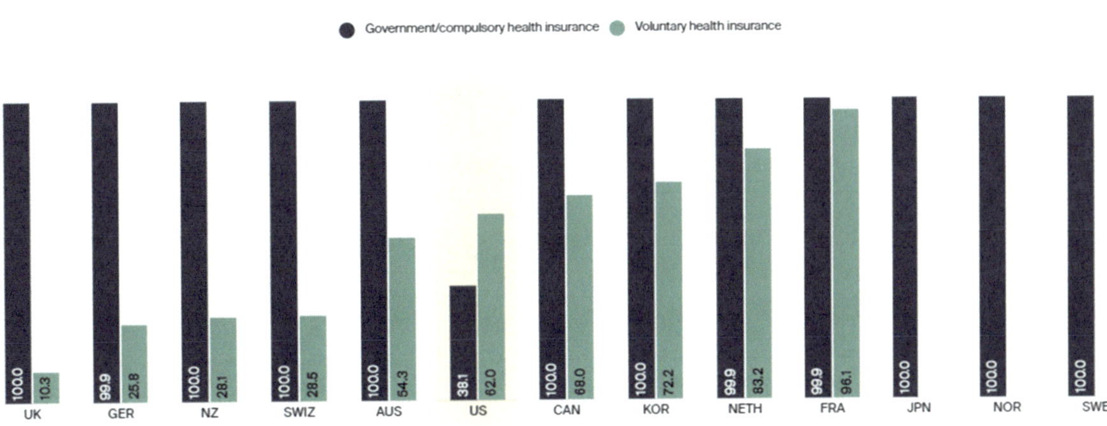

Gunja, M., Gumas, E. and Williams II, R. (2023). *U.S. Health Care from a Global Perspective, 2022: Accelerating Spending, Worsening Outcomes.* [online] The Commonwealth Fund. Available at: https://www.commonwealthfund.org/publications/issue-briefs/2023/jan/us-health-care-global-perspective-2022

With the exception of the Happiness Ranking graph (World Happiness Report, 2023), the data in the figures comes exclusively from the Organization of Economic Co-operation and Development (OECD) either extracted by our authors or reformulated by The Commonwealth Fund (www.commonwealthfund.org) and presented here.

Figures 1, 2, 3 and 4 compare life expectancy at birth, life expectancy at age 65, infant mortality, and maternal mortality amongst several high-income countries. Compared to the other countries graphed, the U.S. has the lowest life expectancy and lowest life expectancy after age 65 for both men and women. Infant mortality and maternal mortality rates reflect greater percentages of mortality than the other linked countries as well.

The United States enjoys a gross domestic product (wealth) that outstrips all other countries by wide margins (Figure 5). The U.S. GDP per capita is third to Switzerland and Norway (Figure 6). Figures 7 and 8 illustrate U.S. healthcare spending, which far exceeds all other high-income countries illustrated. These data beg the issue, "How, what, where, and why is the United States' extraordinary financial resource being allocated toward health spending without delivering on the assertion of world class health outcomes?" In other words, "Where's the money going?" Korea has a GDP ~1/10th the United States, spends 8.8% of its GDP on health care, and life expectancy of 83.5 years compared to the U.S. life expectancy of 77 years spending 17.8% of GDP on health (~ $4.5 trillion) according to the Center for Medicare & Medicaid Services (CMS, 2023).

Figures 9, 10, 11 and 12 embellish the gravity of the outcomes. The United States leads comparable countries in *Potential Years of Lost Life* (premature mortality, Figure 9), *Avoidable Deaths per 100,000 Population* (preventable mortality, Figure 10), *COVID-19 Death Rate* (Figure 11), *and* life expectancy in the U.S. is falling (Figure 12). The question begs, "What's the cause of these abysmal findings?"

Residents in the U.S. vaccinate at rates comparable to other high-income countries, consume alcohol at similar volumes, and smoke less than most (Figures 13,14 and 15), such equivalent behaviors do not contribute to variations in life expectancies. On the other hand, U.S. citizens take the lead in obesity – 67.5% of adults in the United States are overweight or obese (Figure 16), a statistic more probably than not, impacting healthy life expectancy if not life expectancy.

According to the World Happiness Report (2023) and Figure 17, the U.S. ranks 15th in happiness. Scandinavian countries rank highest – Finland, Denmark and Iceland place one, two, three. The U.S. features high rates of suicide, deaths from opioid overdose and deaths by assault – (14.5/100,000 by suicide [CDC, 2023]; 21.6/100,000 by fentanyl overdose [CDC, 2024] and 7.8/100,000 by assault [CDC, (2019]).

According to the CDC (2022), "U.S. Life Expectancy decreased in 2021 for the second consecutive year, according to final mortality data released. The drop was primarily due to increases in COVID-19 and drug overdose deaths." Deaths from suicide and death by homicide (assault) add significantly to the drop in life expectancy as well.

Attributing the root cause of the drop in life expectancy in the U.S. to COVID-19, obesity, drug overdose deaths, suicides and assaults oversimplifies and ignores the social determinates of health crisis in the United States. The decline in life expectancy in the U.S. compared to other high-income countries began long before the pandemic and fentanyl crisis. Data as far back as 1980 -1990 foretold the trajectory (see Figure 12). Shmerling (2022) argues "those with the shortest life expectancies in the U.S. tend to have the most poverty, face the most food insecurity, and have less or no access to healthcare, all factors that contribute to lower life expectancy. Additionally, groups with lower life expectancy tend to have higher-risk jobs that cannot be performed virtually, live in more crowded settings, and have less access to vaccination, which increases the risk of becoming sick with or dying of COVID-19."

Life Expectancy

In the context of policies, politics and governance

In spite of extraordinary national wealth, the policies, politics and governance of the United States shortchange the nation's health. The U.S. dedicates 22.7% of its GDP on social programs (Figure 17), while Sweden (23.7%), Japan (24.9%), Denmark (26.2%), Finland (29.0%), Italy (30.1%) and France (31.6%) allocate more and enjoy solid returns on investment (longer life).

Access to health care constitutes a crucial determinant of health. In 2022, 10.8% of working age adults had no health insurance (CMS, 2023). The U.S. is the only high-income country that does not guarantee health coverage. *It never has.*

Figure 22. ***U.S. Does Not Guarantee Health Coverage***

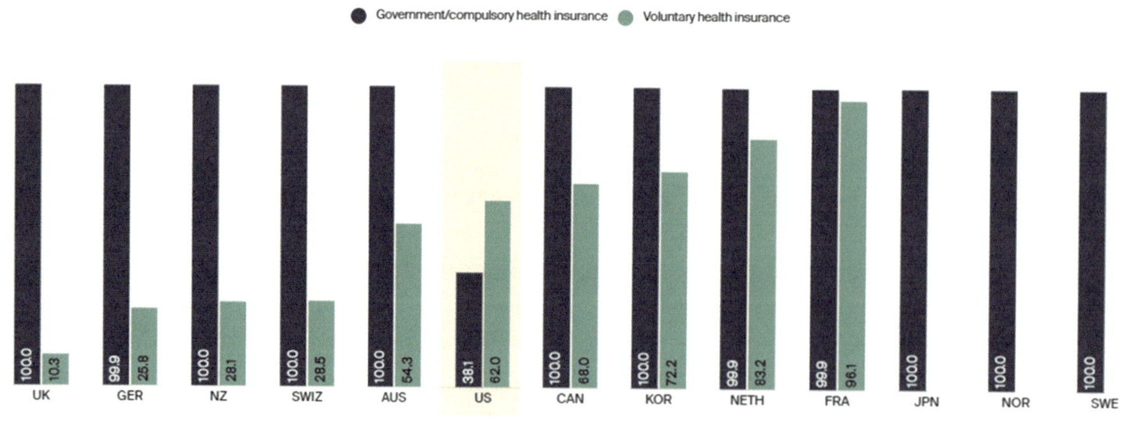

Gunja, M., Gumas, E. and Williams II, R. (2023). *U.S. Health Care from a Global Perspective, 2022: Accelerating Spending, Worsening Outcomes*. [online] The Commonwealth Fund. Available at: https://www.commonwealthfund.org/publications/issue-briefs/2023/jan/us-health-care-global-perspective-2022

So, if the United States does not guarantee health care for everyone but spends far more on healthcare than comparable countries, where *does* the money go?

Analyzing Organization for Economic Cooperation and Development (OECD) data, the Commonwealth Fund identified several factors that counterbalance health care expenditures in the U.S. compared to other high-income countries. The administrative burden associated with health insurance for pre-authorization eligibility, coding, submission and rework of claims represents 15% of excess spending in the United States. Adjusted for cost of living, physicians in the U.S. earn twice as much as physicians in comparable OECD countries – nurses earn 1.5 times as much. The United States spends twice as much per person on retail prescription drugs. U.S. prescription drug prices are two to three times those in other OECD countries. Patients in the U.S. receive greater intensity of treatment per visit or hospital stay, including greater use of advanced diagnostic and treatment technology - 44% higher rates of magnetic resonance imaging exams, 62% higher rates of computed tomography and up to 100% higher rate of coronary artery bypass grafting in patients with acute myocardial infarction. The Commonwealth Fund argues, "The U.S. population is sicker in ways that may increase the intensity of care required. OECD data indicate higher U.S. rates of obesity, diabetes, and heart disease, and a larger share of the population with multiple chronic conditions" (Turner, Miller and Lowry, 2023). Research and development peels off substantial resource to discover novel pharmaceuticals for both generic and rare disorders marketed, prime time advertised and sold in the U.S. at astonishing prices. Health care waste in the form of failed care, failed care coordination, care for over treatment, fraud and abuse and expense due to administrative complexities account for $760 billion to $935 billion annually (Shrank, Rogstad, and Parekh, 2019).

Adding insult to injury, residents of the U.S. pay mightily for their broken system. According to Himmelstein, et al., (2019), more than 60% of individuals in the United States filing for bankruptcy do so because of financially crushing medical expenses.

Early in this treatise (Chapter 2), we revealed the extraordinary profits of big pharma, health insurance conglomerates, health technology giants, and hospital corporations. The Dow Jones Industrial Average constitutes a stock market index of thirty financially powerful companies listed on stock exchanges in the United States – companies like IBM, Visa, Amazon and Microsoft. Healthcare giants like Amgen, Merck, Johnson & Johnson, and UnitedHealth make the list too. Executives and vice executives command outlandish forms of compensation to fund lavish lifestyles and accumulate wealth beyond the wildest imaginations of most individuals. All this accelerates the cost of care in the U.S. and must be defined in the simplest of economic terms.

Make no mistake.

In the United States health care is about profit.

Profits are necessary. Nevertheless, should citizens of the United States pay for a health care system that delivers reduced Life Expectancy, high Avoidable Deaths, and excessive Potential Years Of Life Lost at the expense of enormous corporate profits?

Bending to the influence of corporate America, conservative lawmakers loathe the concepts of healthcare for all. The Affordable Care Act in its initial iteration promised significant reform. Now watered down by the Supreme Court (National Federation of Independent Business v. Sebelius 2012), employer maneuverings, and assault by naysayers to overturn the ACA, the breadth and depth of coverage for eligible participants is significantly diluted.

In chapter 2, Andrea Saunders, JD made the case for the distribution of resource based on *an equal share for all* which ensures basic needs like housing, healthcare, education and food are satisfied for everyone, in contradistinction to distribution by merit, social status or privilege. Dr. Epstein in Chapter 11 argued for a "living wage" – compensation for work performed that provides for basic living essentials. "An equal share for all" and "living wage" constitute the central ethos of distributive justice.

According to the U.S. Department of Labor (2023) and the Office of the Assistant Secretary for Planning and Education (2023), the Federal Minimum Wage (FMW) of $7.25/hour has not been increased since 2009. Although states may legislate higher minimums, 20 states – Alabama, Georgia, Idaho, Indiana, Iowa, Kansas, Kentucky, Louisiana, Mississippi, New Hampshire, North Carolina, North Dakota, Oklahoma, Pennsylvania, South Carolina, Tennessee, Texas, Utah, Wisconsin and Wyoming adhere to the $7.25 Federal wage minimum. Annualized, $7.25/hour equates to $15,080/year based on a forty-hour work week. The HHS Poverty Guideline for a Family of three is $24,860. By any definition, an hourly wage at the FMW constitutes a 21st century brand of slavery served up with chitlins but no health insurance.

Norway sets an astonishing international example of national policies and priorities that deliver on exceptional population health. High GDP per capita; envious life expectancy, healthy life expectancy, infant mortality and maternal mortality; moderate spending on health care and social programs (20.7% GDP); low death rate during COVID-19; comparably low rates of alcohol consumption and smoking; low rates of deaths by assault and opioid use, and high international scores on happiness declare you can have it all – meaningful social programs that deliver on the promise of well-being and life satisfaction, an economy that outshines the U.S. and health outcomes that are second to none.

In 1980 Korea's life expectancy was the lowest of comparable high-income countries at 66.1 years. Strategies were implemented that reversed the trend and in 2021 Korea's life expectancy compares favorably at 83.5 years to other countries (U.S. 77 years). All this on modest health care expenditures of 8.8% of GDP (U.S. 17.8%) sending a clear message that it is not necessary to break the bank to ensure remarkable national health. Factor this too, from 1980 to 2021 Korea's GDP grew from $65.4 billion to $1.82 trillion USD (World Bank, 2022a) and emerged as an international powerhouse in the development and manufacture of high quality, U.S. consumer preferred electronics and EV automobiles. Korea's unemployment rate in 2022 was 2.9% (World Bank, 2022b). Like the Norwegian data, Korea's experience provides probable evidence that population health and economic prosperity can march hand in hand.

We penned this treatise as a call to action. The U.S. Congress, the Supreme Court and the President of the United States bear full responsibility to make this nation not the greatest on earth emblematically, but the greatest on earth factually. Our call establishes a strategic imperative to reverse the U.S. health crisis. It pleads the leaders of our country to dispense with the paralysis of political division and draw upon the examples of Norway, Korea and other high-income nations to implement proven policies that create transformative change and that resuscitate the health of our *entire* nation.

The Family Physicians and Colleagues for Health Justice scream from the rooftops, *"All men and women are created equal regardless of race, religion, color or creed, for we are endowed by our Creator with certain unalienable rights, that among these are life, liberty and the pursuit of happiness."* Advocates, health professionals and lawmakers please heed the call. The nation's health and justice in all policies depend on it.

May peace, too, be with you.

Question for Further Consideration:

1. Do the data on U.S. deaths by suicide, opioid overdose and assault suggest segments of the U.S. population feel an overwhelming burden of despair, self-treat with dangerous drugs to manage despondence and resort to violence to assuage superimposed anger?
2. Should citizens of the United States pay for a health care system that delivers reduced Life Expectancy, high Avoidable Deaths, and excessive Potential Years Of Life Lost in deference to of high corporate profits?
3. Describe the pros and cons of healthcare funded through government provided health insurance opposed to employer provided health insurance as an employee benefit.

Sentinel Readings for a Deeper Dive

Gray, B. (2019). Profits and Health Care: An Introduction to the Issues. [online] Nih.gov. Available at: https://www.ncbi.nlm.nih.gov/books/NBK217897/

Gunja, M., Gumas, E. and Williams II, R. (2023). U.S. Health Care from a Global Perspective, 2022: Accelerating Spending, Worsening Outcomes. [online] Available at: https://www.commonwealthfund.org/publications/issue-briefs/2023/jan/us-health-care-global-perspective-2022

References

CDC (2019). FastStats - Homicide. [online] Available at: https://www.cdc.gov/nchs/fastats/homicide.htm [Accessed 7 Mar. 2024].

CDC (2022). New Report Confirms U.S. Life Expectancy has Declined to Lowest Level Since 1996. [online] Available at: https://www.cdc.gov/nchs/pressroom/nchs_press_releases/2022/20221222.htm [Accessed 7 Mar. 2024].

CDC (2023). Suicide Data and Statistics. [online] Available at: https://www.cdc.gov/suicide/suicide-data-statistics.html [Accessed 7 Mar. 2024].

CDC (2024). Fentanyl Overdose Death Rates More Than Tripled From 2016 to 2021 [online] Available at: https://blogs.cdc.gov/nchs/2023/05/03/7338/ [Accessed 7 Mar. 2024].

CMS (2023). National health expenditures 2022 highlights | CMS. [online] Available at: https://www.cms.gov/newsroom/fact-sheets/national-health-expenditures-2022-highlights [Accessed 7 Mar. 2024].

Gray, B. (2019). Profits and Health Care: An Introduction to the Issues. [online] Nih.gov. Available at: https://www.ncbi.nlm.nih.gov/books/NBK217897/ [Accessed 8 Mar. 2024].

Gunja, M., Gumas, E. and Williams II, R. (2023). U.S. Health Care from a Global Perspective, 2022: Accelerating Spending, Worsening Outcomes. [online] Available at: https://www.commonwealthfund.org/publications/issue-briefs/2023/jan/us-health-care-global-perspective-2022 [Accessed 4 Mar. 2024].

Himmelstein, D., Lawless, R., Thorne, D., Foohey, P. and Woolhandler, S. (2019). Medical Bankruptcy: Still Common Despite the Affordable Care Act. *American Journal of Public Health*, [online] https://doi.org/10.2105/ajph.2018.304901 [Accessed 10 Mar. 2024].

OECD (2017). Health status - Life expectancy at 65 - OECD Data. [online] Available at: https://data.oecd.org/healthstat/life-expectancy-at-65.htm [Accessed 4 Mar. 2024].

OECD (2021a). Health status - Life expectancy at birth - OECD Data. [online] Available at: https://data.oecd.org/healthstat/life-expectancy-at-birth.htm [Accessed 4 Mar. 2024].

OECD (2021b). Health Status : Potential years of life lost. [online] stats.oecd.org. Available at: https://stats.oecd.org/index.aspx?queryid=30124 . [Accessed 4 Mar. 2024].

OECD (2022a). GDP and spending - Gross domestic product (GDP) - OECD Data. [online] Available at: https://data.oecd.org/gdp/gross-domestic-product-gdp.htm [Accessed 4 Mar. 2024].

OECD (2022b). Health care use - Influenza vaccination rates - OECD Data. [online] Available at: https://data.oecd.org/healthcare/influenza-vaccination-rates.htm [Accessed 4 Mar. 2024].

OECD (2022c). Health risks - Alcohol consumption - OECD Data. [online] Available at: https://data.oecd.org/healthrisk/alcohol-consumption.htm [Accessed 4 Mar. 2024].

OECD (2022d). Health risks - Daily smokers - OECD Data. [online] Available at: https://data.oecd.org/healthrisk/daily-smokers.htm [Accessed 4 Mar. 2024].

OECD (2022e). Health Status : Causes of mortality. [online] stats.oecd.org. Available at: https://stats.oecd.org/index.aspx?queryid=30115 [Accessed 4 Mar. 2024].

OECD (2022f). Health Status : Maternal and infant mortality. [online] stats.oecd.org. Available at: https://stats.oecd.org/index.aspx?queryid=30116 [Accessed 4 Mar. 2024].

OECD (2022g). Level of GDP per capita and productivity : GDP per capita levels - most recent year. [online] stats.oecd.org. Available at: https://stats.oecd.org/Index.aspx?QueryId=95894 [Accessed 4 Mar. 2024].

OECD (2022h). Social protection - Social spending - OECD Data. [online] Available at: https://data.oecd.org/socialexp/social-spending.htm [Accessed 4 Mar. 2024].

OECD (2023a). Health Risks - Overweight or Obese Population - OECD Data. [online] Available at: https://data.oecd.org/healthrisk/overweight-or-obese-population.htm [Accessed 4 Mar. 2024].

OECD (2023b). Health status - Infant mortality rates - OECD Data. [online] Available at: https://data.oecd.org/healthstat/infant-mortality-rates.htm [Accessed 4 Mar. 2024].

OECD (2023c). Health Status - Suicide Rates - OECD Data. [online] Available at: https://data.oecd.org/healthstat/suicide-rates.htm [Accessed 4 Mar. 2024].

OECD (2023d). Health Status : Avoidable mortality. [online] stats.oecd.org. Available at: https://stats.oecd.org/Index.aspx?QueryId=96018 [Accessed 4 Mar. 2024].

OECD (2024). Illicit Drug Use. [online] www.oecd-ilibrary.org. Available at: https://www.oecd-ilibrary.org/sites/3f97f180-en/index.html?itemId=/content/component/3f97f180-en [Accessed 4 Mar. 2024].

Office of the Assistant Secretary for Planning and Evaluation (2023). Poverty guidelines. [online] Available at: https://aspe.hhs.gov/topics/poverty-economic-mobility/poverty-guidelines [Accessed 30 March 2024].

Shrank, W., Rogstad, T. and Parekh, N. (2019). Waste in the US Health Care System. Journal of the American Medical Association, [online] https://doi.org/10.1001/jama.2019.13978 [Accessed 8 Mar. 2024].

Shmerling, R. (2022). Why life expectancy in the US is falling. [online] Harvard Health. Available at: https://www.health.harvard.edu/blog/why-life-expectancy-in-the-us-is-falling-202210202835#:~:text=Why%20is%20life%20expectancy%20falling%20in%20the%20US%3F [Accessed 7 Mar. 2024].

Turner, A., Miller, G. and Lowry, E. (2023). High U.S. Health Care Spending: Where Is It All Going? [online] www.commonwealthfund.org. Available at: https://www.commonwealthfund.org/publications/issue-briefs/2023/oct/high-us-health-care-spending-where-is-it-all-going [Accessed 8 Mar. 2024].

U.S. Department of Labor (2023). State Minimum Wage Laws | U.S. Department of Labor. [online] Available at: https://www.dol.gov/agencies/whd/minimum-wage/state [Accessed 30 Mar. 2024].

World Bank (2022a). GDP (current US$) - Korea, Rep. | Data. [online] data.worldbank.org. Available at: https://data.worldbank.org/indicator/NY.GDP.MKTP.CD?locations=KR [Accessed 6 Apr. 2024].

World Bank (2022b). Unemployment, total (% of total labor force) (national estimate) - Korea, Rep. | Data. [online] data.worldbank.org. Available at: https://data.worldbank.org/indicator/SL.UEM.TOTL.NE.ZS?locations=KR [Accessed 6 Apr. 2024].

World Happiness Report (2023). World Happiness Report. [online] Available at: https://worldhappiness.report/ [Accessed 5 Mar. 2024].

Lexicon of Listed Terms and Agencies

- **CDC – Centers for Disease Control** CDC is the nation's leading science-based, data-driven, service organization that protects the public's health. For more than 70 years, we have put science into action to help children stay healthy so they can grow and learn; to help families, businesses, and communities fight disease and stay strong; and to protect the public's health.

- **CMS** – Centers for Medicare & Medicaid Services advances health equity by addressing the health disparities that underlie our health system.

- **OECD** – the Organization for Economic Co-operation and Development is an international organisation that works to build better policies for better lives. Our goal is to shape policies that foster prosperity, equality, opportunity and well-being for all. We draw on 60 years of experience and insights to better prepare the world of tomorrow.

AUTHOR'S BIO SKETCH

James Lenhart. MD, FAAFP, MPH

Dr. Lenhart graduated from the University of New Mexico School of Medicine and took residency in Family Medicine from Brown University Affiliated Hospitals in Pawtucket/Providence, Rhode Island. In 2010, he completed a Master of Public Health degree from the University of Liverpool. He holds the distinction of academic rank of full professor from the University of North Carolina-Chapel Hill, University of Nevada, and University of Arizona.

He now serves as an Associate Program Director for the residency in Family Medicine at Community Health Care in Tacoma, Washington, a University of Washington affiliated program. In that capacity, Dr. Lenhart leads curriculum development including research and scholarship at the residency where he holds academic rank of Associate Clinical Professor.

Glossary

ACEs A validated healthcare questionnaire used to screen for adverse childhood experiences.

Affordable Care Act (ACA) The Patient Protection and Affordable Care Act, referred to as the Affordable Care Act or "ACA" for short, is the comprehensive health care reform law enacted in March 2010. Made affordable health insurance affordable to more people, expanded Medicaid, supported methods to lower healthcare costs.

American Civil Liberties Union (ACLU) the nation's premier defender of the rights enshrined in the U.S. Constitution. The ACLU fights government abuse and vigorously defends individual freedoms including speech and religion, a woman's right to choose, the right to due process, and citizens' rights to privacy.

American Public Health Association (APHA) is the publisher of the American Journal of Public Health and The *Nation's Health* newspaper. Research on public health is shared through the APHA annual meetings. APHA's mission strives to improve the health of the population and to achieve health equity.

American Slavery was a situation or practice in which people were entrapped and exploited in the United States.

AASHTO The American Association of State Highway and Transportation Officials (AASHTO) is a standards setting body which publishes specifications, test protocols, and guidelines that are used in highway design and construction throughout the United States.

Behavioral Risk Factor Surveillance System (BRFSS) is the nation's premier system of health-related telephone surveys that collect state data about U.S. residents regarding their health-related risk behaviors, chronic health conditions, and use of preventive services. Established in 1984 with 15 states, BRFSS now collects data in all 50 states as well as the District of Columbia and three U.S. territories.

Centers for Disease Control (CDC) is the nation's leading science-based, data-driven, service organization that protects the public's health. For more than 70 years, we have put science into action to help children stay healthy so they can grow and learn; to help families, businesses, and communities fight disease and stay strong; and to protect the public's health.

Center for Reproductive Rights is a global human rights organization of lawyers and advocates who ensure reproductive rights are protected in law as fundamental human rights for the dignity, equality, health and well-being of every person.

Civil Rights Act of 1964 is a comprehensive legislation intended to end discrimination based on race, color, religion or national origin.

Community Water Source (CWS) refers to a system that supplies the same population with water year-round and serves at least 25 people or 15 residences.

DALYs Disability-adjusted life years (DALYs) are a measure of overall disease burden, expressed as *the number of years lost due to ill-health, disability, or early death.* Developed as a method evaluate and compare the overall health and life expectancy of different countries.

Department of Justice is a federal executive division responsible for law enforcement and allied programs and services.

Department of Labor is a federal executive division responsible for enforcing labor statutes and promoting the general welfare of U.S. wage earners.

Dwight D. Eisenhower was an American military officer and statesman who became the 34th president of the United States from 1953 to 1961. During World War II, he served as Supreme Commander of the Allied Expeditionary Force in Europe and achieved the five-star rank as General of the Army. The crowning achievement of his presidency was establishment of the Interstate Highway System.

Environmental Policy Innovation Center an organization that helps craft government policies to improve the speed and scale of conservation.

Environmental Protection Agency (EPA) is an American governmental organization that ensures: Americans have access to clean air, water, and land; that scientific evidence shapes environmental policy; federal laws protect human health and the environment; environmental stewardship is factored into US environmental policy; Americans have access to accurate information; contamination is cleaned up; and chemicals in the marketplace are reviewed for safety.

Emergency Provisions: A facility whose primary purpose is to provide temporary shelter for those experiencing homelessness.

Environmental Working Group is an American non-profit group specializing in research and advocacy in the areas of toxic chemicals, drinking water contaminants, and other environmental concerns.

Exposome describes the environmental exposures encountered throughout life and the way in which they impact health and well-being.

Federal Communications Commission (FCC) regulates communications by radio, television, wire, satellite, and cable across the United States.

Federal-Aid Highway Act of 1956 Popularly known as the National Interstate and Defense Highways Act of 1956, the Federal-Aid Highway Act of 1956 established an interstate highway system in the United States.

Frontline Workers are employees who were required to go to their place of employment during the Covid-19 Pandemic.

Functional well-being (FWB): Ability for individual to conduct tasks of daily living including social roles.

GAD-7 A validated medical questionnaire used to screen for generalized anxiety disorder.

Gallup is a global analytic and advice firm that helps leaders and organizations solve thei most pressing problems.

GDP Gross domestic product or the total value of the economies products and services.

Genome all the genetic information (DNA and RNA) of an organism.

Global Burden of Diseases (GBD) is a systematic, scientific effort to quantify the comparative magnitude of health loss due to diseases, injuries, and risk factors by age, sex, and geographies for specific points in time.

Ground Water is a main water source for community water supplies, and is water drawn from subterranean deposits.

Homeless or People Experiencing Homelessness (PEH): A person who lacks fixed, regular, and adequate nighttime residence.

Human Genome Project the Human Genome Project (HGP) is one of the greatest scientific feats in history. The project was a voyage of biological discovery led by an international group of researchers looking to comprehensively study all the DNA (known as a genome) of a select set of organisms.

IRS – Internal Revenue Service the IRS is a bureau of the Department of the Treasury and one of the world's most efficient tax administrators.

Jim Crow Jim Crow segregation was a way of life that combined a system of anti-Black laws and race-prejudiced cultural practices. The term "Jim Crow" is often used as a synonym for racial segregation, particularly in the American South.

John Francis, PhD National Geographic Education Fellow, is nicknamed "the Planetwalker." For 22 years, he did not use motorized transportation. He is the program director for Planetwalk, a nonprofit environmental awareness organization, which aims to educate people not only about the physical environment, but the human environment as well. *Planetwalker: 22 Years of Walking. 17 Years of Silence* frames his autobiography and travels without the use of motorized vehicles for 22 years.

Kaiser Family Foundation KFF is the independent source for health policy research, polling, and journalism. Our mission is to serve as a nonpartisan source of information for policymakers, the media, the health policy community, and the public.

Legal Defense Fund: The Legal Defense Fund (LDF) is America's premier legal organization fighting for racial justice. Using the power of law, narrative, research, and people, we defend and advance the full dignity and citizenship of Black people in America.

Legal Services Corporation (LSC): LSC is the single largest funder of civil legal aid for low-income Americans in the nation. Established in 1974, LSC operates as an independent 501(c)(3) nonprofit corporation that promotes equal access to justice and provides grants for high-quality civil legal assistance to low-income Americans.

March of Dimes: The March of Dimes leads the fight for the health of all moms and babies. We support research, lead programs, and provide education and advocacy so that every family can get the best possible start. Building on a successful 85-year legacy, we support every pregnant person.

Mental Health America is nonprofit who was created to promote mental health, well-being, and illness prevention in the US.

Microbiome the collection of all microbes, such as bacteria, fungi, viruses, and their genes, that naturally live on our bodies and inside us collectively known as microbiota.

Migrant Workers are international migrants who are currently employed or are looking for employed in the country they currently reside in and is not their home country.

National Academies The National Academies of Sciences, Engineering, and Medicine (NASEM), also known as the **National Academies**, is a congressionally chartered organization that serves as the collective scientific national academy of the United States.

National Center for Education Statistics (NCES) is a statistical agency utilized by the United States Department of Education. Through a congressional mandate, this agency collects, analyzes, and reports statistics regarding American education.

National Domestic Workers Alliance (NDWA) is an organization that works to gain labor rights and protections for nannies, housecleaners, and homecare workers.

National Health and Nutrition Examination Survey (NHANES) as an arm of the CDC The National Health and Nutrition Examination Survey is a program of studies designed to assess the health and nutritional status of adults and children in the United States. The survey is unique in that it combines interviews and physical examinations.

National Institutes of Health (NIH): NIH's mission is to seek fundamental knowledge about the nature and behavior of living systems and the application of that knowledge to enhance health, lengthen life, and reduce illness and disability. The NIH provides leadership and direction to programs designed to improve the health of the Nation by conducting and supporting research.

National Resources Defense Council NRDC (the Natural Resources Defense Council) combines the power of more than 3 million members and online activists with the expertise of some 700 scientists, lawyers, and other environmental specialists to confront the climate crisis, protect the planet's wildlife and wild places, and to ensure the rights of all people to clean air, clean water, and healthy communities.

National Survey of Children's Health The National Survey of Children's Health (NSCH) provides rich data on multiple, intersecting aspects of children's lives—including physical and mental health, access to and quality of health care, and the child's family, neighborhood, school, and social context. The National Survey of Children's Health is funded and directed by the Health Resources and Services Administration (HRSA) Maternal and Child Health Bureau.

National Telecommunications and Information Administration (NTIA): a department of the executive branch responsible for advising Presidents on telecommunications an information policy issues.

Occupational Safety and Health Act (OSHA) of 1970 was passed by Congress to ensure all workers have safe working conditions. It provides guidance to employers and employees.

OECD: The Organisation for Economic Co-operation and Development (OECD) is an international organisation that works to build better policies for better lives. Our goal is to shape policies that foster prosperity, equality, opportunity and well-being for all.

Organization for Economic Co-operation and Development (OECD) is an international organization that works with governments, policy makers and citizens to establish international standards that are focused on well-being for all.

Patient Protection and Affordable Care Act (ACA) aims to provide health care coverage to all Americans and prevent escalation of health care costs.

Personal Protective Equipment (PPE) describes equipment worn to minimize exposure to hazards. For healthcare workers, this commonly meant respirators, isolation gowns, gloves, and foot and eye protection.

Point in Time Estimates (PIT): Data that is gathered at one time and used to extrapolate data over a long term.

Roosevelt's New Deal The New Deal established a broad series of programs, public work projects, financial reforms, and regulations enacted by President Franklin D. Roosevelt in the United States between 1933 and 1938 to address the Great Depression

Segregation is the separation or isolation of a race, class, or ethnic group by enforced or voluntary residence in a restricted area, by barriers to social intercourse, by separate educational facilities, or by other discriminatory means.

Social Determinants of Health (SDH or SDOH): non-medical factors or aspects outside the physical and mental body that impact health outcomes.

Socioeconomic status (SES): The collective resources that an individual has. It is often measured as a combination of education, occupation, and income.

Surface Water is water from rivers, lakes, ice, and snow and is one of the two main source types for community water supplies.

The Agency for Healthcare Research and Quality (AHRQ) is an agency under the Department of Health and Human Services whose mission is to produce evidence to make health care safer, higher quality, more accessible, equitable and afordable.

The Agency for Toxic Substances and Disease Registry (ATSDR) is an advisory agency that is part of the US Department of Health and Human Services that creates profiles of toxic substances and conducts research regarding hazardous exposures.

The Centers for Disease Control and Prevention (CDC) is an American governing body that operates under the Department of Health and Human Services to supply information that protects the nation against dangerous health threats.

The Commonwealth Fund is a private foundation thatthat aims to promote a high performing heath care system that achieves better access, improved quality and greater efficiency, particularly for society's most vulnerable.

The Food and Agricultural Organization of the United Nations (FAO) is a specialized agency of the United Nations that leads international efforts to defeat hunger.

The Food Programme (WFP) is a global organization that works to bring life-saving relief in emergencies and use food assistance to build peace, stability, and prosperity for the people of the world. They work with both national agencies and international agencies such as the United Nations, to conduct their goals.

The Healthy People Initiative started as the "Healthy People: The Surgeon General's Report on Health Promotion and Disease Prevention" in 1979. Inspired by Surgeon General Julius Richmond, Healthy People set out to create 10-year objectives focusing on the nation's health and well-being. Healthy People 2030, launched in August 2020, setting out 358 core measurable objectives with an emphasis on social determinants of health, health equity and literacy.

The Institute for Health Metrics and Evaluation (IHME) at the University of Washington engages a large network of individual collaborators with specialties in various topic areas of expertise to conduct the Global Burden of Diseases, Injuries, and Risk Factors Study (GBD) and its affiliated research projects.

The Kaiser Family Foundation (KFF) is a non-profit organization focusing on national health issues, as well as the United State's role in global health policy. KFF serves as a non-partisan source of facts, analysis and journalism for policymakers, the media, the health policy community and the public.

The Human Rights Campaign is an organization based in the United States that works to provide advocacy for LGBTQ+ individuals.

The Library of Congress is a governmental agency that stores vast amounts of historical information and includes numerous articles of the origin of the LGTBQ+ movement and Pride in the United States.

The National Constitution Center is a private, nonprofit organization that serves as America's leading platform for constitutional education and debate.

The Organization for Economic Cooperation and Development, OCED, includes 37 countries that emphasize trade and economic growth. Data is collected through this organization. Data specifically pertaining to education is reported through the NCES.

The Safe Drinking Water Act (SDWA) was passed by the US Congress in 1974 that gives the EPA the authority to set national health-based standards for drinking water.

The State Department of Agriculture (USDA) is an American governing body responsible for supplying leadership on food, agriculture, natural resources, rural development, nutrition, and related issues.

The U.S. Geological Survey is a government agency that studies US landscapes, natural resources, and the hazards that threaten them. **The United Nations (UN)** is an intergovernmental organization whose stated purposes are to support international peace and security, develop friendly relations among nations, achieve international cooperation, and serve as a centre for harmonizing the actions of nations.

United Nations (UN) one place where the world's nations can gather, discuss common problems, and find shared solutions

The United Nations Educational, Scientific and Cultural Organization (UNESCO) is a specialized agency of the United Nations aimed at promoting world peace and security through international cooperation in education, arts, sciences and culture.

The Universal Declaration of Human Rights (UDHR) represents a milestone document in the history of human rights. Drafted by representatives with different legal and cultural backgrounds from all regions of the world, the declaration was proclaimed by the United Nations General Assembly in Paris on 10 December 1948 as a common standard of achievements for all peoples and all nations. It set out, for the first time, fundamental human rights to be universally protected. The UDHR has been translated into over 500 languages. It is widely recognized as having inspired, and paved the way for, the adoption of more than 70 human rights treaties, applied today on a permanent basis at global and regional levels.

The World Economic Forum (WEF) is an independent international organization committed to improving the state of the world by engaging business, political, academic and other leaders of society to shape global, regional and industry agendas.

The World Health Organization (WHO) is the United Nations agency that connects nations, partners and people to promote health, keep the world safe and serve the vulnerable with the goal that everyone, everywhere can attain the highest level of health.

Transportation Research Board The Transportation Research Board (TRB) is a division of the National Academy of Sciences, Engineering, and Medicine, formerly the National Research Council of the United States, which serves as an independent adviser to the President of the United States, the Congress and federal agencies on scientific and technical questions of national importance. It is jointly administered by the National Academy of Sciences, the National Academy of Engineering, and the National Academy of Medicine.

UAW – The International Union, United Automobile, Aerospace and Agricultural Implement Workers of America (UAW) is one of the largest and most diverse unions in North America, with members in every sector of the economy. UAW-represented workplaces range from multinational corporations, small manufacturers and state and local governments to colleges and universities, hospitals, and private non-profit organizations. The UAW has more than 400,000 active members and more than 580,000 retired members in the United States, Canada, and Puerto Rico.

UN – United Nations one place where the world's nations can gather, discuss common problems, and find shared solutions.

UN Women is a branch of the UN that focuses on monitoring and improving gender inequality worldwide.

UNICEF, originally called the United Nations International Children's Emergency Fund in full, now officially **United Nations Children's Fund**, is an agency of the United Nations responsible for supplying humanitarian and developmental aid to children worldwide.

United States Bureau of Labor Statistics is an agency within the United States Department of Labor that serves as part of the United States Federal Statistical System. It is a fact-finding agency for the field of labor economics and statistics.

United States Department of Labor to foster, promote, and develop the welfare of the wage earners, job seekers, and retirees of the United States; improve working conditions; advance opportunities for profitable employment; and assure work-related benefits and rights.

U.S. Consumer Product Safety Commissions (CPSC) is a federal agency formed to protect the public against risks of injury or death from consumer products.

U.S. Department of Health and Human Services (HHS): A cabinet level agency that's goal is to promote the health and well-being of all Americans, by providing for effective health and human services and by fostering sound, sustained advances in the sciences underlying medicine, public health, and social services.

U.S. Department of Housing and Urban Development (HUD): A cabinet level agency that is responsible for policy and programs that address America's housing needs, which improve and develop the Nation's communities, and enforce fair housing laws.

U.S. Department of Transportation The goal of the U.S. Department of Transportation is to deliver the world's leading transportation system, serving the American people and economy through the safe, efficient, sustainable, and equitable movement of people and goods.

U.S. EPA (EPA) The mission of Environmental Protection Agency is to protect human health and the environment. The EPA works to ensure that Americans have clean air, land, and water

U.S. Supreme Court (SCOTUS): The Court is the highest tribunal in the Nation for all cases and controversies arising under the Constitution or the laws of the United States. It seeks to provide "Equal Justice Under the Law"

WaterAid is an international organization that focuses on water, sanitation, and hygiene education founded in 1981.

WHO – World Health Organization an organization of professionals committed to integrity and excellence in health. With a spirit of collaboration and a steadfast commitment to science, we are trusted to care for the world's health.

World Health Organization (WHO) The WHO is an international organization of 194 Member States. The Member States elect the Director-General, who leads the organization in achieving its global health goals.

Index

About the Senior Editor

Inspired by early life experiences, James knew he wanted to be a doctor from an early age. Although adequate for college education, his home state of Montana did not have a medical school, so he relocated to Albuquerque and completed medical studies and the degree of Doctor of Medicine at the University of New Mexico School of Medicine. Dr. Lenhart took residency in Family Medicine at Brown University Affiliated Hospitals in Pawtucket/Providence, Rhode Island and in 2010 completed a Master of Public Health degree from the University of Liverpool. He holds the distinction of academic rank of full professor from the University of North Carolina-Chapel Hill, the University of Nevada, and the University of Arizona Schools of Medicine.

The experiences living in the Southwestern United States amongst Native American and Hispanic peoples during medical school initiated his transition from parochial perspectives to social mindfulness. Eclectic influences toward his full embrace of social progressivism stem from career experiences and life as a family physician in New England, the Pacific Northwest, Las Vegas, Nevada, Southeastern North Carolina and Yuma, Arizona. Emphasizing social medicine while studying for the Master of Public Health degree cemented his ideals.

James now serves as an Associate Program Director for the residency in Family Medicine at Community Health Care in Tacoma, Washington, a University of Washington affiliated program. In that capacity, Dr. Lenhart leads curriculum development including research and scholarship at the residency where he holds the University of Washington academic rank of Clinical Associate Professor.

Dr. Lenhart's other literary works include publication of his master's dissertation *A Comparative Analysis of the Impact of Healthcare Insurance Availability on Health Outcomes in Hawai'i and Mississippi* and a novel, *Conversations for Paco: Why America Needs Healthcare All* an exposé that portrays the people, politics and profits that poison healthcare in America.

About Sleeping Giant Publishing

Sleeping Giant Publishing aims to provide first time authors a streamlined yet eminent vehicle by which to publish their works. We push thoroughly edited manuscripts into high quality printed and electronic formats, market them on our website and YouTube, promote their sales on Amazon and insure accurate accounting of all sales and related transactions.

Ordering

Copies of *The Social Determinants of Health Illustrated: a primer for Advocates • Health Professionals • Lawmakers* may be ordered directly from Amazon or the Sleeping Giant Publishing website "Contact Us" page. It is available in printed and digital formats.

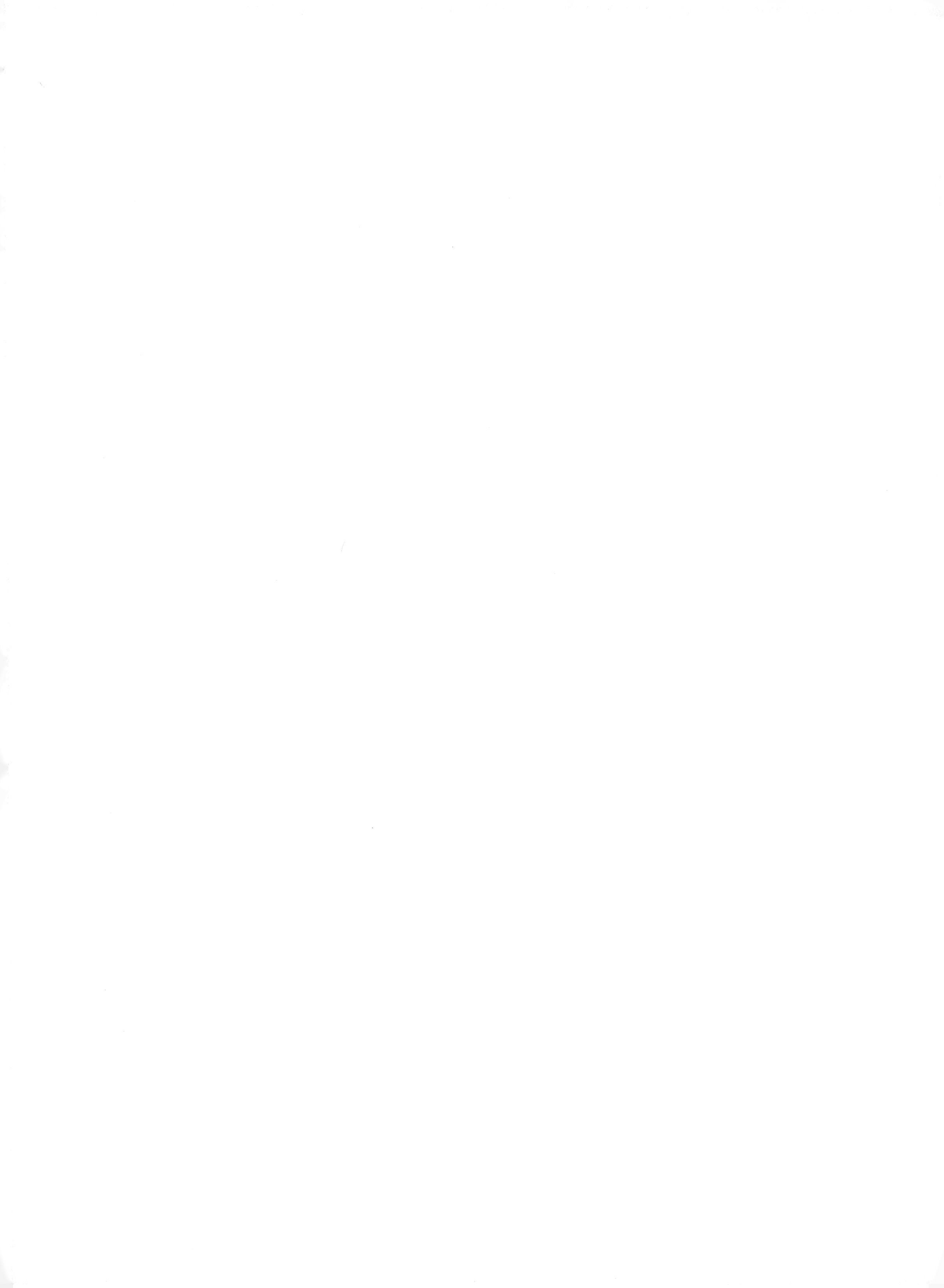

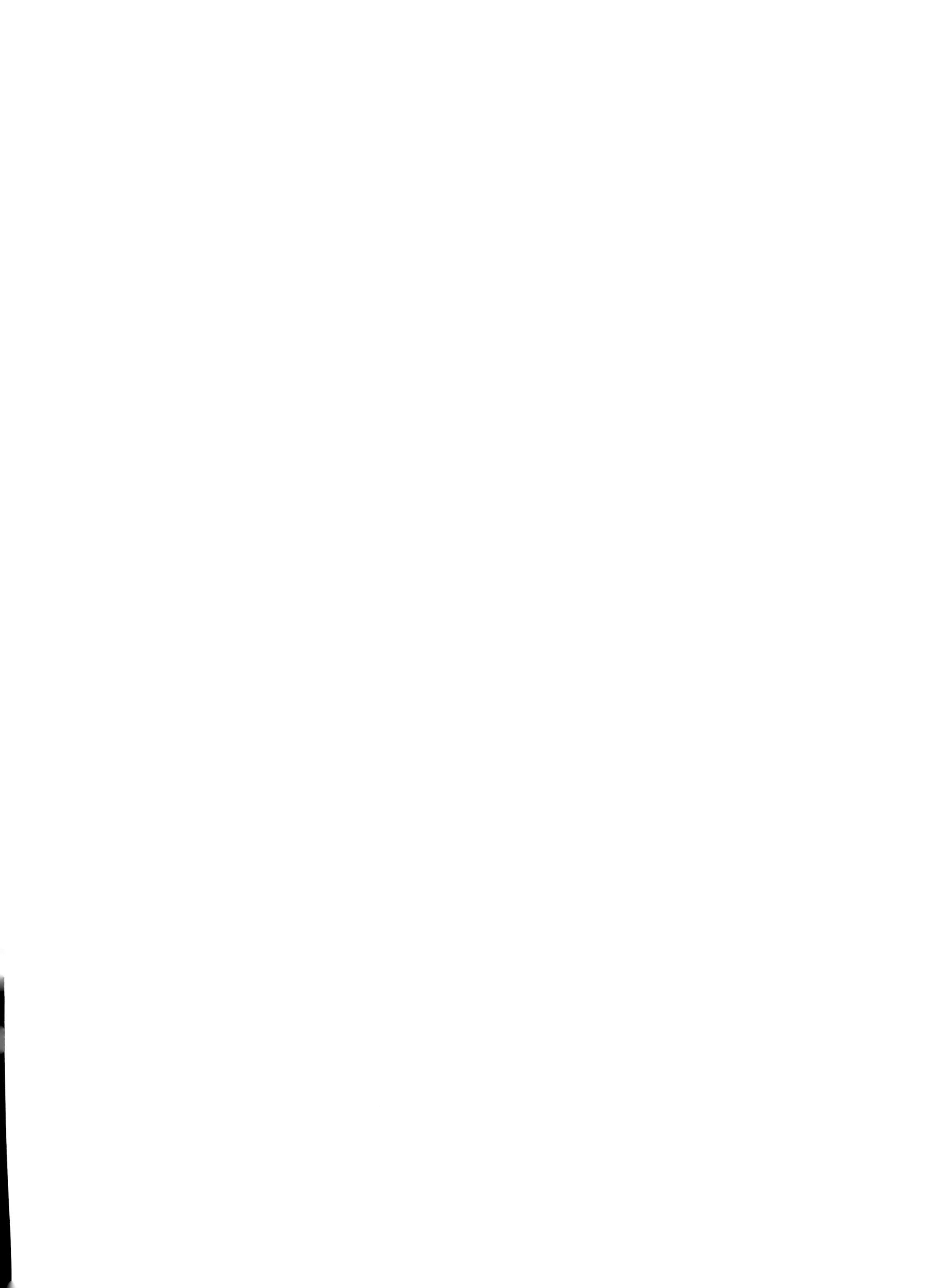

Made in the USA
Columbia, SC
30 April 2024